Caplan's Stroke: A Clinical Approach

Caplan's Stroke: A Clinical Approach

Third Edition

Louis R. Caplan, M.D.

Professor of Neurology, Harvard Medical School;
Senior Neurologist and Director of Stroke Service,
Beth Israel Deaconess Medical Center, Boston

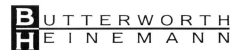

Boston • Oxford • Auckland • Johannesburg • Melbourne • New Delhi

Butterworth–Heinemann supports the efforts of American Forests and the Global ReLeaf program in its campaign for the betterment of trees, forests, and our environment.

Library of Congress Cataloging-in-Publication Data
Caplan, Louis R.
    Caplan's stroke : a clinical approach / Louis R. Caplan.-- 3rd ed.
        p. ; cm.
    Includes bibliographical references and index.
    ISBN 0-7506-9953-1
    1. Cerebrovascular disease. I. Title.
    [DNLM: 1. Cerebrovascular Disorders--diagnosis. 2. Cerebrovascular
Disorders--therapy. WL 355 C244s 2000]
    RC388.5 .C33 2000
    616.8'1--dc21
                                                        99-054757

British Library Cataloguing-in-Publication Data
A catalogue record for this book is available from the British Library.

The publisher offers special discounts on bulk orders of this book.
For information, please contact:
Manager of Special Sales
Butterworth–Heinemann
225 Wildwood Avenue
Woburn, MA 01801-2041
Tel: 781-904-2500
Fax: 781-904-2620

For information on all Butterworth–Heinemann medical publications available,
contact our World Wide Web home page at: http://www.bh.com

10 9 8 7 6 5 4 3 2 1

Printed in the United States of America

Contents

III. PREVENTION, COMPLICATIONS, AND REHABILITATION

Preface to the Third Edition

Seven years have passed since the publication of the second edition of *Stroke: A Clinical Approach*. The first edition was published 14 years ago. Innumerable advances in technology, diagnosis, treatment, and in the understanding and recognition of various cerebrovascular disease processes have occurred, even since the second edition. In this writing, I attempt to bring readers up to date with these advances and still strive to keep this monograph as personal a teaching mode as possible. During the 15 years since the first edition was conceived and written, I have also altered my aims for the book and seek to reflect that change in this edition.

The first edition was originally conceived by Dr. Rob Stein. At the time, Rob was a stroke fellow with Dan Hier and me at the Michael Reese Hospital, University of Chicago. Rob has now been in clinical practice in the Penobscot Bay area of Maine for more than a decade. He remains active in clinical trials and the care of stroke patients. The intent of the first edition was to produce a relatively concise account of the clinical care of stroke patients aimed principally at medical students, trainees in medicine and neurology, general practitioners, internists, and neurologists who were not particularly trained as stroke specialists. Stein and I emphasized fundamentals and a systematic, logical approach to the diagnosis and treatment of individuals with cerebrovascular disease. Diagnostic technology and treatment were not especially advanced in 1985.

To my surprise, the first edition proved popular with stroke specialists as well as with nonneurologists and non–stroke specialist neurologists. I tried to include in the second edition the major technological advances that occurred between 1985 and 1993 while retaining a systematic, personal, integrated approach. The systematic approach was easier in the second edition because I was the sole author. In the first edition, my style and Rob's style were quite different, and the text was not uniform in method or facility of transmittal. Monographs penned by a single individual have the great advantage of providing a planned, well-organized, systematic account of a topic using a uniform writing and teaching style and containing a minimum of redundancies and contradictions. I strove to keep the second edition a personal account in which I shared my own views with the readers. Many books, in striving to present all of the data as fairly as possible, fail to guide the readers through the labyrinth of conflicting ideas and approaches discussed. I attempted to convey the key information and data while continuing to clearly state my views on diagnosis and treatment.

This edition represents an extensive rewriting and elaboration on previous editions. Advances have been so numerous and so far-reaching that I found it impossible not to expand the size of the book considerably. I have continued to try to retain a single consistent approach to stroke diagnosis and care: *The method is more important than the individual details.* I try to explain as clearly as possible my own approach and its rationale. I hope that readers will be able to separate information and data from my own views.

In contrast to the first two editions, this edition is intended for stroke specialists as well as nonexperts. I have included more information about unusual conditions often encountered by stroke specialists (Chapter 11) and have elaborated on the intricacies of the more common stroke syndromes (Chapters 6–13).

I must also make clear what the book is not. I do not include detailed reviews of all stroke clinical trials and so-called evidence-based data. I do review the results of trials and studies that I believe are pertinent to the care of individual stroke patients (e.g., the anticoagulation in atrial fibrillation patients and the carotid surgery trials). Other books are available that review trials in detail. Also, as in the first two editions, I include only relatively brief chapters on prevention, complications, and rehabilitation. These are important topics that deserve full coverage in separate monographs. Excellent books on these topics are available. These are complex subjects about which I have no special experience or expertise. I chose to continue to review these topics eclectically and to share my views concisely on limited aspects.

I have attempted to heed criticisms of the first two editions. I have included more illustrations in the chapters on clinical syndromes, Chapters 6–17. I added discussion and illustrations of venous anatomy in Chapter 2. This topic was omitted previously. In addition, I have added a chapter on venous and dural sinus occlusions, a topic that was previously neglected. I have also added more detail on arterial branch anatomy in Chapter 2. All of the chapters on clinical syndromes have been extensively revised to capture recent information. Rewriting was most extensive in Chapters 11 and 12. Chapter 11, on nonatherosclerotic vascular conditions, is intended to be a ready reference for clinicians to look up conditions with which they may not be familiar. I have also tried to reference this chapter extensively to facilitate further reading. I have included much more extensive coverage of vascular malformations and dural fistulas in Chapter 12. I have updated the references in all of the chapters. Maintaining all of the text on computer has made it possible for me to update all chapters when new information became available; therefore, I believe that all chapters were *en courant* when the book was given to the publisher.

This edition has taken longer than $1^{1}/_{2}$ years to accomplish. I found this edition much more difficult to revise than before. Stroke knowledge and literature have expanded at such a rapid rate that I found it difficult to keep up with all the facets of cerebrovascular disease. I am forever indebted to my wife Brenda for putting up with my early-morning writings and my spousal neglect that, unfortunately, is the price one pays for writing such a book. As always, the help and support of my loyal secretary, Pauline Dawley, has been greatly appreciated. Susan Pioli and her staff at Butterworth–Heinemann have always been helpful, supportive, and encouraging.

Medical students and residents at Tufts and Harvard have asked the questions that guided a search for answers. My stroke fellows and my colleagues at the New England Medical Center and at the Beth Israel Deaconess Medical Center have and continue to remain great resources for information, opinions, and support. Thanks go to Drs. Rafael Llinas and Galen Henderson, who were most helpful in helping me hunt for suitable illustrations, and to Dr. Denise Barbut, who kindly provided the figures for Chapter 16 from her experience in monitoring patients during cardiac surgery. Dr. Michael Alexander offered useful suggestions for revising Chapter 20. Most of all, I thank my patients, who have taught me and others so much about their conditions and about dealing with infirmities. Their insights and courage have been inspirations helping me to weather the disaster that is managed care. I hope and pray that this book in some small measure helps future stroke patients so that past stroke victims will not have suffered completely in vain.

Louis R. Caplan
Boston, Massachusetts
Summer 1999

Preface to the First Edition

Stroke is a very common, yet complex, entity. The third leading cause of death in the United States, it is also an important cause of prolonged morbidity. The past decade has witnessed an explosion of new diagnostic technologies capable of unraveling abnormal cerebral anatomy and function, as well as the structure and function of the brain's vascular supply. New treatment strategies and techniques have proliferated.

Unfortunately, this revolution in technology and neuroscience has left a communication gap between the physician-scientists at academic centers, where the new data are being generated, and the practitioners who care for stroke patients. Most advances have been published in specialty scientific journals. When information is gathered into book form, the result has often been multiauthored compendia that emphasize the complexities, uncertainties, and controversies in stroke diagnosis and treatment. These larger volumes present diverse material from many authors with different views, sometimes without a guiding hand to organize the huge mass of data and lead the clinician through the labyrinth. No wonder many physicians, especially non-neurologists, feel lost in this maze of technology and controversy!

This is a book by clinicians, aimed primarily at physicians who care for patients with stroke. It has three important features that we hope distinguish it from other stroke compendia and legitimize its existence: (1) It is written entirely by two authors and describes a single approach to the stroke patient. (2) It is a "how-to" manual that describes a practical approach to the evaluation, diagnosis, and treatment of the stroke patient. (3) It incorporates, wherever possible, data and strategies gained from our experience with the Harvard and Michael Reese stroke registries and the National Stroke Data Bank. Our goal has been to interpret and organize the newer advances into practical terms referable to the daily care of stroke patients. The book is intended as a manual for the general practitioner, internist, or surgeon confronted with stroke patients and for the medical student and house officer in training. We hope it may prove useful as a general framework or modus operandi for the neurologist, neurosurgeon, or vascular surgeon who does not specialize in stroke.

Part I presents general information and considerations, including bedside and laboratory diagnosis; a brief review of cerebral anatomy, pathology, and pathophysiology; and principles of treatment. Part II, the core of the book, discusses specific stroke and subtypes. The essentials of clinical presentation, diagnosis, and treatment are discussed for the various types of occlusive disease, cerebral embolism, hypoxic-ischemic encephalopathy, and hemorrhagic disorders. Part III briefly considers prevention, complications, and rehabilitation.

The book is pragmatic and details a unified, rational approach to diagnosis and treatment. It is not meant to be a repository of definitive and balanced knowledge, hypotheses, and concepts. Basic science and laboratory data are included only when they contribute to the understanding and practical management of the stroke patient. We briefly introduce the physician to computer logic in an attempt to make the approach to stroke more systematic and measurable. Whenever possible, we include quantitative data from our own stroke registry experience, most of it previously unpublished, to allow estimation of probabilities. Of course, certainty in stroke is the exception and not the rule. Where no solid scientific data exist to guide management in a particular situation, we explain what we do and why. In the chapters on specific stroke syndromes, we use the case analysis method, which closely mimics the usual clinical situation and is easier to digest than didactic exposition. We also translate applications of the newer technologies into simple, pragmatic, utilitarian advice for the clinician. All figures, including illustrations of radiological findings, are presented as drawings rather than photographs, in order to highlight the appearance of the various lesions that occur in stroke patients. References are limited to essential work and are not meant to exhaustive. At times, original classic sources have been chosen, rather than the most recent work, in an effort to acquaint the reader with the richness of the stroke literature.

We wish to thank the teachers, colleagues, and students who made this book possible. Distinction between student and teacher is always artificial, even transparent, since the best teachers are eternal students who ably share their zest and style of learning, and our students teach us more than we know. Drs. Derek Denny-Brown, Walle Nauta, C. Miller Fisher, Raymond D. Adams, Faviau Romanul, and H. Richard Tyler are probably most responsible for kindling and nurturing the senior author's interest in the nervous system and stroke. Many colleagues merit our special thanks: those at Boston's Beth Israel Hospital, especially Drs. Chaim Mayman, Nicholas Zervas, and Arthur Rosenbaum; coworkers in the Harvard Stroke Registry, especially Drs. J.P. Mohr and Howard Bleich; colleagues at the Michael Reese Hospital, especially Drs. Daniel Hier, Allan Burke, James Goodwin, Morris Fisher, Lonnie Amico, Larry Ferguson, Gerry Luken, Gerry Moss, Steve Gould, Dushyant Patel, and Masoud Hemmati; colleagues at the New England Medical Center, especially Drs. Michael Pessin, L. Dana DeWitt, R. Michael Scott, William Shucart, and Samuel Wolpert; former Stroke Fellows Drs. Elizabeth Zaraspe-Yoo, Phil Gorelick, Cathy Helgason, and Michael Kelly, and all the resident physicians who worked with us at the Harvard Medical School, the University of Chicago, and Tufts University.

Louis R. Caplan
Robert W. Stein
Boston, Massachusetts

Caplan's Stroke: A Clinical Approach

Part I
General Principles

Chapter 1
Introduction and Perspective

It was then that it happened. To my shock and incredulity, I could not speak. That is, I could utter nothing intelligible. All that would come from my lips was the sound *ab* which I repeated again and again. . . . Then as I watched it, the telephone handpiece slid slowly from my grasp, and I, in turn, slid slowly from my chair and landed on the floor behind the desk. . . . At 5:15 in that January dusk I had been a person; now at 6:45 I was a case. But I found it easy to accept my altered condition. I felt like a case.

—Eric Hodgins[1]

Cheshire puss . . . Would you tell me please which way I ought to go from here?
That depends a great deal on where you want to get to, said the cat.
I don't much care where, said Alice.
Then it doesn't matter which way you go, said the cat.
So long as I get somewhere, Alice added.
Oh, you're sure to do that, said the cat, if you only walk long enough.

—Lewis Carroll[2]

The past is always with us, never to be escaped; it alone is enduring; but amidst the changes and chances which succeed one another so rapidly in life, we are apt to live too much for the present and too much in the future.

—William Osler[3]

Numbers

In the United States, nearly three-fourths of a million individuals have a stroke and 150,000 (90,000 women and 60,000 men) die from stroke each year.[4] At any one time, there are approximately 2 million stroke survivors living in the United States. In China, approximately 1.5 million people die each year because of stroke.[5] For a long time, stroke has been the third leading cause of death in most countries in the world, surpassed as a killer only by heart disease and cancer. Strokes are an even more important cause of prolonged disability. Survivors of strokes are often unable to return to work or to assume their former effectiveness as citizens, spouses, friends, and parents. The economic, social, and psychological costs of stroke are enormous.

Important Medical and Historical Figures Who Had Strokes

The history of the world has undoubtedly been altered by stroke. Many important leaders in science, medicine, and politics have had their productivity cut prematurely short by stroke. Marcello Malpighi, discoverer of capillaries and the microscopic anatomy of the lungs, kidneys, and spleen, died of an apoplectic right hemiplegia.[6] Louis Pasteur, at age 46 years, had a stroke that caused a left hemiparesis, although he continued to make important advances until additional strokes impaired his function at age 65.[6]

Three important figures in twentieth century neurology—Russell Dejong,[7] the first editor of the journal *Neurology*; Raymond Escourolle, the French neuropathologist; and Houston Merritt, longtime Columbia professor and writer of *Merritt's Textbook of Neurology*—were severely disabled by multiple strokes in their later years. Two important political leaders during the early twentieth century, Vladimir Lenin and Woodrow Wilson, had intellectual impairment caused by stroke while they were at the helms of their countries at critical times in history. Lenin, at age 52 years, had the sudden onset of dysarthria and right hemiparesis. An observer noted that "often as he spoke, the words were slurred, and he paused several times like a man who has lost the thread of his argument."[6] Wilson, the architect of the League of Nations, had a series of small strokes that left him pseudobulbar and with a left hemiparesis at a time when he was ardently working for world peace and cooperation. The heads of state who met at Yalta and elsewhere to divide up the spheres of influence after World War II—Franklin Roosevelt, Winston Churchill, and Josef Stalin—all had severe cerebrovascular disease at the time.[8] Roosevelt subsequently died of a fatal stroke after years of severe hypertension.[9] History might have been different if the brains of these leaders had not been addled by strokes. Public awareness of stroke increased dramatically when President Dwight Eisenhower developed acute dysarthria and when Richard Nixon died after a large embolic cerebral hemisphere infarction.

Personal Tragedy of Stroke

The mortality, morbidity, and economic toll of stroke are impressive. Knowledge that government leaders may have brains damaged and even riddled with brain infarcts and hemorrhages is undoubtedly sobering. Yet even more important, in my own opinion, is the effect of stroke on the individual. What could be worse than the sudden inability to speak, move a limb, stand, walk, see, read, or feel, or become unable to understand spoken language,

write, or remember? Loss of function is often instantaneous and totally unanticipated; impairments may be transient or permanent, slight or devastating. The first common term for stroke, *apoplexy*, literally meant in Greek "struck suddenly with violence."[10] The word *stroke* refers to being suddenly stricken. Stroke patients tell graphically about the personal tragedy of their illness. Eric Hodgins, the popular author of *Mr. Blandings Builds His Dream House*, wrote an autobiographic account of his stroke that he titled *Episode*, from which I quoted at the beginning of this chapter.[1] He changed from a functioning human in one moment to a helpless, dumb invalid, "a case" in the next instant. Imagine an articulate author dependent for his livelihood on his use of language becoming totally unable to speak. Surely, the brain is wholly responsible for intelligence, capability, character, wit, humor, personality, and most of the characteristics that make us recognizable as individuals and as humans. Losing brain function can be dehumanizing and often makes individuals dependent on others. For these reasons, most individuals fear stroke more than any other disease, with the possible exception of cancer. Everyone would like to exit this life with capabilities and mind intact, despite the inevitable aging of our bodies.

When I conjure in my own mind the personal tragedy of stroke, I picture one of my patients, Herman Blumgart, an extremely gifted physician, teacher, and investigator. He was, for many years, physician-in-chief at the Beth Israel Hospital in Boston.[11] His early investigations in coronary artery disease were landmark advances in the understanding of vascular disease of the heart.[12,13] Yearly, he gave the introductory lecture to incoming Harvard Medical School students about the joys and responsibilities of being a physician. I recall his vivid, articulate lectures and bedside demonstrations. He was, in many ways, the model physician. He was also a vocal advocate on behalf of patients. His lecture "Caring for the Patient," presented in 1963 and reported in the *New England Journal of Medicine*, remains a model exposition on doctoring, as valid today as when it was originally delivered.[14] Tragically, this master of communication was rendered, in an instant, severely aphasic. His Wernicke-type aphasia was so severe that he could barely communicate verbally his basic needs and could hardly understand the queries and spoken and written statements of others. He could no longer read, eliminating one of his lifelong joys. As a junior staff neurologist, I was one of his physicians. The angst and frustration of his plight showed clearly on his face each time I saw him. This personal disaster was palpable and dramatic.

Brief History of Stroke

In any human endeavor, the future is heavily influenced by the past. As the dialogue between Alice and the Cheshire Cat (quoted at the beginning of this chapter)[2] teaches, if you want to get somewhere, you must know where you are going. If clinicians are to know where they are headed, they must know where they are and where they and their predecessors have been. History adds an important dimension to knowledge. The past helps focus and broaden the perspective of the present and the future. Osler, and most other important medical innovators, were aware of their debt to history and of their inevitable entanglement with the past as well as the present and future.[3] I begin with a brief review of the early history of stroke. Space necessitates inclusion of only a brief review of some important people and milestones to convey a sense of the historical context of the present state of knowledge about stroke. Of course, the following view of history is eclectic and personal and should be recognized as such.

Hippocrates (circa 400 BC) was probably the first to write about the medical aspects of stroke.[6,10] He and his followers were mostly interested in prognosis, predicting for the patient and family the outcome of an illness.[15] Hippocrates was a keen observer and urged careful observation and recording of phenomenology. Hippocrates wrote in his aphorisms on apoplexy, "persons are most subject to apoplexy between the ages of forty and sixty,"[16] and attacks of numbness might reflect "impending apoplexy."[9] He astutely noted, "when persons in good health are suddenly seized with pains in the head and straightaway are laid down speechless and breathe with stertor, they die in seven days when fever comes on."[6,17] This description of subarachnoid hemorrhage shows the Hippocratic emphasis on observation and prognosis. Hippocrates also observed that there were many blood vessels con-

nected to the brain, most of which were "thin," but two (the carotid arteries) were stout. The Greeks recognized that interruption of these blood vessels to the brain could cause loss of consciousness, and so they named the arteries *carotid*, from the Greek word *karos*, meaning "deep sleep."

A few hundred years after Hippocrates, Galen (131–201 AD) described the anatomy of the brain and its blood vessels from dissections of animals. Although his early writings emphasized observation and experimentation, much of his later works combined mostly theorizing and speculation, in which he attributed disease to a disequilibrium between putative body humors and secretions such as water, blood, phlegm, bile, and so forth.[15] Galen and his voluminous writings dominated the 1,300 years after his death. During the ensuing Dark and Middle Ages, persons who called themselves physicians gained their knowledge solely from studying the Galenic texts, considered at the time to be the epitome of all medical wisdom. Dissection, experimentation, and personal observations were discouraged and not considered scholarly.

Andreas Vesalius (1514–1564) challenged the Galenic tradition by dissecting humans and relying on his own personal observations instead of Galen's writings. Vesalius could not find the rete mirabile of blood vessels that Galen had described (presumably in a lower animal). Vesalius's dissections were published in a volume entitled *De Humani Corpis Fabrica* (usually referred to as the *Fabrica*), which contained the detailed drawings his young artist and collaborator Jan Kalkar reproduced as woodcuts and copper plates.[6,18] The seventh book of the *Fabrica* contains 15 diagrams of a brain. These were the most detailed neuroanatomic studies up to that time.[6] By all accounts, Vesalius had a great flair for lecturing and teaching, and his works and personage stimulated much interest in anatomy.[15]

During the last half of the seventeenth century, two important physicians, Johann Jakob Wepfer (1620–1695) and Thomas Willis (1621–1675), made further anatomic and clinical observations. Wepfer wrote a popular treatise on apoplexy that was originally published in 1658 and had five subsequent editions.[6,19] Wepfer performed meticulous examinations of the brains of patients dying of apoplexy. He described the appearance of the carotid siphon and the course of the middle cerebral artery in the sylvian fissure. Obstruction of the carotid and vertebral arteries was recognized as a cause of apoplexy (the blockage preventing sufficient blood from reaching the brain).[20] Wepfer was the first to show clearly that bleeding into the brain was an important cause of apoplexy. Thomas Willis, a neuroanatomist best known for his *Cerebri Anatome*, which contained a description of a circle of anastomotic vessels at the base of the brain, was also a well-known clinician and an astute observer. Willis recognized transient ischemic attacks and the phenomenology of embolism, as well as the existence of occlusion of the carotid artery.[20,21]

During the eighteenth century, one of the true giants in medical history, Giovanni Battista Morgagni (1682–1771), was able to focus attention on pathology and the cause of disease. Up to that time, anatomy and prognostic formulas had prevailed. Morgagni, a distinguished professor of anatomy at the University of Padua, had a vision that the secret to understanding disease was to carefully perform necropsies on humans with illnesses and then to correlate the pathologic findings with their symptoms during life. Although the clinicopathologic method is now taken for granted, it was a new approach for physicians in the eighteenth century. Morgagni labored his entire career to meticulously collect material for his epic work, *De Sedibus et Causis Morborum per Anatomen Indagatis*, which was published when he was 79 years old.[15,22] *De Sedibus* is a five-volume work organized in the form of 70 letters to a young man describing the cases collected. The first volume was titled *Disease of the Head*. Morgagni's clinical descriptions of patients were detailed but contained no formal physical or neurologic examinations because these were not performed during his lifetime.

One of Morgagni's descriptions illustrates the style and content of the book. "A certain man, who was a native of Genoa, blind of one eye, and liv'd by begging, being drunk, and quarreling with other drunken beggars, receiv'd two blows by their sticks; one on his hand which was slight, and another violent one at the left temple so that blood came out of the left ear. Yet soon after, the quarrel being made up, he sat down at the fire with them . . . and again fill'd himself with a great quantity of wine, by way of pledge of friendship being renewed; and not long after, on the same night, he died."[15] Necropsy showed a large epidural hema-

toma. Morgagni also described cases of intracerebral hemorrhage and recognized that paralysis was on the side of the body opposite to the brain lesion. Morgagni's work shifted the emphasis from anatomy alone to inquiry about diseases and their pathology, causes, and clinical manifestations during life.

During the early years of the nineteenth century, an influential treatise on apoplexy was written by prominent Irish physician John Cheyne (1777–1836). Cheyne's book, which appeared in 1812, was titled *Cases of Apoplexy and Lethargy with Observations upon the Comatose Diseases*.[23] In it, he sought to separate the phenomenology of lethargy and coma from apoplexy. Cheyne's description of the neurologic abnormalities was more detailed than those of his predecessors, and the "morbid appearances" of the patients' brains were emphasized after the example of Morgagni. One illustrative patient was a woman of 32 years who was near the end of her pregnancy. After a headache she became less responsive. Cheyne found that "she preserved the power of voluntary motion of the left side, but the right was completely paralytic. She seemed perfectly conscious, attempted to speak, but could not articulate; she signified by pointing with her left hand that she desired to drink."[23] After a historical review of her case, Cheyne discussed the available treatments (bloodletting, emetics, purges, and external applications) and then described 23 other cases. The pathologic findings included clear descriptions of brain softenings and intracerebral and subarachnoid hemorrhages.[23] After Cheyne, developments were made concurrently in the clinical, anatomic, and pathologic aspects of stroke.

John Abercrombie contributed a more detailed clinical classification of apoplexy in his general text published in 1828.[24] Abercrombie used the presence of headache, stupor, paralysis, and outcome to separate apoplectics into three clinical groups. In the first group, which he termed *primary apoplexy*, the onset was sudden; unilateral paralysis, rigidity and stupor were present. The outcome was poor. These patients probably had large intracerebral hemorrhages or large brain infarcts. In the second group, patients had sudden headache, vomiting, and either faintness or falling but no paralysis. Undoubtedly, these patients had subarachnoid hemorrhages. In the third group, there was unilateral paralysis,

Figure 1-1. Charles Foix in his laboratory at the Salpetriere.

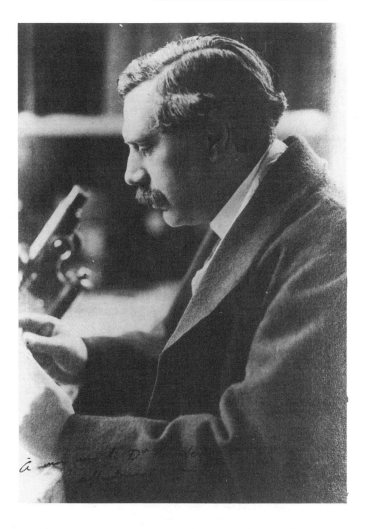

often with abnormal speech, but neither stupor nor headache was present. This group must have had small infarcts or parenchymatous hemorrhages. Abercrombie also speculated on etiologic mechanisms, mentioning spasm of vessels, interruption of the circulation, and rupture of diseased vessels causing hemorrhage.[10,24]

In the middle of the nineteenth century, dissemination of knowledge about the pathology of stroke came with the publication of four atlases, each containing plates of brain and vascular lesions. Hooper's atlas, published in 1828, clearly illustrated pontine and putaminal hemorrhages and a subdural hematoma.[25] Cruveilher (1835–1842),[26] Carswell (1838),[27] and Bright (1831)[28] also published atlases containing lithographs of systemic and neuropathologic lesions. Bright, better known for his work on nephritis, collected more than 200 neuropathologic cases and specimens[10] and included illustrations of 25 nervous system specimens, including cerebrovascular cases, in his volume on nervous system disorders.[28]

During the later part of the nineteenth and the early years of the twentieth centuries, the anatomic details of the cerebral vessels and their supply were studied carefully. Detailed observations of the distribution of the arteries and veins in the cranium were made by Düret, a French neurosurgeon, first working in Charcot's laboratory[29,30]; by Stopford in Britain[31]; and later by Foix, who dissected pathologic specimens at the Salpetriere in France.[32–35] Foix (Figure 1-1) made many key anatomic and clinical observations. Also during this same period, clinicians gathered more information on the clinical findings in patients with strokes that involved various brain regions. The

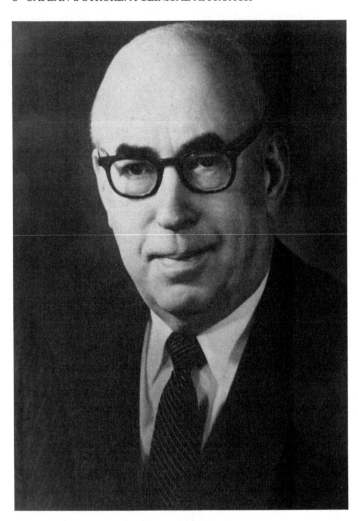

Figure 1-2. C. Miller Fisher.

bulk of these data involved clinical descriptions, with little interest concerning pathogenesis, laboratory confirmation, or treatment. The general medical and neurologic texts of Osler,[36] Gowers,[37] and Wilson[38] contained detailed descriptions of the clinical findings and prognosis of many stroke syndromes. The clinicopathologic method culminated in descriptions by Foix and his colleagues of the syndromes of infarctions in the regions of the middle cerebral artery,[34,35] posterior cerebral artery,[35,39] anterior cerebral artery,[35,40] and vertebrobasilar arteries.[33,35]

Later, reports by C. Miller Fisher (Figure 1-2), who analyzed the findings in patients with internal carotid artery occlusions,[41] cerebellar[42] and basal ganglionic[43] hemorrhages, and lacunar infarcts,[44] and by Kubik and Adams, who described the findings in patients with basilar artery occlusions,[45] carried on the example set by Foix. All of these reports contained meticulous descriptions of the signs and symptoms found in patients with infarcts and hemorrhages in various vascular and brain distributions. Elegant and thorough as these descriptions were, their limitations included (1) reliance on only the fatal cases because precise diagnosis was not possible during life; (2) predominance of anecdotal cases, with few data on the incidence and frequency of findings in large series of patients with the specific described conditions; (3) insufficient availability of technology to allow accurate diagnosis or clarification of the pathogenesis or pathophysiology of the vascular lesions and their effects on the brain; and (4) little information about the effectiveness of various treatments.

During the twentieth century, especially in the 1970s and 1980s, there was an explosive growth of interest in and knowledge about stroke. Advances in technology allowed better visualization of the anatomy and functional aspects of the brain and of vascular lesions during life. New surgical and medical treatments were now possible. Therapeutic trials began to evaluate systematically the efficacy and safety of some of these treatments. Databases and registries of large numbers of well-studied stroke patients helped identify and quantify the most common clinical and laboratory findings in patients with various stroke syndromes. Epidemiologic studies identified more accurately the risk factors for stroke-prevention strategies.

The technological revolution probably began with the work of the Portuguese neurosurgeon Moniz (1874–1955). Moniz surgically exposed and temporarily ligated the internal carotid artery in the neck and then rapidly injected by hand a 30% solution of sodium iodide, taking skull films later at regular intervals.[46] He first used the technique for studying patients suspected of having brain tumors, but he later studied stroke patients. By the time of his monograph on angiography in 1931,[47] Moniz had studied 180 patients; had switched to another opaque-contrast agent, Thorotrast, because of convulsions that had occurred after the injection of sodium iodide; and had demonstrated the occurrence of occlusion of the internal carotid artery during life.[47,48] Modern angiography began with the work of Seldinger in Sweden, who devised a technique by which a small catheter could be inserted into an artery over a flexible guidewire after withdrawing the needle.[49] Catheter angiography of selected vessels in the carotid and vertebral circulations was then possible without surgical incisions. Newer dyes and filming techniques have since made angiography safer and more definitive.

Hounsfield of the research laboratories of Electrical Musical Instruments in Britain originated the concept of computed tomography (CT) during the mid-1960s. The instrument was first tried at the Atkinson-Morley Hospital in London.[6] CT scanners were first introduced to North America in 1973. Films from first-generation scanners were quite primitive, but by the late 1970s, third-generation scanners had made CT a useful, almost indispensable, diagnostic technique. By the mid-1980s, CT was readily available throughout North America and most of Europe. CT allowed clear distinction between brain ischemia and hemorrhage and allowed definition of the size and location of most brain infarcts and hemorrhages. The advent of magnetic resonance imaging (MRI) in clinical medicine in the mid-1980s was a further major advance. MRI proved superior to CT in showing old hemosiderin-containing hemorrhages and in imaging vascular malformations, lesions abutting on bony surfaces, and posterior fossa structures. MRI also made it easier to visualize lesions in different planes by providing sagittal, coronal, and horizontal sections. Improved filming techniques have made it possible to image the brain vasculature through the techniques of magnetic resonance (MR) angiography[50] and CT angiography.[51]

Ultrasound was introduced to medicine in 1961 by Franklin and colleagues, who used Doppler shifts of ultrasound to study blood flow in canine blood vessels.[6,52] B-mode ultrasound was soon used to provide images of the extracranial carotid arteries noninvasively. By the early 1980s, B-mode, continuous-wave, and pulsed-Doppler technology could reliably detect severe extracranial vascular occlusive disease in the carotid and vertebral arteries in the neck. Sequential ultrasound studies allowed physicians to study the natural history of the development and progression of these occlusive lesions and to correlate the occurrence and severity of disease with stroke risk factors, symptoms, and treatment. In 1982, Aaslid and colleagues introduced a high-energy bidirectional pulsed-Doppler system that used low frequencies to study intracranial arteries, termed *transcranial Doppler ultrasound* (TCD).[53] TCD made possible noninvasive detection of severe occlusive disease in the major intracranial arteries during life, as well as sequential study of these lesions.[54]

Introduction of echocardiography and ambulatory cardiac rhythm monitoring in the 1970s and 1980s greatly improved cardiac diagnoses and detection of cardiogenic sources of embolism. By the early 1990s, clinicians could safely define the nature, extent, and localization of most important brain, cardiac, and vascular lesions in stroke patients. Accurate diagnosis using modern technology facilitated clinical-imaging correlations in patients with nonfatal strokes, and this paved the way for monitoring the effects of various treatments. By the end of the twentieth century, advanced brain imaging with CT, MRI, and newer MR modalities, including fluid attenuating inversion recovery images, diffusion, perfusion, and functional MRI, and MR spectroscopy, were able to show clinicians the localization, severity, and potential reversibility of brain ischemia. Vascular lesions could be quickly and safely defined using spiral CT angiography, MR angiography, and extracranial and transcranial ultrasound. Cardiac and aortic sources of stroke were studied using trans-esophageal echocardiography. More sophisticated hematologic testing led to new insights into the role of altered coagulability in causing or contributing to thromboembolism. Clinicians were finally able to recognize and quantify quickly and accurately the key data elements needed to logically treat patients with brain ischemia and hemorrhage.

During the middle of the twentieth century, clinicians had advanced knowledge of clinical phenomenology by personally studying and describing small groups of patients. In 1935, Aring and Meritt studied a group of patients coming to necropsy at the Boston City Hospital to clarify the differential diagnosis between brain hemorrhages and infarcts.[55] Subsequently, Fisher and his colleagues and students studied and described the clinical findings in small numbers of patients with various cerebrovascular syndromes. During the 1970s and 1980s, the technological advances described made it possible to define the clinical and laboratory features of nonfatal, even minor, strokes and prestroke vascular lesions. With better knowledge of clinical and morphologic features, clinicians naturally sought more quantitative data. How often did intracerebral hemorrhages or lacunar infarcts occur? How often did each of the clinical symptoms and signs occur in each subtype of stroke? Clinicians recognized that valid, statistically meaningful data could not be collected unless large numbers of patients with a wide spectrum of representative cases were studied and analyzed. The advent of computers in medicine in the 1970s greatly facilitated the storage and analysis of large quantities of complex data. Collection of data on large numbers of stroke patients began with the series of Dalsgaard-Nielsen in Scandinavia[56] and with a series of patients seen by clinicians at the Mayo Clinic in Rochester, Minnesota.[57,58] The Harvard Cooperative Stroke Registry in the early 1970s was the first computer-based

registry of prospectively studied stroke patients.[59] During the 1970s and 1980s, a number of other stroke registries and databases provided more quantitative information about clinical and laboratory phenomena and diagnoses.[60–64] Community-based studies in South Alabama[65]; Framingham, Massachusetts[66]; Oxfordshire in Great Britain[67]; the Lehigh Valley in Pennsylvania[68]; and various regions in North Carolina, Oregon, and New York[69] generated important epidemiologic data. Computer-based registries and data banks have undoubtedly assisted collection and analysis of a wide variety of clinical, radiologic, pathologic, and epidemiologic information.[70,71] The present text relies heavily on data from these studies, especially those in which I was personally involved.[59,61,63]

During the second half of the twentieth century, there were major advances in therapeutic capabilities, especially in cerebrovascular surgery. In 1951, Fisher suggested the possibility of surgery on stenotic lesions of the extracranial carotid artery: "It is conceivable that some day vascular surgery will find a way to by-pass the occluded portions of the internal carotid artery during the period of ominous fleeting symptoms."[6,41] Carrea, Molins, and Murphy, in Buenos Aires, performed an anastomosis from the external carotid to the internal carotid artery in a patient with severe internal carotid artery stenosis in October 1951, but their report did not appear until 1955.[6,48,72] Eastcott, Pickering, and Rob also performed an anastomosis, this time from the common carotid artery to a segment of the internal carotid artery above an occlusion, in London in May 1953, and their report appeared before that of the Argentine authors.[6,73] DeBakey claimed to have performed the first carotid artery thromboendarterectomy in August 1953, but the case was not reported until many years later.[74] Advances in surgical technique, angiography, and anesthesia led to great improvements in the techniques of endarterectomy during the 1950s and 1960s. By the mid-1960s, carotid endarterectomy became a common, routine surgical procedure. Vascular surgeons also began to operate with technical skill on the extracranial subclavian, vertebral, and innominate arteries for posterior circulation occlusive disease.[6,48,75,76]

The advent of the dissecting microscope and other instrumentation advances led to new capabilities for intracranial surgery. Microsurgery on small and medium-sized arteries facilitated surgical treatment of aneurysms and vascular malformations and made possible anastomoses involving small basal and surface arteries of the brain.[77,78] In the 1970s, bypass procedures using the dissecting microscope created anastomoses between extracranial arteries, such as from the superficial temporal and occipital artery branches of the external carotid artery to the middle cerebral and posterior inferior cerebellar arteries.[77–80] These procedures became popular until a randomized controlled study showed that the anterior circulation bypasses, as then performed, were no better—and were sometimes worse—than medical therapy. Subsequent improvements in neuroanesthesia and intensive care helped reduce the morbidity and mortality of cerebrovascular surgery on the brain and its vasculature.[81] Improvements in brain imaging capabilities now allow stereotactic drainage of some brain hemorrhages.

Medical treatment also changed dramatically during the middle and later portions of the twentieth century. The lack of remedial treatments in the preceding eras was, at least partially, responsible for disinterest in defining the cause of stroke because little could be done in any case. The appearance of effective antihypertensive medicines in the middle years of the twentieth century clearly reduced the incidence of brain parenchymal hemorrhages and also reduced the frequency of ischemic stroke and occlusive vascular disease. Anticoagulant therapy with heparin and dicumarol were introduced as treatments for patients with occlusive cerebrovascular disease in the 1950s. Wright and colleagues at Cornell[82–84] and Millikan, Siekert, and Whisnant at the Mayo Clinic[85] pioneered the use of dicumarol for cerebrovascular indications. The presence of a potentially useful therapy further stimulated interest in stroke and was a factor in generating a meeting of individuals interested in cerebrovascular disease at Princeton, New Jersey, in 1954.[86] This was to be the first of the biennial Princeton conferences that bring together stroke experts and investigators from around the world to discuss problems, advances, and research in stroke. The emergence of stroke as a potentially treatable disease also helped promote the creation in 1967 of a Stroke Council as part of the activities of the American Heart Association (AHA).[87] This council convened its first international stroke conference in Dallas, Texas, in 1976. The journal *Stroke*, also an outgrowth of the AHA, began publication in 1970 with Millikan as its first editor.

If anticoagulants or other treatments are to be effective, therapy should be started in early or premonitory phases of stroke. Fisher had emphasized the presence of temporary short-lived episodes of neurologic symptoms, which he termed *transient ischemic attacks* (TIAs) in his patients with occlusion of the internal carotid artery.[41] Although others, including Hippocrates, Willis, and Gowers,[37] had mentioned the occurrence of these attacks before Fisher, they were generally not well known in the broader medical community. In 1953, Fisher and Cameron reported a patient with multiple TIAs and basilar artery disease, in whom the attacks ceased after introduction of heparin and the anticoagulant phenylindandione.[6,88] The authors commented, "Transient phenomena preceding the onset of a stroke are much more frequent than is commonly believed, for the patient often neglects them while his physician does not inquire about their occurrence once paralysis has occurred."[88] Analysis of the usual time-sequence features of stroke by physicians at the Mayo Clinic and elsewhere led to the introduction and popularization of terms that described the tempo of the symptoms and signs. These designations included progressing stroke, reversible ischemic neurologic deficits, completed strokes, and so forth. It was hoped that these designations would be simple and easy to distinguish by physicians not sophisticated in neurology and that the designations would predict prognosis and response to various treatments. These terms proved difficult to define. Furthermore, experience showed that they did not predict whether the patient would show a brain infarct on neuroimaging studies; nor did they predict the prognosis, the nature of the vascular process causing the ischemia, or the response to various treatments.[89,90] Their use now is solely for descriptive purposes. These terms do not represent diagnoses or the basis for treatment selection.

In 1950, Craven commented on the use of aspirin as an agent that might prevent thrombosis. Craven had observed that dental patients who took aspirin often bled after tooth extractions, and he reasoned that aspirin might be interfering with the normal clotting process.[6,91] Only later was aspirin shown to affect platelet adhesion and aggregability. Aspirin was not used for the treatment of cerebrovascular symptoms until the early 1970s.[92] By the mid-1970s, however, aspirin use was so widespread that therapeutic trials of its effectiveness were designed and reported.[93,94] During the 1980s and 1990s, other drugs that affected platelet functions by inactivating platelet receptors for adenosine diphosphate and inactivating the glycoprotein IIa/IIIb fibrinogen receptor[95] were developed and introduced into practice, including ticlopidine[96,97] and clopidogrel.[98] Other potentially effective pharmacologic agents became available after 1950. Corticosteroids, mannitol, and glycerol, which are osmotically active agents that reduce brain edema, were used to control increased intracranial pressure. Beta-adrenergic blocking agents, angiotensin-converting enzyme inhibitors, and calcium channel blocking agents afforded better control of arterial hypertension. Basic research on the mechanisms of nerve cell injury led physicians during the 1990s to test so-called neuroprotective drugs that were posited to ameliorate the cellular metabolic consequences of ischemic injury.[99,100]

Thrombolytic therapy to lyse occlusive thromboemboli in stroke patients was tried briefly in the early 1960s, but was abandoned because of an unacceptably high rate of brain hemorrhage.[101] During the 1980s, streptokinase and recombinant tissue plasminogen activator (rt-PA) were shown to be effective in the treatment of acute coronary artery thrombosis, and these drugs were first introduced as investigational agents to treat patients with cerebrovascular thrombi.[102,103] During the next decade and a half, knowledge gradually accumulated about the effectiveness and safety of various thrombolytic drugs in patients with angiographically defined vascular occlusive lesions.[104] After reports of the European Cooperative Acute Stroke Study[105] and the National Institute of Neurological Disorders and Stroke rt-PA Study[106] concerning the use of intravenous rt-PA were published in 1995, the U.S. Food and Drug Administration released rt-PA for stroke and the AHA[107] and American Academy of Neurology[108] committees published guidelines endorsing rt-PA use. Although the results of these trials and the need for vascular diagnostic testing were debated,[109] the treatment of acute stroke patients dramatically changed after the approval of thrombolytic treatment in the United States. Stroke was now seen as an emergency—time = brain. Doctors, hospitals, and emergency services had to prepare to treat patients with acute stroke urgently and more systematically.

Physicians' armamentaria of surgical and medical treatments grew impressively, but before 1970 there were few objective data on the effectiveness, safety, and use of the various treatments. Reliance on anecdotal reports of treatment responses in selected, small samples of patients clearly was not satisfactory. During the 1970s and 1980s, methods were developed and improved for more systematic, planned, scientific, statistically based studies and analyses, and even meta-analyses of large series of representative patients prospectively entered in multicenter, randomized, controlled therapeutic trials.[110] Therapeutic trials of the effect of aspirin and other agents that alter platelet functions were helpful in suggesting the use of these drugs in some patients.[93–97,111] Trials have also shown the effectiveness of anticoagulation in preventing brain embolism in patients with atrial fibrillation.[112–115] Trials have been and are being used to evaluate the effectiveness of various surgical procedures, such as carotid endarterectomy[116–120] and extracranial to intracranial bypass procedures.[121] Trial methodology, design, and statistical analysis have improved with experience. Well-conceived therapeutic trials, meta-analyses, and systematic reviews of these therapeutic trials offer promise for clarifying some aspects of the treatment of common cerebrovascular conditions in the future. Barnett, Fields, and Toole have been pioneers in the introduction and performance of stroke treatment trials. However, the expense, requirements for large numbers of patients, need for clearly verifiable, commonly occurring end points, and other practical considerations make these multicenter trials unsatisfactory for studying the treatment of many cerebrovascular conditions.

Stroke as a Model Example of Brain and Vascular Disease

Stroke is the prototype of a focal, well-circumscribed brain lesion. Fisher is fond of saying that neurology is learned "stroke by stroke." Knowledge of the symptoms and signs in patients with focal brain infarcts and hemorrhages has been instrumental in developing an understanding of the functioning of various brain structures and regions. Awareness of the clinical findings in patients with frontal lobe hemorrhages has undoubtedly helped clinicians to recognize tumors, focal infections, atrophies, and other disease processes located in the frontal lobes. The ability to localize infarcts and hemorrhages precisely with CT and MRI has greatly facilitated study of anatomic-physiologic correlations. Study of stroke patients and stroke animal models has improved understanding of brain electrophysiology, chemistry, pharmacology, and overall physiology.

Stroke also provides a model for the study of vascular diseases. Atherosclerosis, embolism, and thrombosis are all usually systemic disorders that affect many critical organs in addition to the brain. Information about the morphology, development, and etiology of lesions in the cerebrovascular bed has undoubtedly influenced knowledge of vascular conditions that affect the coronary, renal, and limb arteries. Of course, the corollary is also true; stroke clinicians clearly can and should gain from clinicians and researchers who study vascular diseases affecting these other body regions. Similarly, study of patients with cardioembolic strokes has advanced knowledge about the heart and its diseases. Stroke patients often have abnormalities of blood coagulation. Elucidation of clotting and bleeding dysfunction underlying stroke has advanced general knowledge about the formed and serologic elements of the blood and the vascular endothelium and about their functions in coagulation.

Stroke Care

It is not possible to overemphasize that the care of strokes is not the same as the care of stroke patients. Most strokes result from systemic illnesses such as hypertension, atherosclerosis, cardiac diseases, and coagulopathies. These conditions profoundly affect other body organs and general health, as well as the brain and central nervous system. Specialists sometimes only see and treat one portion of the body and ignore the general problem, similar to the proverbial blind men feeling isolated parts of the elephant. As physicians, we must be sure that the general systemic disorders, such as hypertension and atherosclerosis, receive deserved detailed and long-term attention. As entry portals into the health care system, clinicians seeing stroke patients can and should become key figures in preventing disease and in correcting unhealthy practices.

Strokes create other health problems. These include not only the acute complications that are discussed in Chapter 19, but also problems such as increased wear and tear on the joint structures of the hip, knee, and ankle because of altered gait; aspiration and recurrent bronchopulmonary infections; and poor bladder emptying, with an increased frequency of urinary-tract infections. Strokes also have profound social, psychological, and economic effects on stroke patients and their families and friends. Physicians caring for stroke patients must consider all of the multiple facets of the condition and must liberally use other medical and ancillary health personnel. The family often needs as much attention, education, and compassion as the patient. In another book, I have devoted considerable attention to the general approach toward and care of patients, especially those with neurologic illnesses.[122]

The other organs exist to keep the brain functioning normally. Any change in the brain's function and activity profoundly affects living. No medical task exists that is more complex, more multifaceted, more important, and potentially more rewarding than caring for a stroke patient.

References

1. Hodgins E. Episode: Report on the Accident Inside My Skull. New York: Atheneum, 1964;7–14.
2. Carroll L. Alice's Adventures in Wonderland. New York: Dutton, 1929;93–94.
3. Osler W. Aequanimitas. In Aequanimitas with Other Addresses to Medical Students, Nurses and Practitioners of Medicine. Philadelphia: Blakiston, 1932;8–9.
4. Broderick J, Brott T, Kothari R, et al. The Greater Cincinnati/Northern Kentucky Stroke Study. Preliminary first-ever and total incidence rates of strokes among blacks. Stroke 1998;29:415–421.
5. Chen ZM, Xu Z, Coillins R, Li WX, Peto R. Blood pressure, blood cholesterol and stroke mortality in a population with low mean cholesterol level. Cerebrovasc Dis 1998;8(Suppl 4):1.
6. Fields WS, Lemak NA. A History of Stroke: Its Recognition and Treatment. New York: Oxford University Press, 1989.
7. Gilman S, Russell N. DeJong, 1907–1990. Ann Neurol 1991;29:108–109.
8. Friedlander, WJ. About three old men: an inquiry into how cerebral atherosclerosis has altered world politics. Stroke 1972;3:467–473.

9. Bruenn HG. Clinical notes on the illness and death of president Franklin D. Roosevelt. Ann Intern Med 1970; 72:579–591.

10. McHenry LC Jr. Garrison's History of Neurology. Springfield, IL: Charles C. Thomas, 1969.

11. Linenthal AJ. First a Dream: The History of Boston's Jewish Hospitals, 1896 to 1928. Boston: Beth Israel Hospital, 1990;276–294.

12. Blumgart HL, Schlesinger MJ, Davis D. Studies on the relation of the clinical manifestations of angina pectoris, coronary thrombosis, and myocardial infarction to the pathological findings. Am Heart J 1940;19:1–9.

13. Blumgart HL, Schlesinger MJ, Zoll PM. Angina pectoris, coronary failure, and acute myocardial infarction. JAMA 1941;116:91–97.

14. Blumgart HL. Caring for the patient. N Engl J Med 1964; 270:449–456.

15. Nuland S. Doctors, Bibliography of Medicine. Birmingham, AL: Libraries of Gryphon Editions, 1988.

16. Adams F. The Genuine Works of Hippocrates: Translated from the Greek. Baltimore: Williams and Wilkins, 1939.

17. Clark E. Apoplexy in the Hippocratic writings. Bull Hist Med 1963;37:301–314.

18. Vesalius A. De Humani Corporis Fabrica. Basileae, Italy: J Oporini, 1543.

19. Wepfler JJ. Observationes Anatomicae, ex Cadaveribus Eorum, quos Sustulit Apoplexia, cum Exercitatione de Ejus Loco Affecto. Schaffhausen, Germany: Joh. Caspari Suteri, 1658.

20. Gurdjian ES, Gurdjian ES. History of occlusive cerebrovascular disease: I. From Wepfer to Moniz. Arch Neurol 1979;36:340–343.

21. Toole JF. The Willis lecture: transient ischemic attacks, scientific method, and new realities. Stroke 1991;22: 99–104.

22. Morgagni GB. The seats and causes of disease investigated by anatomy. Translated by B Alexander. London: Millar and Cadell, 1769. Birmingham: Classics of Medicine Library.

23. Cheyne J. Cases of Apoplexy and Lethargy with Observations upon the Comatose Diseases. London: J Moyes Printer, 1812.

24. Abercrombie J. Pathological and Practical Researches on Diseases of the Brain and Spinal Cord. Edinburgh: Waugh and Innes, 1828.

25. Hooper R. The Morbid Anatomy of the Human Brain Illustrated by Coloured Engravings of the Most Frequent and Important Organic Diseases to which that Viscus is Subject. London: Rees, Orme, Brown, and Green, 1831.

26. Cruveilhier J. Anatomie Pathologique du Corps Humain: Descriptions Avec Figures Lithographiées et Caloriées des Diverses Alterations Morbides Dont le Corps Humain Est Susceptible. Paris: J.B. Bailliere, 1835–1842.

27. Carswell R. Pathological Anatomy: Illustrations of the Elementary Forms of Disease. London: Longman, 1838.

28. Bright R. Reports of Medical Cases, Selected with a View of Illustrating the Symptoms and Cures of Diseases by a Reference to Morbid Anatomy. London: Longman, Rees, Orme, Brown, and Green, 1831.

29. Duret H. Sur la distribution des arteres nouricieres du bulbe rachidien. Arch Physiol Norm Pathol 1873;2:97–113.

30. Duret H. Recherches anatomiques sur la circulation de l'encephale. Arch Physiol Norm Pathol 1874;3:60–91,316–353.

31. Stopford JS. The anatomy of the pons and medulla oblongata. J Anat Physiol 1928;50:225–280.

32. Foix C, Hillemand P. Irrigation de la protuberance. C R Soc Biol (Paris) 1925;92:35–36.

33. Foix C, Hillemand P. les Arteres de l'axe encephalique jusqu'au diencephale inclusivement. Rev Neurol (Paris) 1925;41:705–739.

34. Foix C, Levy M. Les ramollissements sylviens. Rev Neurol (Paris) 1927;43:1–51.

35. Caplan LR. Charles Foix–the first modern stroke neurologist. Stroke 1990;21:348–356.

36. Osler W. The Principles and Practice of Medicine (5th ed). New York: D Appleton, 1903.

37. Gowers WR. A Manual of Disease of the Nervous System. London: J and A Churchill, 1893.

38. Wilson SAK, Bruce AN. Neurology (2nd ed). London: Butterworth–Heinemann, 1955.

39. Foix C, Masson A. Le Syndrome de l'artere cerebrale posterieure. Presse Med 1923;31:361–365.

40. Foix C, Hillemand P. Les Syndromes de l'artere cerebrale anterieure. Encephale 1925;20:209–232.

41. Fisher CM. Occlusion of the internal carotid artery. Arch Neurol 1951;65:346–377.

42. Fisher CM, Picard E, Polak A, et al. Acute hypertensive cerebellar hemorrhage: diagnosis and surgical treatment. J Nerv Ment Dis 1965;140:38–57.

43. Fisher CM. Clinical Syndromes in Cerebral Hemorrhage. In: W Fields (ed), Pathogenesis and Treatment of Cerebrovascular Disease. Springfield, IL: Charles C Thomas, 1961;318–342.

44. Fisher CM. Lacunes: small, deep cerebral infarcts. Neurology 1965;15:774–784.

45. Kubik CS, Adams RD. Occlusion of the basilar artery: a clinical and pathological study. Brain 1946;69:73–121.

46. Moniz E. L'encephalographie artèrielle, son importance dans la localisation des tumeurs cérébrales. Rev Neurol (Paris) 1927;2:72–90.

47. Moniz E. L'angiographie Cérébrale. Paris: Masson, 1931.

48. Gurdjian ES, Gurdjian ES. History of occlusive cerebrovascular disease: II. After Moniz with special reference to surgical treatment. Arch Neurol 1979;36:427–432.

49. Seldinger SI. Catheter replacement of the needle in percutaneous arteriography. Acta Radiol 1953;39:368–376.

50. Edelman RC, Mattle HP, O'Reilly GV, et al. Magnetic resonance imaging of flow dynamics in the circle of Willis. Stroke 1990;21:56–65.

51. Knauth M, von Kummer R, Jansen O, et al. Potential of CT angiography in acute ischemic stroke. Am J Neuroradiol 1997;18:1001–1010.

52. Franklin DL, Schlegel WA, Rushner RF. Blood flow measured by Doppler frequency shift of back-scattered ultrasound. Science 1961;134:564–565.

53. Aaslid R, Markwalder TM, Nornes H. Non-invasive transcranial Doppler ultrasound recording of flow velocity in basal cerebral arteries. J Neurosurg 1982;57:769–774.

54. Caplan LR, Brass LM, DeWitt LD, et al. Transcranial Doppler ultrasound: present status. Neurology 1990;40: 696–700.

55. Aring CD, Meritt HH. Differential diagnosis between cerebral hemorrhage and cerebral thrombosis. Arch Intern Med 1935;56:435–456.
56. Dalsgaard-Nielsen T. Survey of 1000 cases of apoplexia cerebri. Acta Psychiatr Neurol Scand 1955;30:169–185.
57. Whisnant JP, Fitzgibbons JP, Kurland LT, et al. Natural history of stroke in Rochester, Minnesota, 1945 through 1954. Stroke 1971;2:11–22.
58. Matsumoto N, Whisnant JP, Kurland LT, et al. Natural history of stroke in Rochester, Minnesota, 1955 through 1969: an extension of a previous study 1945 through 1954. Stroke 1973;4:20–29.
59. Mohr JP, Caplan LR, Melski JW, et al. The Harvard Cooperative Stroke Registry: a prospective registry. Neurology 1978;28:754–762.
60. Kunitz S, Gross CR, Heyman A, et al. The Pilot Stroke Data Bank: definition, design, and data. Stroke 1984;15:740–746.
61. Caplan LR, Hier DB, D'Cruz I. Cerebral embolism in the Michael Reese Stroke Registry. Stroke 1983;14:530–536.
62. Chambers BR, Donnan GA, Bladin PF. Patterns of stroke: an analysis of the first 700 consecutive admissions to the Austin Hospital Stroke Unit. Aust N Z J Med 1983;13:57–64.
63. Foulkes MA, Wolf PA, Price TR, et al. The Stroke Data Bank: design, methods, and baseline characteristics. Stroke 1988;19:547–554.
64. Bogousslavsky J, Mille GV, Regli F. The Lausanne Stroke Registry: an analysis of 1,000 consecutive patients with first stroke. Stroke 1988;19:1083–1092.
65. Gross CR, Kase CS, Mohr JP, et al. Stroke in south Alabama: incidence and diagnostic features—a population based study. Stroke 1984;15:249–255.
66. Wolf PA, Kannel WB, Dauber TR. Prospective investigations: the Framingham study and the epidemiology of stroke. Adv Neurol 1978;19:107–120.
67. Oxfordshire Community Stroke Project. Incidence of stroke in Oxfordshire: first year's experience of a community stroke registry. BMJ 1983;287:713–717.
68. Alter M, Sobel E, McCoy RC, et al. Stroke in the Lehigh Valley: incidence based on a community-wide hospital registry. Neuroepidemiology 1985;4:1–15.
69. Yatsu FM, Becker C, McLeroy K, et al. Community hospital-based stroke programs: North Carolina, Oregon, and New York: I. Goals, objectives, and data collection procedures. Stroke 1986;17:276–284.
70. Mohr JP. Stroke data banks [editorial]. Stroke 1986;17:171–172.
71. Caplan LR. Stroke Data Banks, Then and Now. In R Courbier (ed), Basis for a Classification of Cerebrovascular Disease. Amsterdam: Excerpta Medica, 1985;152–162.
72. Carrea R, Molins M, Murphy G. Surgical treatment of spontaneous thrombosis of the internal carotid artery in the neck. Carotid-carotideal anastomosis. Acta Neurol Latinoamer 1955;1:71–78.
73. Eastcott HHG, Pickering GW, Rob CG. Reconstruction of internal carotid artery in a patient with intermittent attacks of hemiplegia. Lancet 1954;2:994–996.
74. DeBakey ME. Successful carotid endarterectomy for cerebrovascular insufficiency: nineteen year follow-up. JAMA 1975;233:1083–1085.
75. Crawford ES, DeBakey ME, Fields WS. Roentgenographic diagnosis and surgical treatment of basilar artery insufficiency. JAMA 1958;168:509–514.
76. DeBakey ME, Crawford ES, Cooley DA, et al. Cerebral arterial insufficiency: one to 11 year results following arterial reconstructive operation. Ann Surg 1965;161:921–945.
77. Jaccobson JH, Wallman LJ, Schumacher GA, et al. Microsurgery as an aid to middle cerebral artery endarterectomy. J Neurosurg 1962;19:108–115.
78. Yasargil MG. Microsurgery Applied to Neurosurgery. Stuttgart, Germany: Georg Thieme Verlag, 1969;108–109.
79. Yasargil MG, Krayenbuhl HA, Jacobson JH. Microneurosurgical arterial reconstruction. Surgery 1970;67:221–233.
80. Maroon JK, Donaghy RMP. Experimental cerebral revascularization with autogenous grafts. J Neurosurg 1973;38:172–179.
81. Ropper AH, Kennedy SF (eds). Neurological and Neurosurgical Intensive Care. Rockville, MD: Aspen, 1988.
82. Wright IS, McDevitt E. Cerebral vascular disease: significance, diagnosis, and present treatment, including selective use of anticoagulant substances. Ann Intern Med 1954;41:682–698.
83. McDevitt E, Carter SA, Gatje BW, et al. Use of anticoagulants in treatment of cerebral vascular disease. JAMA 1958;166:592–596.
84. Groch SN, McDevitt E, Wright IS. A long-term study of cerebral vascular disease. Ann Intern Med 1961;55:358–367.
85. Millikan CH, Siekert RG, Whisnant JP. Anticoagulant therapy in cerebral vascular disease: current status. JAMA 1958;166:587–592.
86. Millikan CH (ed). Cerebral Vascular Diseases. In Transactions of the Second Conference Held under the Auspices of the American Heart Association. Princeton, NJ, Jan 16-18, 1957. New York: Grune & Stratton, 1958.
87. Caplan LR. The stroke council and the young investigator award. Mayo Clin Proc 1989;64:125–128.
88. Fisher CM, Cameron DG. Concerning cerebral vasospasm. Neurology 1953;3:468–473.
89. Caplan LR. Are terms such as *completed stroke* or *RIND* of continued usefulness? Stroke 1983;14:431–433.
90. Caplan LR. TIAs—we need to return to the question, what is wrong with Mr. Jones? Neurology 1988;38:791–793.
91. Craven LL. Experiences with aspirin [acetylsalicylic acid] in the nonspecific prophylaxis of coronary thrombosis. Mississippi Valley MJ 1953;75:38–44.
92. Harrison MJG, Marshall J, Meadows JC, et al. Effect of aspirin in amaurosis fugax. Lancet 1971;2:743–744.
93. Fields WS, Lemak NA, Frankowski RF, et al. Controlled trial of aspirin in cerebral ischemia. Stroke 1977;8:301–316.
94. Canadian Cooperative Study Group. A randomized trial of aspirin and sulfinpyrazone in threatened stroke. N Engl J Med 1978;299:53–59.
95. Coller BS. Blockade of platelet GPIIb/IIIa receptors as an antithrombotic strategy. Circulation 1995;92:2373–2380.
96. Hass WK, Easton JD, Adams HP Jr, et al. A randomized trial comparing ticlopidine hydrochloride with aspirin for the prevention of stroke in high-risk patients. Ticlopidine

Aspirin Stroke Study Group. N Engl J Med 1989;321: 501–507.

97. Gent M, Blakeley JA, Easton JD, et al. The Canadian American Ticlopidine Study (CATS) in thromboembolic stroke. Lancet 1989;1:1215–1220.

98. The CAPRIE Steering Committee. A randomized trial of clopidogrel vs aspirin in patients at risk of ischemic events (CAPRIE). Lancet 1996;348:1329–1339.

99. Fisher M. Prophylactic Neuroprotection. In M Fisher (ed), Stroke Therapy. Boston: Butterworth–Heinemann, 1995; 233–245.

100. The European Ad Hoc Consensus Group. Neuroprotection as an initial therapy in acute stroke. Cerebrovasc Dis 1998;8:59–72.

101. Meyer JS, Gilroy J, Barnhart ME, et al. Therapeutic Thrombolysis in Cerebral Thromboembolism: Randomized Evaluation of Intravenous Streptokinase. In CH Millikan, R Siekert, JP Whisnant (eds), Cerebrovascular Diseases. New York: Grune & Stratton, 1964;200–213.

102. Del Zoppo GJ, Zeumer H, Harker LA. Thrombolytic therapy in stroke: possibilities and hazards. Stroke 1986;17: 595–607.

103. Sloan MA. Thrombolysis and stroke: past and future. Arch Neurol 1987;44:748–768.

104. Pessin MS, del Zoppo G, Furlan AJ. Thrombolytic Treatment in Acute Stroke: Review and Update of Selective Topics. In M Moscowitz, LR Caplan (eds), Cerebrovascular Diseases, 19th Princeton Conference. Boston: Butterworth–Heinemann, 1995;409–418.

105. Hacke W, Kaste M, Fieschi C, et al. Intravenous thrombolysis with recombinant tissue plasminogen activator for acute hemispheric stroke. The European Cooperative Acute Stroke Study (ECASS). JAMA 1995;274:1017–1025.

106. The National Institute of Neurological Disorders and Stroke rt-PA Study Group. Tissue plasminogen activator for acute ischemic stroke. N Engl J Med 1995;333:1581–1587.

107. Adams HP, Brott TG, Furlan AJ, et al. Use of thrombolytic drugs. A supplement to the guidelines for the management of patients with acute ischemic stroke. A statement for Health Care Professionals from a special writing group of the Stroke Council American Heart Association. Stroke 1996;27:1711–1718.

108. Quality Standards Subcommittee of the American Academy of Neurology. Practice advisory: thrombolytic therapy for acute ischemic stroke—summary statement. Neurology 1996;47:835–839.

109. Caplan LR, Mohr JP, Kistler JP, et al. Should thrombolytic therapy be the first line treatment for acute ischemic stroke? N Engl J Med 1997;337:1309–1313.

110. Beaudry MA, Hachinski VC. Cerebrovascular Disease. In RJ Porter, BS Schoenberg (eds), Controlled Clinical Trials in Neurological Disease. Boston: Kluwer Academic, 1990;113–129.

111. Sivenius J, Puranen J. Antiplatelet therapy in secondary prevention of stroke. A review of efficacy and tolerability. CNS Drugs 1997;8:38–50.

112. Peterson P, Godtfredsen J, Boysen G, et al. Placebo—controlled randomized trial of warfarin and aspirin for prevention of thromboembolic complications of chronic atrial fibrillation: the Copenhagen AFASAK Study. Lancet 1989;1:175–179.

113. The Boston Area Anticoagulation Trial for Atrial Fibrillation Investigators. The effect of low-dose warfarin on risk of stroke in patients with nonrheumatic atrial fibrillation. N Engl J Med 1990;323:1505–1511.

114. Stroke Prevention in Atrial Fibrillation Study Group Investigators. Preliminary report of the stroke prevention in atrial fibrillation study. N Engl J Med 1990;322: 863–868.

115. The European Atrial Fibrillation Trial Study Group. Optimal oral anticoagulation therapy in patients with nonrheumatic atrial fibrillation and recent cerebral ischemia. N Engl J Med 1995;333:5–10.

116. Fields WS, North RR, Hass WK, et al. Joint study of extracranial arterial occlusion as a cause of stroke: organization of study and survey of patient population. JAMA 1968;203:955–960.

117. Veterans Administration Cooperative Study. Role of carotid endarterectomy in asymptomatic carotid stenosis. Stroke 1986;17:534–539.

118. North American Symptomatic Carotid Endarterectomy Study Group. Carotid endarterectomy: three critical evaluations. Stroke 1987;18:987–989.

119. Asymptomatic Carotid Atherosclerosis Study Group. Study design for randomized prospective trial of carotid endarterectomy for asymptomatic atherosclerosis. Stroke 1989;20:844–849.

120. European Carotid Surgery Trialists Collaborative Group. Randomised trial of endarterectomy for recently symptomatic carotid stenosis: final results of the MRC European Carotid Surgery Trial (ECST). Lancet 1998;351: 1379–1387.

121. EC/IC Bypass Study Group. Failure of extracranial-intracranial bypass to reduce the risk of ischemic stroke. N Engl J Med 1985;313:1191–1200.

122. Caplan LR. The Effective Clinical Neurologist. Boston: Blackwell, 1990.

Chapter 2
Basic Pathology, Anatomy, and Pathophysiology of Stroke

Stroke is anything but a homogeneous entity. Disorders as different as rupture of a large blood vessel that causes flooding of the brain with blood and occlusion of a tiny artery with softening in a small but strategic brain site both qualify as strokes. These two pathologic caricatures of stroke subtypes are as divergent as grapes and watermelons, two obviously dissimilar substances that are included together under the large category of fruit. *Stroke* refers to any damage to the brain or the spinal cord caused by an abnormality of the blood supply. The term *stroke* is usually used when the symptoms begin abruptly, whereas cerebrovascular disease is a more general term that carries no connotation as to the tempo of brain injury. Of course, many patients with severely diseased blood vessels have had no injury to brain tissue. A blood or cardiovascular abnormality precedes and subsequently leads to the brain injury. Recognition of the cardiovascular lesion or hematologic disorder before the brain becomes damaged offers clinicians a window of opportunity during which brain damage can be prevented. At times, even when brain injury has occurred, the patient is unaware of any symptoms and neurologists may not be able to detect any abnormality on neurologic examination. Sophisticated neuroimaging techniques have taught clinicians that such "silent strokes" are common.

Diagnosis and treatment of stroke patients require a basic understanding of the anatomy, physiology, and pathology of the two major structures involved—the brain and spinal cord— and of the blood vessels that supply blood to these structures. To be effective, clinicians caring for stroke patients must have an intimate familiarity with (1) the appearance of the normal brain and its various lobes and regions; (2) the appearance of brain tissue damaged by various vascular disorders; (3) the usual locations and course of arteries supplying the brain and spinal cord, and veins that drain blood from these regions; and (4) the frequency, location, and appearance of diseases of the cerebrovascular system. Note that this discussion includes a number of words related to vision. Many of the diagnostic tests used, especially imaging of the brain and blood vessels, produce pictures. Clinicians must be able to visualize what the structures and diseases look like. For this reason, this chapter relies heavily on illustrations.

This chapter offers succinct and basic coverage of the topics just mentioned. I begin the chapter by introducing the different mechanisms of brain damage in stroke. These stroke mechanisms are the major players, the key actors in the drama of stroke. Their characterization, recognition, and treatment form the core of this book. Normal vascular anatomy and distribution are then described and illustrated. Next, the usual distribution and frequency of these different mechanisms in the blood vessels and in the brain are discussed and diagrammed. The chapter closes with a discussion of stroke pathophysiology, the dynamics of the functional response of the vascular system and brain to the primary injuries.

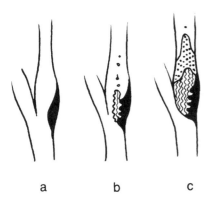

a   b   c

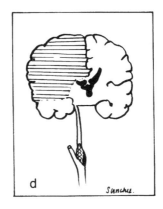

d

Figure 2-1. Internal carotid artery atherosclerotic lesions: (**a**) plaque; (**c**) plaque with platelet-fibrin emboli; (**c**) plaque with occlusive thrombus; (**d**) recent ischemic cerebral infarct caused by internal carotid artery occlusion.

Pathology: Mechanisms of Cerebrovascular Damage to Brain Tissue

The first questions the clinician should ask about a stroke patient are "What caused the brain dysfunction?" and "What pathologic process is active in this patient?" There are two major categories of brain damage in stroke patients: (1) ischemia—a lack of blood flow depriving brain tissue of needed fuel and oxygen and (2) hemorrhage—the release of blood into the brain and into extravascular spaces within the cranium. Bleeding damages the brain by cutting off connecting pathways and by causing localized or generalized pressure injury to brain tissue; biochemical substances released during and after hemorrhage also may adversely affect nearby vascular or brain tissues.[1,2]

Ischemia

Ischemia can be further subdivided into three different mechanisms: thrombosis, embolism, and decreased systemic perfusion. An analogy to a simple plumbing situation illustrates the difference among the three major mechanisms of ischemia. Suppose that a woman calls a plumber and tells him that when she turns on the faucet in the second floor bathroom on the right she gets no water. The plumber finds that the pipe that feeds the sink has rusted badly and is blocked. He repairs the local pipe and water flow is restored. That local occlusive process in the pipe, in vascular terms, would qualify as thrombosis, meaning a process that occurs in situ within a blood vessel. Suppose instead that the pipe had been blocked by material that originated in the water tank and simply stopped in the pipe to that sink, occluding the pipe. This obstruction by material originating from afar is embolism. Fixing the local pipe would not prevent further material from getting into the system and blocking other pipes. Suppose instead that the plumber finds that the water pressure is intermittently low and flow to all the sinks and showers is deficient because of a leak in the water tank or low water pressure in the house's entire plumbing. This situation is akin to systemic hypoperfusion; there is no local problem with the pipe to one sink but instead a general circulatory problem. Clearly, these three different situations dictate different management by the plumber and that is the main reason for separating these three mechanisms. I return to this analogy when treatment is discussed in Chapter 5.

Thrombosis

By convention, *thrombosis* refers to an obstruction of blood flow due to a localized occlusive process within one or more blood vessels. The lumen of the vessel is narrowed or occluded by an alteration in the vessel wall or by superimposed clot formation (Figure 2-1). The most common type of vascular pathology is atherosclerosis, in which fibrous and muscular tissues overgrow in the subintima and fatty materials form plaques that can encroach on the lumen. Next, platelets adhere to plaque crevices and form clumps that serve as nidi for the deposition of fibrin, thrombin, and clot.[3,4] Atherosclerosis affects chiefly the larger extracranial and intracranial vessels.[5,6] Occasionally, a clot forms within the lumen because of a primary hematologic problem, such as polycythemia, thrombocytosis, or a systemic hypercoagulable state. The smaller, penetrating intracranial vessels are more often damaged by hypertension than by atherosclerotic processes.[7,8] In such cases, increased arterial tension leads to hypertrophy of the media and deposition of fibrinoid material into the vessel wall, a process that gradually encroaches on the already small lumen. Atheromatous plaques, often referred to as *micoatheromas*, can obstruct the orifices of penetrating arteries.

Less common vascular pathologies leading to obstruction include (1) fibromuscular dysplasia,[9] an overgrowth of medial and intimal elements that compromises vessel contractility and luminal size; (2) arteritis, especially of the Takayasu[10] or giant-cell type[11]; (3) dissection of the vessel wall,[12] often with a luminal or extraluminal clot temporarily obstructing the vessel; and (4) hemorrhage into a plaque,[13] leading to acute or chronic luminal compromise. At times, the focal vascular abnormality is a functional change in the contractility of blood vessels. Intense focal vasoconstriction can lead to decreased blood flow and thrombosis. Dilatation of blood vessels also alters local blood flow and clots often form in dilated segments.

Embolism

In embolism, material formed elsewhere within the vascular system lodges in a vessel and blocks the blood flow. In contrast to thrombosis, embolic luminal blockage is not caused by a localized process originating within the blocked vessel. The material arises proximally, most commonly from the heart; from major arteries such as the aorta, carotid, and vertebral arteries; and from systemic veins (Figure 2-2). Cardiac sources of embolism include the heart valves, endocardium, and clots or tumors within the atrial or ventricular cavities.[14] Artery-to-artery emboli are composed of clot, platelet clumps, or fragments of plaques that break off from the proximal vessels.[15] Clots originating in systemic veins travel to the brain through cardiac defects such as an atrial septal defect or a patent foramen ovale, a process termed *paradoxical embolism*.[16] Also, occasionally air, fat,[17] plaque material,[18] particulate matter from injected drugs,[19] bacteria,[20] and tumor cells enter the vascular system and embolize to brain vessels.

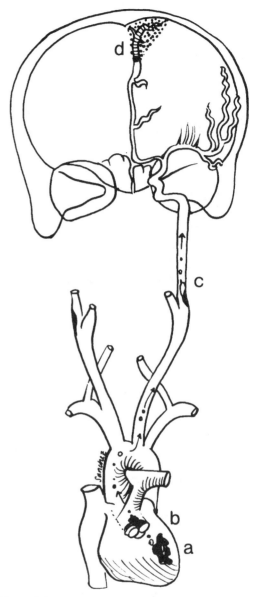

Figure 2-2. Examples of potential sources of embolism: (**a**) cardiac mural thrombus; (**b**) vegetations on heart valve; (**c**) emboli from carotid plaque. Also shown: (**d**) infarcted cortex in area supplied by terminal anterior cerebral artery caused by embolism.

Decreased Systemic Perfusion

In decreased systemic perfusion, diminished flow to brain tissue is caused by low systemic perfusion pressure. The most common causes are cardiac

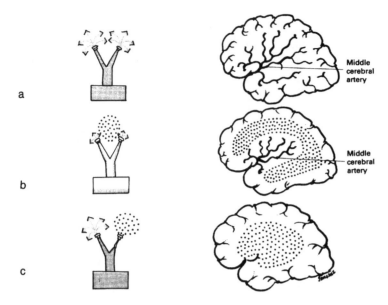

Figure 2-3. In heart (pump) failure and watershed infarction, (**a**) normal pump and arterial circulation do not occur; instead, due to (**b**) low pump pressure and border-zone ischemia, water goes to the center of hoses (arteries), and stippled areas show poor flow. In contrast, with (**c**) "blocked hose" and middle cerebral artery infarction, water flow is deficient in the center of supply (stippled area).

pump failure (most often due to myocardial infarction or arrhythmia) and systemic hypotension (due to blood loss or hypovolemia). In such cases, the lack of perfusion is more generalized than in localized thrombosis or embolism and affects the brain diffusely and bilaterally. Poor perfusion is most critical in border zone or so-called watershed regions at the periphery of the major vascular supply territories (Figure 2-3, compare B with A and C).[21,22] Asymmetric effects can result from preexisting vascular lesions causing an uneven distribution of underperfusion.

Damage Caused by Ischemia

All three mechanisms of ischemia lead to temporary or permanent tissue injury. Permanent injury is termed *infarction*. Capillaries or other vessels within the ischemic tissue may also be injured, so that reperfusion can lead to leakage of blood into the ischemic tissue, resulting in a hemorrhagic infarct. The extent of brain damage depends on the location and duration of the poor perfusion and the ability of collateral vessels to perfuse the tissues at risk. Brain and vascular injuries may lead during the hours and days after stroke to brain edema. In the chronic phase, glial scars form, and macrophages gradually ingest the necrotic tissue debris within the infarct, leading to shrinkage of the volume of the infarcted tissue or to formation of a frank cavity.

Hemorrhage

Hemorrhage can be further subdivided into two subtypes: subarachnoid and intracerebral. These two subtypes have different causes, pose different clinical problems, and have different management.

Subarachnoid Hemorrhage

In subarachnoid hemorrhage, blood leaks out of the vascular bed onto the brain's surface and is disseminated quickly via the spinal fluid pathways into the spaces around the brain (Figure 2-4).[23] Bleeding most often originates from aneurysms or arteriovenous malformations, but bleeding diatheses or trauma can also cause subarachnoid bleeding. A ruptured aneurysm releases blood rapidly at systemic blood pressure, suddenly increasing intracranial pressure, whereas bleeding from other causes is usually slower and at lower pressures.

Intracerebral Hemorrhage

The terms *intracerebral* and *parenchymal hemorrhage* describe bleeding directly into the brain substance. The cause is most often hypertension, with leakage of blood from small intracerebral arterioles damaged by the elevated blood pressure.[24–28] Bleeding diatheses, especially from the iatrogenic prescription of anticoagulants or from trauma,

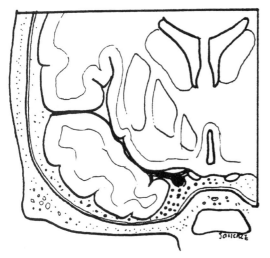

Figure 2-4. Subarachnoid hemorrhage: Blood is seen spreading from a ruptured aneurysm into the subarachnoid space.

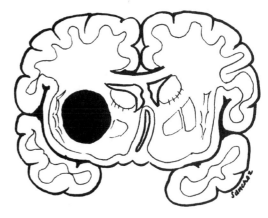

Figure 2-5. Intracerebral or intraparenchymal (putaminal) hemorrhage: Note mass effect and shift of cerebral midline.

drugs, vascular malformations, and vasculopathies (e.g., amyloid degeneration), can also cause bleeding into the brain. Parenchymatous hemorrhages occur in a localized region of the brain (Figure 2-5). The degree of damage depends on the location, rapidity, volume, and pressure of the bleeding.

Intracerebral hemorrhages are at first soft and dissect along white matter fiber tracts. When bleeding dissects into the ventricles or onto the surface of the brain, blood is introduced into the cerebrospinal fluid. The blood clots and solidifies, causing swelling of adjacent brain tissues. Later, blood is absorbed, and after macrophages clear the debris, a cavity or slit forms that may disconnect brain pathways. The intracranial cavity is a closed system. The bony skull and dura act as a fortress protecting the brain from outside injury. In adverse situations, such as swelling or hemorrhage arising inside the fortress, these structures may constitute a prison, restricting and strangulating their enclosed contents and forcing herniation of tissue from one compartment to another.[29–31]

Stroke Mechanism Guides Treatment

The problems in these five major subtypes of strokes—thrombosis, embolism, decreased systemic perfusion, subarachnoid hemorrhage, and intracerebral hemorrhage—are quite distinct and require different treatment strategies. Some therapies suitable for ischemia would be disastrous if the problem were hemorrhage (e.g., using anticoagulants or opening a blood vessel to diminish supposed ischemia would augment hemorrhage). Even within the various subcategories of ischemia, treatment depends on the subtype. Other major subtypes also require differing treatments (e.g., operating on a blood vessel for supposed local thrombosis might be unnecessary if the problem were embolism and would certainly be ineffective in preventing subsequent emboli from arising proximally). The origin of the embolism also affects treatment: Embolism arising from the heart requires different therapeutic strategies than embolism arising from localized vessel plaques. In regard to systemic hypoperfusion, pump failure or hypovolemia caused by intestinal bleeding needs urgent attention, which would be needlessly delayed by inappropriate angiography or a futile search for a localized extracranial vascular lesion. In subarachnoid hemorrhage, the major aim of treatment is to prevent the next aneurysmal leak, whereas in intracerebral hemorrhage, rebleeding is rare and treatment is aimed at controlling and limiting the local bleeding and pressure effects of the hemorrhage.

To treat the stroke patient optimally, the physician must identify the correct mechanism of stroke. Because it is not always possible to be absolutely certain of the single true mechanism, the clinician often must consider the possibility of more than one mechanism, such as thrombosis or embolism, and must evaluate for each. At times, more than one mechanism is operant (e.g., in subarachnoid hemorrhage the blood may cause spasm of blood vessels and thus induce local ischemia). A thrombus obstructing a carotid artery can also fragment and lead to distal artery-to-artery embolism.

Anatomy: Common Anatomic Sites of Vascular and Brain Lesions

Clinical neurology differs from most medical specialties in its emphasis on, and even obsession with, anatomy. To localize and repair damage to water pipes, the effective plumber must be aware of exactly where the pipes are, what they supply, and where they are most likely to be damaged by various hazards. Abnormal neurologic signs and symptoms depend more on the localization of the brain injury than on its mechanism. Although all portions of the lung or liver look and function identically, different regions within the brain appear and act differently. The nervous system is a world of uncountable individual nerve cells and networks, each with quite different and unique characteristics and chemical messengers. Each of the various mechanisms of stroke just reviewed has its own preferences for anatomic brain loci. Identification of the location of the stroke depends on analysis of the abnormal neurologic symptoms and signs and on interpretation of brain imaging. This section of this chapter reviews the important anatomic facts about the extracranial and intracranial arteries,[32] their normal regions of supply, and the most common loci for various vascular pathologies. Next, the anatomic predilections of the major stroke mechanisms within the brain are outlined. This subject is discussed more extensively in the second part of this book, where specific stroke syndromes are addressed.

Normal Vascular Anatomy

Arterial Circulation

The common carotid arteries (CCAs) bifurcate in the neck, usually opposite the upper border of the thyroid cartilage, into the internal carotid arteries (ICAs), which run posteriorly as a direct extension of the CCA, and the external carotid arteries (ECAs), which course more anteriorly and laterally. The ICAs travel behind the pharynx and give off no neck branches. The ICAs then enter the skull through the carotid canal within the petrous bone and form an S-shaped curve, first coursing within the petrous temporal bone and then within the cavernous sinus. This intracavernous portion of the ICAs is called the *carotid siphon* because of the shape. The siphon portion of the ICAs gives rise to ophthalmic artery branches that exit anteriorly. The ICAs then penetrate the dura and from their supraclinoid portions give off anterior choroidal and posterior communicating arteries before bifurcating into the anterior cerebral arteries (ACAs), which course medially, and the middle cerebral arteries (MCAs), which course laterally (Figure 2-6).

The ECAs have two major vascular channels that ordinarily supply the face that can act as collateral circulation if the ICAs occlude: the facial arteries, which course along the cheek toward the nasal bridge, where they are termed the *angular arteries*, and the *preauricular arteries*, which terminate as the superficial temporal arteries. The other important arterial supply of the face involves the frontal and supratrochlear branches from the ophthalmic arteries (ICA system), which supply the medial forehead above the brow. When an ICA occludes, these ECA branches can be an important source of collateral blood supply. The patterns of collateral circulation from the ECAs to the ICAs are illustrated in Figure 3-2.

The ACAs course medially until they reach the longitudinal fissures and then run posteriorly over the corpus callosum. They supply the anterior medial portions of the cerebral hemispheres and give off deep branches to the caudate nuclei and the basal frontal lobes. The first portion of the ACA is sometimes hypoplastic on one side, in which case the ACA from the other side supplies both medial frontal lobes. The anterior communicating artery connects the right and left ACAs and provides a means of collateral circulation from the anterior circulation of the opposite side when one ACA is hypoplastic or occludes.

The main stem of the MCAs courses laterally, giving off lenticulostriate artery branches to the basal ganglia and internal capsule. As they near the sylvian fissures, the MCAs trifurcate into

Figure 2-6. Lateral **(a)** and antero-posterior **(b)** views of branches of the internal carotid artery (ICA). (ACA = anterior cerebral artery; MCA = middle cerebral artery; PCA = posterior cerebral artery.)

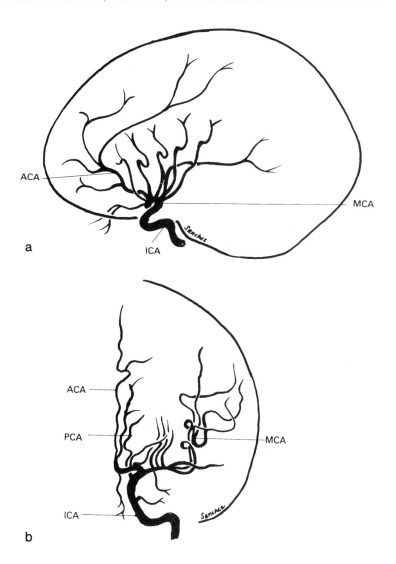

small anterior temporal branches and large superior and inferior trunks. The superior trunks supply the lateral portions of the cerebral hemispheres above the sylvian fissures, and the inferior trunks supply the temporal and inferior parietal lobes below the sylvian fissures.

The anterior choroidal arteries (AChAs) are relatively small arteries that originate from the internal carotid arteries after the origins of the ophthalmic and posterior communicating arteries. The ophthalmic artery projects anteriorly into the back of the orbit whereas the anterior choroidal and posterior communicating arteries project posteriorly from the ICA. The AChAs course posteriorly and laterally running along the optic tract. They straddle

territory between components of the anterior (internal carotid) and posterior circulations (vertebrobasilar system).[33] The AChAs give off penetrating artery branches to the globus pallidus and posterior limb of the internal capsule. They then give branches laterally to the medial temporal lobe, and medial branches supply a portion of the midbrain and the thalamus. The AChAs end in the lateral geniculate body where they anastomose with lateral posterior choroidal artery branches of the posterior cerebral arteries and in the choroid plexus of the lateral ventricles near the temporal horns. Figure 2-7 is a drawing of the course of the AChA. Figures 2-8 and 2-9 show the courses of the main cerebral arteries—the ACAs, MCAs, and posterior

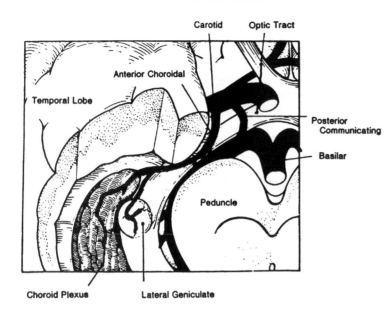

Carotid   Optic Tract

Anterior Choroidal

Temporal Lobe

Posterior
Communicating

Basilar

Peduncle

Choroid Plexus   Lateral Geniculate

Figure 2-7. The vascular supply of the anterior choroidal artery. (Reprinted with permission from C Helgason, LR Caplan, J Goodwin, T Hedges. Anterior choroidal artery-territory infarction. Arch Neurol 1986;43:681–686. Copyright © American Medical Association.)

cerebral arteries (PCAs). Figure 2-10 shows a cut section of the cerebral hemispheres showing the distribution of the supply of these cerebral arteries and the AChAs.

Traditionally, by convention, the carotid artery territories just described are referred to as the *anterior circulation* (front of the brain), whereas the vertebral and basilar arteries and their branches are termed the *posterior circulation* (because they supply the back of the brain). Each ICA supplies roughly two-fifths of the brain by volume, whereas the posterior circulation accounts for approximately one-fifth of the total. Despite its much smaller size, the posterior circulation contains the brain stem, a midline strategically critical structure without which consciousness, movement, and sensations cannot be preserved. The posterior circulation is constructed quite differently from the anterior circulation and consists of vessels from each side (the vertebral and anterior spinal artery branches), which unite to form midline arteries that supply the brain stem and spinal cord. Within the posterior circulation, there is a much higher incidence of asymmetric, hypoplastic arteries; of variability of supply; and of retention of fetal circulatory patterns.[34–36] The proximal portions of the posterior circulation on the two sides differ. On the right, the subclavian artery arises from the

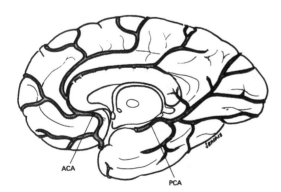

ACA

PCA

Figure 2-8. Anterior (ACA) and posterior (PCA) cerebral arteries: medial view of sagittal section.

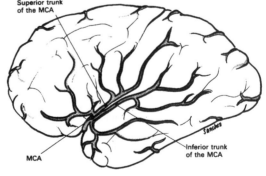

Superior trunk
of the MCA

MCA

Inferior trunk
of the MCA

Figure 2-9. Middle cerebral artery (MCA): lateral view, with superior and inferior trunk branches.

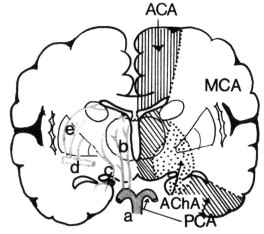

Figure 2-10. Coronal view: The right side depicts territories supplied by the anterior cerebral artery (ACA), middle cerebral artery (MCA), posterior cerebral artery (PCA), and anterior choroidal artery (AChA). The left side depicts individual vessels: (a) basilar artery; (b) thalamoperforators, which originate in the PCA; (c) AChA; (d) MCA; (e) lenticulostriate arteries.

Figure 2-11. Lateral view depicting the vertebral and carotid arteries in the neck, the brain stem, and the cerebellum. (CCA = common carotid artery; ECA = external carotid artery; ICA = internal carotid artery)

innominate artery, a common channel supplying the anterior and posterior circulations. On the left side, the subclavian artery usually arises directly from the aortic arch after the origin of the left CCA.

The first branch of each subclavian artery is the vertebral artery (VA) (Figure 2-11). The VAs course upward and backward until they enter the transverse foramens of C6 or C5 (sixth or fifth cervical vertebra) and run within the intravertebral foramina, exiting to course behind the atlas before piercing the dura mater to enter the foramen magnum. Their intracranial portions end at the medullopontine junction, where the two VAs join to form the basilar artery. Figure 2-12 shows the divisions of the VAs: the first portion before entry into the bony vertebral column (V1), the portion within the vertebral columns (V2), the portion of the artery after exit from the vertebral column that arches behind the atlas and before entry into the cranium

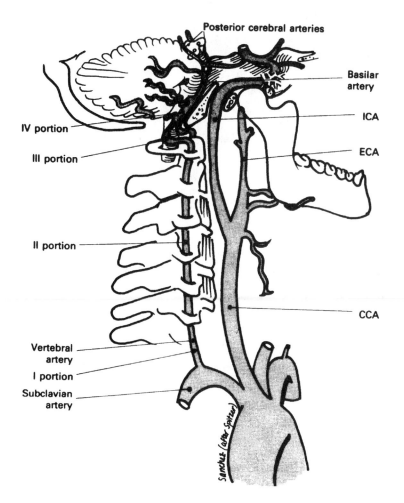

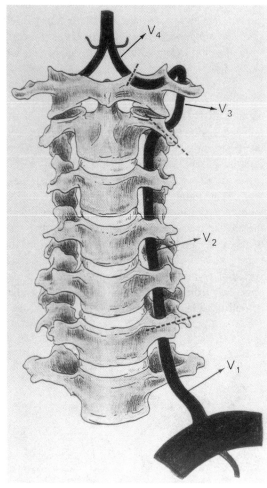

Figure 2-12. The portions of the vertebral artery and their relation to the bony vertebral column. (Reprinted with permission from LR Caplan. Posterior Circulation Disease: Clinical Findings, Diagnosis, and Management. Boston: Blackwell, 1996.)

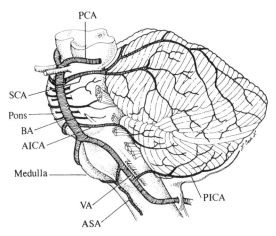

Figure 2-13. Drawing of the intracranial vertebral and basilar arteries and their major branches in oblique view. (VA = vertebral artery, BA = basilar artery, ASA = anterior spinal artery, PCA = posterior cerebral artery, PICA = posterior inferior cerebellar artery, AICA = anterior inferior cerebellar artery, SCA = superior cerebellar artery.) (Reprinted with permission from C Chaves, LR Caplan, CS Chung, et al. Cerebellar infarcts in the New England Medical Center Posterior Circulation Registry. Neurology 1994;44:1385–1390.)

(V3), and the intracranial portion (V4). In the neck, the VAs have many small muscular and spinal branches.

The intracranial portions of the VAs give off posterior and anterior spinal artery branches, penetrating arteries to the medulla, and the large posterior inferior cerebellar arteries (PICAs). The basilar artery runs in the midline along the clivus, giving off bilateral anterior inferior cerebellar artery (AICA) and superior cerebellar artery (SCA) branches before dividing at the pontomesencephalic junction into terminal PCA branches (Figures 2-13 and 2-14). The vascular supply of the brain stem has been worked out by Foix,[37–39] Stopford,[40] and Gillilan[41] and is illustrated in Figure 2-15. Large paramedian arteries and smaller, short circumferential arteries penetrate through the basal portions of the brain stem into the tegmentum. Long circumferential arteries course around the brain stem giving off branches to the lateral tegmentum. The PCAs give off penetrating arteries to the midbrain and thalamus, course around the cerebral peduncles, and then supply the occipital lobes and inferior surface of the temporal lobes (Figure 2-16; see Figure 2-8).

The circle of Willis allows for connections between the anterior circulations of each side, through the anterior communicating artery, and between the posterior and anterior circulations of each side through the posterior communicating artery (Figure 2-17).

Venous and Dural Sinus Anatomy

The veins within the cranium contain approximately 70% of the cerebral blood volume. The intracranial veins are usually divided into the venous dural sinuses and the superficial and deep venous drainage systems.

The dural venous sinuses are trabeculated, endothelial-lined channels whose fibrous walls are formed by the inner and outer layers of the dura mater. The sinuses are situated at the junctions and edges of the falx cerebri and the tentorium cerebelli. The intracranial veins drain into the dural sinuses, which in turn empty into the neck veins to drain into the superior vena cava. A system of venous lakes within the skull also drains into the dural sinuses.

The paired cavernous sinuses are located on the lateral surface of the body of the sphenoid bone and are connected with each other by the anterior and posterior intercavernous sinuses. The cavernous sinuses reach the superior orbital fissure anteriorly and posteriorly extend to the petrous apices. The ophthalmic and facial veins drain into the cavernous sinuses. The internal carotid arteries lie on the medial walls of the cavernous sinuses.

The superior sagittal sinus courses in an arc from anteriorly to far posteriorly in the superior margin of the falx cerebri and ends at the internal occipital protuberance by draining into the confluence of the sinuses (torcula herophili). The superior sagittal sinuses drain most of the blood from the cerebral hemispheres. The inferior sagittal sinus is smaller and shorter than the superior sagittal sinus and runs in the inferior margin of the falx until it joins with the great cerebral vein of Galen to form the straight sinus. The paired transverse sinuses originate at the torcula and course anterolaterally along the skull between the attachments of the tentorium cerebelli. At the petrous portion of the temporal bones, the transverse sinuses empty into the sigmoid sinuses, which course medially and inferiorly to reach the jugular foramina where they become the jugular veins. One of the transverse sinuses (most often the left) is sometimes hypoplastic or absent. The superior and inferior petrosal sinuses begin at the cavernous sinuses and drain into the sigmoid sinuses and the jugular veins. The majority of the venous blood within the cranium flows posteriorly and drains into the sigmoid sinuses into the jugular veins and from there into the superior vena cava. Figure 2-18 shows the major venous dural sinuses and some of the large draining veins.

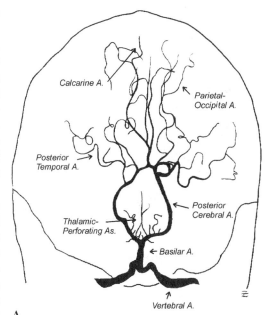

A

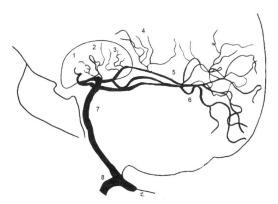

B

Figure 2-14. Large intracranial posterior circulation arteries as they appear on arteriograms. The drawing above (**A**) is a posteroanterior view and the drawing below (**B**) shows a lateral projection. (1 = thalamosubthalamic [thalmoperforating] arteries; 2 = thalamogeniculate arteries; 3 = posterior choroidal arteries; 4 = parieto-occipital arteries; 5 = posterior temporal arteries; 6 = posterior cerebral artery; 7 = basilar artery; 8 = intracranial vertebral artery.) (Reprinted with permission from LR Caplan. Posterior Circulation Disease: Clinical Findings, Diagnosis, and Management. Boston: Blackwell, 1996.)

The superior group of cerebral veins drain most of the medial surface, the superior parts of the lateral surfaces, and the anterior portions of the ventral surfaces of the cerebral hemispheres. They

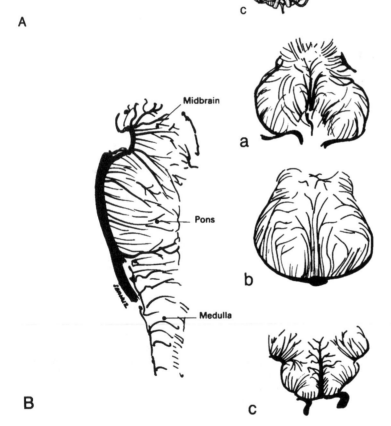

Figure 2-15. The vascular supply of the brainstem. (**A**) Penetrating brainstem arteries. (**B**) Drawing based on angiographic postmortem opacification of arteries: (**a**) midbrain; (**b**) pons; (**c**) medulla. (PICA = posterior inferior cerebellar artery.) (Adapted from MB Carpenter. Core Text of Neuroanatomy. Baltimore, MD: Williams & Wilkins, 1978;333.)

empty into the frontal and parietal regions of the superior sagittal sinus. The middle cerebral veins consist of a superficial and a deep vein. The superficial middle cerebral veins drain the sylvian fissures and the opercula and empty into the cavernous sinuses. The deep middle cerebral veins form on the insular surfaces and drain into the basal veins of Rosenthal. The basal veins arise on the ventral surface of the brain lateral to the optic chiasm and course posteriorly to the cerebral peduncles where the interpeduncular vein connects the two basal veins. The basal veins then course around the peduncles with the posterior cerebral arteries and empty into the great cerebral vein of Galen.

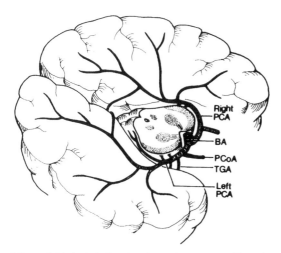

Figure 2-16. Artist's drawing shows the course and branching of the posterior cerebral arteries (PCAs) as they course around the midbrain, and their temporal and parieto-occipital branches. (BA = basilar artery; PCoA= posterior communicating artery; TGA = thalamogeniculate artery.) (Reprinted with permission from LR Caplan. Posterior Circulation Disease: Clinical Findings, Diagnosis, and Management. Boston: Blackwell, 1996.)

The inferior cerebral veins drain from the inferior and lateral surfaces of the temporal and occipital lobes into the transverse sinuses. The paired internal cerebral veins originate behind the foramina of Monro and course posteriorly side by side near the midline. The thalamostriate veins course with the stria terminalis between the caudate nucleus and the thalamus on each side to drain into the internal cerebral veins. The two internal cerebral veins and the basal veins of Rosenthal join below or behind the splenium of the corpus callosum to form the great cerebral vein of Galen.

The veins that drain the brain stem and cerebellum are divided into three groups. The superior group drain the superior portions of the cerebellum and the rostral and dorsal brain stem. They empty into the vein of Galen, the basal veins of Rosenthal, or the petrosal veins, which drain into the petrosal sinuses. One of the superior veins, the precentral vein, is an important anatomic landmark because it separates the pons below the vein from the midbrain above. The petrosal group of veins drain the ventral surface of the brain stem, the superior and inferior surfaces of the cerebellar hemispheres, and the lateral recesses of the fourth ventricle. They drain into the superior petrosal sinuses or their tributaries. The tentorial group of veins are posteriorly located and drain the inferior vermis and the medial portions of the cerebellar hemispheres. They drain into the straight sinus or lateral sinuses near the torcula.[32,36]

Figure 2-17. Internal surface of the skull, showing exit of the cranial nerves and their relationship to the arteries of the circle of Willis. (ACA = anterior communicating artery; AICA = anterior inferior cerebellar artery; MCA = middle cerebral artery; PCA = posterior cerebral artery; SCA = superior cerebellar artery; VA = vertebral artery.)

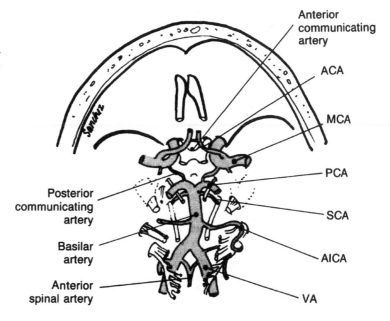

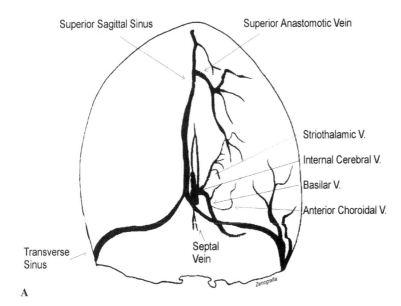

Superior Sagittal Sinus

Superior Anastomotic Vein

Striothalamic V.

Internal Cerebral V.

Basilar V.

Anterior Choroidal V.

Transverse Sinus

Septal Vein

A

Figure 2-18. Major dural venous sinuses and some of the large draining veins. (**A**) A view at the level of the base of the skull. (**B**) Lateral view. (Reprinted with permission from LR Caplan. Posterior Circulation Disease: Clinical Findings, Diagnosis, and Management. Boston: Blackwell, 1996.)

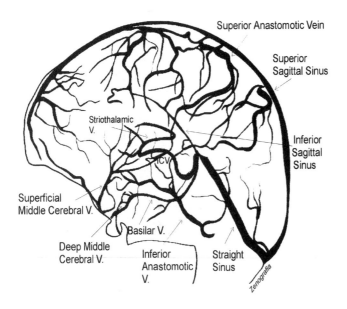

Superior Anastomotic Vein

Superior Sagittal Sinus

Striothalamic V.

ICV.

Inferior Sagittal Sinus

Superficial Middle Cerebral V.

Basilar V.

Deep Middle Cerebral V.

Inferior Anastomotic V.

Straight Sinus

B

Distribution of Vascular Pathology

Thrombosis

Atherosclerotic narrowing most commonly occurs at the origins of the ICAs in the neck. The remainder of the nuchal ICAs are seldom affected, but the carotid siphon is a frequent site for atheromas. The supraclinoid carotid arteries and the main stem MCAs and ACAs are affected less often than the ICAs in the neck and the siphon in the general population,[42–44] although in black, Chinese, and Japanese patients, MCA disease is more common than disease of the ICAs.[44–48]

Sites of predilection for atherosclerotic narrowing in the posterior circulation include the proximal origins of the VAs and the subclavian arteries, the proximal and distal ends of the intracranial vertebral arteries, the basilar artery, and the origins of the PCAs.[36,44–49] Figure 2-19 shows the most frequent loci of atherosclerosis. Atherosclerotic narrowing rarely affects the distal superficial branches of the cerebral (ACA, MCA, PCA) or cerebellar (PICA, AICA, SCA) arteries.

Lipohyalinosis and medial hypertrophy secondary to hypertension affect mainly (1) penetrating lenticulostriate branches of the MCAs; (2) anterior perforating vessels of the ACA; (3) penetrating arteries originating from the AChAs; (4) thalamogeniculate penetrators from the PCAs; and (5) paramedian perforating vessels to the pons, midbrain, and thalamus from the basilar artery [36,50] (Figure 2-20). At times, atheromatous plaques within parent arteries or microatheromas within the orifices of branches cause blockage of penetrating arteries.[36,51] The distribution of atheromatous branch disease is the same as that of lipohyalinosis except that atheromatous branch disease may also obstruct larger branches (e.g., the anterior choroidal artery branches of the ICAs and the thalamogeniculate pedicles from the PCAs).

Dissection—traumatic or spontaneous tearing of a vessel wall with intramural bleeding—usually involves the distal extracranial carotid and vertebral arteries.[12,36,52] Less common are dissections of the intracranial ICAs, MCAs, VAs, and basilar arteries.[36,53,54] Temporal arteritis characteristically affects the ICAs and VAs just before they pierce the dura to enter the cranial cavity, as well as the branches of the ophthalmic arteries before they pierce the globe.[11,55]

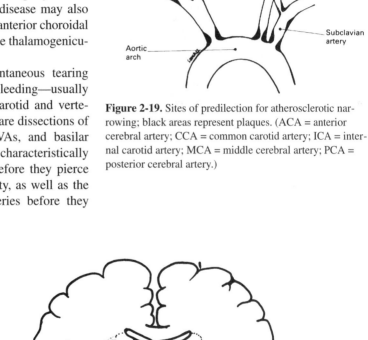

Figure 2-19. Sites of predilection for atherosclerotic narrowing; black areas represent plaques. (ACA = anterior cerebral artery; CCA = common carotid artery; ICA = internal carotid artery; MCA = middle cerebral artery; PCA = posterior cerebral artery.)

Figure 2-20. Penetrating arteries prone to lipohyalinosis and microaneurysms: the thalamogeniculate and lenticulostriate vessels and arteries to the pons.

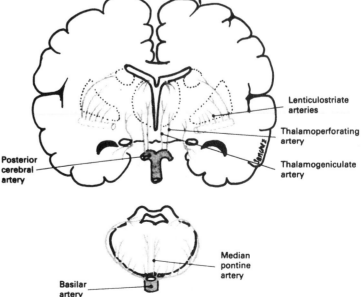

Embolism

Emboli can block any artery depending on the size and nature of the embolic material. Large emboli, often clots formed within the heart, can block even large extracranial arteries, such as the innominate, subclavian, carotid, and vertebral arteries in the neck. More often, smaller thrombi formed in the heart or the proximal arteries embolize to block intracranial arteries, such as the ICAs, ACAs, VAs, basilar artery, PCAs, and especially the MCAs and their superior and inferior trunks. Within the anterior circulation, there is a strong predilection for emboli to go to the MCAs and their branches. Small balloons released into the ICAs in experimental animals consistently follow flow patterns to travel to MCA branches.[56] Within the posterior circulation, emboli preferentially block the intracranial VA, the distal basilar artery, and the PCAs.[36] Smaller fragments—such as tiny or fragmented thrombi, platelet-fibrin clumps, cholesterol crystals or other fragments from atheromatous plaques, and calcified fragments from valve and vessel surfaces—tend to embolize to superficial small branches of the cerebral and cerebellar arteries and the ophthalmic and retinal arteries.

Intracerebral Hemorrhage

Intracerebral hemorrhage is often caused by hypertensive damage to small penetrating vessels and has the same vascular distribution as lipohyalinosis (see Figures 2-20 and 2-21).[28,57] Charcot and Bouchard originally described in 1872 microaneurysms, which they believed ruptured, causing intracerebral hemorrhage.[25,26] Studies indicate that sudden increases in blood pressure and blood flow can also cause these same penetrating arteries to break, even in the absence of chronic hypertensive changes.[27,28] Vascular malformations can occur anywhere within the brain.

Subarachnoid Hemorrhage

Aneurysms most often affect junctional regions of the larger vessels of the circle of Willis. The ICA-posterior communicating artery junction, anterior communicating artery–ACA junction, and the MCA trifurcations are the most common sites. The supraclinoid ICAs, pericallosal arteries, vertebral-PICA junctions, and apex of the basilar artery are also frequent sites (Figure 2-22).[36,58,59] Vascular malformations that cause the syndrome of subarachnoid hemorrhage are either located in the brain, abutting on pial or ventricular surfaces, or situated within the ventricular system or the subarachnoid space. Some large malformations are located entirely within the subarachnoid cerebrospinal fluid compartment.

Distribution of Brain Pathology

Ischemia

Brain lesions caused by thrombosis are not easily distinguished from those caused by embolism because in many patients thrombosis of a vessel can lead to distal artery-to-artery embolism. Usually, the region of ischemia tends to lie in the center of the supply of the occluded artery. The extent and size of the infarct depend on the rate of occlusion, adequacy of collateral circulation, and resistance of brain structures to ischemia. In patients with angiographically documented occlusion of the ICA in the neck, Ringelstein and colleagues separated those patients with an intra-arterial embolus to the MCA and its branches ("occlusio supra occlusionem") from those who had cortical and subcortical infarcts that were considered related to diminished blood flow secondary to the ICA occlusion.[60] Figure 2-23 shows some of the patterns of infarction in patients with ICA occlusions. In a separate study, Ringelstein and his colleagues studied the distribution of lesions in the brain in patients with cardiogenic cerebral embolism.[61] Figure 2-24, derived from their report, illustrates their findings.

In patients who have systemic hypoperfusion, in contrast, the regions most vulnerable to ischemia are located in the border zones between major vessel supply zones (see Figure 2-3). The situation has been likened to a watering system for a field.[62] If a hose is blocked and the pressure of water in the pump remains constant, the portion of the field least well supplied is at the center of the blocked hose (see Figure 2-3B). More water flows through the open hoses to supply the edges of territory sup-

Figure 2-21. Horizontal cerebral section and sagittal brain stem section show the most common sites of intracerebral hemorrhage.

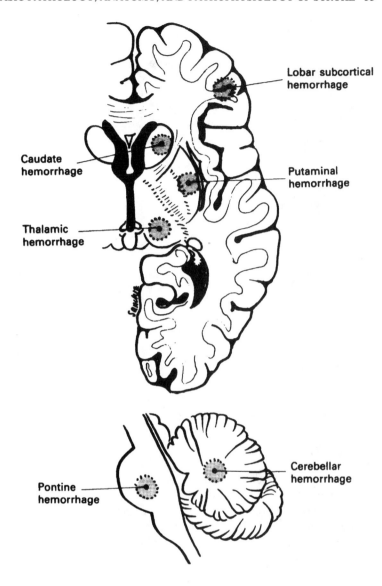

plied by the blocked hose. However, if pump pressure is reduced, water trickles out each hose, and only the center of supply of each hose receives water (see Figure 2-3C). Low pressure reduces flow to the border-zone regions or watersheds between hoses. Another way to consider the distribution of damage in patients with low flow is the concept of distal fields.[21] The regions that receive the least blood are those farthest from the center of the longest vessels. These distal fields are situated at the edges of the major vessel distributions and most often are located in the posterior portions of the cerebral hemispheres.

Intracerebral Hemorrhage

The most common brain locations for hypertensive intracerebral hemorrhages are as follows: lateral ganglionic and capsular (40%), thalamus (12%), lobar white matter (15% to 20%), caudate nucleus (8%), pons (8%), and cerebellum (8%)[28] (see Figure 2-21). Hemorrhages owing to vascular malformations have no special predilection sites but are most often either subcortical or near the brain surface. Hemorrhages caused by amyloid angiopathy also are usually lobar and seldom affect the basal ganglia or posterior fossa structures.

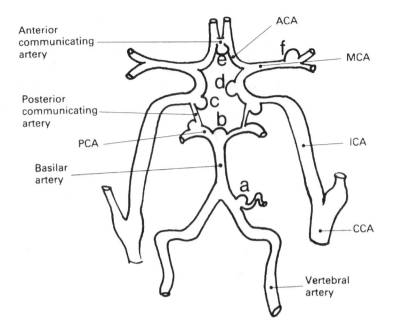

Figure 2-22. The most common sites of intracranial aneurysms: (a) posterior inferior cerebellar artery; (b) basilar artery; (c) posterior communicating artery (PCA); (d) internal carotid artery (ICA); (e) anterior communicating artery (ACA); and (f) bifurcation of the middle cerebral artery (MCA). (CCA = common carotid artery.)

Hemorrhages caused by illicit drugs, especially cocaine and amphetamines, have the same general distribution as hypertensive hemorrhages, probably because the mechanism of bleeding is an acute increase in blood pressure. Patients who develop intracranial hemorrhages after using cocaine have a much higher frequency of aneurysms and vascular malformations than hemorrhages that develop after amphetamine use.[28] Hemorrhages in patients who are being treated with anticoagulants preferentially involve the cerebral white matter and the cerebellum.[28,63]

Physiology and Pathophysiology of Brain Ischemia and Hemorrhage

Ischemia

Normal Metabolism and Blood Flow

The brain is a metabolically active organ. Unlike other body organs, the brain uses glucose as its sole substrate for energy metabolism. Glucose is oxidized to carbon dioxide (CO_2) and water (H_2O). Glucose metabolism leads to conversion of adenosine diphosphate (ADP) into adenosine triphosphate (ATP). A constant supply of ATP is needed to maintain neuronal integrity and to keep the major extracellular cations Ca^{++} (calcium ions) and Na^+ (sodium ions) outside the cells, and the intracellular cation K^+ (potassium ions) within the cells. Production of ATP is much more efficient in the presence of oxygen. Although in the absence of oxygen anaerobic glycolysis leads to formation of ATP and lactate, the energy yield is relatively small, and lactic acid accumulates within and outside of cells.[64] The brain requires and uses approximately 500 cc of oxygen and 75–100 mg of glucose each minute, a total of 125 g of glucose each day.[65]

These requirements for oxygen and glucose translate into a need for lots of oxygenated blood containing adequate sugar. Even though the brain is a relatively small organ, accounting for only 2% of adult body weight, the brain uses approximately 20% of the cardiac output when the body is resting.[65] Cerebral blood flow (CBF) is normally approximately 50 ml for each 100 g of brain tissue per minute, and cerebral oxygen consumption, usually measured as the cerebral metabolic rate for oxygen ($CMRO_2$), is normally approximately 3.5 cc/100 g per minute.[62] By increasing oxygen extraction from the bloodstream, compensation can be made to maintain $CMRO_2$ until CBF is reduced to a level of 20 to 25 ml/100 g per minute.[64] Positron emission tomography (PET) can measure CBF, $CMRO_2$, and oxygen extraction fraction (OEF), and the cerebral

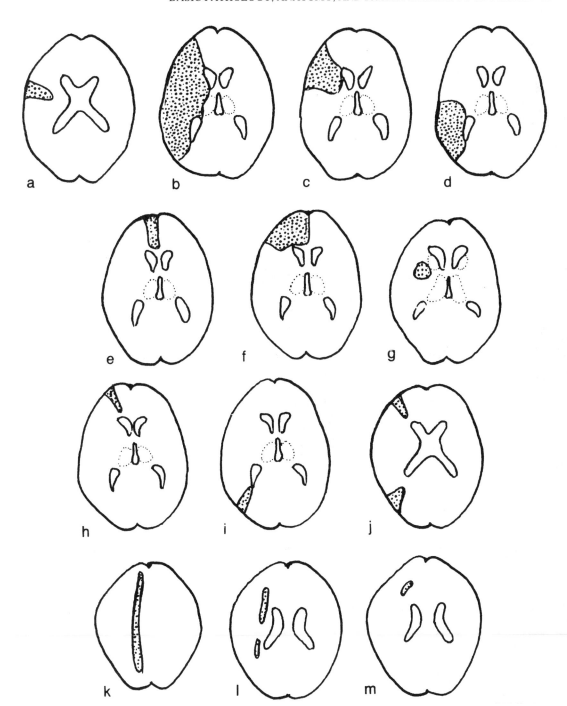

Figure 2-23. Most common computed tomography locations of infarcts in the anterior circulation infarcts are shown by hatched gray: **(a)** wedge-shaped middle cerebral artery (MCA) infarct, **(b)** entire MCA territory, **(c)** superior division MCA, **(d)** inferior division MCA, **(e)** anterior cerebral artery, **(f)** anterior cerebral artery and MCA, **(g)** striatocapsular infarct, **(h)** wedge-shaped anterior watershed infarct, **(i)** wedge-shaped posterior watershed infarct, **(j)** anterior and posterior watershed infarcts, **(k)** linear watershed infarct, **(l)** oval-shaped deep watershed infarct, **(m)** small white matter watershed infarct. (Reprinted with permission from LR Caplan. Cerebrovascular Disease: Larger Artery Occlusive Disease. In: S Appel [ed], Current Neurology, Vol 8. Chicago Yearbook Medical,1988;179–226.)

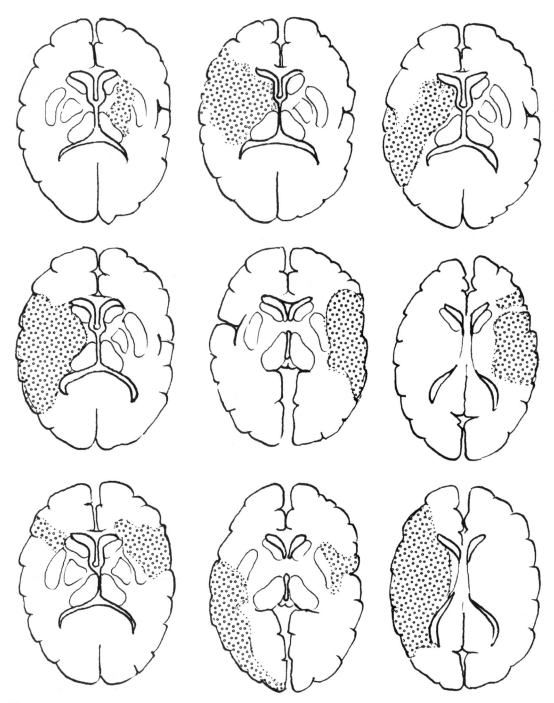

Figure 2-24. Infarctions in patients with embolic strokes. (Reprinted with permission from EB Ringelstein, S Koschorke, A Holling, et al. Computed tomographic pattern of proven embolic infarctions. Ann Neurol 1989;26:759–765.)

Figure 2-25. Thresholds of ischemia. (CBF = cerebral blood flow.)

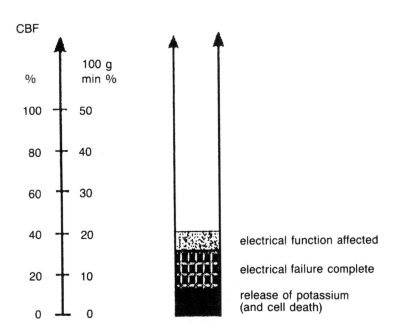

metabolic rate for glucose (CMRgl) in various brain regions of interest.[66] PET scanning is discussed in more detail in Chapter 4.

Brain energy use and blood flow depend on the degree of neuronal activity. In 1890, Roy and Sherrington first demonstrated the ability of the brain to increase local blood flow in response to regional changes in neuronal activity.[67–68] PET and functional magnetic resonance imaging (MRI) show that using the right hand increases metabolism and CBF in the left motor cortex. Clearly, it is critical for survival of brain tissue that there be systems to maintain CBF despite changes in systemic blood pressure. The capacity of the cerebral circulation to maintain relatively constant levels of CBF despite changing blood pressure has traditionally been termed *autoregulation.* CBF remains relatively constant when mean arterial blood pressures are between 50 and 150 mm Hg.[64] When blood pressure is chronically raised, both the upper and lower levels of autoregulation are raised, indicating a higher tolerance to hypertension but also increased sensitivity to hypotension.[69]

Blood flow velocities within the intracranial arteries vary from 40 to 70 cm per second.[65] When CBF increases or an artery narrows, the velocity in that segment of artery increases. At first glance, increased velocity in response to a reduction in luminal diameter seems paradoxical. One must try,

however, to visualize a simple example of velocity of liquid flow—an ordinary garden hose. When using a hose to wash off a pavement or a patio, to generate a high pressure jet of water, the nozzle is turned to reduce the luminal diameter. The more narrow the nozzle lumen, the more pressure in the stream until the lumen is nearly effaced, at which time water dribbles out, and velocity becomes greatly reduced. This analogy will be useful in Chapter 4 when considering transcranial Doppler, an ultrasound device that can measure blood flow velocities in segments of the major basal intracranial arteries.

Local Brain Effects of Ischemia

When blood flow to a brain region is reduced, survival of the at-risk tissue depends on the intensity and duration of the ischemia and the availability of collateral blood flow. Animal experiments provide estimates of thresholds of brain ischemia (Figure 2-25).[64] At blood flow levels of approximately 20 ml/100 g per minute, electroencephalographic (EEG) activity is affected. $CMRO_2$ also begins to fall when CBF is diminished below 20 ml/100 g per minute. At levels below 10 ml/100 g per minute, cell membranes and functions are severely affected. Neurons cannot survive for long at blood flows below 5 ml/100 g per minute.

When neurons become ischemic, a number of biochemical changes potentiate and enhance cell death: K^+ moves across the cell membrane into the extracellular space, and Ca^{++} moves into the cell, where it greatly compromises the ability of intracellular membranes to control subsequent ion fluxes and causes mitochondrial failure[66]; normally, there is a 10-fold gradient difference between extracellular and intracellular (cytosolic) Ca^{++}. Decreased oxygen availability leads to production of oxygen molecules with unpaired electrons, termed *oxygen-free radicals*. These free radicals cause peroxidation of fatty acids in cell organelles and plasma membranes, causing severe cell dysfunction.[70] With decreased oxygen availability, anaerobic glycolysis leads to an accumulation of lactic acid and a decrease in pH. The resulting acidosis also greatly impairs cell metabolic functions.

The activity of neurotransmitters, often referred to as *excitatory neurotransmitters*[70–72] (glutamate, aspartate, and kainic acid), is significantly increased in regions of brain ischemia.[70,71] Hypoxia, hypoglycemia, and ischemia all contribute to cause energy depletion and an increase in glutamate release but a decrease in glutamate uptake. This increased availability of glutamate causes vulnerable neurons to receive toxic exposure to glutamate, thereby increasing the likelihood of cell death. Glutamate entry opens membranes and increases Na^+ and Ca^{++} influx into cells. Large influxes of Na^+ are followed by entry of chloride ions and water, causing cell swelling and edema. Glutamate is an agonist at both *N*-methyl-D-aspartate (NMDA) and non-NMDA (kainate and quisqualate) receptor types, but only NMDA receptors are linked to membrane channels with high calcium permeability.[72] Knowledge of these changes in the neuronal and extracellular spaces is important to recall when treatment of acute stroke patients is discussed in Chapter 5.

These aforementioned local metabolic changes cause a self-perpetuating cycle of changes that lead to increasing neuronal damage and cell death. Changes in ionic concentrations of Na^+, K^+, and Ca^{++}; release of oxygen-free radicals; acidosis; and release of excitatory neurotransmitters further damage cells, leading to more local biochemical changes, which in turn cause more neuronal damage.[73] At some time, the process of ischemia becomes irreversible, despite reperfusion of tissues with adequate oxygen and glucose-rich blood. At times, although the severity of ischemia is insufficient to cause neuronal necrosis, ischemia may nevertheless set in motion a process of programmed cell death referred to as *apoptosis*.[74]

The degree of ischemia caused by blockage of an artery varies in different zones supplied by that artery. In the center of the zone, blood flow is lowest and ischemic damage is most severe. This region of the most severe damage is often referred to as the *core* of the infarct. On the periphery of blood supply, collateral blood flow allows continued delivery of blood, although at a rate lower than normal. Referring to Figure 2-25, metabolism at the center of supply may be reduced sufficiently to cause cell necrosis (0–10 ml/100 g per minute), whereas at the periphery, supplies of 10 to 20 ml/100 g per minute might stun the brain, causing electrical failure but not permanent cell damage. The zone of dysfunctional, but not dead, brain surrounding the center of infarction has traditionally been referred to as the *ischemic penumbra*. Garcia and Anderson eloquently describe this region as follows: "Penumbral neurons are thought to be paralyzed in a shadowy state between life and death, merely awaiting the restoration of either adequate blood flow or other as yet unknown conditions before resuming full life."[70] Some neurons are thought to be more vulnerable to hypoxia and decreased fuel supply than other neurons, termed *selective vulnerability*.

Arterial Occlusion and Reaction to the Occlusive Process

Brain ischemia should not be viewed as a static anatomic-pathologic process. It is a dynamic, often unstable, condition. Brain tissue, in imminent danger of irreversible death, nevertheless often recovers remarkably well, leaving no trace of its previous precarious situation. To treat patients optimally, physicians must understand the various factors that affect outcome. The discussion of pathophysiology so far has centered on the function and metabolism of local regions of brain tissue. To understand the variety of factors affecting outcome, I now turn to a more macroscopic view of both the process of arterial occlusion and the way in which occlusive changes are handled by the body.

Vascular occlusion most often begins with formation of atherosclerotic plaques within extracranial and large intracranial arteries. Atherosclerotic plaques cause brain ischemia in a variety of ways. Progressive intimal thickening leads to stenosis or occlusion of the vessel, resulting in reduced distal blood flow. Plaques often interrupt the endothelium and then ulcerate. A breach of the vascular endothelium disrupts the smooth vascular lining and initiates a process of platelet adherence to the vessel wall. The tiny hemostatic plug then enlarges by aggregation of platelets to each other. ADP, epinephrine, and collagen can all increase platelet aggregation.[75] Activated platelets release ADP and arachidonic acid. In the presence of the enzyme cyclooxygenase, arachidonic acid is metabolized to prostaglandin endoperoxides, which can be converted by thromboxane synthetase to thromboxane A_2, a potent vasoconstrictor and inducer of further platelet aggregation and secretion.[3] At the same time, the vascular endothelium may secrete prostacyclin, a potent vasodilator and inhibitor of platelet aggregation.[76] Both vascular patency and the formation of platelet fibrin clots may be determined by the balance between thromboxane A_2, prostacyclin, and other factors.

Atherosclerotic plaques thus interact with blood platelets to form nidi of loosely adherent platelets and fibrin that can break off and embolize distally. The platelet nidus can initiate the coagulation cascade leading to formation of an occlusive thrombus. Plaque hemorrhage also can lead to rapid reduction in the vascular lumen and may predispose to thrombus formation with subsequent embolization. When a critical plaque size and reduction in luminal area are reached, the occlusive process often accelerates. Reduced luminal size and plaque bulk change the physical-mechanical properties of blood flow and local turbulence.[77,78] Cracking, ulceration, and clot formation are promoted and accelerated by these changes in flow dynamics.[77,78] Studies of plaques removed at endarterectomy in patients with severe ICA stenosis often show platelet-fibrin and erythrocyte-fibrin thrombi attached to ulcerated atheromas.[79] Cracking of the endothelium and arterial intima can lead to direct contact between the luminal contents and the material within the plaque. Tissue factor within the plaque can activate the coagulation cascade and lead to formation of a red, erythrocyte-fibrin thrombus within the lumen.

The occlusive lesion is often an embolus formed more proximally, in which case vascular occlusion is quite sudden. Thrombi can also form in situ when the body's coagulation system has been activated and the blood is hypercoagulable. In some patients with hypercoagulability, thrombi form simultaneously or sequentially in multiple, systemic extracranial and intracranial arteries and veins. In other patients with arterial lesions (e.g., arterial atherosclerotic plaques or dissections), the process of occlusive thrombosis is accelerated at sites of vascular disease. Hypercoagulability can be a lifelong hereditary problem. Systemic diseases, such as cancer, regional enteritis, and thrombocytosis, can cause increased clotting. The process of atherothrombosis (e.g., in the coronary or cerebrovascular systems) can also activate serologic coagulation factors that promote further thrombosis.[80–82]

Much of the treatment of patients with thromboembolic stroke concerns attempts to affect or reverse the coagulation process or to facilitate clot lysis or removal. Clinicians treating patients with ischemia should be familiar with the general features of blood coagulation to effectively choose and monitor antithrombotic and thrombolytic therapies.

The final step in the coagulation cascade is the conversion of the soluble protein fibrinogen into insoluble polymers termed *fibrin*. These strands of fibrin form a network of fibers that entangle formed blood elements (i.e., platelets and erythrocytes) into a clot. Fibrin is quite adhesive and has the capability of contracting. The fibrinogen-to-fibrin reaction occurs when factor II, prothrombin, is converted to thrombin. The amounts of circulating fibrinogen and prothrombin are important in these reactions.

Prothrombin can be activated in two different ways: In the so-called extrinsic system of coagulation, a tissue or endothelial injury releases thromboplastic substances, tissue factors, which in turn cause both platelet activation and activation of some of the blood serine protease coagulation factors, especially factors V, VII, and X. Activation of factor X catalyzes the reaction of prothrombin to thrombin. Activation of platelets causes them to agglutinate, to adhere to the injured vessel wall, and to release various intracellular substances, which in turn activate the coagulation system.[82–85]

The complementary intrinsic coagulation system refers to blood-coagulation factors that circulate in inactive forms (factors V, VIII [antihemophilic globulin], IX, X, XI, XII) and are

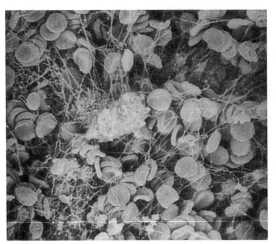

Figure 2-26. Phase microscope image of a red thrombus composed of fibrin and erythrocytes formed in a thrombogenic system, in a vessel with a low flow rate. (Courtesy of SH Hanson and CH Kessler, Emory University, Division of Hematology.)

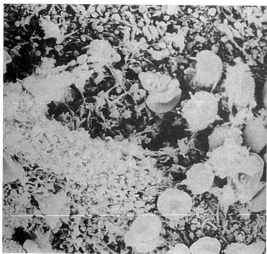

Figure 2-27. Phase microscope image of a white fibrin-platelet thrombus formed in a high-flow system. (Courtesy of SH Hanson and CH Kessler, Emory University, Division of Hematology.)

intrinsic to the blood. Activation of factor XII from an inert precursor form to an activated form triggers a series of reactions, described as the *coagulation cascade* in which the various blood-clotting factors are sequentially converted to their active enzymatic forms. Ultimately, these reactions lead to activation of factor X, which catalyzes the prothrombin (thrombin reaction).[82–85] Thrombin, in turn, in addition to converting fibrinogen to fibrin, has an important influence on blood platelets, causing them to swell, aggregate, and release substances that affect vascular tone and blood coagulability.[82–84]

Also important are various natural inhibitors of coagulation: antithrombin III, protein C, and protein S. Deficiencies in any of these serum proteins can cause increased coagulability. Genetically transmitted disorders can also lead to hypercoagulability. One common inherited disorder leads to functional resistance to the anticoagulant effects of activated protein C.[86] This genetic defect is termed the *Leiden factor V mutation* and is caused by a point mutation in factor V.[87] Another genetic disorder that predisposes to thrombosis is caused by a mutation in the prothrombin gene.[88] These mutations in the prothrombin and factor V genes are common in patients who develop cerebral venous thrombosis and phlebothromboses especially if they also take oral contraceptives.[89]

Naturally occurring factors also exist that act to lyse clots once they are formed. Tissue plasminogen activator and other substances activate plasminogen to form plasmin, a potent fibrinolytic enzyme. Plasminogen is also activated by various coagulation factors, such as factor XII, so that the process of coagulation itself activates the thrombolytic system. Various plasmin inhibitors ("antiplasmins") are also present.[90]

Pathologists and hematologists recognize and describe three different types of thrombi[83]:

1. Red thrombi are composed mostly of red blood cells and fibrin, and they form in areas of slowed blood flow. Their formation does not require an abnormal vessel wall or tissue thromboplastin (Figure 2-26).

2. White thrombi, in contrast, are composed of platelets and fibrin and do not contain red blood cells (Figure 2-27). White clots form almost exclusively in areas in which the vessel wall or endothelial surface is abnormal, characteristically in fast-moving bloodstreams.

3. Disseminated fibrin deposition in small vessels.

These types of thrombi are distinct and are affected by different therapeutic agents. In many cases, the thrombus begins as a white platelet fibrin clot and then a red thrombus is laid down as a cap over the initial platelet mass.[83,84]

When a major artery occludes, a crisis is created. Pressure drops distal to the occlusion and the brain region supplied by that vessel is acutely deprived of blood. Diminished blood flow in turn activates protective mechanisms that help restore needed blood flow to the ischemic region. Low pressure helps to draw blood from higher pressure regions. Collateral circulation increases. Ischemic cell damage causes release of lactic acid and other metabolites. The resulting local tissue acidosis leads to vasodilation, augmenting regional CBF.[91] If brain tissue is deprived of blood and needed nourishment for too long it dies. At times, there are varying grades of ischemia, ranging from irreversible cell death in the most deprived zone to a reversible situation of diminished electrical activity but normal or only slightly elevated extracellular potassium concentration in the threatened ischemic penumbral zone.[70,71,91,92] The severity of the ischemic crisis depends on the rate of vascular occlusion. A vessel that gradually occludes may already have stimulated abundant collateral circulation so that final occlusion produces less stress on the system.

Factors Affecting Tissue Survival

The survival of the brain regions at risk depends on a number of factors: (1) the adequacy of collateral circulation, (2) the state of the systemic circulation, (3) serologic factors, (4) changes within the obstructing vascular lesion, and (5) resistance within the microcirculatory bed.

Adequacy of Collateral Circulation. Congenital deficiencies in the circle of Willis and prior occlusion of potential collateral vessels decrease the available collateral supply. Hypertension or diabetes diminishes blood flow in smaller arteries and arterioles and thus reduces the potential of the vascular system to supply blood flow to the needy region.

State of the Systemic Circulation. Cardiac pump failure, hypovolemia, and increased blood viscosity all reduce CBF. The two most important determinants of blood viscosity are the hematocrit and the fibrinogen levels.[93–95] In patients with hematocrits in the range of 47–53%, lowering of the hematocrit by phlebotomy to below 40% can increase cerebral blood flow by as much as 50%.[95] Blood pressure is also very important. Elevation of blood pressure except at malignant ranges increases CBF. Surgeons take advantage of this fact by injecting catecholamines to raise blood pressure and flow during the clamping phase of carotid endarterectomy. Low blood pressure significantly reduces flow. In some patients, the balance is so tenuous that simply sitting in bed or standing lowers collateral pressure enough to induce symptoms.[96,97]

Serologic Factors. The blood functions as a carrier of needed oxygen and other nutrients. Hypoxia is clearly detrimental because each milliliter of blood delivers a less-than-normal oxygen supply. Low blood sugar similarly increases the risk of cell death. Higher-than-normal blood sugar also can be detrimental to the ischemic brain.[98,99] Elevated serum calcium levels[100,101] and high blood-alcohol content[102] may also be important detrimental variables.

Changes within the Obstructing Vascular Lesion. Embolic occlusive thrombi do not adhere to the vessel wall of the recipient artery and frequently move on. The moving embolus can block a more distal intracranial artery, causing added or new ischemia, or it may fragment and pass through the vascular bed. Clot formation activates an endogenous thrombolytic system that includes tissue plasminogen activator (t-PA).[90] Inhibitors of t-PA are also present. Sudden obstruction of a vascular lumen can cause reactive vasoconstriction (spasm), which in turn causes further luminal compromise. Thrombolysis, passage of clots, and reversal of vasoconstriction all promote reperfusion of the ischemic zone. If reperfusion occurs quickly enough, the stunned, reversibly ischemic brain may recover quickly. The occlusive clot may propagate further proximally or distally along the vessel, blocking potential collateral channels. The distal end of the thrombus can also break loose and embolize to an intracranial receptive site. Hypercoagulable states promote such extension of thrombi.

Resistance within the Microcirculatory Bed.
The vast majority of CBF does not occur in the large macroscopic arteries at the base of the brain or along the surface. Most flow occurs through microscopic vessels: the arterioles, capillaries, and venules. Resistance to flow in these small vessels is affected by prior diseases, such as hypertension and diabetes, which often cause thickening of vessel walls. Experimental animals and patients that have been hypertensive before a vascular occlusion fare worse than individuals previously normotensive, presumably because of these microcirculatory changes. Both hyperviscosity and diffuse thromboses within the capillaries and microvessel bed greatly reduce flow through the microcirculation. Ischemic insults may produce biochemical changes that lead to platelet activation, clumping of erythrocytes, and plugging of the microcirculation. Ames referred to these changes as causing a "no reflow" state in the microvascular bed, even when large arteries are reperfused.[103] In general, studies of CBF are sensitive to changes in resistance in the microcirculatory bed. Remember that flow is inversely proportional to resistance in the vascular bed, the majority of which is microcirculatory.

Edema and pressure changes within the brain and cranial cavity also influence survival of brain tissue and patient recovery after vascular occlusions. There are two types of brain edemas: (1) water accumulation inside cells, termed *cytotoxic edema*; and (2) fluid within the extracellular space, often termed *vasogenic edema*.[104] Extracellular edema is also often referred to as "wet edema" because in such cases, the cut surface of the brain oozes edema fluid, whereas intracellular (cytotoxic) edema is termed *dry edema*.[104] Cytotoxic edema is caused by energy failure, with movement of ions and water across the cell membranes into cells. Extracellular edema is influenced by hydrostatic pressure factors, especially increased blood pressure and blood flow, and by osmotic factors. When proteins and other macromolecules enter the brain extracellular space because of breakdown of the blood-brain barrier, they exert an osmotic gradient pulling water into the extracellular space. This vasogenic edema accumulates more in the cerebral and cerebellar white matter because of the difference in compliance between gray and white matter.[102]

Brain swelling caused by cytotoxic edema means a large volume of dead or dying brain cells, which implies a bad outcome. On the other hand, edema within the extracellular space does not necessarily require severe neuronal injury, and fluid in the extracellular compartment can potentially be mobilized and removed. In any case, severe edema may cause gross swelling of the brain; shifts in position of brain tissue, with potential pressure damage; and herniation of brain contents from one compartment to another.

Intracranial pressure may also be increased, leading to increased morbidity and decreased CBF. When intracranial pressure is increased, the pressure in the venous sinuses and draining veins must also increase if blood is to be drained normally from the cranium. There must be a gradient between venous pressure and intracranial pressure for drainage to occur. Also, for tissue perfusion to occur, arterial pressure must exceed venous pressure. Blood flow is already compromised in the presence of vascular occlusion. Increased intracranial pressure places an additional stress on the system, forcing even higher the flow values required for tissue survival. Brain edema and increased intracranial pressure also cause headache, decreased consciousness, and vomiting.[105] Pressure shifts and herniation cause pressure-related damage to adjacent tissues and signs of dysfunction of the compressed structures.[31,106] Because pressure shifts and herniations are more common after intracerebral hemorrhage, due to the additional presence in the brain of an extra mass of tissue (hematoma), I discuss herniations further in the discussion of intracerebral hemorrhage.

Events During the First Three Weeks
after Vascular Occlusion

Experience shows that the tenuous balance created by occlusion of a major artery is temporary and usually resolves in 2–3 weeks at most. During this period, any systemic changes, such as decrease in fluid volume or positional or pharmacologically mediated drops in blood pressure, can cause worsening of symptoms. By 3 weeks, either the brain tissue has died, causing a brain infarct, or collateral sources of blood flow develop, which adequately supply the region at risk. By 2–3 weeks, collateral circulation stabilizes, and the patient is less vulnerable to positional or circulatory changes. In addition to causing ischemia through low perfusion, the occlusive thrombus, which at first loosely adheres to the vessel wall, can propagate distally or can fragment and embolize to a distal artery. By 2–3 weeks, the clot has become more adherent and has much less tendency to embolize. Most studies of patients with anterior[107,108] and posterior circulation ischemia [36,109,110] document a low frequency of progression of acute ischemic deficits after 2 weeks.

During the hours, days, and early weeks after a vascular occlusion, the question of death or survival of at-risk brain tissue can be viewed as a clash between factors acting to worsen ischemia and natural body responses that prevent or limit ischemia. Table 2-1 summarizes these "good guys" versus "bad guys" responses, which are useful to keep in mind when treatment is discussed. Clinicians hope to build on the body's natural defenses and counteract the factors that promote ischemia.

This process of shifting vulnerability translates clinically into fluctuating variable symptoms and signs during the early period after a vascular occlusion. Acute blockage of an artery often translates into the sudden onset of symptoms. After vascular occlusion, a weighing of the balance of positive and adverse factors toward the adverse side causes transient deficits or fluctuating, stepwise, or gradual worsening of neurologic symptoms and signs. Sudden worsening is often related to distal embolization.

Intracerebral Hemorrhage

Hemorrhage into the brain parenchyma is often preceded by hypertensive damage to small cerebral penetrating arteries and arterioles. Small aneurysmal dilatations, first hypothesized by Charcot and Bouchard in the 1870s, pepper the penetrating vascular territories of hypertensive patients[25,26,28] and in some patients represent weak points that rupture under increased arterial tension. In the majority of patients, abrupt elevation in blood pressure causes rupture of small penetrating arteries that had no prior vascular damage.[27,28] Leakage from these small vessels produces a sudden but local pressure effect on

Table 2-1. Balancing of Factors after Vascular Occlusion

Factors Promoting Ischemia	Body Responses Acting to Limit Ischemia
Decreased blood flow due to occlusion	Opening of collateral vascular channels
Embolization of clot	Passing and fragmentation of emboli
Activation of coagulation factors and inhibitors of thrombolysis	Activation of thrombolytic factors
Propagation of clot	Lysis of clot
Decreased blood flow caused by hypotension, hypovolemia, low cardiac output	Improvement in general medical condition, especially after correction of abnormalities

surrounding capillaries and arterioles, causing them in turn to break.[111] An avalanche-type effect ensues, in which vessels at the circumference break, adding volume to the gradually enlarging hemorrhage (Figure 2-28). The accumulation of hematoma at the periphery can be likened to a snowball rolling downhill, gathering volume along its circumference as it descends. High blood pressure and this avalanche effect enlarge the hemorrhage, while mounting local tissue pressure acts as a tamponade to the bleeding.

Trauma, bleeding disorders, and degenerative changes in congenitally abnormal blood vessels within vascular malformations also may initiate intracerebral bleeding, which then progresses in a manner similar to hypertensive intracerebral hemorrhage. The gradual increase in size of the hematoma translates clinically into gradual worsening of symptoms and signs until the hematoma attains its final size. Hematomas can stop enlarging and may drain themselves by emptying into the ventricular system or the cerebrospinal fluid (CSF) at the pial surface.

If the hemorrhage becomes sizable, the increase in intracranial volume must increase intracranial pressure. When intracranial pressure rises, the venous pressure in the draining dural sinuses increases pari passu. To perfuse the brain, the arterial pressure must rise to produce an effective arteriovenous difference. Thus, the patient with intracerebral hemorrhage may have a mark-

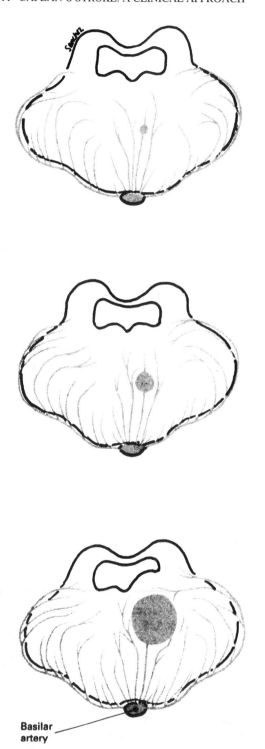

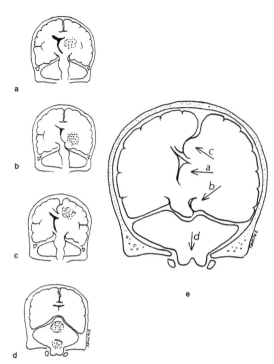

Figure 2-29. Shifts and herniations: Displacement of brain tissues caused by mass-producing strokes are illustrated by patients with hematomas. **(a)** Basal ganglionic hematoma causes compression of the ipsilateral ventricle and shift of the midline to the opposite side. **(b)** Deep hematoma causes uncal herniation. The medial temporal lobe exerts pressure on the upper brainstem. **(c)** Frontal hematoma causes herniations of the cingulum under the falx cerebri. **(d)** Cerebellum hematoma causes increased posterior fossa pressure with herniation of the cerebellum through the foramen magnum. These patterns are also illustrated on the larger figure to the right **(e)**.

Figure 2-28. Avalanche-type effect in pontine hemorrhage, showing gradual development of hemorrhage caused by rupture of small vessels on the periphery of the hemorrhage.

edly elevated blood pressure merely because of the hemorrhage, not necessarily reflecting the true level of premorbid blood pressure. Although lowering this pressure does help to stop bleeding, caution must be exercised because the elevated pressure also serves to perfuse the areas of brain not damaged by the hemorrhage.

Patients with intracerebral hemorrhage often worsen during the first 24–48 hours after their initial symptoms. This worsening can be explained by continued bleeding but most often is related to the development of edema around the lesion,[111,112] to the effects of the lesion on blood flow and metabolism, and—in large hemorrhages—to shifts in brain contents and herniations. Effects caused by masses in patients with hematomas are more common than in patients with ischemia because an extra volume of substance has been added (blood in the hematoma), in addition to the surrounding edema. Most often, pressure effects in hemispheral hematomas result in a shift of the midline without herniation of brain contents. The brain is compartmentalized by bony fortresses (anterior, middle, and posterior fossas) and by dural structures (falx cerebri and tentorium cerebelli), which, under normal circumstances, contain their usual contents. When mass effects are severe, brain tissue bulges or spills out of its usual abode into a different compartment—a process called *herniation*.[28,31,106]

Brain shifts and herniations and their effects are depicted in Figure 2-29. The most common are (1) herniation of the temporal lobe through the tentorial notch, to compress the midbrain (see Figure 2-29A); (2) symmetric, downward pressure by the swollen cerebral hemispheres on the rostral brain stem, causing elongation (see Figure 2-29B); (3) herniation of the anterior medial frontal lobe, usually of the cingulate gyrus, under the falx cerebri (see Figure 2-29C); (4) herniation of the cerebellum upward through the tentorial notch, to compress the brain stem (see Figure 2-29D); and (5) downward herniation of the cerebellar tonsils through the foramen magnum, compressing the medulla and upper cervical spinal cord (see Figure 2-29E).

Shifts in brain contents can also lead to compression or stretch of arteries and infarction in areas of supply and secondary hemorrhages. The most common loci of secondary vascular changes leading to infarction involve the PCAs where they pass between the tentorium and the medial temporal lobe and the ACAs adjacent to the falx (Figure 2-30). Distortion of the upper brain stem at the tentorial opening often leads to secondary hemorrhages in the brain stem. These usually involve the midline and paramedian vessels and are called *Düret hemorrhages*, after the French clinician and researcher who first described them.[28,113] Düret hemorrhages are illustrated in Figure 2-31.

The ventricular system may also be compressed at variable sites. Hematomas in the puta-

men or cerebral lobes may distort the foramen of Monro, causing dilatation of the contralateral lateral ventricle. Thalamic hematomas often obstruct and compress the third ventricle, leading to hydrocephalus of both lateral ventricles. Cerebellar hemorrhages can compress the forth ventricle or cerebral aqueduct, leading to obstructive hydrocephalus of the third and lateral ventricles. These examples of hydrocephalus are depicted in Figure 2-32.

Shifts in brain contents, herniations, and secondary infarctions, as well as Düret hemorrhages and hydrocephalus, all cause clinical worsening of signs and symptoms.

Subarachnoid Hemorrhage

Subarachnoid bleeding nearly always abruptly increases intracranial pressure (ICP). Systemic blood pressure and volume must be maintained or augmented to preserve brain perfusion in the face of the increased ICP. After the initial bleeding, three major risks affect subsequent events: rebleeding, vasoconstriction, and hydrocephalus. Once the outer wall of abnormal blood vessels, most often aneurysms and vascular malformations, has been breached, the vessels are vulnerable to rebleeding. Clearly, a second or third bleed poses substantial threats for survival because each bleed increases ICP and the amount of blood in the CSF. Arteries bathed in bloody CSF often become constricted. Vasoconstriction can be local or more diffuse, and frequently leads to ischemia, brain edema, and infarction.[114,115] Blood within the CSF can clog the absorptive membranes, leading to communicating hydrocephalus—dilation of all of the ventricular system. At times, the initial bleed or subsequent bleeds are into the brain, as well as on its surface. In these patients, the discussion of intracerebral hemorrhage also applies because they have both intracerebral and subarachnoid hemorrhages.

Having laid the basic building blocks for understanding the mechanisms of stroke, I proceed directly to clinical diagnosis at the bedside and then laboratory diagnosis in the following chapters.

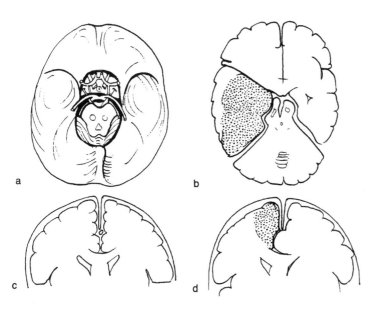

Figure 2-30. Infarcts caused by compression of arteries: **(a)** normal anatomy showing the posterior cerebral artery (PCA) crossing up and over the edge of the tentorium; **(b)** infarction of medial temporal lobe owing to compression of PCA between herniated uncus and tentorium; **(c)** anatomy showing the anterior cerebral artery (ACA) in relation to falx; **(d)** infarction of medial frontal lobe owing to compression of ACA against falx.

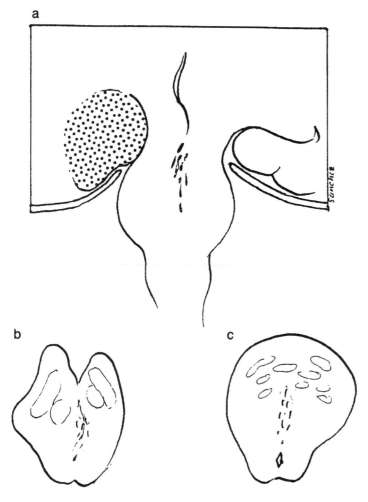

Figure 2-31. Düret hemorrhages: **(a)** herniation with compression of midbrain (longitudinal view); **(b)** midbrain cross section; **(c)** pons cross section.

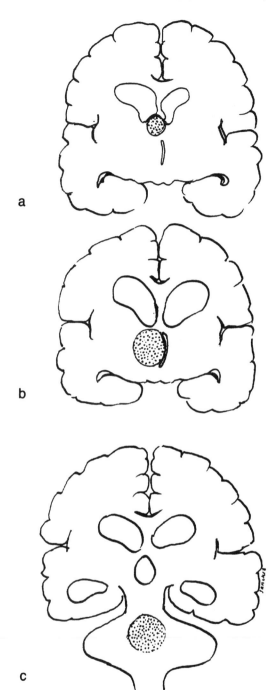

Figure 2-32. Strokes causing hydrocephalus: **(a)** hematoma blocking foramen of Monro, causing dilatation of the ventricle on the left; **(b)** thalamic hematoma compressing the third ventricle, causing dilatation of the lateral ventricles; **(c)** cerebellar hematoma compressing the fourth ventricle, causing dilatation of the third ventricle and lateral ventricles.

References

1. Kapp J, Mahaley M, Odom G. Cerebral arterial spasm: III. Partial purification and characterization of spasmogenic substances in feline platelets. J Neurosurg 1968;29:350–356.
2. Ropper A, Zervas N. Cerebral blood flow after experimental basal ganglia hemorrhage. Ann Neurol 1982;11:266–271.
3. Weiss H. Platelet physiology and abnormalities of platelet function. N Engl J Med 1975;293:531–540,580–588.
4. Ashby B, Daniel JL, Smith JB. Mechanisms of platelet activation and inhibition. Hematol Oncol Clin North Am 1990;4:1–26.
5. Baker A, Iannone A. Cerebrovascular disease: I. The large arteries of the circle of Willis. Neurology 1959;9:321–332.
6. Fisher CM, Gore I, Okabe N, et al. Atherosclerosis of the carotid and vertebral arteries—extracranial and intracranial. J Neuropathol Exp Neurol 1965;24:455–476.
7. Fisher CM. Lacunes: small deep cerebral infarcts. Neurology 1965;15:774–784.
8. Fisher CM. The arterial lesions underlying lacunes. Acta Neuropathol 1969;12:1–15.
9. Houser O, Baker H, Sandok B, et al. Cephalic arterial fibromuscular dysplasia. Radiology 1971;101:605–611.
10. Vinijchalkul L. Primary arteritis of the aorta and its main branches (Takayasu's arteriopathy). Am J Med 1967;43:15–27.
11. Goodwin J. Temporal Arteritis. In P Vinken, G Bruyn (eds), Handbook of Clinical Neurology, Vol 39. Amsterdam: North Holland, 1980:13–342.
12. Fisher CM, Ojemann R, Roberson G. Spontaneous dissection of cervico-cerebral arteries. Can J Neurol Sci 1978;5:9–19.
13. Imparato A, Riles T, Mintzer R, et al. The importance of hemorrhage in the relationship between gross morphologic characteristics and cerebral symptoms in 376 carotid artery plaques. Ann Surg 1983;197:195–203.
14. Caplan LR, Hier DB, D'Cruz I. Cerebral embolism in the Michael Reese Stroke Registry. Stroke 1983;14:530–536.
15. Fisher CM. Observations of the fundus oculi in transient monocular blindness. Neurology 1959;9:333–347.
16. Jones H, Caplan LR, Come P, et al. Paradoxical cerebral emboli: an occult cause of stroke. Ann Neurol 1983;13:314–319.
17. Dines D, Linscheid R, Didier E. Fat embolism syndrome. Mayo Clin Proc 1972;47:237–241.
18. Beal M, Williams R, Richardson E, et al. Cholesterol embolism as a cause of transient ischemic attacks and cerebral infarction. Neurology 1981;31:860–865.
19. Atlee W. Talc and cornstarch emboli in eyes of drug users. JAMA 1972;219:49–51.
20. Hart RG, Foster JW, Luther MF, et al. Stroke in infective endocarditis. Stroke 1990;21:695–700.
21. Mohr J. Neurological Complications of Cardiac Valvular Disease and Cardiac Surgery Including Systemic Hypotension. In P Vinken, G Bruyn (eds), Handbook of Clinical Neurology, Vol 38. Amsterdam: North Holland, 1979:143–171.

22. Romanul F, Abramowicz A. Changes in brain and pial vessels in arterial boundary zones. Arch Neurol 1964;11: 40–65.

23. Symonds C. Spontaneous subarachnoid hemorrhage. Q J Med 1924;18:93.

24. Caplan LR. Intracerebral Hemorrhage. In H Tyler, D Dawson (eds), Current Neurology, Vol 2. Boston: Houghton Mifflin, 1979;185–205.

25. Cole F, Yates P. Intracerebral microaneurysms and small cerebrovascular lesions. Brain 1967;90:759–768.

26. Rosenblum W. Miliary aneurysms and "fibrinoid" degeneration of cerebral blood vessels. Hum Pathol 1977;8: 133–139.

27. Caplan LR. Intracerebral hemorrhage revisited. Neurology 1988;38:624–627.

28. Kase CS, Caplan LR. Intracerebral Hemorrhage. Boston: Butterworth, 1993.

29. Finney L, Walker A. Transtentorial Herniation. Springfield, IL: Thomas, 1962.

30. Fisher CM. Observations concerning brain herniation. Ann Neurol 1983;14:110.

31. Ropper AH. Lateral displacement of brain and level of consciousness in patients with acute hemispheral mass. N Engl J Med 1986;314:953–958.

32. Stephens R, Stilwell D. Arteries and Veins of the Human Brain. Springfield, IL: Thomas, 1969.

33. Helgason C, Caplan LR, Goodwin J, Hedges T. Anterior choroidal artery-territory infarction. Arch Neurol 1986; 43:681–686.

34. Lie T. Congenital Malformations of the Carotid and Vertebral Arterial Systems, Including the Persistent Anastomoses. In P Vinken, G Bruyn (eds), Handbook of Clinical Neurology, Vol 12. Amsterdam: North Holland, 1972; 289–339.

35. Caplan LR. Vertebrobasilar Occlusive Disease. In HJM Barnett, J Mohr, B Stein, F Yatsu (eds), Stroke: Pathophysiology, Diagnosis and Management. New York: Churchill Livingstone, 1986;549–619.

36. Caplan LR. Posterior Circulation Disease: Clinical Findings, Diagnosis, and Management. Boston: Blackwell, 1996.

37. Foix C, Hillemand P. Contributions a l'etude des ramollissements protuberentiels. Rev Med 1926;43:287–305.

38. Foix C, Hillemand P. Les arteres de l'axe encephalique jusqu'a diencephale inclusivement. Rev Neurol 1925;32: 705–739.

39. Caplan LR. Charles Foix—the first modern stroke neurologist. Stroke 1990;21:348–356.

40. Stopford J. The arteries of the pons and medulla oblongata. J Anat Physiol 1915,1916;50:131–164,255–280.

41. Gillilan L. Anatomy and Embryology of the Arterial System of the Brainstem and Cerebellum. In P Vinken, G Bruyn (eds), Handbook of Clinical Neurology, Vol 11. Amsterdam: North Holland, 1972;24–44.

42. Fisher CM. Clinical Syndromes in Cerebral Arterial Occlusion. In W Fields (ed), Pathogenesis and Treatment of Cerebrovascular Disease. Springfield, IL: Thomas, 1961;151–181.

43. Castaigne P, Lhermitte F, Gautier JC, et al. Internal carotid artery occlusion: a study of 61 instances in 50 patients with postmortem data. Brain 1970;93:231–258.

44. Caplan LR. Cerebrovascular Disease: Large Artery Occlusive Disease. In S Appel (ed), Current Neurology, Vol 8. Chicago: Yearbook Medical, 1988;179–226.

45. Gorelick PB, Caplan LR, Hier DB, et al. Racial differences in the distribution of anterior circulation occlusive cerebrovascular disease. Neurology 1984;34:54–59.

46. Caplan LR, Gorelick PB, Hier DB. Race, sex, and occlusive cerebrovascular disease: a review. Stroke 1986;17: 648–655.

47. Kieffer S, Takeya Y, Resch J, et al. Racial differences in cerebrovascular disease: angiographic evaluation of Japanese and American populations. AJR Am J Roentgenol 1967;101:94–99.

48. Feldmann E, Daneault N, Kwan E, et al. Chinese–white differences in the distribution of occlusive cerebrovascular disease. Neurology 1990;40:1541–1545.

49. Moossy J. Morphology, sites, and epidemiology of cerebral atherosclerosis. Res Publ Assoc Res Nerv Ment Dis 1966;51:1–22.

50. Mohr JP. Lacunes. Stroke 1982;13:3–11.

51. Caplan LR. Intracranial branch atheromatous disease. Neurology 1989;39:1246–1250.

52. Caplan LR, Zarins C, Hemmatti M. Spontaneous dissection of the extracranial vertebral artery. Stroke 1985;16: 1030–1038.

53. O'Connell BF, Towfighi J, Brennan RW, et al. Dissecting aneurysms of head and neck. Neurology 1985;35:993–997.

54. Caplan LR, Baquis GD, Pessin MS, et al. Dissection of the intracranial vertebral artery. Neurology 1988;38: 868–877.

55. Wilkinson I, Russell R. Arteries of the head and neck in giant cell arteritis. Arch Neurol 1972;27:378–391.

56. Gacs G, Merei FT, Bodosi M. Balloon catheter as a model of cerebral emboli in humans. Stroke 1982;13:39–42.

57. Fisher CM. Clinical Syndromes in Cerebral Hemorrhage. In WS Fields (ed), Pathogenesis and Treatment of Cerebrovascular Disease. Springfield, IL: Thomas, 1961;318–342.

58. Bull J. Contribution of radiology to the study of intracranial aneurysms. BMJ 1922;2:1701–1708.

59. Alpers B. Aneurysms of the Circle of Willis. In WS Fields (ed), Intracranial Aneurysms and Subarachnoid Hemorrhage. Springfield, IL: Thomas, 1965;5–24.

60. Ringelstein E, Zeumer H, Angelou D. The pathogenesis of strokes from internal carotid artery occlusion. Stroke 1983;14:867–875.

61. Ringelstein EB, Koschorke S, Holling A, et al. Computed tomographic pattern of proven embolic brain infarctions. Ann Neurol 1989;26:759–765.

62. Zulch K, Behrends R. The Pathogenesis and Topography of Anoxia, Hypoxia, and Ischemia of the Brain in Man. In J Meyer, H Gastant (eds), Cerebral Anoxia and the EEG. Springfield, IL: Thomas, 1961;144–163.

63. Kase C, Robinson K, Stein R, et al. Anticoagulant-related intracerebral hemorrhage. Neurology 1985;35:943–948.

64. Jafar JJ, Crowell RM. Focal Ischemic Thresholds. In JH Wood (ed), Cerebral Blood Flow. New York: McGraw-Hill, 1987;449–457.

65. Toole JF. Cerebrovascular Disorders (4th ed). New York: Raven Press, 1990.

66. Frackowiak R, Lenzi G, Jones T, et al. Quantitative measurements of regional cerebral blood flow and oxygen metabolism in man using ^{15}O and positron emission tomography: therapy, procedure, and normal values. J Comput Assist Tomogr 1980;4:722–736.

67. Roy CS, Sherrington CS. On the regulation of the blood-supply of the brain. J Physiol (London) 1890;11: 85–108.

68. Friedland RP, Iadecola C. Roy and Sherrington (1890): a centennial reexamination of "On the regulation of the blood-supply of the brain." Neurology 1991;41:10–14.

69. Symon L. Pathological Regulation in Cerebral Ischemia. In JH Wood (ed), Cerebral Blood Flow. New York: McGraw-Hill, 1987;413–424.

70. Garcia JH, Anderson ML. Pathophysiology of cerebral ischemia. Crit Rev Neurobiol 1989;4:303–324.

71. Collins RC, Dobkin BH, Choi DW. Selective vulnerability of the brain: new insights into the pathophysiology of stroke. Ann Intern Med 1989;110:992–1000.

72. Choi DW. Excitotoxicity and Stroke. In LR Caplan (ed), Brain Ischemia, Basic Concepts and Clinical Relevance, London: Springer, 1995;29–36.

73. Garcia JH. Mechanisms of Cell Death in Ischemia. In LR Caplan (ed), Brain Ischemia, Basic Concepts and Clinical Relevance. London: Springer, 1995;7–18.

74. Mattson MP, Barger SW. Programmed Cell Life: Neuroprotective Signal Transduction and Ischemic Brain Injury. In MA Moskowitz, LR Caplan (eds). Cerebrovascular Diseases, Nineteenth Princeton Stroke Conference, Moskowitz MA. Boston: Butterworth–Heinemann, 1995;271–290.

75. Nurden AT, Duperat V-G, Nurden P. Platelet function and pharmacology of antiplatelet drugs. Cerebrovasc Dis 1997 (Suppl 6):2–9.

76. Moncada S, Higgs E, Vane J. Human arterial and venous tissues generate prostacyclin (prostaglandin 4) a potent inhibitor of platelet aggregation. Lancet 1977;1:18–20.

77. Hennerici M, Sitzer G, Weger H-D. Carotid Artery Plaques. Basel: Karger, 1987.

78. Schmid-Schonbein H, Perktold K. Physical Factors in the Pathogenesis of Atheroma Formation. In LR Caplan (ed), Brain Ischemia, Basic Concepts and Clinical Relevance. London: Springer, 1995;185–213.

79. Fisher CM, Ojemann RG. A clinico-pathologic study of carotid endarterectomy plaques. Rev Neurol (Paris) 1986; 142:573–589.

80. Fisher M, Francis R. Altered coagulation in cerebral ischemia. Arch Neurol 1990;47:1075–1079.

81. Tohgi H, Kawashima M, Tamura K, et al. Coagulation-fibrinolysis abnormalities in acute and chronic phases of cerebral thrombosis and embolism. Stroke 1990;21:1663–1667.

82. Feinberg WM. Coagulation. In LR Caplan (ed), Brain Ischemia, Basic Concepts and Clinical Relevance. London: Springer, 1995;85–96.

83. Deykin D. Thrombogenesis. N Engl J Med 1967;276: 622–628.

84. Mustard JF, Murphy EA, Rowsell HC, et al. Factors influencing thrombus formations in vivo. Am J Med 1962; 33:621–647.

85. Rybak ME. Disorders of Hemostasis. In J Noble (ed), Textbook of General Medicine and Primary Care. Boston: Little, Brown, 1987;535–552.

86. Svensson PJ, Dahlback B. Resistance to activated protein C as a basis to venous thrombosis. N Engl J Med 1994; 330:517–522.

87. Bertina RM, Koelman BPC, Rosendall FR, et al. Mutation in the blood coagulation factor V associated with resistance to activated protein C. Nature 1994;369:64–67.

88. Poort SR, Rosendaal FR, Reitsma PH, Bertina RM. A common genetic variation in the 3'-untranslated region of the prothrombin gene is associated with elevated plasma prothrombin levels and an increase in venous thrombosis. Blood 1996;88:3698–3703.

89. Martinelli I, Sacchi E, Landi G, et al. High risk of cerebral vein thrombosis in carriers of a prothrombin-gene mutation and in users of oral contraceptives. N Engl J Med 1998;338:1793–1797.

90. Sloan M. Thrombolysis and stroke. Arch Neurol 1987;44: 748–768.

91. Raichle M. The pathophysiology of brain ischemia. Ann Neurol 1983;13:2–10.

92. Astrup J, Siesjo B, Simon L. Thresholds in cerebral ischemia: the ischemic penumbra. Stroke 1981;12:723–725.

93. Thomas D, du Boulay G, Marshall J, et al. Effect of hematocrit on cerebral blood flow in man. Lancet 1977; 2:941–943.

94. Thomas D, Marshall J, Russell RW, et al. Cerebral blood flow in polycythemia. Lancet 1977;2:161–163.

95. Tohgi H, Yasmanouchi H, Murakami M, et al. Importance of the hematocrit as a risk factor in cerebral infarction. Stroke 1978;9:369–374.

96. Caplan LR, Sergay S. Positional cerebral ischemia. J Neurol Neurosurg Psychiatry 1976;39:385–391.

97. Toole J. Effects of change of head, limb, and body position on cephalic circulation. N Engl J Med 1968;279:307–311.

98. Ginsberg M, Welsh F, Budd W. Deleterious effect of glucose pretreatment on recovery from diffuse cerebral ischemia in the cat. Stroke 1980;11:347–354.

99. Plum F. What causes infarction in ischemic brain? Neurology 1983;33:222–233.

100. Siesjo BK, Kristian T, Katsura K. The Role of Calcium in Delayed Postischemic Brain Damage. In LR Caplan (ed), Cerebrovascular Diseases, the Nineteenth Princeton Stroke Conference, Moskowitz MA. Boston: Butterworth–Heinemann, 1995;353–370.

101. Gorelick PB, Caplan LR. Calcium, hypercalcemia and stroke. Current concepts of cerebrovascular disease. Stroke 1985;20:13–17.

102. Hillbom M, Kaste M. Ethanol intoxication: a risk factor for ischemic brain infarction in adolescents and young adults. Stroke 1981;12:422–425.

103. Ames A III, Wright RL, Kouada M, et al. Cerebral ischemia: II. The no-reflow phenomenon. Am J Pathol 1968;52:437–453.

104. O'Brien MD. Ischemic Cerebral Edema. In LR Caplan (ed), Brain Ischemia, Basic Concepts and Clinical Relevance. London: Springer, 1995;43–50.

105. Ropper AH. Brain edema after stroke, clinical syndrome and intracranial pressure. Arch Neurol 1984;41:26–29.

106. Ropper AH. A preliminary MRI study of the geometry of brain displacement and level of consciousness with acute intracranial masses. Neurology 1989;39:622–627.

107. Barnett H. Delayed cerebral ischemic episodes distal to occlusion of major cerebral arteries. Neurology 1978;28:7 69–774.

108. Fisher CM. Occlusion of the internal carotid artery. Arch Neurol Psychiatry 1951;65:346–377.

109. Caplan LR. Occlusion of the vertebral or basilar artery. Stroke 1979;10:277–282.

110. Jones H, Millikan C, Sandok B. Temporal profile of acute vertebrobasilar system infarction. Stroke 1980;11: 173–177.

111. Fisher CM. Pathological observations in hypertensive cerebral hemorrhage. J Neuropathol Exp Neurol 1971;30: 536–550.

112. Herbstein D, Schaumberg H. Hypertensive intracerebral hematoma: an investigation of the initial hemorrhage and rebleeding using Cr 51 labeled erythrocytes. Arch Neurol 1974;30:412–414.

113. Duret H. Traumatismes Cranio-Cerebaux. Paris: Librarie Felix Alcan, 1919.

114. MacDonald RL. Cerebral Vasospasm. In KMA Welch, DJ Reis, LR Caplan, et al. (eds), Primer on Cerebrovascular Diseases. San Diego: Academic Press, 1997;490–497.

115. Hijdra A, van Gijn J, Nagelkerke NJD, et al. Prediction of delayed cerebral ischemia, rebleeding, and outcome after aneurysmal subarachnoid hemorrhage. Stroke 1988;19: 1250–1256.

Chapter 3
Diagnosis and the Clinical Encounter

For when the cause of the complaint is unsure, 'twould be a miracle to find a cure.
—Miguel de Cervantes

A 36-year-old man, JH, becomes confused at work and is brought to the hospital. On arrival, it is obvious that his left limbs are weak. He is very sleepy and at times barely arousable. The nurse in the emergency ward at the hospital calls you, his physician, and relates that your patient is having a stroke.

Information Used for Stroke Diagnosis

The preceding patient vignette describes a seriously ill man; the clinician's first task is to decide what is the matter with him. This chapter follows the process of diagnosis by a stepwise consideration of the facts in his case. Before proceeding with the specific case example, however, the general process of stroke diagnosis is reviewed. Clinical diagnosis is often difficult, but the process becomes easier and more logical if approached systematically. I routinely follow several steps and rules and urge each individual clinician to become familiar with the diagnostic methods that he or she uses. Routines and thoroughness prevent errors made by snap guesses or impulsive diagnoses. I have elaborated elsewhere in much more detail on the subject of clinical neurologic diagnoses[1,2] and only summarize briefly the main points here.

First, the clinician must decide on the key questions to be asked. Answers are difficult unless the questions are clearly framed. The most general questions should be asked first, followed by the more specific ones. In neurology, two diagnostic questions always require an answer: (1) What is the disease mechanism—the pathology and pathophysiology? and (2) Where is the lesion(s)—the anatomy of the disorder? In regard to the stroke patient, the "what" question concerns which of the five stroke mechanisms (hemorrhage—subarachnoid or intracerebral; ischemia—thrombotic, embolic, or decreased global perfusion) is present. Of course, before distinguishing among stroke mechanisms, clinicians should first ask whether the findings could be caused by a nonvascular process, such as a brain tumor, metabolic disorder, infection, intoxication, or traumatic injury that mimics stroke. The "where" question concerns the anatomic location of the disorder, both in the brain and in the vascular system.

Usually, different data are used to answer these two quite different questions. In determining stroke mechanism, the following clinical bedside data are helpful:

1. Ecology—the past and present personal and family illnesses of the patient
2. Presence and nature of past strokes or transient ischemic attacks (TIAs)
3. Time of the onset of the symptoms
4. Activity at the onset of the stroke
5. Temporal course and progression of the findings (Was the stroke onset sudden with the deficit maximal at onset? Did it progress in a stepwise, remitting, or progressive fashion? Were there fluctuations between normal and abnormal?)
6. Accompanying symptoms such as headache, vomiting, and decreased level of consciousness

Responses to these items can all be gleaned from a careful history from the patient, a review of physicians' and medical records, and data collected from observers, family members, and friends. These data are primarily historical and require little sophisticated knowledge of neurology. The general physical examination, which uncovers disorders not known from the history, adds to the data used for diagnosing the stroke mechanism. Elevated blood pressure, cardiac enlargement or murmurs, and vascular bruits are examples of physical findings that influence the identification of the stroke mechanism.

Diagnosis of stroke location is made using different data:

1. Analysis of the neurologic symptoms and their distribution
2. Findings on neurologic examination

The history and knowledge of general systemic diseases tell the clinician what is wrong; the neurologic examination tells more where the disease process is located.

Mechanism and anatomic diagnoses are not absolute. More realistic are estimates of probability. In one patient, intracerebral hemorrhage may be the most likely diagnosis, by far, but embolism and thrombosis are also possible and should not be eliminated from consideration. In another patient, there might be an apparent toss-up between thrombosis and embolism.

The process of diagnosis involves two basic techniques: (1) hypothesis generation and testing and (2) pattern matching. As the patient relates the history, the clinician should be thinking of possible diagnoses and testing hypotheses by asking additional questions that help confirm or refute the hypotheses. For example, an elderly patient with known coronary and peripheral limb atherosclerosis has a left hemiparesis noted on awakening. In such a case, considering the ecology, I would first think of thrombosis because that would be a common stroke mechanism. I would then ask whether there had been prior transient episodes of left limb symptoms. Their presence would strongly favor thrombosis.

Anatomic hypotheses are also generated. A left hemiparesis raises the possibility of a right cerebral or brain stem lesion, so I ask about accompanying visual, sensory, or brain stem symptoms that would help generate a more specific anatomic localization. The process of anatomic diagnosis is much like locating a missing person. First, the clinician must determine whether the person is in the United States before limiting the whereabouts to Massachusetts, then the Boston vicinity, then to a specific street in the Brookline neighborhood. Similarly, regarding the diagnosis of mechanism, the physician must decide on ischemia versus hemorrhage before hypothesizing about subtypes of ischemia. The physician must identify thrombosis versus embolism versus global hypoperfusion before distinguishing subtypes of thrombosis, such as lacunar or large artery, anterior or posterior circulation. Thus, the clinician proceeds systematically from the more general to the more specific. Clearly, the amount of available data may limit reasonable hypotheses to the most general inferences. In some patients, few historical data are available.

The other technique used by most clinicians is pattern matching. For example, I recognize the person I call "Jim" by comparing the individual in front of me with a mental image of Jim that I conjure in my mind. I do not ordinarily list individual features (e.g., height, glasses, hair style). Similarly, clinicians try to identify a constellation of findings that match their mental images of patterns of stroke mechanisms and pathology and anatomy.

Although the preceding description indicates a sequence of analysis, diagnosis of "what" and "where" should proceed concurrently as well as sequentially. While obtaining the patient's history, have the patient elucidate information that allows prediction of the probability of various stroke mechanisms and locations. At the end of the history, be prepared to list these and to assign rough probability estimates. Next, think about and plan the examination. In this patient, what additional findings are important and help to confirm or refute the preliminary diagnoses? What data allow more specificity? In the patient with left hemiparesis, the presence of a left visual field deficit or left visual neglect would localize the lesion to the right cerebral hemisphere. Nystagmus or a gaze palsy to the right would favor a brain stem site. A right carotid bruit or a cholesterol crystal in the right ocular fundus would favor a right carotid artery site. After the general and neurologic examinations, re-examine the original hypotheses and their probabilities. New or unexpected findings from the examinations might stimulate new hypotheses or might confirm or refute prior hypotheses. A blood pressure of 260/140 mm Hg would clearly increase the likelihood of hemorrhage. The absence of a pulse or presence of papilledema on examination would change prior estimated probabilities.

Next, proceed to ask what laboratory tests might help refine the hypotheses generated at the end of the history and the examinations. Also, initial laboratory test results help determine the need for other tests. Laboratory tests should also be planned, reviewed, and ordered sequentially (this topic is elaborated in Chapter 4). Overall, the process of diagnosis should be logical, systematic, and sequential.

Procedure for Diagnosis of Stroke Mechanism and Brain Localization

Mimicking a Computer

Computers have taught clinicians to be more aware of the process and mechanics of diagnosis. In an individual patient, how would a computer estimate the most likely stroke mechanism diagnosis? Physicians may not always have ready access to a computer and the necessary software to take advantage of computer diagnosis. They can, however, emulate the logic and methodology of the computer process for a more systematic diagnostic strategy. One technique of computer diagnosis is the use of Bayes's theorem.[3,4] Needed for this methodology are (1) the incidence of each illness (in this case, stroke mechanism) in the population studied and (2) the incidence of a given finding in each illness (stroke mechanism). Armed with this information and the findings in the individual patient, the computer calculates the probability of a given stroke mechanism. The use of probabilities mimics the way clinicians usually approach a diagnostic problem. Seldom is a single diagnosis absolutely certain (100%). More often, a given diagnosis (e.g., cerebral embolisms) is considered most likely (perhaps 70% probable); but thrombotic occlusion also should be considered (perhaps 20%); and intracerebral hemorrhage, although unlikely (10%), still enters into the differential diagnosis.

Knowing the frequencies of the various stroke mechanisms provides what is usually called *a priori odds*. An analysis of data from large stroke studies and registries[5–19] (Table 3-1) shows that approximately 80% of all strokes are ischemic and 20% are hemorrhagic. Therefore, if no other specific information were available about a stroke patient, the diagnosis of ischemic stroke would be correct four out of five times, but subarachnoid hemorrhage would be correct for fewer than 1 patient in 10. The remainder of the computer prediction uses individual factors (e.g., headache preceding stroke, activity at onset, prior evidence of atherosclerosis) to predict the mechanism. For example, Table 3-2 presents the relative frequency of headache during the days or weeks preceding stroke. Relatively few patients had headaches preceding stroke, but the finding was slightly more common in patients with thrombotic stroke and intracerebral hemorrhage and less common in patients with either subarachnoid hemorrhage or cerebral embolism. In this example, the difference in frequency is small. By contrast, headache at or near the onset of stroke (Table 3-3) invariably occurred in patients with subarachnoid hemorrhage but was clearly less often present in patients with other mechanisms of stroke.

These data can also be presented in graphic form: Figure 3-1, from a study of patients seen on the stroke service at the Michael Reese Hospital and the University of Illinois,[20] depicts the frequency—by stroke subtype—of headache preceeding stroke (often called *sentinel headache*) and headache at onset of stroke. The computer and the alert physician sum the individual data items, factor in the a priori odds, and arrive at a total probability for a given stroke mechanism in each stroke patient. During the discussion of individual data items in the remainder of this chapter, I include important data results from stroke registry experience.

Ecology

Included within ecology are prior medical diseases and demographic data that might predispose the patient to have one or more of the stroke mechanisms. When called to see a patient with stroke, the physician usually has available some background information from the family, another physician, or the clinician's own knowledge. For example, a call from the hospital emergency room might describe a "65-year-old man with angina pectoris, two prior

Table 3-1. Frequency and Types of Strokes in Various Studies

Study	Year	n	T	LA	Lac	ICU	Emb	ICH	SAH	Isch total	Hem total
Aring-Merritt[5]	1935	407	81	—	—	—	3	—	—	84	15
Whisnant et al.[6]	1971	548	75	—	—	—	3	10	5	78	15
Matsumoto et al.[7]	1973	993	71	—	—	—	8	10	6	79	16
Kannell et al.[8.]	1965	90	63	—	—	—	15	4	18	78	22
Harvard Stroke Registry[9]	1978	694	53	34	19	—	31	10	6	84	16
Michael Reese Stroke Registry[10]	1983	472	31	18	13	30	17	14	8	78	22
Austin Hospital[11]	1983	700	68	45	23	18	8	6	Excl	94	6
South Alabama[12]	1984	160	19	6	13	40	26	8	6	85	14
Pilot Stroke Data Bank[13]	1984	928	30	19	11	25	22	11	13	77	24
Lausanne Stroke Registry[14]	1988	1,000	56	43	13	8	20	11	Excl	89	11
Stroke Data Bank [15]	1988	1,805	25	6	19	32	14	13	13	71	26
Lehigh Valley Stroke Registry[16]	1989	2,639	60	—	9	—	20	9	Excl	91	9
Oxfordshire Community Stroke Project[17]	1990	675	—	—	—	—	—	10	5	81	15
Taiwan Stroke Registry[18]	1997	676	46	17	29	20	29	Excl	Excl	100	Excl
Community Hospital Stroke Program[19]	1990	4,129	32	—	—	—	11	5	2	60	10

Emb = embolism; Excl = excluded from study; Hem = hemorrhage; ICH = intracerebral hemorrhage; ICU = infarct cause unknown; Isch = ischemia; LA = large artery; Lac = lacune; n = number of cases; SAH = subarachnoid hemorrhage; T = thrombosis.

Table 3-2. Headache Preceding Stroke

	Thrombosis	Embolus	ICH	SAH
Yes	27 (8.2%)	8 (4%)	6 (8%)	1 (3%)
No	291 (89%)	177 (87%)	61 (77%)	27 (87%)
Other	9 (2%)	18 (9%)	12 (15%)	3 (10%)
Total	**327**	**203**	**79**	**31**

ICH = intracerebral hemorrhage; Other = no data—patient, aphasic, stuporous, or information not available; SAH = subarachnoid hemorrhage.
Source: Reprinted with permission from J Mohr, LR Caplan, J Melski, et al. The Harvard Cooperative Stroke Registry: a prospective registry. Neurology 1978;28:754–762.

Table 3-3. Headache at Onset of Stroke

Registry	Thrombosis	Lacune	Embolus	SAH	ICH	ICU
HSR	12%	3%	9%	78%	33%	—
MRSR	29%	16%	17%	98%	80%	13%

HSR = Harvard Stroke Registry; ICH = intracerebral hemorrhage; ICU = infarct cause unknown; MRSR = Michael Reese Stroke Registry; SAH = subarachnoid hemorrhage.

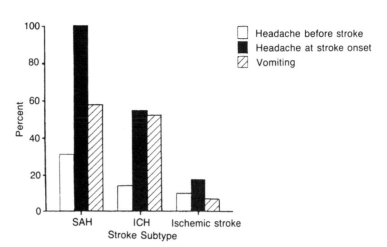

Figure 3-1. Graph shows frequency of headache patterns and vomiting in patients with ischemic strokes and hemorrhages in the Michael Reese and University of Illinois stroke registries. (Reprinted with permission from PB Gorelick, DB Hier, LR Caplan, et al. Headache in acute cerebrovascular disease. Neurology 1986;36:1445–1450.)

heart attacks, diabetes, and hypertension who arrived here today with. . . ." This information leads the physician to consider the probability of particular stroke mechanisms in the patient who is about to be seen. In the preceding example, the presence of diabetes and coronary artery disease strongly favors a diagnosis of associated atherosclerosis of the extracranial cervical vessels and a thrombotic (or artery-to-artery embolus) mechanism of stroke. The presence of prior heart disease raises the possibility of arrhythmia, mural thrombosis, ventricular aneurysm, and valvular heart disease—all potential sources of cerebral embolism. The presence of hypertension increases the probability of intracerebral hemorrhage (ICH), especially if the hypertension is severe, a determination that can be made quickly. An alert physician would also be sure to inquire whether the patient was being treated with anticoagulants for the cardiac disease, a factor that would greatly increase the chance of ICH.

The clinician uses the presence of individual risk factors to alter the likelihood that an individual patient has a particular stroke mechanism. Perhaps another example will help clarify this statement. I have said that, on average, 60% of strokes are considered thrombotic, 20% are embolic, 12% are ICH, and 8% are due to subarachnoid hemorrhage (SAH). The presence of severe hypertension (e.g., 220/130 mm Hg) would certainly make hemorrhage, especially ICH, much more likely. This factor would significantly shift the odds toward ICH and slightly to SAH. If another factor, such as age, is then added (e.g., if the severely hypertensive

patient were a 23-year-old woman) this would make the major alternative diagnosis, thrombotic stroke, much less likely and would further increase the likelihood of a hemorrhagic mechanism. This shift of probabilities can be described as "loading on" or "detracting from" a specific diagnosis: For example, severe hypertension loads heavily on ICH (+ + + +); youthfulness detracts from thrombosis. Data from prior experience, such as those found in registries, can help determine quantitatively the relative shift of odds.

Table 3-4 lists the incidence of diabetes, hypertension, and coronary artery disease in the various subtypes of stroke in the Harvard Stroke Registry (HSR) and the incidence of other similar variables in the Michael Reese Stroke Registry (MRSR). Note that hypertension was more common in all groups in the MRSR and atherosclerosis more prominent in the HSR. The populations in these two registries were quite different: the HSR included a predominantly white, middle- and upper-class population with a high incidence of atherosclerosis, whereas the MRSR had more young, black, hypertensive individuals with a lower prevalence of atherosclerosis. Black, Chinese, and Japanese populations have a higher incidence of ICH and intracranial occlusive disease than white populations.[21–28] Table 3-5 lists estimated loading weights that could be assigned to the various risk factors. At times, the effect of a condition is indirect; for example, the presence of diabetes increases the chance of myocardial infarction, which in turn increases the likelihood of a cardiac-origin embolism.

Table 3-4. Incidence of Various Risk Factors in Each Type of Stroke

	Thrombosis (%)	Lacune (%)	Embolus (%)	ICH (%)	SAH (%)
HSR					
Atherosclerosis*	56	37	34	11	5
Diabetes	26	28	13	15	2
Past hypertension	55	75	40	72	19
MRSR					
Angina pectoris	13	8	20	5	0
Past MI	23	16	40	12	0
Recent MI	7	12	12	3	0
Past hypertension	75	55	55	68	44

HSR = Harvard Stroke Registry; ICH = intracerebral hemorrhage; MI = myocardial infarction; MRSR = Michael Reese Stroke Registry; SAH = subarachnoid hemorrhage.
*Includes peripheral vascular disease, coronary artery disease, and neck bruits.

Table 3-5. Weighting of Ecological Factors

	Thrombosis	Lacune	Embolus	ICH	SAH
Hypertension	++	+++	—	++	+
Hypertension +++	—	+	—	++++	++
Coronary disease	+++	—	++	—	—
Claudication	+++	—	+	—	—
Atrial fibrillation	—	—	++++	—	—
Sick sinus syndrome	—	—	++	—	—
Valvular heart disease	—	—	+++	—	—
Diabetes	+++	+	+	—	—
Bleeding diathesis	—	—	—	++++	+
Smoking	+++	—	+	—	+
Cancer	++	—	++	—	—
Old age	+++	+	+	+	—
Black or Asian origin	+	+	—	++	—

Hypertension +++ = severe hypertension; ICH = intracerebral hemorrhage; SAH = subarachnoid hemorrhage; + = slight loading; ++ = moderate loading; +++ = heavy loading; ++++ = maximal loading.

I now return to the patient JH discussed at the beginning of this chapter. I continue to discuss his case and its analysis during the remainder of the discussion of clinical diagnosis.

After the call from the emergency room, before leaving for the hospital, the secretary is asked to pull JH's office chart. He had last been seen 1 year ago, at age 35 years, because of bronchitis. Notes indicate that he smoked three packs of cigarettes a day, had always had normal blood pressures, and had no history of cardiac or neurologic symptoms. He had described, however, a high incidence of heart attacks in his family. He had been overweight, and his blood cholesterol level last year was 295. He was advised to pursue a weight-reduction program, to reduce his intake of fats and cholesterol-containing foods, to stop smoking, and to return for a recheck. He had not returned.

When leaving for the hospital, think about the information known, based on the emergency room nurse's call and on JH's records. The illness was said to have begun rather suddenly, and the brain lesion must be focal because he has an obvious left limb paralysis. Abrupt-onset focal brain lesions are most often strokes, but his youth serves as a reminder to be certain to consider focal brain lesions other than stroke. Brain tumors, abscesses, trauma, and encephalitis can cause focal findings, and without other information, it is not yet certain how abruptly the symptoms began and progressed. If the process is a stroke, as would be statistically most likely, review the background information regarding risks for the different stroke mechanisms. His past smoking, family history of cardiac disease, and high blood cholesterol level suggest to you the possibility of premature atherosclerosis, with large artery occlusive disease as the mechanism of the stroke. An unusual type of cardiac disease with cerebral embolism is another mechanism that is suggested by the family history of cardiac disease. ICH could also cause left-sided paralysis and sleepiness, but the absence of past hypertension makes this less likely. Make a mental note to quickly check his blood pressure and seek signs of organ damage due to hypertension on examination. The first hypothesis regarding preliminary stroke mechanism is large artery atherosclerosis with embolism, and ICH is also to be seriously considered. Systemic hypoperfusion and SAH seldom cause severe hemiplegia at outset.

So far, few neurologic data are available that could help localize the lesion. The patient has a left-sided paralysis, and so the right cerebral hemisphere and right pons are the most likely sites of pathology. The report of confusion at work favors a cerebral hemispheric lesion. Plan to ask questions that will promote more precise localization.

Having used the ecologic data to shift the usual stroke mechanism probabilities, carry these probabilities into an investigation of the next data items, such as prior cerebrovascular symptoms, course of illness, accompanying symptoms, and so on—each of which then further modifies the probabilities.

When you arrive at the emergency room, the nurse says that the patient's pulse and blood pressure are normal. The patient is awake but cannot give any account of his illness. He seems unaware that his left limbs are paralyzed. The coworker who was with him when he became ill says that he suddenly seemed dazed and quickly became hemiplegic, falling to the ground. His wife says that he did not follow previous dietary advice and was still smoking heavily. She said he had not been ill, but a week before he told her that for 10 minutes one morning, his left arm and face had temporarily felt numb, symptoms he attributed to a draft from an air conditioner in the office.

Prior Cerebrovascular Symptoms

Although not especially common, prior cerebrovascular events so heavily load probabilities that they should be given considerable importance. TIAs in the same vascular territory are frequent precursors of thrombotic stroke, so their presence, especially when multiple, is virtually diagnostic of that stroke mechanism. If a patient presenting to the hospital with aphasia and right limb weakness had had an attack of transient right-handed weakness 3 weeks earlier and an attack of right face and right hand numbness and weakness 1 week earlier, the clinician could be relatively certain that the stroke was a result of thrombotic occlusive disease within the left anterior circulation. If, in addition, that same individual had also had a black shade descending over the left eye, causing temporary blindness, the location could be further refined, and it would seem certain that the occlusive lesion involved the carotid artery before its ophthalmic artery branch. The presence, nature, and duration of TIAs are important. Information about the presence of TIAs must be vigorously and repeatedly sought.

Patients are often naive about the functions of the body, especially the nervous system. Most stroke patients attribute their weakness, lack of feeling, and visual deficits to the local limbs or to the eyes; they often do not understand that the central nervous system (CNS) control of these functions has been damaged. They often wonder why the head is being studied and imaged rather than the arm or leg, where surely the trouble resides. Patients usually do not volunteer information they think is unrelated to their present trouble. A woman with visual difficulty will not tell her eye doctor about a vaginal discharge, considering the latter problem in the province of her gynecologist. Similarly, a patient with hand weakness might not tell the physician about prior leg weakness, not realizing that the conditions are related. The same individual will surely not tell the doctor about temporary visual dysfunction, considering the eye problem to belong to the ophthalmologist. Patients often attribute their temporary symptoms to banal

Table 3-6. Transient Ischemic Attacks (TIAs) in Patients with Severe Carotid Artery Occlusive Disease

Time	First TIA n = 59	Last TIA n = 56*
<1 day	2	16
1 day –1 wk	9	25
1 wk –1 mo	14	7
>1 mo	34	8

*In three patients, the timing of the last TIA was unknown.
Source: Reprinted with permission from J Mohr, LR Caplan, JMelski, et al. The Harvard Cooperative Stroke Registry: a prospective registry. Neurology 1978;28:754–762.

causes in the environment (e.g., an air conditioner draft, as in the case of JH). Symptoms of TIA must be elicited specifically: "Have you ever had temporary weakness of your right hand, your right leg, your face? Have you had difficulty speaking, seeing, and so forth?" On entry to the hospital, or during the first physician encounter, patients are often not at their optimum performance levels. They may be sick, frightened, or worried and therefore suboptimal observers and witnesses. Many patients have told me on the third or even seventh day of stroke about prior TIAs, having denied their presence when queried on admission.

Some patients cannot provide information about a TIA because of aphasia, altered level of consciousness, amnesia, and so on. Other observers, such as family, hospital visitors, and friends, should be queried because the patient may have told them about prior symptoms, or these individuals may have observed altered function in the patient. Caution must be exercised in exploring symptoms at the patient's work site, because knowledge about a patient's neurologic problem might adversely affect job status. Clearly, permission should be sought before approaching employers or coworkers for health information. In this case, the coworker and wife were present and could provide useful data when the patient could not.

In patients with small vessel disease (lacunar infarction), TIAs occur but are less common. In the HSR, TIAs occurred in 23% of patients with lacunar disease, compared with 50% of patients with large vessel arteriosclerosis.[9] When present, TIAs are more likely to be stereotyped (e.g., weakness of face, arm, and leg in each attack) and are usually limited to a period of days. In contrast, patients with occlusion of larger blood vessels, such as the internal carotid artery (ICA) in the neck, may have TIAs during a period of weeks or months. It takes longer for a large vessel (8–15 mm in diameter) to occlude than for a small vessel (several hundred microns in diameter) to do so. In large vessel disease, the TIAs may be less stereotyped, with weakness of a hand in one attack and aphasia and facial numbness in another. The larger the vascular territory, the more opportunity there is for variety. Note, in Table 3-6, that in carotid artery occlusion, the initial TIA most often occurred months before the stroke, whereas the last TIA often preceded the stroke by less than a week. As a vessel occludes, TIAs can become more frequent. Thus, a TIA occurring yesterday is much more ominous than a single TIA that occurred 3 months ago, and the recent TIA would demand more urgent evaluation and treatment.

The term *TIA* designates ischemia, but it does not differentiate between an embolic and a thrombotic mechanism, or between a small vessel and a large vessel site. Cerebral embolism can produce a transient disorder that would qualify as a TIA. Some evidence supports the notion that embolism is more likely to produce less frequent but longer attacks, whereas low flow states produce briefer but more frequent attacks. Shotgun-like repeated episodes of ischemia in the same vascular territory virtually always indicate a critical degree of vessel narrowing. Single but longer attacks are more often associated with an ulcerated plaque or other embolic source.

Occasionally, a patient gives a history of transient deficits in different vascular territories. Such a patient was DB, who awakened one night with numbness of his left arm and leg, symptoms that were gone by morning, when he told his wife. Two nights later, while on his way to the bathroom, he noted weakness and numbness of his right limbs. In the morning, his physician could still document slight weakness of the right hand but noted no other abnormalities on examination.

Had this patient confused his left and right sides and mislocalized the initial symptoms? A week later, the same patient suddenly developed a cold, painful right leg, and investigations confirmed bacterial endocarditis as the source of his multiple embolizations.

Table 3-7. Activity at Onset in Subtypes of Stroke

Activity at Onset	Thrombosis (%)	Embolus (%)	Lacune (%)	ICU (%)	ICH (%)	SAH (%)
On arising	40	17	50	31	13	15
Stress	1	5	1	5	10	15
ADL	54	68	47	50	64	64
Unknown	5	10	2	14	13	6

ADL = activities of daily living; ICH = intracerebral hemorrhage; ICU = infarct cause unknown; SAH = subarachnoid hemorrhage.
Source: Reprinted with permission from LR Caplan, D Hier, I D'Cruz. Cerebral embolism in the Michael Reese Stroke Registry. Stroke 1983;14:530–536.

In our patient, JH, the single TIA provided an important clue in predicting the most probable stroke mechanism. The symptoms involved the left arm and face, making it unlikely that the cause was a local disturbance in these parts of the body. This must have been a transient brain event and one localized to the same side of the brain, probably the same vascular territory as the stroke. A thrombotic event seems the likely mechanism. TIAs do not usually precede ICH. If the mechanism was cardiac-origin embolism, emboli would have hit the same general target twice in a row. It would help if he were alert enough to tell whether there had been more transient attacks because many attacks in the same territory make cardiac-origin embolism quite unlikely.

In addition to TIA, past strokes may also help the alert clinician pinpoint a stroke mechanism. A patient with three prior strokes during the past year involving the vertebrobasilar, left carotid, and right carotid systems has a high probability of cerebral embolism. A normotensive patient with several prior ICHs in different loci has a high probability of having a bleeding diathesis or amyloid angiopathy as the cause of a propensity for ICH. JH had no history of a stroke.

Activity at Onset

Traditional teaching states that most thrombotic strokes occur when the circulation is least active and most sluggish (e.g., during the night or during a nap, with the deficit usually noticed on arising). Embolism and hemorrhage, in contrast, would be more likely to occur when the circulation is more active or when blood pressure rises. New data show that most ischemic[29] and hemorrhagic

strokes[30] actually occur during the morning hours, especially between 10 AM and noon after the patient has awakened and begun daily activities. Table 3-7 contains data from the MRSR on the frequencies of the various stroke mechanisms in relationship to activity at onset. A significant number of hemorrhages do occur at night, and thrombotic deficits can occur during activity. It is, however, unusual for a thrombotic stroke or a lacune to develop during vigorous physical activity or coition. A particularly common time for embolism to occur is on arising at night to urinate, the so-called *matudinal* (morning) embolus. Coughing or a vigorous sneeze can also shake loose an embolic particle, resulting in brain embolism. The onset in JH was during relatively sedentary activities at work.

Early Course of Development of the Deficit

Table 3-8 contains data from the HSR, MRSR, and Lausanne Stroke Registries concerning the temporal course of the neurologic deficit. Often, the early course gives important information about the stroke mechanism. A few examples may serve to illustrate.

WC, a previously hypertensive man, suddenly became aphasic and hemiplegic while eating lunch with his family. When initially examined in the emergency room, he was mute and had a severe right hemiplegia. Two hours later, he was much improved and could lift his right leg and say a few words.

The improvement shortly after onset of the deficit argues strongly against an ICH. The deficit,

Table 3-8. Early Course of Deficit in Various Registries (%)

	Thrombosis			Lacune			Embolus			ICH			SAH	
	HSR	MRS	LSR	HSR	MRS	LSR	HSR	MRS	LSR	HSR	MRS	LSR	HSR	MRS
Maximal at onset	40	45	66	38	40	54	79	89	82	34	38	44	80	64
Stepwise/ stutter	34	30	—	32	28	—	11	10	—	3	9	—	3	14
Gradual, smooth	13	14	27	20	24	40	5	1	13	63	51	52	14	18
Fluctuating	13	11	7	10	8	5	5	0	5	0	2	4	3	4

HSR = Harvard Stroke Registry; ICH = intracerebral hemorrhage; LSR = Lausanne Stroke Registry; MSR = Michael Reese Stroke Registry; SAH = subarachnoid hemorrhage.

which was maximal at onset and was unassociated with headache, is most compatible with an embolic mechanism. The next case illustrates a different scenario.

> RP was admitted to the hospital, and the intern called to say that RP had developed a gradually progressive hemiplegia throughout the day. On closer questioning, RP related the following account: At 9:30 AM, while eating breakfast, her left hand became clumsy, and she dropped a piece of bread. When she climbed the stairs to go to her room, she noticed a slight limp in her left foot. Worried about her problem, she rested for an hour and was comforted when, on rising, she could walk down the stairs without any difficulty and clear the table without a trace of left hand awkwardness. At midday, while sitting on the couch, her left limbs became weak and she could lift neither her arm nor her leg.

RP's account was typical of a stuttering onset, with improvement in the deficit, followed by worsening. Again, this course would be difficult to understand if the initial deficit had been caused by ICH; the tempo was most compatible with a thrombotic process.

I call the process of eliciting the historical details from RP "walking through" the course of illness with the patient. Most patients have difficulty quantifying their deficits and estimating the course of their illness. When patients are asked to describe their activities, an alert observer can often better gauge the course of development of the deficit. I encourage clinicians to construct a "course of illness" graph, which depicts the temporal pattern of the findings.[1,31] Inspection of this graph helps to predict stroke mechanism.[31] Such a graph would aid diagnosis in the following case.

> BK was admitted to the hospital with a note that stated she had sudden onset of left hemiplegia while shopping. While the patient was trying on a hat in a store, the shopkeeper had noted a droop of the face and had called for an ambulance, against the patient's wishes. The shopkeeper recalled the patient walking to the next room and gesturing with both hands. When the ambulance arrived 10 minutes later, the patient could walk to the ambulance but had a limp and less swing of the left arm. On arrival at the hospital, she had a severe left hemiplegia, eyes and head were deviated to the right, and she vomited and complained of headache.

The gradual development of a progressive focal deficit, accompanied by gradually developing symptoms of increased intracranial pressure (ICP), suggested ICH, a diagnosis confirmed by computed tomography (CT). In this case, a call to the shop clarified the early course of illness and helped suggest the correct diagnosis.

In patient JH, the onset was abrupt and presumably maximal at onset because he fell with a hemiplegia. Among the two stroke mechanisms with the

Table 3-9. Frequency of Accompanying Symptoms at or near Onset by Stroke Subtype (%)

	Thrombosis			Embolism			Lacune			ICH			SAH	
	HSR	LSR	SDB	HSR	LSR	SDB	HSR	LSR	SDB	HSR	LSR	SDB	HSR	SDB
Decreased consciousness	15	13	14	20	12	29	3	3	2	39	50	57	68	48
Vomiting	11	—	8	6	—	5	3	—	1	46	—	29	48	45
Seizures	0.3	1	3	4	0	3	0	0	0.1	7	7	9	7	7
Headache	12	17	11	9	18	10	3	7	5	33	40	41	78	87

HSR = Harvard Stroke Registry; ICH = intracerebral hemorrhage; LSR = Lausanne Stroke Registry; SAH = subarachnoid hemorrhage; SDB = Stroke Data Bank.

highest probability so far—embolism and atherosclerosis with thrombosis—each often has a tendency to begin abruptly and to have maximal deficit at or near onset. Recall from the discussion in Chapter 2 that when atherosclerotic large artery lesions critically reduce the size of the residual lumen, occlusive thrombosis often develops. Because the thrombus is initially not adherent, portions may break loose and embolize. Sudden, maximal-at-onset deficits in patients with large artery occlusions are presumed to be caused by artery-to-artery embolism from the donor site of thrombosis to a recipient intracranial artery. Thus, the onset and course to date of JH do not help choose between the two mechanisms being considered most strongly.

Accompanying Symptoms

Headache is an invariable symptom of SAH. Sudden release of blood into the subarachnoid space increases ICP and usually leads to severe headache, vomiting, and a decrease in the level of consciousness. In ICH, the focal deficit usually develops progressively, and only later, when there has been enlargement of the hematoma, do headache, vomiting, and decreased consciousness develop. Loss of consciousness is common in SAH and is rare in ischemic stroke unless the ischemia involves the brain stem bilaterally. Seizures are rare in the early period of stroke; their presence argues for embolic stroke or ICH. Table 3-9 lists the frequency of accompanying features by stroke mechanism.

Combining two pieces of information often adds greatly to the accuracy of the probabilities. An example of this is seen in Table 3-10, which analyzes the presence of vomiting for each stroke mechanism in relation to the stroke's location in the anterior or posterior circulation. Vomiting is common in posterior circulation strokes, presumably because of involvement of the so-called vomiting center in the floor of the fourth ventricle. Vomiting is rare in ischemic strokes in the anterior circulation, however, whether thrombotic or embolic. In the anterior circulation, ICH was accompanied by vomiting, presumably because of the associated increase in ICP. Thus, vomiting and anterior circulation location usually equal ICH. A patient with a right hemiparesis and aphasia who vomits early during the stroke has a high likelihood of harboring an ICH.

Patient JH denied headache but did have lethargy, qualifying as some decrease in level of consciousness. Decrease in level of consciousness is unusual in lacunar infarction, one subtype of thrombotic stroke. He had not vomited. These features do not, in his case, help differentiate between thrombosis and embolism.

Table 3-10. Vomiting and Location and Type of Stroke

ICH	
Anterior circulation	19/29 (48.5%)
Posterior circulation	8/12 (67%)
Thrombosis	
Anterior circulation	3/141 (2%)
Posterior circulation	24/83 (29%)
Embolism	
Anterior circulation	4/198 (2%)
Posterior circulation	6/21 (29%)

ICH = intracerebral hemorrhage.
Source: Reprinted with permission from J Mohr, LR Caplan, J Melski, et al. The Harvard Cooperative Stroke Registry: a prospective registry. Neurology 1978;28:754–762.

Localization and Detection
of the Vascular Lesion

Having pursued the historical features as thoroughly as possible, the clinician should be ready to perform a general and neurologic examination. While proceeding, the principal aims should be kept in mind. They are (1) to detect vascular and cardiac abnormalities that aid in determining stroke mechanism and localization of vascular lesions and (2) to localize the process within the CNS. Once the clinician knows where the lesion is in the brain, a knowledge about the anatomy of the vascular supply, about the risk factors in the patient, and about the results of the vascular examination help the clinician predict the most likely vascular location and process in the patient.

Findings from Examination of the Heart

The diagnosis of cardiogenic embolism is important because its evaluation and treatment differ from intrinsic disease of the extracranial and intracranial vessels. A careful detailed history of possible cardiac symptoms, angina, myocardial infarction, palpitations or arrhythmia, congestive heart failure, and rheumatic heart disease is as important as the neurologic history. The heart should be examined thoroughly, taking time to estimate size, character, and quality of heart sounds and gallops; listening for murmurs is not enough.

Findings from Examination of the Vascular System

Examination of the available systemic and extracranial arteries may give clues to the presence of atherosclerosis or diminished flow not detectable by history. Note the pulse for at least a minute, seeking any irregularities. Feel the radial pulses simultaneously, looking for a significant difference in the strength of the pulse or a delay on one side. In all reported examples of subclavian steal, the diminished blood flow to the arm produced a definite pulse alteration.[32,33] If the pulses are equal and synchronous, it is probably not necessary to check blood pressure in each arm. Feel the femoral and foot pulses and listen to the femoral region for an arterial bruit. Remember that some patients with hyperdynamic circulation (e.g., fever, anemia, or hyperthyroidism) have bruits over many peripheral vessels. When a femoral bruit is present, listen over the antecubital and supraclavicular fossas to determine whether bruits are a generalized phenomenon and not necessarily indicative of focal disease.

Next, gently palpate the carotid artery in the neck. Recall that you are feeling the common carotid artery (CCA) until you reach the bifurcation high in the neck. The ICA then proceeds posteriorly and usually cannot be felt; the external carotid artery (ECA) projects slightly forward and laterally and can be traced. The left carotid artery is positioned more posteriorly and deeper, so that the carotid pulses rarely feel equal. Feeling a carotid pulse in the neck tells the examiner that the CCA is patent; it gives absolutely no information about the ICA. Even if the proximal ICA is occluded, a pulse can often be seen and felt along the ICA because of propagation of the pulse wave from the CCA. All too often, a bounding carotid pulse is falsely considered evidence against an ICA occlusion. Listening to the carotid artery beginning low in the neck and progressing cranially is important.

Recall that many nonstenosing processes can cause carotid bruits. The most common of these are transmitted cardiac murmurs, especially aortic stenosis, tortuous vessels, and hyperdynamic circulatory states. Transmitted heart murmurs and hyperdynamic states produce bruits usually heard over the entire vessel, often loudest at the base of the neck. These bruits are usually low-pitched, relatively short, and are invariably heard best over the supraclavicular fossa, perhaps because of the presence of lung tissue just beneath this region, which better transmits the sound. The auscultatory features of a focal vascular constriction can be compared with those of mitral stenosis because each impedes flow and creates a pressure differential beyond the area of blockage. The bruit caused by local constriction of a carotid or vertebral artery is usually:

1. Focal in location, often loudest at the bifurcation high in the neck and not audible at the base—Osler said that the murmur of mitral stenosis is often limited to the region of a dime; the same explanation is valid for the focality of a focal carotid artery stenosis.

Figure 3-2. Lateral view showing internal (ICA) and external (ECA) carotid arteries. ECA branches supply collateral circulation after ICA occlusion. Inset shows palpation points for angular (A), brow (B), cheek (C), and frontal pulses (F).

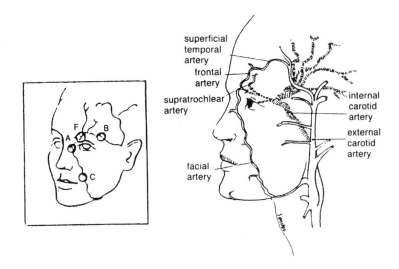

2. Long—It takes longer for blood to course across a constricted vessel; the diastolic murmur of tight mitral stenosis is also long.
3. High-pitched—The blood flow velocity is often increased in regions of arterial stenosis. The increased velocity is associated with a high-pitched sound.

After listening to the carotid arteries in a similar way, auscultate over the supraclavicular fossa and then follow the course of each vertebral artery (VA), first within the posterior cervical triangle and then up the sternocleidomastoid muscle to the mastoid region. Sometimes, a unilateral vertebral artery bruit is a reflection of augmented flow to compensate for a contralateral VA occlusion; the bruit is then on the "wrong side" for the symptoms. The bell of an old-fashioned stethoscope is usually superior to the diaphragm or flat bell of the newer stethoscopes for bruit detection and analysis.

Clues to the patency of the carotid system arteries can also be obtained by careful palpation of the ECA branches on the face. The most readily palpable arteries in normal individuals are the facial artery along the edge of the lower jaw; the preauricular artery just anterior to the ear; and the superficial temporal artery in the temple region. It is important to feel both sides simultaneously to detect a delay or asymmetry of the pulses. When the ECA or CCA on one side is occluded or severely stenosed, the facial, preauricular, and superficial temporal pulses are diminished on that side, and the regions of supply may feel cool to the touch. When the ICA is occluded before its ophthalmic artery branch, the ECA may supply critical collateral vessels, usually about the orbit.

The augmented flow can often be felt as brisk increased pulsation at the cheek, brow, or inner angle of the eye. Fisher designated these pulses *ABC* (angular, brow, cheek) for easy recall (Figure 3-2).[34] At times, the superficial temporal artery provides collateral supply to the supraorbital and supratrochlear branches of the ophthalmic artery feeding the low pressure ophthalmic-carotid system.[35] In the normal situation, blood flows from the ICA to the ophthalmic artery to the supraorbital (frontal artery) and supratrochlear branches cephalad up the brow. In the normal situation, obliteration of these arteries at the brow blocks the distal pulse above it. When there is low pressure in the ophthalmic system, flow goes down these vessels from superficial temporal artery collaterals into the orbit. In that circumstance, obliteration of the brow pulse does not block the forehead pulses, but a finger on the forehead pulses stops the pulsation in the brow, a reversal of the usual normal pattern of flow. This finding is called the *frontal artery sign.*[35]

Remember that there is alternative rich collateral circulation at the circle of Willis, especially through the anterior communicating and posterior communicating arteries, which brings collaterals from the opposite cerebral hemisphere and posterior circulation, respectively. Thus, the absence of augmented facial collateral vessels does not mean that the ICA system is not obstructed. On the other hand, the presence of collateral flow through the orbit is diagnostic of a low pressure ophthalmic-carotid system and thus is important clinically. The technique for detecting this is easy to master at the bedside.

Also feel for the occipital artery behind the mastoid process. This branch of the ECA often provides collateral circulation to the distal extracranial VA in the neck when the VA is occluded at its origin. A bounding occipital artery pulse on one side provides some evidence of VA occlusive disease. In temporal arteritis, the superficial temporal and occipital arteries are often tender, nodular, and pulseless. Compression of these arteries in temporal arteritis often reveals firm arterial walls in contrast to the normal situation.

At times, stenosis of the origin of the ECA produces a bruit that could be confused with an ICA-origin lesion. When the lesion is in the ECA, the bruit can sometimes be traced forward toward the area of the facial artery. Also, blockage of the major ECA branches reduces or obliterates an ECA bruit but does not alter a bruit of ICA origin.[36]

Be sure to feel the femoral and pedal pulses and to inspect the fingers and toes. Claudication and peripheral vascular occlusive disease highly correlate with atherostenosis of the carotid and vertebral arteries in the neck.[9] Cyanosis, coldness, or frank gangrene of digits usually means either embolism from the heart or the aorto-iliac region blocking the distal digital arteries, or in situ thrombosis of digital arteries owing to a coagulopathy or severe occlusive peripheral vascular disease. Endocarditis is often associated with tender small nodules in the pulp of the fingers and toes.

> JH had a normal-sized heart and normal rhythm. There were no cardiac murmurs. Blood pressure was 130/70 mm Hg. All pulses were palpable, and there were no vascular bruits. The facial pulses were normal and symmetric.

The results of the cardiac and vascular examinations provided no new clues in JH. The absence of a carotid artery bruit and the presence of normal facial pulses does not exclude severe carotid artery disease in the neck but offers no positive evidence for its occurrence.

Findings from Examination of the Eyes

The eyes provide a window into the body's vascular system and can yield clues concerning stroke mechanism. Subhyaloid hemorrhages, large round hemorrhages with a fluid level, represent sudden bleeding below the retina and almost always reflect a sudden change in ICP. They are frequently seen in patients with SAH and also occur in suddenly developing large ICHs. The severity of hypertensive retinopathy and arteriosclerotic changes is important to note. In long-standing stenosis of the ICA, the reduced pressure in the ophthalmic artery tributaries may minimize hypertensive changes ipsilateral to the stenosis. The same phenomenon is well known as the Goldblatt phenomenon in experimental renal artery stenosis. The kidney arteries on the side of the ligature are spared the systemic hypertensive effects, whereas the opposite renal vessels and systemic vessels show advanced hypertension. Cholesterol emboli (Figure 3-3), small fluffy retinal infarcts, white platelet plugs,[37] and venous stasis retinopathy [38,39] all provide clues to the presence of low pressure in the ophthalmic-ICA system and are discussed in more detail in the section on ICA disease in Chapter 6. The iris is also supplied by tributaries of the ophthalmic artery and can reveal ischemic damage in patients with ICA disease.[40]

Stroke Localization

Findings from the Neurologic Examination

Clinical localization of the brain lesion is primarily from the findings on neurologic examination. It would be impossible and probably unprofitable to review here the full details of the neurologic examination. In fact, many non-neurologists feel uncomfortable when confronted with a stroke patient because they feel ill-equipped to detect neurologic signs and to explain them in anatomic detail. Actually, the neurologic findings do not have a heavy impact on the diagnosis of stroke mechanism, although the findings do help with the anatomic location of the lesion. Useful anatomic data for practical diagnosis can, in fact, be summarized rather briefly. Rather than systematically reviewing the examination, I comment here only on important, practical, useful features. A more detailed dis-

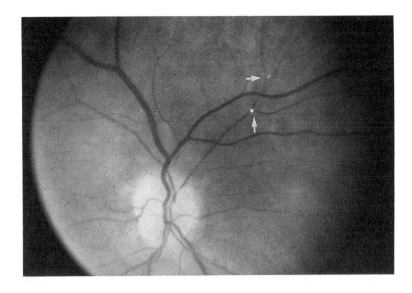

Figure 3-3. Cholesterol crystal (*vertical white arrow*) impacted in branch point of a retinal artery. Above it (*horizontal white arrow*) is smaller crystal possibly derived from more proximal one.

cussion of the neurologic examination is published elsewhere.[41]

I have been impressed that the most important and most frequently missed signs of brain dysfunction involve abnormalities of (1) higher cortical function, (2) level of alertness, (3) the visual and oculomotor systems, and (4) gait.[1,2,41] These are parts of the examination most often overlooked by non-neurologists, which provide key clues to anatomic localization.

Tests of High-Level Cortical Function

Higher cortical function testing should always include examination of language function, especially if the patient has symptoms or signs referable to the right limbs or the right visual field. A good screening test is the writing of a brief paragraph describing the stroke or TIA. Asking the patient to read a paragraph from a newspaper or a magazine is also helpful. Ask the patient to name objects in the environment and to repeat spoken language. Remember that there is a large difference between dysarthria (an abnormality of speech articulation and pronunciation) and aphasia (altered content, expression, and understanding of language). If patients are mute and do not write, it is often difficult to be sure whether they are aphasic unless they follow commands or select objects or words from choices in a clearly erroneous manner.

When symptoms or signs of dysfunction are present in the left limbs or visual field, it is especially important to test visuospatial functions and to look for neglect of the left side of space.[41,42] Ask the patient to draw a clock or a house and to copy a single two-dimensional figure. Patients with right hemispheral cortical lesions will often omit the left side of their figures and their drawings contain abnormal angles and proportions. Ask the patient to read a brief paragraph or headline or to look at a picture with the examiner. Left neglect is manifested by omitting words, phrases, or people on the left side of the page. Also notice how the patient heeds environmental stimuli to the right and left sides.

Memory can also be affected by a focal CNS lesion, usually involving the posterior cerebral artery (PCA) territories. The clinician can test memory by asking patients to recall the material contained in the paragraph they read, a picture they were shown, or what they wrote in their own paragraph description. Alternatively, patients may be asked to recall three items that they were shown or were told about. I have discussed the examination of higher cortical functions in more detail elsewhere.[1,41]

Level of Alertness

Decreased level of consciousness is an important sign of increased ICP or lesions of the brain stem reticular activating system or bilateral cerebral hemispheres.[2,43–46] Nonetheless, often there is no comment in the record regarding whether the patient was bright and alert or drowsy or delirious. Does the patient require frequent prodding to stay alert? Often, the nurses on the floor or the family who are with the patient for much of the day can better answer this question. They should always be interrogated about the patient's alertness and the appropriateness of mental performance or deviations from premorbid behavior.

Visual and Oculomotor Function

Much of the mammalian brain is concerned with visual interpretation and exploration, looking and seeing. Large lesions of the posterior hemispheres may produce only visual dysfunction and may leave speech, movement, and other sensations unscathed. Not to test the visual fields in a stroke patient is a cardinal sin, similar to failing to palpate the abdomen in a patient with unexplained shock. Test the visual fields by presenting a visual stimulus, usually a finger or pin in the peripheral portion of each visual field in each eye, and determine on confrontation when the patient sees it. Also ask the patient to look at something—a picture, a paragraph, or the scene outside the window. Is there consistent omission of objects on one side?

Probably the most common eye movement abnormality in patients with stroke is a conjugate-gaze paralysis. The eyes may be deviated to one side, usually the side of the hemispheral lesion, and both eyes fail to look toward the opposite side. This abnormality usually means a frontal or deep hemispheral lesion in the hemisphere opposite to the gaze palsy[41,47] or a lesion in the pons on the same side as the gaze palsy. Nystagmus, a rhythmic oscillation of the eyes on horizontal or vertical gaze, is usually diagnostic of a vertebrobasilar location of the stroke, as are dysconjugate palsies or paralysis of movement of one eye or one eye muscle.

Gait

Some patients with cerebellar lesions have a normal examination when recumbent or seated but cannot walk. These patients are too often discharged from the emergency room only to return later, desperately ill from cerebellar hemorrhage or infarction. Observation of gait also gives a great deal of information about motor function and its symmetry. Is there dragging of one foot, delay in hip flexion on one side, or less arm swing on one side? Are adventitious tremors or odd posturing of a limb seen as the patient walks?

Aspects of Motor Function

Having covered the usual omissions, I now turn to an evaluation of the motor system. Be sure to test each limb proximally and distally. In central lesions, the most important weakness is usually in the shoulder abductors, arm extensors, finger extensors and abductors, thigh flexors, leg flexors, and foot and toe dorsiflexors and everters. Check for drift of the outstretched hands. Try to estimate the relative motor strength in face, arms, hands, and legs. In hemiparetic patients, are any of these regions disproportionately affected or preserved? Test coordination of each limb by the finger-nose, toe-object maneuvers. Deep tendon reflexes are of little importance in central lesions during the acute stroke, but it is informative to elicit the Babinski response.

Somatosensory Functions

In patients with cerebral lesions, higher sensory functions—such as position sense, object recognition, and extinction—are more often affected than elementary pin or touch perception. A useful single screening test is (1) have the patient close the eyes; (2) touch a specific spot on the patient's fingers, hand, or foot; and then (3) direct the patient to touch precisely the same spot with the opposite hand. This test requires no equipment and is an excellent measure of point-position localization, a good reflection of higher sensory tactile function. Of course, at the same time, you are also testing fine touch because if patients cannot feel the touch, they fail the test. Also, with the patient's eyes still closed, touch both arms, both hands, and then both legs simultaneously, to see whether the patient ignores the touch consistently on one side of the body. Again, try to assess the relative sensory involvement in face, arms, hands, and legs for disproportionately severe involvement or sparing.

When you have tabulated in your mind the neurologic findings, step back from the bedside and think. Where is the lesion likely to be? If there is more than one possible or probable location, you may think of further bedside testing that could distinguish among these possibilities. Do not leave the bedside before you feel confident in your clinical localization.

Common Localization Patterns

Neuroanatomic findings can usually be placed in one of seven general categories. The process is simply one of pattern recognition—that is, matching the patient's clinical deficit with that of patients with known lesions in one of the following regions. Also, are there expected findings that are absent or unexpected added findings beyond those described among these patterns?

1. Left hemisphere lesion (in the anterior hemisphere in the territory of the ICA and its middle cerebral artery [MCA] and anterior cerebral artery [ACA] tributaries): aphasia, right limb weakness, right limb sensory loss, right visual field defect, poor right conjugate gaze, difficulty reading, writing, and calculating

2. Right hemisphere lesion (in ICA-ACA-MCA distribution): neglect of the left visual space, difficulty drawing and copying, left visual field defect, left limb motor weakness, left limb sensory loss, poor left conjugate gaze, extinction of the left stimulus of two simultaneously given visual or tactile stimuli

3. Left PCA lesion: right visual field defect, difficulty reading with retained writing ability, difficulty naming colors and objects presented visually, normal repetition of spoken language, numbness and sensory loss in the right limbs

4. Right PCA lesion: left visual field defect, often with neglect, left limb numbness and sensory loss

5. Vertebrobasilar territory infarction: spinning dizziness; diplopia; weakness or numbness of all four limbs or bilateral regions; crossed motor or sensory findings (e.g., numbness or weakness of one side of the face and the opposite side of the body); ataxia; vomiting; headache in the occiput, mastoid, or neck; bilateral blindness or dim vision; on examination, nystagmus or dysconjugate gaze, gait or limb ataxia out of proportion to weakness, bilateral recently acquired weakness or numbness (i.e., one

side not due to an old stroke or other defect), crossed signs, bilateral visual-field defects, amnesia

6. Pure motor stroke (internal capsule or basis pontis): weakness of face, arm, and leg on one side of the body, without abnormalities of higher cortical function, sensory or visual dysfunction, or reduced alertness

7. Pure sensory stroke (Thalamus): numbness or decreased sensibility of face, arm, and leg on one side of the body, without weakness, incoordination, visual or higher cortical function abnormalities

In some patients, the findings are quite limited and do not represent the full clinical syndrome. For example, the abnormality may be limited to aphasia, yet this is sufficient to place the patient in the category of left hemisphere anterior circulation disease because no other pattern includes aphasia. Similarly, nystagmus and ataxia are diagnostic of a brain stem or cerebellar process in the category of vertebrobasilar disease. In other patients, the findings are not sufficient to allow definite localization but suggest a number of possibilities. Sudden abnormalities of behavior are found in patients with caudate nucleus,[48,49] thalamic,[50,51] and frontal lobe infarction. Weakness limited to a single limb could fit into a number of these categories (numbers 1, 2, 3, 4, 5, or 6 in the preceeding list).

The neurologic findings also may help predict the stroke mechanism. An example would be a hypertensive patient with pure motor stroke on the right. This lesion is invariably due to a small lacunar infarct in the internal capsule or pons or a small hemorrhage in these areas. A patient with sudden onset of Wernicke-type fluent aphasia without accompanying weakness or motor signs has a left temporal embolus or a small posterior putaminal hemorrhage undercutting the left temporal lobe. We now return to the patient JH who had a different presentation.

> JH was very sleepy. He could not cooperate for tests of drawing or copying. He was not aware of his left limb paralysis. He did not notice visual stimuli to his left. His eyes were deviated to the right but moved fully to the left with passive head rotation. There was severe paralysis of the left face, arm, and leg, with virtually no

movement to pinch or other stimulation. He did not feel touch on his left limbs and could not reliably tell which way his fingers and toes were moved. Pin and pinch were felt as a general discomfort, which he could not localize. Deep tendon reflexes were reduced on the left, and the left plantar response was extensor.

The neurologic findings in JH clearly localize the process to the right cerebral hemisphere. The severe motor, somatosensory, and vision loss and lack of awareness of the deficit point to a large lesion involving the frontal and paracentral regions. The decreased level of alertness and the involvement of multiple systems (motor, somatosensory, visual) suggest a large zone of brain abnormality or a deep lesion involving subcortical structures and the internal capsule. Conjugate eye deviation is especially common in deep lesions.

I now review my hypotheses about stroke mechanisms and localization in JH. The site of brain dysfunction is surely the frontal and central portions of the right cerebral hemisphere. The vascular pathway supplying this region involves blood coming from the heart to the aorta to the right innominate, internal carotid, and middle cerebral arteries. Vascular examination has offered no evidence for disease at any of these locations. The ecology suggests the possibility of large artery occlusive disease, which would be statistically most commonly located at the origin of the ICA in the neck. Atherostenosis at the ICA within the siphon and within the proximal MCA are less likely but possible sites of disease.

Probable stroke mechanisms can be listed, in order of likelihood, as (1) premature atherosclerotic occlusive disease with thrombosis and distal intra-arterial embolization of clot, (2) cardiogenic embolism, and (3) ICH. The clinical findings on neurologic examination exclude the possibility of lacunar infarction. The focality of findings and absence of headache exclude SAH. ICH is possible, given the reduction in alertness and the likelihood of a large deep hemispheral lesion, but the absence of risk factors (e.g., hypertension, bleeding abnormality, anticoagulation, and drug use) and the presence of a preceding TIA argue strongly against ICH. The absence of any history of cardiac disease and the normal cardiac findings place cardiogenic embolism below thrombosis as a probable stroke

mechanism. I am now ready to test and refine these hypotheses by laboratory and imaging investigations, which are discussed in the next chapter.

Using Information from a Stroke Registry or Data Bank

Early in the discussion of clinical diagnosis, I introduced the computer so that the clinician could emulate computer logic. I now return to the computer. Suppose that data were available from detailed analyses of patients with stroke. The registry could be the clinician's own data, collected from patients seen at a single institution, or it could be data gleaned by others or pooled from many registries. I have cited information from such registries throughout this chapter.[5–19] Ideally, these registries should include information from each of the categories discussed so far (i.e., demography, risk factors, past TIAs and strokes, onset and course of the deficit, accompanying symptoms, cardiac and vascular abnormalities on examination, and localization from the clinical and imaging tests). The clinician could then search the registry data for patients with characteristics matching his or her cases. The final diagnosis in these matching cases would help the clinician to estimate more accurately the probability of particular stroke mechanisms and causative vascular lesions in his or her own patients.

I now illustrate the use of such a registry. First is a patient who is agitated and has Wernicke's aphasia as the only abnormality on neurologic examination. Tables 3-11 through 3-13 document a search on a patient with Wernicke's aphasia, using data from the HSR.[9] From among all testable patients with information about aphasia (469 patients), 54 had Wernicke's aphasia. The distribution of diagnoses in patients with and without Wernicke's aphasia is tabulated in Table 3-11. The Wernicke's aphasia group differs from patients without Wernicke's aphasia because they include more patients with emboli and ICH and fewer examples of thrombosis. However, there are significant numbers of patients showing all stroke mechanisms, so that these data only suggest probabilities. Next, I think of a way to make the groups more specifically like our patient: This patient had no motor weakness. I search the group with Wernicke's aphasia again but now stipulate the absence of

Table 3-11. Diagnosis in Patients with and without Wernicke's Aphasia

	Thrombosis	Embolism	ICH	SAH	Total
With Wernicke's aphasia	8 (15%)	35 (65%)	8 (15%)	3 (6%)	54
Without Wernicke's aphasia	222 (53%)	124 (30%)	39 (9%)	30 (7%)	415

ICH = intracerebral hemorrhage; SAH = subarachnoid hemorrhage.
Source: Reprinted with permission from J Mohr, LR Caplan, J Melski, et al. The Harvard Cooperative Stroke Registry: a prospective registry. Neurology 1978;28:754–762.

Table 3-12. Diagnosis: No Motor Weakness with and without Wernicke's Aphasia

	Thrombosis	Embolism	ICH	SAH	Total
With Wernicke's aphasia	0 (0%)	12 (75%)	3 (19%)	1 (6%)	16
Without Wernicke's aphasia	56 (58%)	24 (25%)	2 (2%)	14 (15%)	96

ICH = intracerebral hemorrhage, SAH = subarachnoid hemorrhage.
Source: Reprinted with permission from J Mohr, LR Caplan, J Melski, et al. The Harvard Cooperative Stroke Registry: a prospective registry. Neurology 1978;28:754–762.

Table 3-13. Diagnosis: No Motor Weakness and No Hypertension with and without Wernicke's Aphasia

	Thrombosis	Embolism	ICH	SAH	Total
With Wernicke's aphasia	0 (0%)	5 (100%)	0 (0%)	0 (0%)	5
Without Wernicke's aphasia	16 (41%)	15 (38%)	1 (3%)	7 (18%)	39

ICH = intracerebral hemorrhage; SAH = subarachnoid hemorrhage.
Source: Reprinted with permission from J Mohr, LR Caplan, J Melski, et al. The Harvard Cooperative Stroke Registry: a prospective registry. Neurology 1978;28:754–762.

motor weakness, so the findings might be more useful. I then look at patients with Wernicke's aphasia with no motor weakness, comparing patients who have Wernicke's aphasia but no weakness with patients who have no Wernicke's aphasia and no weakness (see Table 3-12). Now the figures are more impressive because the registry does not contain a single example of thrombosis with Wernicke's aphasia and no weakness. There are, however, a significant number of patients with ICH. From these data, the major differential diagnosis using the past experience of the HSR would be embolus versus ICH.

I now think harder and ask whether there is any other factor that could be added that would differentiate these two conditions: This patient had no history of hypertension and was not hypertensive in the hospital. Hypertension is, of course, common in ICH. If no hypertension is added to the list of search criteria (see Table 3-13), only five patients remain who have Wernicke's aphasia, no

weakness, and no hypertension, and all had cerebral embolism. Using the past experience of the HSR, this patient probably has a cerebral embolus. Of course, the odds would be much higher if the number of patients with Wernicke's aphasia, no weakness, and no hypertension were 100 rather than five, but the computer has allowed quick and precise comparison of this patient with the experience of the registry.

References

1. Caplan LR. The Effective Clinical Neurologist. Boston: Blackwell, 1990.
2. Caplan LR, Kelly JJ. Consultations in Neurology. Toronto: BC Decker, 1988.
3. Bayes T. An essay towards solving a problem in the doctrine of chances. Philos Trans R Soc Lond 1763;53:270–418. Reprinted in Biometrika 1935;45:296–315.
4. Winkler RL. Introduction to Bayesian Inference and Decision. New York: Holt, Rinehart and Winston, 1972.

5. Aring C, Merritt H. Differential diagnosis between cerebral hemorrhage and cerebral thrombosis. Arch Intern Med 1935;56:435–456.

6. Whisnant J, Fitzgibbons J, Kurland L, et al. Natural history of stroke in Rochester, Minnesota, 1945–1954. Stroke 1971;2:11–22.

7. Matsumoto N, Whisnant J, Kurland L, et al. Natural history of stroke in Rochester, Minnesota, 1955-1969. Stroke 1973;4:20–29.

8. Kannel W, Dawber T, Cohen M, et al. Vascular disease of the brain—epidemiologic aspects. Am J Public Health 1965;55:1355–1356.

9. Mohr J, Caplan LR, Melski J, et al. The Harvard Cooperative Stroke Registry: a prospective registry. Neurology 1978;28:754–762.

10. Caplan LR, Hier D, D'Cruz I. Cerebral embolism in the Michael Reese Stroke Registry. Stroke 1983;14:530–536.

11. Chambers B, Donnan G, Bladin P. Patterns of stroke: an analysis of the first 700 consecutive admissions to the Austin Hospital stroke unit. Aust N Z J Med 1983;13:57–64.

12. Gross C, Kase C, Mohr J, et al. Stroke in south Alabama: incidence and diagnostic features—population-based study. Stroke 1984;15:249–255.

13. Kunitz S, Gross C, Heymann A, et al. The Pilot Stroke Data Bank: definition, design, and data. Stroke 1984;15:740–746.

14. Bogousslavsky J, Van Melle G, Regli F. The Lausanne Stroke Registry: analysis of 1000 consecutive patients with first stroke. Stroke 1988;19:1083–1092.

15. Foulkes MA, Wolf PA, Price TR, et al. The Stroke Data Bank: design, methods, and baseline characteristics. Stroke 1988;19:547–554.

16. Friday G, Lai SM, Alter M, et al. Stroke in the Lehigh Valley: racial/ethnic difference. Neurology 1989;39:1165–1168.

17. Bamford J, Sandercock P, Dennis M, et al. A prospective study of acute cerebrovascular disease in the community: the Oxfordshire Community Stroke Project: 1981–1986. J Neurol Neurosurg Psychiatry 1990;53:16–22.

18. Yip P-K, Jeng JS, Lee T-K, et al. Subtypes of ischemic stroke in hospital-based stroke registry in Taiwan. Stroke 1997;28:2507–2512.

19. Coull BM, Brockschmidt JK, Howard G, et al. Community hospital-based stroke programs in North Carolina, Oregon and New York: IV. Stroke diagnosis and its relation to demographics, risk factors, and clinical status after stroke. Stroke 1990;21:867–873.

20. Gorelick PB, Hier DB, Caplan LR, et al. Headache in acute cerebrovascular disease. Neurology 1986;36:1445–1450.

21. Gorelick PB, Caplan LR, Hier DB, et al. Racial differences in the distribution of anterior circulation occlusive disease. Neurology 1984;34:54–59.

22. Kieffer S, Takeya Y, Resch J, et al. Racial differences in cerebrovascular disease: angiographic evaluation of Japanese and American populations. AJR Am J Roentgenol 1967;101:94–99.

23. Heyman A, Fields WS, Keating RD. Joint study of extracranial arterial occlusion: VI. Racial differences in hospitalized patients with ischemic stroke. JAMA 1972; 222:285–289.

24. Russo LS. Carotid system transient ischemic attacks, clinical, racial, and angiographic correlations. Stroke 1981;12:470–473.

25. Heyden S, Heyman A, Goree J. Nonembolic occlusion of the middle cerebral and carotid arteries: a comparison of predisposing factors. Stroke 1970;1:363–369.

26. Barnett HJM. The International Collaborative Study of Superficial Temporal Artery–Middle Cerebral Artery Anastomosis. In FC Rose (ed), Advances in Stroke Therapy. New York: Raven Press, 1982;179–182.

27. Huang CY, Chan FL, Yu YL, et al. Cerebrovascular disease in Hong Kong Chinese. Stroke 1990;21:230–235.

28. Feldmann E, Daneault N, Kwan E, et al. Chinese-white differences in the distribution of occlusive cerebrovascular disease. Neurology 1990;40:1541–1545.

29. Marler J, Price TR, Clark GL, et al. Morning increase in onset of ischemic stroke. Stroke 1989;20:473–476.

30. Sloan M, Price TR, Foukes MA, et al. Circadian rhythmicity of stroke onset: intracerebral and subarachnoid hemorrhage. Ann Neurol 1990;28:226–227.

31. Caplan, LR. Course-of-illness graphs. Hosp Pract 1985;20:125–136.

32. Baker R, Rosenbaum A, Caplan LR. Subclavian steal syndrome. Contemp Surg 1974;4:96–104.

33. Caplan LR. Vertebrobasilar Occlusive Disease. In HJM Barnett, JP Mohr, B Stein, P Yatsu (eds), Stroke: Pathophysiology, Diagnosis, and Management. New York: Churchill Livingstone, 1986;549–619.

34. Fisher CM. Facial pulses in internal carotid artery occlusion. Neurology 1970;20:476–478.

35. Caplan LR. The frontal artery sign: a bedside indicator of internal carotid occlusive disease. N Engl J Med 1973;288:1008–1009.

36. Reed C, Toole J. Clinical technique for identification of external carotid bruits. Neurology 1981;31:744–746.

37. Fisher CM. Observations of the fundus oculi in transient monocular blindness. Neurology 1959;9:333–347.

38. Kearns T, Hollenhorst R. Venous stasis retinopathy of occlusive disease of the carotid artery. Mayo Clin Proc 1963;38:304–312.

39. Carter JE. Chronic Ocular Ischemia and Carotid Vascular Disease. In EF Bernstein (ed), Amaurosis Fugax. New York: Springer, 1988;118–134.

40. Fisher CM. Dilated pupil in carotid occlusion. Trans Am Neurol Assoc 1966;91:230–231.

41. Caplan LR. The Neurological Examination in Textbook of Neurology. In M Fisher, J Bogousslavsky (eds), Boston, Butterworth–Heinemann, 1998;3–18.

42. Heir D, Mondlock J, Caplan L. Behavioral deficits after right hemisphere stroke. Neurology 1983;33:337–344.

43. Caplan LR. The Patient with Reduced Consciousness or Coma. In Skillman J (ed), Intensive Care. Boston: Little, Brown, 1975;559–567.

44. Plum F, Posner J. Diagnosis of Stupor and Coma (3rd ed). Philadelphia: Davis, 1980.

45. Young GB, Ropper AH, Bolton CFB. Coma and Impaired Consciousness: A Clinical Perspective. New York, McGraw-Hill, 1998.

46. Fisher CM. The neurologic examination of the comatose patient. Acta Neurol Scand 1969;45(Suppl 36):1–56.

47. Mohr J, Rubinstein L, Kase C, et al. Gaze palsy in hemispheral stroke: the NINCDS Stroke Data Bank. Neurology 1984;34:199.
48. Caplan LR, Schmahmann JD, Kase CS, et al. Caudate infarcts. Arch Neurol 1990;47:133–143.
49. Mendez MF, Adams NL, Skoog-Lewandowski K. Neurobehavioral changes associated with caudate lesions. Neurology 1989;39:349–354.
50. Graff-Radford NR, Eslinger PJ, Damasio AR, et al. Non-hemorrhage infarction of the thalamus: behavioral, anatomic and physiologic correlates. Neurology 1984;34:14–23.
51. Barth A, Bogousslavsky J, Caplan LR. Thalamic Infarcts and Hemorrhages. In J Bogousslavsky, LR Caplan (eds), Stroke Syndromes. Cambridge: Cambridge University Press, 1995;276–283.

Chapter 4
Laboratory Diagnosis

Having reviewed the basic elements on which diagnosis is based and the preliminary diagnostic impressions from the clinical encounter, I now turn to the laboratory. Laboratory investigations should be planned to test, confirm, and elaborate on the hypotheses of stroke mechanism and anatomic localization generated from the clinical encounter. A shotgun approach to laboratory tests is discouraged. Instead, an individualized and eclectic program of tests should be tailored to the individual patient's problems. Whenever possible, tests should be selected and interpreted sequentially. Results of the initial investigations should help determine the next step in testing.

In this chapter, I consider various tests in relation to the following series of questions, which clinicians should ask sequentially:

1. Is the brain lesion(s) caused by ischemia or hemorrhage, or is it related to a nonvascular stroke mimic?
2. Where is the lesion(s)? What is its size, shape, and extent?
3. What is the nature, site, and severity of the vascular lesion(s)?
4. Are abnormalities of blood constituents causing or contributing to brain ischemia or hemorrhage?
5. Are there abnormalities of brain function and metabolism in regions not shown to be damaged by computed tomography (CT) or magnetic resonance imaging (MRI)? Are there abnormalities of blood flow not detected by the tests of large artery vascular imaging?

With these questions in mind, I continue to follow JH, the 36-year-old patient with left hemipare-sis introduced in Chapter 3, as he proceeds through the diagnostic laboratory tests.

Question 1: Is the Brain Lesion Caused by Ischemia or Hemorrhage, or Is It Related to a Nonvascular Stroke Mimic?

Computed Tomography

In 36-year-old JH, the most likely stroke mechanism diagnoses after the clinical encounter are large artery occlusive disease and cardiogenic embolism, with infarction of the right frontal and central regions. Hemorrhage from an unusual cause and even nonstroke etiologies are much less likely but possible causes. The next step is a brain-imaging procedure that allows the clinician to distinguish among these possibilities. A CT scan in this patient (Figure 4-1) shows a large, hypodense lesion in the right cerebral hemisphere. This clearly identifies the process as ischemic. A non-vascular lesion large enough to cause a hemiplegia should be readily visible on CT. This lesion conforms well to the middle cerebral artery (MCA) territory and involves the surface and depth in a triangular configuration quite typical for infarction.

CT is readily available in most hospitals and can reliably show intracerebral hemorrhage (ICH). When the mechanism is ischemic, CT may show infarction as a low-density lesion or may initially remain normal.[1] The signs of infarction on CT scans can be quite subtle in patients who are imaged within several hours of the onset of symptoms. Loss of distinction between grey and white matter, obscuring of the basal ganglia density, loss

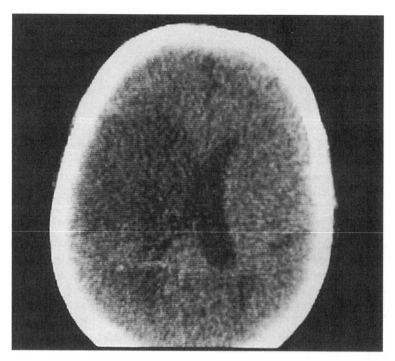

Figure 4-1. Computed tomography scan, nonenhanced: large, superficial, and deep infarct in the right middle cerebral artery territory (on left of figure). The right lateral ventricle is compressed by the swollen brain.

of definition of the insula, and slight hypodensity within the infarcted zone are often visible in patients with acute brain infarcts.[2]

Subarachnoid hemorrhage (SAH) is not as reliably diagnosed by CT, especially if the bleeding is minor or has occurred days previously. Increased density is in the cerebrospinal fluid (CSF) adjacent to bone. Visualization depends more on the hematocrit (Hct) in the CSF than on the iron content.[3] Because contrast infusions make this meningeal area bright on CT, SAH is particularly difficult to diagnose if there has not been an unenhanced scan. In those circumstances when SAH is suspected from the clinical findings of headache and restlessness, lumbar puncture (LP) may be required to confirm or exclude SAH.[4]

Magnetic Resonance Imaging

MRI is probably more sensitive than CT in detecting early ischemic changes. MRI can also accurately show ICH, especially when echo-planar and gradient-echo susceptibility–weighted images are performed.[5] MRI shows tomographic sections in multiple planes of proton distribution modified by spin-lattice (T1) and spin-spin (T2) relaxation times.[6,7] Inversion recovery pulse sequences exploit tissue T1 variations to provide contrast, while T2 information is obtained from spin-echo sequences. Infarction prolongs the T1 and T2 relaxation constants and appears as a dark, hypointense image on T1-weighted sequences and as a bright, hyperintense lesion on T2-weighted films.[6,7] Ischemia alters water content in the cells, changing their response to a magnetic field. Fluid-attenuated inversion recovery (FLAIR) images[8] and diffusion-weighted images[9,10] are especially sensitive for detection of acute brain infarcts.

The appearances of ICH are quite different from ischemia; they are complex, depend on the duration of time since the bleed, and the choice of MRI imaging technique.[11] Hemoglobin derivatives have paramagnetic effects. Imaging appearance depends on the nature of the compound, oxyhemoglobin, methemoglobin, hemosiderin, or ferritin. Its appearance is also dependent on whether the substances are present inside cells or in the interstitial extracellular spaces. During the first 12 hours after intracerebral bleeding, hematomas contain mostly oxyhemoglobin, which is not paramagnetic. The hematoma appearance during that time reflects mostly protein and water content. On T1-weighted images, the acute hematoma appears as isointense or slightly hypointense (dark), with a surrounding hypointense darker rim. T2-weighted images are often hyperin-

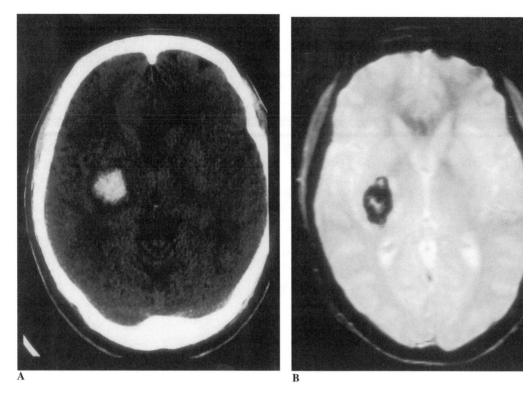

Figure 4-2. Acute intracerebral hemorrhage imaged by computed tomography and magnetic resonance imaging. **(A)** CT shows a recent putaminal hemorrhage on the left of the scan that is imaged as a well-circumscribed hyperdense lesion surrounded by a small dark rim that represents edema. **(B)** A susceptibility-weighted MRI that shows the same lesion now imaged as a black area.

tense (bright), reflecting water content. Between 12 and 48 hours after the onset of hemorrhage, deoxyhemoglobin is formed within extravascular red blood cells (RBCs), especially within the depth of the hematoma. During the next week, oxidation to methemoglobin occurs, beginning at the periphery of the lesion. By day 5 or 6, T1-weighted images show a central area of bright signal due to short T1, and a darker signal around the hematoma due to edema. On T2-weighted images, the center often becomes dark and is surrounded by bright images. Chronic bleeds contain hemosiderin within macrophages and tissues and show as bright, intense areas on T2-weighted images.[11] Table 4-1 reviews the MRI findings in patients with hematomas at various times after bleeding. Susceptibility-weighted gradient echo images are particularly sensitive to blood and calcium and have the capability of showing even hyperacute hemorrhages.[5] In summary, MRI shows hemorrhage less dramatically than CT and requires careful scrutiny of serial images using different acquisition techniques by experienced observers. The presence of mass effects and the location and shape of the lesion can help in the differentiation of hemorrhage from ischemia on MRI. One study comparing CT and MRI found that neither was superior in detecting early hemorrhages or infarcts.[12] Another study found that MRI performed 24 hours or later after symptom onset was superior compared to CT in defining the ultimate location of brain infarcts.[13] Figures 4-2 and 4-3 show hematomas imaged by CT and MRI.

Patients with SAH are not easy to study by MRI. Restless, ill patients often have difficulty holding still for the time required to produce high-quality images. The relaxation times of blood admixed with CSF approximate the signal from normal brain parenchyma, especially in T1-weighted images. T2 images often do show a bright signal. FLAIR images can often show subarachnoid hemorrhages as a bright signal adjacent to the nulled low-signal intensity CSF.

Table 4-1. Magnetic Resonance Imaging Findings in Patients with Brain Hematomas

Stage	Time	Hemoglobin Form	T1*	T2*	Hemosiderin rim (T2)*	Edema (T2)*
Hyperacute	Hours	Oxyhemoglobin	Equal or decreased	Increased	—	Increased
Acute	Days	Deoxyhemoglobin	Equal or decreased	Decreased	—	Increased
Early subacute	Weeks	Methemoglobin-intracellular	Increased	Decreased	Decreased	Increased
Late subacute	Weeks–months	Methemoglobin-extracellular	Increased	Increased	Decreased	—
Chronic	Years	Hemosiderin	Equal or decreased	Decreased	Decreased	—

T1 = spin-lattice relaxation times; T2 = spin-spin relaxation times.
*Signal intensity relative to normal brain.
Source: Modified from K Dul, BP Drayer. CT and MR Imaging of Intracerebral Hemorrhage. In CS Kase, LR Caplan (eds), Intracerebral Hemorrhage. Boston: Butterworth–Heinemann, 1994;73–93.

Computed Tomography versus Magnetic Resonance Imaging

Brain imaging has become an absolutely integral part of the evaluation of all patients with cerebrovascular disease. Stroke is such a potentially devastating disease that clinicians need all of the objective data available to prognosticate, diagnose, and treat individual stroke patients. CT and MRI are noninvasive and safe, and new-generation scanners produce an enormous amount of clinically useful information. I am not convinced at all by the economists who want to save some pennies—not at the expense of the brains of patients.

With improvement in MRI, MR has, for the most part, replaced CT in most instances. There are, however, still some advantages of CT. I believe that either a CT or an MRI scan should be performed at least once during the course of stroke in each patient.

In regard to imaging of brain lesions, CT has the following advantages:

1. At present, CT is more readily available. It is generally easier to obtain an acute CT scan in most hospitals than an urgent MRI.
2. CT is less expensive than MRI.
3. CT imaging and its interpretation is much less dependent than MRI on selection of technique and filming planes. More experience with CT interpretation makes these scans easier to read by most clinicians who are not neuroradiologists.
4. CT scans of ICH are easier to interpret than MRI scans and, in most circumstances, yield adequate data for clinical decision making without the need for MRI scanning.
5. CT images subarachnoid blood as well as MRI, and the shorter scanning time of CT is important in restless patients whom you do not want to heavily sedate.

CT has the following disadvantages:

1. CT is not as sensitive as MRI in detecting and imaging acute infarcts.
2. CT is not accurate in delineating lesions adjacent to bony surfaces (e.g., in the orbital, frontal, and temporal lobes). CT is quite inferior to MRI in imaging brain stem and cerebellar infarcts and hemorrhages.
3. CT is mostly a one-plane technique for routine examinations; multiple planes require longer imaging time for reconstruction. MR, by using multiple planes (horizontal, transaxial, coronal, sagittal) shows the three-dimensional location of lesions far better than CT reconstructions.
4. CT is not as useful in detecting and delineating spinal cord strokes.

Figure 4-3. Computed tomography scan shows a hypertensive intracerebral hemorrhage on the left of the scan. The white center is surrounded by a large rim of edema.

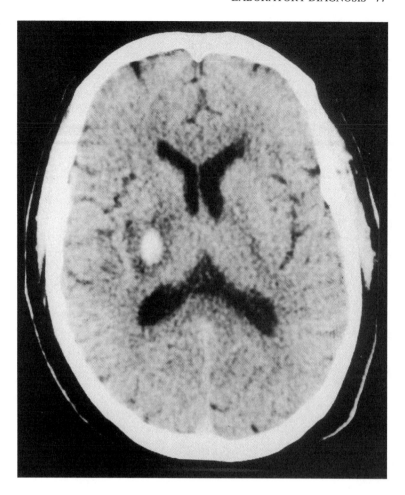

CT and MRI results depend on the time of the scan in relation to the clinical event. In patients with ischemia, early CT scans are often normal or contain only subtle abnormalities. Contrast enhancement, in my experience, has not been helpful. During the first days after stroke onset, infarcts are usually round or oval and have poorly defined margins. Later, infarcts become more hypodense and dark, and are more wedge-like and circumscribed. Some infarcts that had been hypodense become isodense during the second and third weeks after stroke onset.[14] This so-called fogging effect may obscure the lesion for some time.[1,14] Later, infarcts become hypodense again. Edema also begins to develop within the first days in patients with large infarcts. Edema is manifested by low density surrounding the lesion and mass effect with displacement of adjacent structures.

FLAIR and diffusion-weighted MRI images show infarcts as bright signals even during the first hours after symptom onset. T1-weighted MRI images performed during the first day show infarcts as a loss of gray-white contrast and decreased image intensity (darkness). T2-weighted sequences show hyperintensive bright foci of ischemia. During the next days, lesions become darker on T1-weighted and brighter on T2-weighted images. Increased signal on T2-weighted images may be evident years after the stroke.

Despite the fact that a patient clinically has had a transient ischemic attack (TIA) and has no residual symptoms or signs at the time of scanning, imaging often shows a brain infarct. Nicolaides and colleagues studied 149 patients with hemispheral TIAs and found that 48% had an infarct on CT, most often in the symptomatic hemisphere.[15] MRI is clearly more sensitive than CT in detecting infarcts in patients with TIAs.[16] Among three studies that included brain-imaging results in 103 patients with TIAs, 27% had infarcts on CT scans whereas 73% had infarcts on MRI.[16]

Immediately after the onset of bleeding, intracerebral hematomas are seen on CT as well-circumscribed areas of high density with smooth borders. Sequential scans in some patients have shown continued bleeding with enlargement of the hematomas in later scans. In one study, substantial growth in the volume of hematomas occurred in 26% of patients between the admission CT scan and a scan performed an hour later.[17] Another 12% of patients showed enlargement of hematoma between CT scans taken 1 hour and 20 hours after admission.[17] Occasionally, a blood-fluid level is seen within acute hematomas. Edema develops within the first days and is seen as a dark rim around the white hematoma. As absorption of blood proceeds, the white image becomes more irregular and hypodense, and edema subsides. Ring enhancement of the outer dark zone may occur and may remain evident for weeks after the bleeding. In patients with low Hcts, or those scanned initially weeks after stroke onset, hematomas can appear as solely hypodense lesions. I have discussed the evolution of hematomas on MRI in the section on differentiation of hemorrhage from infarction.

In JH, the CT had shown the lesion quite well and had indicated without a doubt that the lesion was ischemic. I saw no reason to order MRI.

Lumbar Puncture

LP, introduced into clinical medicine by Quincke in 1891, is still an important diagnostic test. LP is especially important in the diagnosis and management of patients with SAH. As has been emphasized, CT and MRI are not sensitive tests for the detection of SAH, especially if bleeding is minor in degree and occurred days before scanning. The accuracy of CT in documenting subarachnoid blood diminishes after 24 hours.[18] Large SAHs are often preceded by small warning leaks that are easily overlooked by CT but readily diagnosed by LP. By definition, subarachnoid blood rapidly disseminates and is present in the lumbar theca within minutes. The absence of blood on LP excludes the diagnosis of SAH. When blood

is present, the quantity of blood and the pressure of CSF can also be measured and followed by later spinal taps. Counting the number of erythrocytes in the first and third or fourth tubes of CSF, measurement of the CSF Hct, and spectrophotometric analysis of the CSF give an accurate quantitative database. When RBCs lyse, oxyhemoglobin is released into the CSF, reaches a maximum level in approximately 36 hours, and gradually disappears between days 7 and 10.[3,19] Bilirubin is first detectable approximately 10 hours after SAH, reaches a maximum at 48 hours, and persists for approximately 2–4 weeks after large hemorrhages.[3,19] Oxyhemoglobin and methemoglobin are detected at maximal light-absorption peaks at 415 μ on spectrophotometry. The bilirubin peak is approximately 460 μ.[3,20] Sequential LPs with measurement of CSF pressure, quantity of blood, and relative quantities of oxyhemoglobin and bilirubin help to determine the time since the last bleeding and can show evidence of fresh bleeding.

The CSF findings can also help differentiate ICH from ischemia. LPs in most patients with ICH show blood-tinged or xanthochromatic fluid under increased pressure, with an increased number of polymorphonuclear leukocytes, and an increased protein content.[3,19–23] Using spectrophotometric analysis, oxyhemoglobin and bilirubin can also be detected in higher-than-normal amounts. Some deep hemorrhages do not communicate with the CSF, however, and LP in these patients can remain normal. CT and MRI are much better diagnostic tests than LP in separating brain infarction from hemorrhage. However, LP is quite helpful in patients with brain infarcts and hemorrhages related to various infectious and neoplastic diseases.[23]

Question 2: What Is the Nature, Location, and Morphology of the Brain Lesion?

The next important questions the clinician must ask concern the characteristics of the brain lesion found. Where is the lesion? How large is it? What is its extent? What is the effect of the lesion on intracranial structures? Do the location and characteristics of this lesion correlate well with the clinical findings and explain the patient's symptoms and signs? Are there other lesions, and if so, do they have similar or different characteristics from the symptomatic lesion?

Having differentiated ischemia from hemorrhage, the clinician needs to know more about the lesion to predict the most likely stroke mechanism, localize the underlying vessels involved, prognosticate the probable future course, and select optimal treatment. The laboratory answers to the delineation of the morphology of the brain process usually come from neuroimaging with CT or MRI or both. FLAIR and diffusion-weighted MRI scans[24] are especially helpful when patients are tested soon after stroke onset. Tests of brain function, metabolism, and blood flow such as positron emission tomography (PET), single-photon emission CT (SPECT), xenon-enhanced CT (XeCT), electroencephalogram (EEG), and quantitative neurophysiology can be helpful in localization of the fundamental abnormality in the brain in some patients in whom the results of standard CT and MRI scans are normal or equivocal. Most of these tests will probably be superseded by the newer MRI capabilities when diffusion-weighted and perfusion MRI become widely available. Clinicians are fortunate to have available clinical data from the neurologic examination before neuroimaging. Having already made hypotheses about lesion localization, clinicians can match these hypotheses with the imaging results. Does the location of the lesion(s) on CT or MRI explain the clinical signs? Could the lesion(s) be an asymptomatic, incidental finding not related to the recent event? Are the clinical signs more severe than would be expected from the imaging studies? A discrepancy might indicate that some tissue, although not morphologically damaged enough to show on scans, is not functioning normally.

What if the Lesion Is an Infarct?

Brain ischemia occurs in 80% of stroke patients. In these patients, CT or MRI do not show a hematoma. Hemorrhagic stippling (hemorrhagic infarction) may be present. Lumbar puncture does not show the findings of SAH. Analysis of the neuroimaging findings should allow useful information about the lesion location and morphology.

What Vascular Territory Is Involved?

Identification of the vessels supplying an area of symptomatic infarction is the first step toward identifying the causative vascular lesion. Ultrasound and vascular imaging tests can then be planned to show the vessels involved. Once a plumber has pinpointed a blocked sink, the plumber can examine the water tank, the pump, and the pipes that lead to that blocked region, knowing that mischief must be located within the water delivery system. In 36-year-old JH with left hemiparesis, CT has shown an infarct that involves the deep and superficial territory of the right MCA. Infarction is present above and below the sylvian fissure. The responsible vascular lesion must involve the vascular tree proximal to the origin of the lenticulostriate arteries, which supply the deep territory that is infarcted. These vessels branch from the main stem of the MCA. The vascular process probably involves the proximal right MCA. Possibilities from viewing only the imaging data include (1) in situ occlusive disease of the MCA; (2) cardiogenic embolism to the MCA; (3) an intra-arterial embolus from the aorta, right common carotid artery, or internal carotid artery (ICA); and (4) propagation of clot or embolism from the ICA in the siphon.

Suppose that the infarct had involved the paramedian frontal lobe cortex in the supply region of the anterior cerebral artery (ACA), in addition to the MCA territory. Clearly, the vascular process would then have had to originate proximal to the ICA intracranial bifurcation into the ACA and MCA. Similarly, within the posterior circulation, the location of infarction yields important clues to the location of the vascular process. In a patient with quadriparesis, MRI shows an infarct in the paramedian basis pontis bilaterally. Careful scrutiny of the films also shows a small infarct in the right cerebellum in the territory of the anterior inferior cerebellar artery, which originates from the lower to midportion of the basilar artery. The lesion must involve the basilar artery proximal to the anterior inferior cerebellar artery branches. The vascular process could be an in situ occlusive lesion within the basilar artery or an embolus to this region arising from the heart, the aorta, the innominate or subclavian arteries, or the cervical or intracranial portion of one of the vertebral arteries. If the cerebellar lesion had involved the posterior inferior cerebellar artery territory, the clinician would know that the vascular lesion must have affected the intracranial vertebral artery from which the posterior inferior cerebellar artery branches. A knowledge of vascular distribution and supply is essential to localizing the vascular abnormality. Chapter 2 includes diagrams and descriptions of the vascular territories and examples of anterior circulation infarct distributions (see Figures 2-6 through 2-9, 2-17, and 2-18).

How Large Is the Infarct?

The size of the lesion is helpful in prognosis. Although the severity of the clinical deficit is not directly proportional to infarct size, larger lesions in the same anatomic area cause more severe deficits than small lesions in the same location. The infarct size, as shown on CT or MRI, should be matched in the clinician's mind with the size of the vascular territory involved. The noninfarcted tissue (entire vascular territory minus the infarct) represents the tissue at risk for further ischemia. To determine the at-risk tissue, the vascular lesion must be known. For example, a small infarct in the territorial supply of a lenticulostriate branch might represent the entire supply of that small penetrating branch. If the vascular lesion were in the MCA proximal to that lenticulostriate branch, a large area of brain tissue would still be at risk for spread of the ischemic damage. Diffusion-weighted and perfusion MRI studies can give more direct information about the brain tissue at risk for infarction by a given vascular lesion. When the perfusion defect is larger than the diffusion-weighted zone of infarction, the remainder of the brain showing the perfusion deficit is at imminent risk if blood flow to that zone is not improved. Large lesions often exert mass effect and displace normal intracranial contents, especially if edema develops. Large lesions are also more often accompanied by a reduced level of alertness. Mass effect and stupor often dictate treatment strategies aimed at these problems. Large infarcts also represent a relative contraindication for anticoagulant treatment because brain hemorrhages develop much more often in large infarcts than in small ones.

Does the Location and Extent of the Infarct Correlate with the Clinical Findings? Are Other Ischemic Lesions Present?

Clinicians should decide if the lesion found is appropriate to the patient's clinical symptoms and signs. In JH, the right cerebral hemisphere lesion explains quite well his left hemiplegia. A lesion in the left cerebral hemisphere or cerebellum would not have correlated with the clinical findings. In the case of JH, the clinicians could be quite confident that the symptomatic lesion was identified. In some other patients—especially those with TIAs or minor clinical symptoms and signs, and those patients with minor or equivocal brain-imaging findings—it may be more difficult to determine if a brain-imaging lesion relates to the clinical findings. It is also useful to match the extent of the infarct with the severity of the neurologic deficit. When the clinical findings outweigh the brain-imaging lesion, there may be considerable brain tissue that is not functioning normally but is not yet infarcted. This "stunned" brain often retains the ability to return to normal when reperfused.

Many patients have brain infarcts that do not relate to their symptoms. These so-called silent infarcts are common[15,16]; in these patients, clinical manifestations were absent, minor, or forgotten. The presence of silent and symptomatic infarcts can yield clues as to the mechanism of the present symptomatic infarction. Guilt by association—identification by the company it keeps—is an important, but by no means an infallible, strategy. For example, suppose that a patient is admitted with a pure motor hemiparesis involving his left limbs. CT and MRI do not show a lesion involving the right descending corticospinal system, but five small lacunes in other regions are noted. The likelihood is high that the symptomatic vascular process is also lacunar infarction. Data from the Lausanne Stroke Registry indicate that 62% of recurrent strokes have the same stroke mechanism as the first stroke.[25] If CT shows multiple scattered cortical infarcts in different vascular territories, then cardiogenic embolism, multiple large artery occlusive disease, and a hypercoagulable state are the most likely stroke mechanisms.

Are Edema or Mass Effect Present?

Edema can develop around infarcts and may even be potentiated by reperfusion of a blocked artery.[26] Sometimes the zone of actual infarction is quite small, but the surrounding edema zone is large. In young patients, edema may be more threatening than in geriatric patients in whom brain atrophy might allow room for brain expansion. Displacement of midline structures,[27,28] effacement of gyri, encroachment on cisternal spaces, and brain stem displacement can often be judged well on diagnostic-quality CT and MRI scans.

What Is the Age of the Infarct?

There are some general rules for identifying the age of an ischemic lesion. In the beginning of this chapter, I noted some sequential changes that occur in brain infarcts, and these sequential changes are discussed in more detail elsewhere.[1,6,7,29] On CT, well-defined borders, severe hypodensity, and shrinkage of the infarcted brain region all suggest a chronic infarct that is months old. Poor definition from the surrounding brain, edema, mass effect, and contrast enhancement all suggest an acute process. In practice, however, these rules are not often as helpful as clinicians would like them to be. Diffusion-weighted images usually only show bright signal in infarcts that are less than 1 week old.

Usually, the history gives the clinician a relatively accurate time of reference. Surprisingly, some acute lesions quickly become well delineated and defined and appear to be older than they actually are. Also, lesions that are months old are not appreciably different by imaging than those that are years old.

What if the Imaging Lesion Represents an Intracerebral Hemorrhage?

The presence of a brain hematoma prompts quite different queries.

Does the Location Provide a Clue as to Etiology of the Hemorrhage?

In Chapter 2, I indicated the usual loci of hypertensive brain hemorrhages. These are usually deep and are most often located in the lateral ganglionic region, subcortex, thalamus, caudate nucleus, pons, and cerebellum. In a hypertensive patient with a hematoma confined to one of these regions, the likelihood of an etiology other than hypertension is quite low. Angiography in patients with hypertension and deep hematomas has a low yield for showing aneurysms, arteriovenous malformations (AVMs), or other vascular lesions.[30] Hematomas resulting from aneurysms, so-called meningocerebral bleeds, are invariably contiguous to the aneurysms at the brain base or surface. In amyloid angiopathy, hemorrhages are lobar, often multiple, and can be accompanied by small infarcts.[31,32] Anticoagulant-related ICHs are most often lobar or cerebellar, evolve gradually, and enlarge.[33,34] AVMs may be located anywhere in the brain, especially in subependymal locations. Calcifications and heterogeneity within the hematoma raise suspicion of an underlying AVM.

How Large Is the Hematoma?

Is there mass effect? By definition, a hematoma represents an extra volume of material in the cranium. Mass effect is more common and more serious in hematomas than in brain infarction. Large size correlates with poor outcome in hematomas at any location. Both mass effect and displacement of adjacent structures are readily analyzed on CT and MRI images.[27,28]

Does the Hematoma Drain Into the Cerebrospinal Fluid Pathways?

Is the hemorrhage causing hydrocephalus? Hematomas decompress themselves by draining into the CSF on the surface of the brain and into the ventricular system. In the past, ventricular drainage was considered an ominous sign, but now it is recognized that ventricular drainage is not always bad. The alternative to drainage is an increase in the mass of blood within the brain parenchyma. Nature might have already accomplished decompression of the lesion—a goal that the surgeon hopes to gain by operative drainage.

The mass effect produced by the hematoma and blood within the ventricular system can obstruct the flow of CSF. Blockage of the ventricular system is most common at the foramen of Munro (putaminal bleeds) and at the level of the third (thalamic hemorrhage) and fourth ventricle (cerebellar hemorrhage). Dilatation of the ventricular system (hydrocephalus) augments the mass effect of the hematoma and is often amenable to surgical decompression by temporary drainage or permanent shunting of CSF fluid.

What if Imaging Studies Show Subarachnoid Hemorrhage?

Location of Blood

What is the location of the blood? Blood may accumulate around a bleeding aneurysm or in the adjacent subarachnoid spaces and cisterns, thus yielding a clue as to the site of bleeding. Blood in the suprasellar cisterns and frontal interhemispheric fissure predicts an anterior communicating artery aneurysm.[35,36] Blood localized predominantly in one sylvian fissure suggests an MCA bifurcation aneurysm on that side.[35,36] Thick blood in the pontine and cerebellopontine angle cisterns predicts a posterior fossa aneurysm. Since the early 1980s, Van Gijn and colleagues have identified a pattern of perimesencephalic hemorrhage that does not seem to reflect aneurysmal rupture and has a benign prognosis.[37–39]

How much bleeding has occurred generally or locally? The thickness of blood on CT or MRI correlates roughly with the degree of bleeding. Large subarachnoid bleeds are more often complicated by hydrocephalus and delayed cerebral infarction owing to vasoconstriction than are smaller leaks. Vertical layers of blood clot more than 1 mm thick, or local clots larger than 5 × 3 mm are often associated with angiographically documented vasoconstriction.[40,41] Repeated LPs, washing away of the blood at the time of aneurysm surgery, and installation of thrombolytic agents such as recombinant tissue plasminogen activator (rt-PA), are strategies that have been used to deal with large subarachnoid bleeds.

Are There Regions of Infarction?

SAH is often complicated by vasoconstriction and delayed ischemic damage. Infarction is most often localized to the territory supplied by the artery harboring the aneurysm but can be located elsewhere. The presence of acute ischemia clearly suggests that vasoconstriction is present. Vasoconstriction can also produce a pattern of generalized brain ischemia without focal infarction.

Is Hydrocephalus Present?

Blood within the subarachnoid space can diminish the absorptive capability of the arachnoid granulations. Communicating hydrocephalus develops because CSF production exceeds absorption. This complication can be managed by repeated LPs to remove CSF or by temporary or permanent CSF drainage or shunting.

What if Computed Tomography and Magnetic Resonance Are Negative?

Normal neuroimaging is common in patients with transient ischemia and early after ischemia develops.

FLAIR and diffusion-weighted MRI scans are often helpful in those patients who later show infarcts on T2-weighted MRI scans.[8–10,24] In those patients who have only transient ischemia, or persistent ischemia without infarction, the clinical symptoms and signs provide some clues as to localization. EEG, quantitative EEG mapping, PET, SPECT, and XeCT also help generally to localize the lesion, but they give information about brain electrical and metabolic function and blood flow rather than morphology.

Question 3: What Is the Nature, Site, and Severity of the Vascular Lesion(s)?

Having localized and quantified the process in the brain, the clinician is now ready to turn to the identification of the vascular lesion(s). The clinical findings and brain neuroimaging results have usually narrowed down the vascular region of interest in the individual stroke patient. In patient JH, it is known that the vascular process must be within the right carotid artery system or lie more proximally in the heart, aorta, or innominate artery.

What if the Stroke Mechanism Is Ischemia?

Ultrasound

Although Christian Doppler discovered the principal idea that underlies ultrasound in 1842, the first clinically applicable devices used to study blood flow were not introduced until the early 1960s. During the 1970s, amplitude modulation and brightness modulation (B-mode) pulse echo ultrasound were introduced into clinical examinations of the extracranial arteries to detect atherosclerotic changes. The duplex scanner that produced a B-mode image of the extracranial artery being insonated, combined with a pulsed Doppler spectrum analysis, was first introduced in 1979. During the 1980s, Duplex scanning became widely used in clinics throughout the world as a means of detecting and quantifying disease of the carotid arteries. Since the early 1980s, major advances in computer technology and electronics have made ultrasound an important tool for identifying occlusive vascular lesions within the neck and basal intracranial cerebral arteries. Ultrasound energy is used to detect interfaces among structures of different densities

Figure 4-4. B-mode ultrasound of carotid artery bifurcation region. On the left is a small plaque near the origin of the internal carotid artery (ICA). (CCA = common carotid artery; ECA = external carotid artery.)

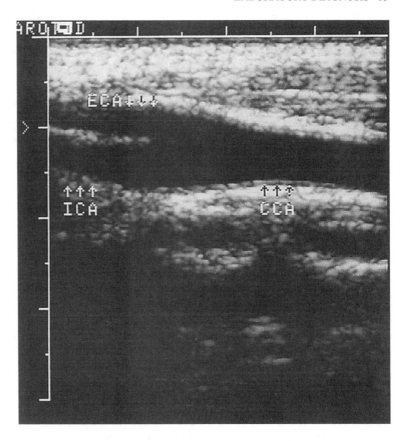

and to detect moving targets such as RBCs. The ultrasonic information is received through a probe or transducer held over the artery being studied, and the information is converted into electrical energy, either for developing an image or for generating Doppler curves of blood-flow velocity.

B-Mode Imaging

High-resolution B-mode ultrasound scanning of the neck provides images in several planes of the neck arteries. Figure 4-4 shows a B-mode image of the carotid bifurcation in the neck, showing a plaque. Advances in technology can show these lesions in different planes (Figures 4-5 and 4-6) and allow three-dimensional reconstruction of the arterial lesions (Figure 4-7). B-mode scanning is quite accurate at the carotid bifurcation in the neck and at the origin of the vertebral artery (VA) from the subclavian artery. Lesions higher in the neck and more proximally located are technically harder to image well. Figure 4-8 is a B-mode picture of a normal subclavian and proximal vertebral artery.

Figure 4-9 shows a B-mode image of an occluded vertebral artery.

B-mode is quite accurate for assessment of the degree of luminal narrowing, in the identification of ulcerations and intraplaque hemorrhages, and for delineating the gross surface-wall characteristics of the carotid arteries. When compared with angiography and pathologic study of the arteries at endarterectomy, B-mode generally has good sensitivity and specificity (80%) for detection of significant occlusive lesions.[42,43] Figure 4-10 is a composite B-mode ultrasound image that shows the great potential of the technique for imaging all of the major proximal cervical arteries. However, B-mode performed by itself has limitations.[44] The large size of the ultrasound probe and sharp angulation of the vessels sometimes prevent adequate display of the vessels, especially at the VA origin. Calcifications and clots are not imaged.

Often the sonographer can distinguish soft, irregular, ulcerated plaques from firm, fibrous, or calcified plaques. Echolucent plaques are usually rich in cholesterol[45] and are susceptible to reduction in size

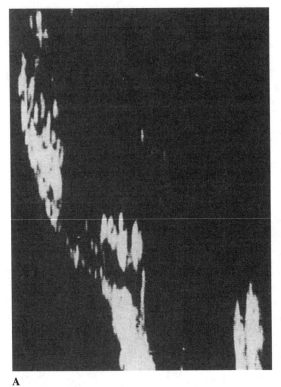
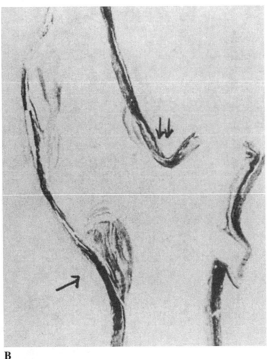

A   B

Figure 4-5. (A) B-mode view of the carotid artery. **(B)** Picture of the stained carotid artery specimen: The two arrows point to the flow divider between the internal carotid artery on the left and the external carotid artery on the right. The single arrow points to a plaque in the characteristic location along the posterior wall of the internal carotid artery opposite the flow divider. (Reprinted with permission from M Hennerici, W Steinke. Durchblutungsstorungen des Gehirns—neue diagnostische Moglichkeiten. Gütersloh: Verlag Bertelsmann Stiftung, 1987.)

as well as progression. Calcified, hard echodense plaques in contrast usually do not change much with time.[45] Echolucent plaques with an irregular surface are more likely than echogenic plaques to progress and cause brain infarction.[46]

Thrombi within the arterial lumen can usually be detected using a combination of the Doppler flow spectra and B-mode ultrasound images. B-mode is quite accurate at separating normal arteries and those with minor plaques from those arteries with severe stenosing lesions (>70% narrowed). More difficult is the separation of arteries with severe pre-occlusive stenosis from those in whom the artery is occluded. Analysis of B-mode images

Figure 4-6. Transverse sections through various types of plaques. The plaque on the upper right has had an intramural hemorrhage. (Reprinted with permission from M Hennerici, W Steinke. Durchblutungsstorungen des Gehirns— neue diagnostische Moglichkeiten. Gütersloh: Verlag Bertelsmann Stiftung, 1987.)

also requires experience and familiarity with the vascular anatomy. Arteries can be misidentified, especially from analyzing only one view. Experience has shown that B-mode imaging is enhanced by the addition of multigated, pulsed-Doppler apparatus. The combined B-mode and Doppler diagnostic systems are called *duplex systems*. The pulsed-Doppler in this duplex system helps identify the arteries and orientation of B-mode images. The analysis of flow-velocity patterns by Doppler, recorded from different positions within the arterial lumen, provides qualitative and quantitative information about hemodynamic changes. The B-mode images help show the location of the velocity changes. The duplex system offers advantages over either B-mode scanning or Doppler analysis alone. Figure 4-11 shows a duplex scan of a normal VA.

Doppler Sonography Systems

Continuous Wave and Pulsed-Doppler Systems. There are two main Doppler systems: Continuous wave Doppler measures an average velocity for blood moving through an artery or vein beneath the probe; pulsed-Doppler is range gated to measure the velocity of blood in small volumes at specific selected sites within the vessel lumen. The continuous wave Doppler device can readily determine

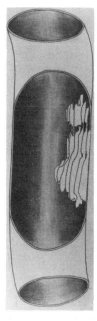

Figure 4-7. Three-dimensional reconstruction of a plaque. (Reprinted with permission from M Hennerici, W Steinke. Durchblutungsstorungen des Gehirns—neue diagnostische Moglichkeiten. Gütersloh: Verlag Bertelsmann Stiftung, 1987.)

mean-flow velocities of the periorbital arteries, the carotid arteries in the neck, and the VAs at their origins and at the cervical region near the skull base (C_1–C_2). Moving the Doppler probe along the

Figure 4-8. B-mode ultrasound figure that shows the subclavian artery on the right and the origin and proximal portion of the right vertebral artery that courses from right to left on the figure.

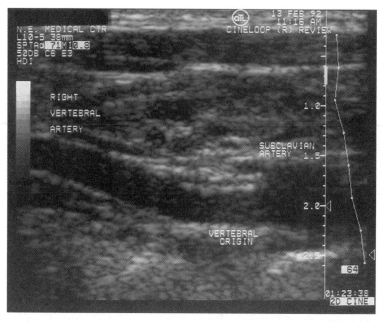

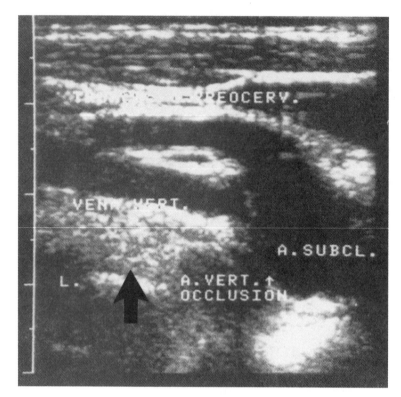

Figure 4-9. B-mode ultrasound with the same orientation as Figure 4-8. The left vertebral artery is occluded. The vascular structures above the occluded artery are the vertebral vein and the thyrocervical artery. (Reprinted with permission from LR Caplan. Posterior Circulation Disease: Clinical Findings, Diagnosis, and Management. Boston: Blackwell, 1996.)

course of the carotid and vertebral arteries allows identification of the bifurcation of the carotid arteries and major changes in audible blood-flow signals. Doppler curves can be analyzed using fast Fourier transform spectral analysis to detect peak frequencies and broadening of the spectrum.[47]

Figures 4-11 and 4-12 include various Doppler curves. The severity of stenosis is estimated by the

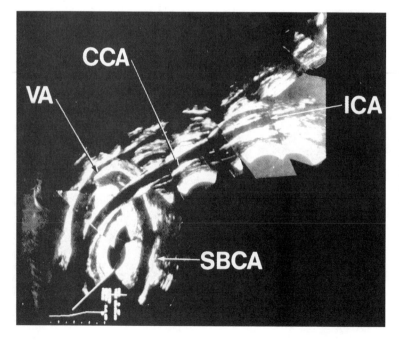

Figure 4-10. Composite B-mode ultrasound image shows the innominate artery and its subclavian, carotid, and vertebral artery branches in the neck. (Courtesy of Drs. Burt Eikelboom and Rob Ackerstaff.) (CCA = common carotid artery; ICA = internal carotid artery; SBCA = subclavian artery; VA = vertebral artery.) (Reprinted with permission from LR Caplan. Posterior Circulation Disease: Clinical Findings, Diagnosis, and Management. Boston: Blackwell, 1996.)

Figure 4-11. Duplex scan of a normal vertebral artery (VA): Top panel shows a brightness modulation of the VA (white lines mark the lumen). Bottom panel shows the Doppler spectrum from this artery.

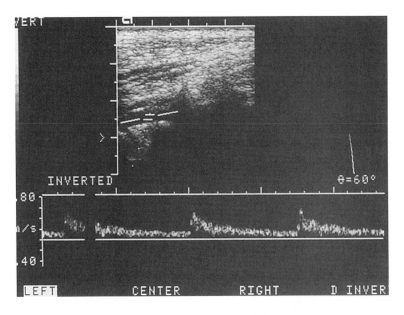

increase in peak systolic frequency, the presence and severity of poststenotic turbulence, and an increase in diastolic blood-flow velocity.[47] Most readers are familiar with the task of washing off a pavement by using a hose. Turning the adjustable end of the hose changes the diameter of the lumen of the nozzle. When the nozzle is tightened, the jet stream of the water is under higher velocity and is more effective in washing the surface. If the nozzle is tightened too much, however, the stream dribbles out or stops altogether. Similarly, in regions of luminal narrowing, blood velocity increases in an inverse proportion to the size of the lumen until a critical reduction in lumen size severely limits flow.

In patients with suspected occlusive disease of the subclavian and innominate arteries, a variety of noninvasive tests can measure blood flow in the arm. The relative velocity of pulsed-wave propagation in the two arms then can be compared. Forearm blood flow can also be studied by oscillography and venous occlusive plethysmography.

Color Doppler Flow Imaging and Power Doppler. Color Doppler flow imaging (CDFI) represents an advance in technology. In this technique, the spatial and temporal distribution of color-coded Doppler signals are visualized in real time and displayed as color images superimposed on gray-scale images of the surrounding tissues.[48] This technique is especially good for showing changes in blood-flow patterns near small plaques. This technique has an extremely high sensitivity and accuracy for detecting minor, moderate, and severe degrees of carotid artery stenosis.[48–51] CDFI improves evaluation of the extent of carotid artery plaques by the simultaneous two-dimensional display of tissue structure and flow-velocity profile. Real-time images are easier to see and interpret than are curves of velocity. The technology also helps differentiate smooth from irregular surfaces and from ulcerative niches.[49] Severe stenosis cannot always be differentiated from complete occlusion by CDFI.[49] This technique shows great promise for showing VA lesions in the neck.

Power Doppler is a system based on the display of the integrated power of the Doppler signal obtained from an insonated artery.[52,53] This technique is able to remove some of the artefacts and improve some limitations of CDFI. The color display on power Doppler imaging is independent of the angle of insonation. The intravascular surface is better shown using power Doppler. Calcification within plaques can also be visualized with this sytem. Power Doppler improves the assessment of the severity of carotid artery stenosis and plaque morphology compared with CDFI.[52]

Transcranial Doppler Ultrasound. One of the major advances in the field of analysis of vascular lesions has been the introduction of the transcranial Doppler (TCD) system, which permits study of the

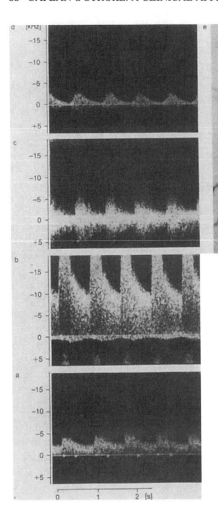

Figure 4-12. Doppler spectra taken from various sites from patient with the arteriogram shown on the right. At **a**, the maximal systolic frequency is reduced to 5 kHz; at **b**, there is increased velocity at the region of stenosis to a maximum of 20 kHz, with an endiastolic velocity of 10 kHz; **c** and **d** show velocities within the distal artery. The spectra are broadened and show decreased antegrade velocities. (Reprinted with permission from G von Reutern, HJ Budingen. Ultraschalldiagnostik der hirnversorgenden Arterien. Stuttgart: Georg Thieme Verlag, 1989.)

intracranial arteries. Extracranial ultrasound examinations use pulse frequencies ranging from 3 to 10 MHz. These ultrasound frequencies cannot penetrate bone sufficiently to reflect signals from the intracranial arteries.[47,54–56] Aaslid and colleagues showed that signals could be obtained from the MCA and ACA, using a 2-MHz probe directed intracranially from the temporal bone just above the zygomatic arch.[54] Now, three separate windows are used for probe placement, taking advantage of natural skull foramina or soft-tissue regions.[47,54–56] The temporal window is used for insonating the MCA and its major branches, the proximal ACA, and the ICA bifurcation as well as the posterior cerebral arteries. A transorbital probe is placed near the eye and is used for studying blood velocities in the ICA siphon and ophthalmic arteries. A suboccipital win-

dow through the foramen magnum allows recording of frequencies from the intracranial VAs and the proximal portion of the basilar artery.[47,54–56] Figure 4-13 shows these ultrasonic windows.

Early studies using TCD confirmed normal values and techniques and showed that the technology was useful in detecting severe stenosis or occlusion of basal cerebral arteries.[54–59] A microprocessor-controlled directional pulsed-wave adjustable probe is placed at one of the windows and moved until maximal signals are obtained; velocities are then recorded at different depths along the arteries. The introduction of three-dimensional display vascular maps helps orient the insonation to the location of the artery being studied. Specially designed helmets and headbands can be used to hold the probes in place, facilitating monitoring of arteries over time. These

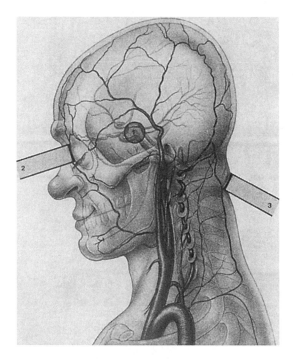

Figure 4-13. Diagram shows locations for transcranial Doppler probes: (1) temporal window, (2) orbital window, (3) suboccipital foramen magnum window. (Reprinted with permission from G von Reutern, HJ Budingen. Ultraschall-diagnostik der hirnversorgenden Arterien. Stuttgart: Georg Thieme Verlag, 1989.)

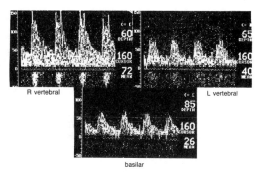

Figure 4-14. Transcranial Doppler spectra: The velocities in the right intracranial vertebral artery (VA) are much higher than in the left VA and the basilar artery. Arteriography showed a region of severe stenosis in the intracranial right VA.

improvements allowed the introduction of Duplex scanning of intracranial arteries. Power Doppler technology has also been applied to transcranial Duplex scanning.[53] B-mode images of the intracranial arteries can be produced and color coded scans can be obtained from intracranial arteries during transcranial sonography.[48] Solutions that contain microbubbles can be injected intravenously to obtain contrast-enhancement of the transcranial ultrasound signals. Contrast-enhancement improves the diagnostic capability of the transcranial ultrasound scans.[60–62] Interpretation of the results of TCD depends on integrating information from extracranial and intracranial ultrasound and from study of all of the major intracranial arteries at various depths.

TCD has revolutionized the study of stroke patients at the bedside. TCD can accurately detect important atherostenotic lesions within the major basal cerebral arteries—the intracranial ICAs, MCAs, intracranial vertebral arteries, and the proximal and middle portions of the basilar artery. TCD is also helpful in showing the hemodynamic effects of extracranial occlusive lesions on velocities in the intracranial branches. The combination of continuous-wave Doppler, color-flow Doppler, and TCD is effective in screening for major occlusive lesions within the extracranial and intracranial arteries within the posterior circulation.[48,63,64] Vascular narrowing due to vasoconstriction and augmented flow through collateral channels and through AVMs all increase blood-flow velocity. TCD can be used to monitor vasoconstriction in patients with SAH. Figures 4-14 and 4-15 show TCD velocity curves in patients with an intracranial and an extracranial lesion, respectively.

Reserve capacity for augmenting blood flow can be studied using TCD and various vasodilator stimuli.[65] Emboli of all kinds can be detected as sudden alterations in flow, with characteristic sound signals.[66–71] TCD can also be used to detect paradoxical emboli.[72–76] Bubbles are injected into an arm vein while the TCD probe is held over a temporal window. In patients without cardiac shunts, no change is noted over the probe. In the presence of cardiac defects with shunting, air emboli are heard and can be recorded.[72–76] Emboli monitoring is discussed in more detail in Chapter 9.

> In patient JH, ultrasound examinations were quite helpful. Duplex scanning of the ICAs in the neck suggested an occlusion of the right ICA at its origin. The left ICA had only minor disease. TCD showed an inability to detect blood flow in the right MCA. Collateral flow was detected through the

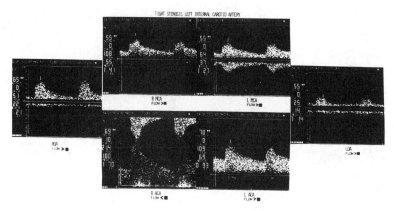

Figure 4-15. Transcranial Doppler spectra from a patient with severe stenosis of the left internal carotid artery (ICA) in the neck, showing decreased left middle cerebral artery (MCA) velocity and a delta flow velocity >25 cm per second (*delta* refers to difference between MCA peak systolic flow velocities on the two sides at 55-mm depth); reversal of flow with slightly increased velocities in the left anterior cerebral artery (ACA); increased velocity in the right ACA; and decreased left ophthalmic-artery-flow velocities, compared with the right side. (LOA = left ophthalmic artery; ROA = right ophthalmic artery.)

right ACA and posterior cerebral artery (PCA). There was also some damping of flow in the ICA siphon, presumably due to the proximal ICA obstruction in the neck. The left MCA showed normal velocities.

Computed Tomography and Magnetic Resonance Imaging

Some information about the brain vessels can often be gleaned from careful scrutiny of CT and MRI scans, especially after contrast enhancement. On plain CT, an acutely thrombosed artery can sometimes be seen as a hyperdense image that has the shape and distribution of an artery or vein. The MCA is the most frequently involved artery. The hyperdense MCA sign is virtually diagnostic of the presence of a clot within the MCA. Occasionally, the basilar artery and the PCAs can show similar hyperdensity on unenhanced scans indicating thromboembolic occlusion of these vessels. Calcific particles arising from calcific material in heart valves or a calcified atherostenotic plaque can also sometimes be identified within brain arteries on plain CT scans. Contrast enhancement can show large berry aneurysms and dolichoectatic fusiform aneurysms; absence of opacification of an artery can indicate the high probability of occlusion of that vessel. CT can also suggest dural sinus thrombosis by showing thrombosed serpiginous cortical veins the superior sagittal, or other sinuses as high-density

clots on plain CT scans. After contrast enhancement, CT may show a filling defect, representing a clot within the sagittal sinus, the so-called empty delta sign. Serial cross sectional CT images of the neck after contrast infusion can also yield information about carotid artery plaques, occlusions, and plaque hemorrhages.[77] CT of the neck can also show spontaneous, traumatic arterial dissections.

Flow within brain arteries can also be studied with MRI. Vessels with high-velocity flow appear black (signal void) on MRI images, whereas arteries with slower flow may show as white hyperintensities. Occlusions can be inferred when a flow void is not seen on images that show cross section views of arteries. Aneurysms and dissections can also frequently be identified and followed by MRI scanning. Cross section views of dissections often show intramural hematomas and luminal encroachment. Enhancement of arteries can be seen after intravenous injection of gadopentetate dimeglumine-diethylenetriaminepentaacetic acid in patients with brain ischemia and infarction.[78,79] Enhancement best correlates with slow flow and is often found in collateral arteries in patients with brain infarction and proximal vascular occlusions.

Magnetic Resonance Angiography

Magnetic resonance angiography (MRA) offers many advantages over other noninvasive methods of vascular imaging. MRA films can be acquired with and immediately after MRI. MRA examinations are noninvasive and quite safe. High-quality MRAs of the extracranial and intracranial arteries can be achieved by using gradient-echo techniques and short echo times.[80–82] Not all of the arteries can be imaged at the same time. The arch and extracranial arteries require a different technique and different views than the intracranial arteries. Knowledge of the likely location of the vascular lesions helps the examiner focus on particular regions, improving the yield of the examination. Veins can also be studied; the imaging of veins is referred to as *MR venography*. MRA can be performed using a variety of different techniques, including two-dimensional and three-dimensional time-of-flight and phase contrast imaging. MRA is a functional process that creates an image of flow in blood vessels. Unlike standard contrast injection angiograms, the images do not show anatomy. At times, contrast infusion of gadolinium solutions are needed to obtain better images of the arterial circulation.[83,84] To obtain diagnostic-quality images, patients must be cooperative and be able to hold still during the examinations. Patient positioning is critical.

Within the anterior circulation, the ICA origins are usually well visualized but at times MRA overestimates the severity of luminal narrowing.[85,86] MRA is quite accurate in patients with complete ICA occlusions and has similar sensitivity and specificity to Duplex ultrasound in screening for the presence of severe ICA stenotic lesions.[86] The changing angles and curvature of the ICA in the siphon often make interpretation of this region more difficult than the straight portions of the artery. The horizontal segment of the MCA is usually well shown.

MRA of the vertebral artery origins from the subclavian arteries is often suboptimal because of the overlapping of arteries. Superimposition of arteries sometimes make images difficult to interpret, a problem most older clinicians are aware of in interpreting arch-contrast angiography. Special views often must be taken to see the origins of the VAs. The second portion of the VA within the intervertebral foramina is well shown on MRA. The third portion of the VA, that section of the artery that curves around the rostral cervical vertebrae, is often not well seen on MRA because of the sharp angulation and curvature of the artery. The intracranial vertebral arteries and the basilar artery are usually well shown on intracranial MRA, especially the

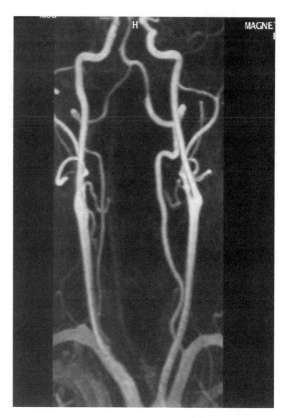

Figure 4-16. Gadolinium-enhanced magnetic resonance angiography image of the neck and proximal intracranial arteries. The innominate, subclavian, carotid, and vertebral arteries are shown quite well.

rostral bifurcation of the basilar artery into the PCAs. Quereshi and colleagues evaluated the ability of MRA to detect significant occlusive lesions among 118 patients with brain infarcts.[87] Among the 176 large arteries visualized by both MRA and conventional angiography, angiography confirmed 9 out of 10 (90%) extracranial and 32 out of 40 (80%) of intracranial abnormalities shown by MRA. There were few false-negative or false-positive abnormalities.[87] Figure 4-16 shows a gadolinium-enhanced MRA examination of the neck arteries, and Figures 4-17 and 4-18 are MRA intracranial examinations. Figure 4-17 shows bilateral MCA stenosis, and Figure 4-18 is normal except for basilar artery plaques.

MRA has proven to be an excellent screening technique for occlusive disease. Standard angiography may still be needed in some patients to better delineate the vascular lesions.[88] In patient JH,

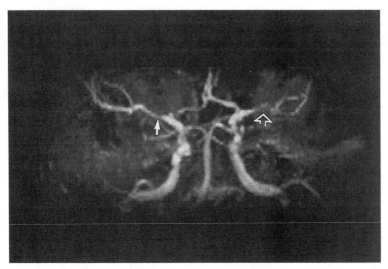

Figure 4-17. Magnetic resonance angiography: The outlined arrowhead points to a severe stenosis of the left middle cerebral artery (MCA); the right MCA has a less severe stenosis (*solid arrow*).

MRA confirmed a right ICA occlusion in the neck. Intracranial views also showed occlusion of the proximal MCA.

Computed Tomography Angiography

Development of more rapid spiral (helical) computed tomography scanners has enabled the development of computed tomography angiography (CTA).[89–93] This technique involves intravenous injection of a bolus of dye followed by helical scanning. Volumetric data acquisition and improved computerized image manipulation have improved the CTA image display into three-dimensional reformations. CTA is based on anatomic imaging, and when blood flow is severely reduced, CTA has theoretical advantages over MRA, which is a functional imaging technique. The ICAs are well shown in the neck, and the results of CTA for quantification of carotid stenosis are comparable to those obtained with MRA.[89] Compared with conventional angiography there are few false-positive and false-negative results. CTA also provides useful images of intracranial arteries and can show regions of intracranial stenosis, dolichoectasia, and aneurysms. Figure 4-19 is a CTA that shows hypoplasia or severe stenosis of the distal portion of an intracranial VA. Bolus injection of contrast followed by sequential imaging using helical CT can yield rapid information about regions of brain ischemia and blockage of intracranial arteries.[94] Occlusion of the MCA or its branches can be detected from the images even without reformation, allowing a rapid

decision about thrombolysis. The contrast dye infusion also enhances the brain CT images, yielding a perfusion CT scan that is somewhat comparable to a perfusion image MR scan.

New technology and improvements in older techniques now provide clinicians with a menu of different strategies for brain and vascular studies in patients with ischemia. All the investigations— MRI, FLAIR images, MRA, diffusion and perfusion MRI—can be performed using MR technology within a few minutes. Alternatively, if MR is not readily available or cannot be used, spiral CT can be used to create brain images and CTA of the cervicocranial arteries. Extracranial and transcranial ultrasound can be used as the diagnostic vascular tests in patients who have only had brain imaging or can be used to corroborate and quantify the blood-flow effects of vascular lesions found by CTA and MRA. Ultrasound is also used effectively to monitor the progression and regression of vascular occlusive lesions once they are identified.

Standard Contrast Catheterization
Cerebral Angiography

MRA and CTA have the advantage of being able to be performed at the same time as brain imaging and are noninvasive. The advent of high-quality CTA, MRA, and cervical and transcranial ultrasonography have led to a marked decrease in the indications for standard catheter angiography. Standard catheter angiography is indicated when the preliminary tests do not satisfactorily clarify the nature of vas-

Figure 4-18. Intracranial magnetic resonance angiography. The carotid arteries and their intracranial branches and the vertebral and basilar arteries are well seen. The left A1 segment of the internal carotid artery is hypoplastic (*arrows*). The basilar artery shows some irregularities owing to plaques but there are no important stenotic lesions.

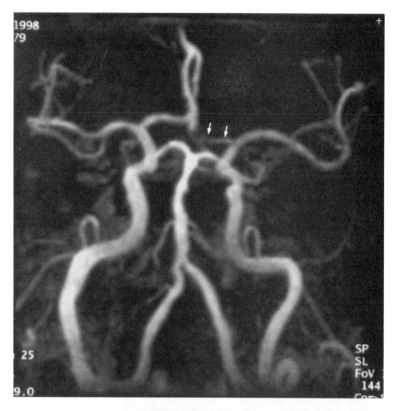

cular lesions and when treatment depends on the nature and severity of those vascular lesions. For example, angiography is used in patients in whom carotid artery stenosis has been shown by MRA and Duplex sonography, but these two tests give conflicting estimates of the severity of stenosis. Angiography is often required to better define cerebral aneurysms and vascular malformations. Catheter angiography is used as a prelude to intravascular interventions such as intra-arterial thrombolysis and angioplasty because the treatment is given directly within the artery. In experienced hands, angiography reveals valuable information and has a relatively low incidence of serious complications. Complications depend on (1) the equipment, dye, and catheters used; (2) the amount of dye; (3) the number of injections; (4) the experience of the angiographer; and (5) whether a large volume of contrast is injected into the aortic arch. The general medical and psychological state of the patient, adequacy of hydration, renal function, and nature and severity of vascular disease are also important factors that affect the complication rate.

Angiography should be tailored to the clinical question and therapeutic alternatives. Neuroimaging (CT or MRI) or ultrasonography, or both,

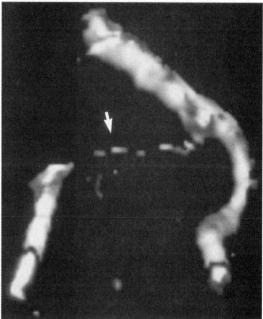

Figure 4-19. Computed tomography angiography reformatted shows hypoplasia or severe stenosis of the distal portion of the intracranial vertebral artery on the left (*arrow*). (Reprinted with permission from LR Caplan. Posterior Circulation Disease: Clinical Findings, Diagnosis, and Management. Boston: Blackwell, 1996.)

should precede angiography. These tests help the angiographer focus on the particular regions of interest. Screening of other arterial regions by noninvasive techniques allows the angiographer to limit the angiographic procedure, thus helping reduce morbidity, time, and expense. The clinician and the angiographer should decide together on the important data clinically needed, considering the clinical context of the study.

I use and teach several critical angiography "rules"[88,95]:

1. Tailor angiography to the patient and the individual problem. Avoid extra injections, catheterization, and dye because they increase the risk of the procedure.

2. Follow Sutton's law. Sutton robbed banks because that is where the money is—go after the highest-yield information first. I have seen angiographers, after a catheter had flipped unexpectedly into a vessel that was not the primary focus of attention, take several films "while they were there," believing that the films might be necessary anyway. Too often, a complication or other unforeseen exigency curtails the procedure before the important data are obtained. First things first.

3. The clinician responsible for the patient and the angiographer should plan and discuss the procedure together. Ideally, the procedure should be performed with both present, choosing together the next shot as the data accumulate. Because of time constraints and other commitments, this is not always possible. Telephone contact at critical decision points often is an acceptable substitute. If a clinician cannot be reached during the procedure, discussion of the plan of attack and treatment choices with the angiographer is a minimum requirement. In some circumstances, the relationship between angiographer and clinician is so well oiled by shared past experiences that the angiographer learns how the clinician approaches most common situations. In that case, consultation during the procedure would occur only if unexpected or unusual findings were uncovered. Ideally, if the responsible clinician is not the surgeon who will perform an operative procedure, the surgeon also should be contacted when findings are uncovered that would dictate an operation. Surgeons may have their own demands for studies before surgery, and this is best accomplished during the angiography. Communication between clinicians and neuroradiologists is also important for the performance and interpretation of MRAs and CTAs, because neuroradiologists should monitor the studies as they are performed to be sure that the information derived answers the queries raised by the clinicians caring for the patient.

4. Avoid an aortic arch injection whenever possible. The yield of arch opacification studies is low. Akers and colleagues reviewed the results of 1,000 consecutive patients who had arch angiography, followed by selective catheterization of both carotid and vertebral arteries.[96] Only six (0.6%) had intrathoracic vascular pathology that was hemodynamically important, including four lesions at the common carotid artery origin and two at the innominate artery origin. Three of these lesions (two common carotid arteries and one innominate) would have been discovered if only selective catheterization were performed. Inability to selectively catheterize these arteries and fluoroscopy identify most cases requiring arch injection. The absence of a significant lesion in the head or neck should alert the angiographer to opacify the origin of the artery on the way out. Arch injections usually require 40–50 ml of contrast material injected under pressure, so cardiac overload and renal toxicity do occur. A large bolus of dye used for filming the arch limits the amount of dye that should be used during selective catheterization. Arch films are also not easy to read because of overlapping of vessels. In my opinion, there is no reason to perform routine arch angiography. Only the major arteries of interest should be studied using the Seldinger technique of selective catheterization. In addition, intra-arterial digital subtraction filming techniques allow use of less dye while retaining high-quality films.

5. Use the least amount of dye and injections to arrive at a therapeutic decision. Often, the initial opacification provides enough information so that other injections are not needed.

6. Talk to and examine the patient at least briefly after each dye injection, to detect any complication that might dictate stopping the procedure. The neurologic examination depends on the vessels studied. For example, after posterior circulation opacification, check vision and memory; after carotid artery injection, check speech and arm movement.

In JH, I did not perform contrast angiography. The concordance of the MRA, ultrasound data, and the unlikelihood of a treatable lesion persuaded me not to pursue angiography. His clinical deficit was also severe and not reversible.

Cardiac Evaluation

Cardioembolic mechanisms of ischemic stroke are common. The proportion of ischemic strokes generally considered to have originated from cardioembolic sources has increased dramatically with the development of sophisticated technology that has the capability of defining cardiac and vascular lesions. A wide variety of different cardiac lesions are now known to be potential sources of embolism, while in the past, only acute myocardial infarction and rheumatic mitral stenosis with atrial fibrillation were generally accepted cardiac sources.

Cardiac emboli arise from a heterogeneous assortment of diseases that affect the heart valves, heart rhythm, endocardial surface, and myocardium. Pump failure can cause general cerebral hypoperfusion. In addition, many patients with cerebral ischemia owing to atherosclerosis have coexisting coronary artery atherosclerosis. Late deaths in series of patients with ischemic stroke are most often caused by coronary artery disease and myocardial infarction rather than to cerebrovascular disease. These facts should direct the physician's attention to the stroke patient's heart, as well as to the brain and its vascular supply.

The question is not whether to look at the heart but how thoroughly to do so. What is the yield of intensive cardiac investigation? Is it worth the cost? Most clinicians agree that it is important to take a careful cardiac history, particularly seeking symptoms of arrhythmia, congestive heart failure, angina pectoris, and prior myocardial infarctions. The heart should be carefully examined, noting heart size, quality of sounds, rhythm, and presence of gallops, in addition to seeking and characterizing murmurs. An electrocardiogram and chest x-ray should also be obtained routinely because of their high screening value, safety, and low cost.

Echocardiography has a high yield in patients with ischemic stroke, in whom there is

1. Known prior heart disease
2. A clinical course suggestive of brain embolism—that is, sudden onset of neurologic deficit, while active, without prior TIAs
3. A history of peripheral embolism in the limbs or abdominal viscera

4. Absence of a definite extracranial or intracranial vascular lesion that explains the brain ischemia

The fourth group is particularly important to emphasize. Young patients who have no known risk factors for atherosclerosis often harbor unexpected cardiac sources, such as cardiac tumors, intra-atrial defects, or cardiomyopathy. In other patients, the results of preliminary investigations include:

1. Absence of extracranial and intracranial vascular disease on noninvasive testing
2. A superficial infarct on CT or MRI in the distribution of a peripheral branch of the MCA or PCA
3. CT or MRI showing infarcts in multiple vascular territories
4. Normal arteriography in a patient whose clinical deficit and CT are not compatible with lacunar infarction
5. Angiography (CTA, MRA, or standard catheter) that shows distal cutoff of a cerebral artery branch or a luminal filling defect without severe proximal arterial stenosis

In these circumstances, intensive cardiac testing is essential. Transthoracic echocardiography (TTE) is usually performed first, and the results may be definitive, and thus transesophageal echocardiography (TEE) would not be required. Because the left atrium is directly anterior to the esophagus, atrial lesions, occult valvular disorders, and ulcerative lesions of the proximal aorta, often missed by transthoracic echocardiography, are detected by the TEE approach. TEE shows many abnormalities not revealed by TTE. The use of TEE in patients with strokes and TIAs has been extensively reviewed.[97–100] TEE is more accurate than TTE in showing atrial and ventricular thrombi, in detecting and quantifying intracardiac shunts, and more often shows spontaneous echo contrast than TTE.

TEE may not be able to identify some cardiac sources of emboli. Some thromboemboli are too small to be detected. An embolus that is 1–2 mm can produce a devastating neurologic deficit, and this size particle is often beyond the resolution of echocardiography.[101,102] The other major reason for failure of echocardiography to show a thrombus is that thrombosis and embolism are dynamic processes. When a thrombus leaves the heart to go to the brain, echocardiography may not show a residual thrombus within the heart if performed soon

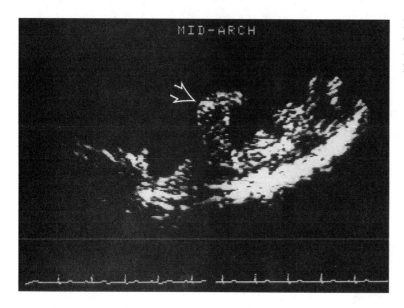

Figure 4-20. Transesophageal echocardiography of the mid aortic arch shows a large protruding plaque that was mobile (*arrow*).

after the clinical event.[101,102] Later, the thrombus may reform.

TEE also yields important information about the proximal aorta, a region not imaged by TTE. Figure 4-20 shows a large protruding aortic plaque detected by TEE. TEE is important in all patients in whom TTE suggests, but does not adequately define, the cardiac pathology, and in all patients in whom other studies (cerebrovascular, hematologic, and other cardiac investigations) do not satisfactorily show the cause of brain embolism and brain ischemia. Radionuclide testing, including gated blood pool imaging (multigated acquisition scans), also may be helpful in selected patients as might other cardiac imaging techniques.[103]

The aorta is an important potential source of embolism, especially during angiography and cardiac surgery. Presently, TEE is the most effective method of imaging the aorta for plaques and thrombi. The ascending aorta can also be insonated using a Duplex ultrasound probe placed in the right supraclavicular fossa. The arch and proximal descending thoracic aorta can be imaged using a left supraclavicular probe.[104] The results so far are preliminary but promising. Most plaques are located in the curvature of the arch from the distal ascending aorta to the proximal descending aorta, regions shown by B-mode ultrasound.[104]

When clinical suspicion is high and echocardiography is not diagnostic, CT,[105] MRI, or ultrafast CT[106] of the heart might image cardiac clots. Platelet scintigraphy using radionuclides[107] might also indicate pooling of platelets on the surface of a mural thrombus or other cardiac lesion. Remember also that documentation of a possible cardioembolic source—such as mitral valve prolapse, mitral annulus calcification, or akinetic zones—does not mean per se that the patient has brain embolism. Coexistent atherosclerotic disease may be the cause.

Many patients with atherosclerosis of the carotid and vertebral arteries in the neck have coexistent peripheral vascular occlusive disease and coronary artery disease. Because coronary artery disease, even when silent, can be life-threatening, screening of these patients for silent myocardial ischemia is important, especially if surgery is considered.[108] A variety of different radionuclide techniques can detect regions of poor myocardial perfusion.[109–112] Imaging of the heart after the patient has been given dipyridamole (dipyridamole-thallium myocardial imaging) and some exercise often shows regions of silent ischemia.[110–112] In one study, among 38 patients with severe cerebrovascular occlusive disease, 60% had reversible or fixed myocardial perfusion deficits using this radionuclide scintigraphic test.[112] Treadmill or supine exercise testing with electrocardiographic monitoring is another commonly used screening technique. Radionuclide angiography can also be helpful in assessing left ventricular function and perfusion at rest and with exercise. If severe coronary artery disease is suggested by screening tests, coronary angiography may be needed to localize and quantify the coronary artery disease to guide treatment.

The use of routine ambulatory monitoring for cardiac rhythm disturbances is not clear. In patients suspected of brain embolism, the yield is probably high enough to dictate the use of monitoring. In patients with lacunar infarcts and those with a well-defined atherosclerotic extracranial vascular cause for their stroke, the yield is probably low. Cardiac rhythm monitoring should probably be done in any patient whose initial EEG suggests a cardiac rhythm abnormality.

Other Investigations

A wide variety of other tests have been used in the past to study arterial flow in the brain vessels. Most of these investigations have been superseded by newer ultrasound technology and neuroimaging techniques. These include oculoplethysmography and ophthalmodynamometry, techniques that were described in the first two editions of this book but have now been superseded by TCD. A new ultrasound technology, color Doppler imaging of the vessels that supply the eye, has become available and can accurately image and define vascular lesions that involve the ophthalmic and central retinal arteries.[113,114]

What if the Neuroimaging Tests Have Shown Intracerebral Hemorrhage?

The most common cause of ICH is hypertension, either acute or chronic. When the blood pressure is high and CT or MRI shows a hematoma in a typical location for hypertensive ICH, a search for AVMs or aneurysms has a low yield. In young patients with no hypertension or with intraventricular or lobar hematomas, however, studies of the intracerebral arteries often show vascular lesions. Patients with ICH after use of cocaine, especially the hydrochloride form, have a relatively high incidence of underlying vascular malformations.[115]

MR can often show AVMs and cavernous angiomas. Vascular channels, serpiginous arteries, mixed-density heterogeneous signals, and the presence of old bleeds containing hemosiderin are clues to the presence of vascular malformations. Contrast-enhanced CT and MR, plain or enhanced with gadopentetate dimeglumine-diethylenetriaminepentaacetic acid, can show large aneurysms if they are in the plane of the sections taken. MRA effectively shows AVMs and aneurysms. In some patients, angiography using selective arterial catheterization by the Seldinger technique, with opacification of the arteries supplying the ICH, is needed for definitive exclusion of small AVMs and aneurysms. Cavernous and veinous angiomas are usually not detected by cerebral angiography.

What if Neuroimaging or Lumbar Puncture Show Subarachnoid Hemorrhage?

Cerebral angiography is still often required for the study of patients with SAH not explainable by trauma or a known bleeding diathesis. Aneurysmal rerupture is such a potentially lethal event that clinicians must be sure an aneurysm is not present in patients with SAH. MRA and CTA[116] are useful in screening for aneurysms, but at present, these techniques are probably not definitive enough in many patients for surgical exploration, and dye opacification is still often required. MR is helpful in detecting small vascular malformations near the ependymal and pial surfaces. MRA and CTA may be useful in following patients after surgical or endovascular treatment of aneurysms and AVMs, and in following unruptured aneurysms and AVMs not treated surgically. TCD is helpful in following patients with aneurysmal SAH in detecting and monitoring vasoconstriction in the basal intracranial arteries.[57,117,118]

Question 4: Are Abnormalities in the Blood Causing or Adding to Brain Ischemia or Hemorrhage?

Once the clinician has determined the nature, site, and severity of the vascular lesion, it is important to find out whether abnormalities of blood constituents are causing or contributing to brain ischemia or hemorrhage. Clinicians must not forget the blood. Abnormalities of the clotting system can lead to hypercoagulability and thrombosis. Even in patients with lesions known to predispose to thromboembolism and brain ischemia, the acute event is often precipitated by a change in the blood and its coagulability. Infections, cancer, and inflammatory bowel disease are examples of conditions that are associated with release of acute phase reactants that may alter coagulability sufficiently to promote thromboembolism—especially if there is a pre-existing lesion that affects an endothelial surface. Bleeding diatheses often cause intracranial bleeding. Abnormalities of the viscosity of blood can alter blood flow, especially in small arterioles and capillaries of the brain, and in patients with occlusive lesions. Increased viscosity can cause or contribute to regional decreases in CBF and potentiate ischemia. Autoimmunity, which can be detected and monitored by blood tests, can lead to occlusive cerebrovascular disease.

What if the Problem Is Ischemia?

The formed cellular elements of the blood—erythrocytes, leukocytes, and platelets—should always be studied. Screening tests of coagulation functions should also be a part of the routine evaluation of patients with brain ischemia. In addition, other blood components may be analyzed, such as serum proteins, coagulation factors, antiphospholipid antibodies, and blood viscosity.

Erythrocytes

Quantitative and qualitative RBC abnormalities can affect blood flow and clotting. The level of Hct clearly affects blood viscosity and the rheologic properties of blood. Physicians have long been aware that high Hct levels, such as 60% or more, can cause clotting in normal young adults. In older patients with pre-existing atherosclerosis and small-vessel disease, high Hcts that are still within the normal range can compound the vascular disease and limit perfusion. Studies in animals[119] and humans[120–122] confirm that the Hct level can affect blood flow and prognosis even when Hct levels are not frankly polycythemic. The Hct level also has a heavy impact on blood viscosity.[123–124] Lowering the Hct from 45 to 32 results in doubling of CBF.[125]

Sickle cell disease and other hemoglobinopathies can lead to altered flow and hypercoagulability. Sickle cell disease and spherocytosis are associated with multifocal brain infarcts. TCD documents abnormalities of flow velocities even in young patients with sickle cell disease.[126] These abnormalities correlate well with regions of arterial narrowing and with the occurrence of strokes[127,128] and help select patients for prophylactic blood transfusions.[129] Hemoglobin and Hct certainly should be measured in every patient with stroke. Hemodilution has been advocated as a measure to augment blood flow during acute ischemia. Lowering of relatively high Hct levels by blood donations has been advocated as a measure to prophylactically reduce the risk of stroke in stroke-prone individuals. Hemoglobin electrophoresis is important in those with racial and genetic predispositions to hemoglobinopathies, especially if anemia is present. Careful examination of a stained blood smear for the morphology of RBCs can suggest the possibility of a hemoglobinopathy. Severe anemia also can compound brain ischemia, but low Hct levels are rare in stroke patients.

Leukocytes

The white blood cell (WBC) count is often elevated in patients with myocardial infarction and is also often slightly elevated in patients with brain infarcts. Some have even correlated a high WBC count with the severity of carotid atherosclerosis,[130] but the issue is complicated by the fact that cigarette smokers have high WBC counts. Leukemia with high WBC counts can cause packing of capillaries and small arterioles with aggregates of large WBCs, causing multiple small infarcts and hemorrhages. This is suggested, obviously, by a high leukocrit in the capillary tube used to measure Hct. Measurement of WBC count is usually a routine part of a complete blood cell count, which should be ordered on each stroke patient.

Platelets

Platelets are critical structures active in the initiation of blood coagulation. Quantitative and qualitative platelet abnormalities can cause hypercoagulability and bleeding. Thrombocytosis, especially with platelet counts greater than 1 million, can cause hypercoagulability.[131] Platelet counts should be a routine part of the initial evaluation of patients with ischemic stroke because thrombocytosis can potentiate thrombosis. Low platelet counts can suggest the presence of other disorders, such as the antiphospholipid antibody syndrome,[132–134] consumptive coagulopathies, lupus erythematosus, and thrombotic thrombocytopenic purpura—all of which are often complicated by brain ischemia. Platelet counts can fall during the course of illness (e.g., after use of heparin),[135] so that a baseline count before treatment is occasionally useful for later comparison. Some patients with platelet counts in the normal range have increased platelet aggregation, abnormal secretory function of their platelets, or qualitative abnormalities of platelet morphology and function. In vitro platelet function tests are usually performed in hematologic research laboratories, and even experts disagree on their applicability to the in vivo state. Platelet aggregation is usually measured after the addition of various agents known to increase aggregation, such as arachidonic acid, adenosine diphosphate, epinephrine, and collagen.[136,137] The extent of platelet activation can also be studied by measuring the levels of β-thromboglobulin in the blood.[138,139] β-Thromboglobulin is secreted during platelet-release reactions, and, when optimal venipuncture technique is used, the levels are good markers of in vivo platelet activation and secretion. Simultaneous measurement of platelet factor 4, which has a short half-life, can help control for in vitro platelet changes.[137] Platelet production of thromboxane B_2 can be performed by radioimmunoassays and von Willebrand factor antigen can also be quantified.[140] Polymorphisms in the platelet glycoprotein II/III fibrinogen receptor have been described; these may also predispose to hypercoagulability and brain and myocardial ischemia.[141]

Serum Proteins

Fibrinogen is an important part of the coagulation system because fibrinogen is converted to fibrin monomers by the action of thrombin. Fibrin is an essential component of red and white thrombi. Fibrinogen also contributes to blood viscosity because high levels of fibrinogen can increase blood viscosity. Under ordinary circumstances, the Hct and fibrinogen levels are the two most important single predictors of whole blood viscosity.[123,124]

Normal fibrinogen levels usually range from 250 to 400 mg/dl. High levels of fibrinogen have been shown to be risk factors for stroke in several prospective studies.[142–145] Fibrinogen levels can also rise as acute-phase reactants in the early period after stroke.

Ancrod (a defibrogenating enzyme of Malayan pit-viper venom), has been used to lower fibrinogen levels and to decrease fibrin formation, potentially lyse thrombi, and increase blood flow.[146,147] Omega-3 fish oil preparations containing eicosapentaenoic acid may also act to decrease fibrinogen content.[148] Fibrinogen can also be mechanically removed from the blood. Heparin-mediated extracorporeal low-density lipoprotein precipitation is a system devised by Austrian physicians that removes fibrinogen as well as low-density lipoproteins from the blood and has the capability of quickly and significantly reducing fibrinogen blood levels.[149]

Patients with a predisposition to stroke recurrence have a slightly lower serum albumin level and albumin to globulin ratio than those without recurrence.[143,144] Abnormally high levels of immunoglobulins (Ig) A, IgG, and IgM can indicate autoimmune disease and can be a clue to diagnosis in patients with unexplained brain ischemia. Macroglobulins found in Waldenström's macroglobulinemia and multiple myeloma also can increase blood viscosity and cause or potentiate multiple loci of ischemia. At present, immunoglobulin measurements are not part of the routine evaluation of stroke patients because of their low yield. In selected patients with clinical and ophthalmoscopic suggestions of hyperviscosity, however, and in those with a high serum globulin level, serum immunoelectrophoresis can be helpful.

Studies of Coagulation Factors and Coagulation

The prothrombin time (PT) and the activated partial thromboplastin time (aPTT) are excellent screening tests of coagulation function and are routinely available in nearly all hospital laboratories. Measurement of the PT and the aPTT should be a part of the evaluation of all stroke patients. Other tests are ordered if (1) a hypercoagulable state is suspected by acceleration of the PT or aPTT; (2) multiple vascular occlusions are present; (3) there is a past history of recurrent thrombophlebitis or miscarriages; or (4) known neoplastic, collagen vascular, rheumatologic, or inflammatory diseases are present. Some serum proteins—such as antithrombin III, protein C, and protein S—are natural inhibitors of coagulation. A decrease in the level of these substances because of a familial inherited disorder or an acquired disease can cause hypercoagulability. An inherited coagulation deficit, usually referred to as *resistance to activated protein C,* has been described by Dutch investigators from Leiden.[150,151] In most instances, resistance to activated protein C is caused by a point mutation in the gene that encodes for coagulation factor V.[151] The presence of this mutation, called *factor V Leiden,* is accompanied by a threefold to fivefold increase in the frequency of venous thromboembolism in the lower extremities[152] and an increased frequency of cerebral venous thrombosis. Factor V Leiden is the most common recognized genetic disorder that leads to hypercoagulability. The second most common genetic mutation that leads to a prothrombotic state is a mutation in the gene encoding prothrombin.[153] This mutation involves a transition from guanine to adenine at position 20210 in the sequence of the 3' untranslated region of the prothrombin gene.[153] The frequency of cerebral and peripheral venous thrombosis is greatly increased in carriers of the prothrombin gene mutation, especially if they also take oral contraceptive pills.[154] Genetic analysis is warranted in patients with unexplained hypercoagulability, especially those with cerebral venous thrombosis and recurrent peripheral venous thromboembolism.

The level of coagulation factors VII, VIII, IX, and X can be measured in most hematologic laboratories but have not been well studied in large groups of stroke patients. Abnormal levels of Factor VIII can cause hypercoagulability and recurrent strokes.[155,156] Factor VIII elevation can be chronic, precede and predispose to stroke,[155] elevate as an acute-phase reactant in systemic illnesses such as ulcerative colitis, and can elevate secondary to thrombosis. In the latter case, it is a marker and not the cause of the thrombosis.[156]

Hemostatic markers of coagulation activity have been used to detect and monitor hypercoagulability.[157] Thrombin acts as a catalyst of the proteolysis of fibrinogen to fibrin. During this reaction, fibrinopeptide A is generated. The level of fibrin D-dimer is also an index of fibrin generation. The level of the prothrombin activation fragment F1.2 is a measure of in vivo thrombin generation. Increasing intensity of anticoagulation is accompanied by decreasing thrombin generation as measured by the F1.2 levels.[158] Fibrinolysis involves the dissolution of fibrin by endogenous fibrinolytic mechanisms. Fibrinolytic activity can be estimated by the levels of fibrinopeptide B-B1-42 and of tissue plasminogen activator and its inhibitor. Thrombosis is favored when thrombin proteolysis of fibrinogen (increased fibrinopeptide A and D-dimer levels) exceeds plasmin proteolysis (increased fibrinopeptide B-B1-42 and tissue plasminogen activator to its inhibitor ratio).[139,159–162] Several studies have monitored the levels of these substances in acute stroke patients and during follow-up.[139,159,162]

Antiphospholipid Antibodies

Antiphospholipid antibodies (APLAs) are usually IgG or IgM antibodies that bind to negatively charged phospholipids. Phospholipids are important constituents of vascular endothelium, heart proteins, platelets, and other cells. The two most commonly measured APLAs are anticardiolipin antibody and the so-called lupus anticoagulant (LA). LAs are acquired immunoglobulins that are associated clinically with thrombosis, not bleeding; most patients with LA do not have systemic lupus erythematosus. The laboratory hallmark of LA is a prolonged aPTT that does not correct when normal plasma is added. This indicates the presence of an inhibitor of clotting rather than a deficiency of a necessary coagulation factor.

LA can be sought using a sensitive phospholipid reagent, the kaolin clotting time, or the Russell viper venom time.[132] Anticardiolipin antibodies of the IgG or IgM types can be measured. IgG antibody levels, especially those greater than 40 GPL (IgG phospholipid) units, correlate with a relatively high risk of stroke and recurrent stroke.[163] The screening tests for syphilis—the VDRL and Reiter protein reaction—depend on the activity of APLAs. False-positive serologic tests for syphilis are often found in patients with APLAs, and thrombocytopenia is present in a third of APLA-positive patients. The clinical syndrome consists of frequent venous and arterial thrombotic events, such as thrombophlebitis, pulmonary embolism, TIAs, strokes, myocardial infarctions, and recurrent fetal loss in women.[132–134] It is likely that the mechanism of recurrent brain ischemia is excessive clotting. APLAs may be directed against the endothelium or platelet membranes and may alter coagulability and vascular functions. APLAs should be measured in situations in which the usual risk factors for ischemic stroke are not present, and certainly in patients with livedo reticularis, strokes (Sneddon's syndrome), and those patients with clinical features matching the primary APLA syndrome.[132–134,157]

Other Blood Measurements

An elevated erythrocyte sedimentation rate can be an important clue to the presence of a systemic inflammatory disease or unsuspected vasculitis. It should be ordered in patients with suspected temporal arteritis and in young and elderly patients with unexplained strokes.

After the demonstration that sugar administration could worsen experimentally induced brain ischemia,[164,165] Plum and colleagues[166,167] noted a poorer prognosis in stroke patients with elevated blood sugars. Because blood sugar is a critical metabolite for the brain, there is no doubt that abnormal levels can be deleterious to patients with stroke. Blood sugar elevation can also be triggered by tissue damage with release of catecholamines and mobilization of sugar. Large infarcts and hemorrhages are often associated with elevations in the blood sugar level. Patients with hypercalcemia due to hyperparathyroidism also have a higher frequency of stroke, probably due to the vascular or platelet effects of calcium.[168–170] Dehydration diminishes blood volume, thus potentially decreasing blood flow. Measurements of blood urea nitrogen and electrolytes are useful in determining the presence and degree of dehydration and would demonstrate important electrolyte imbalance. Blood lipids, including total cholesterol and fractionation into high-density lipoprotein and low-density lipoprotein components, should be measured in each patient with brain ischemia. Markedly increased levels of triglycerides, low-density lipoproteins, and chylomicra can increase blood viscosity. These levels are useful to analyze in patients with known familial hyperlipidemia, premature atherosclerosis, and patients who have clinical hyperviscosity syndromes. A clue to the presence of chylomicra is the presence of milky, lipemic serum, especially after a meal.

Every patient with an ischemic stroke or TIA should have, at the minimum, measurements of the following before proceeding with aggressive diagnostic or therapeutic intervention: hemoglobin, Hct, WBC count, platelet count, aPTT, PT, fibrinogen, blood sugar, calcium, total and high-density

lipoprotein and low-density lipoprotein cholesterol, blood urea nitrogen, sodium, chloride, potassium, and carbon dioxide.

> Patient JH had an Hct of 41 and had normal WBC and platelet counts. The PT and aPTT were also normal. Blood sugar on admission was 145, but levels returned to normal after a few days.

What if the Patient Has Hemorrhage—Either Intracerebral Hemorrhage or Subarachnoid Hemorrhage?

Bleeding diatheses are important causes of intracranial bleeding. Probably the most common bleeding disorders are now iatrogenic, including the use of heparins, warfarin compounds, rt-PA and other fibrinolytic compounds, and possibly aspirin use. Usually, these clinical situations are known and are not diagnostic dilemmas. Measurement of the PT and partial thromboplastin time (PTT) are usually sufficient to screen for these disorders. Platelet counts detect thrombocytopenia, and the bleeding time is a useful screening procedure measuring platelet function, among other conditions. Hemophilia and other lifelong bleeding diatheses are usually known before the intracranial bleed occurs. Measurement of antihemophilic globulin and other coagulation factors is helpful in patients with previously uncharacterized bleeding disorders. A history of prior bleeding episodes (vaginal, dental, postoperative, and so forth) and the presence of systemic purpura are the best clues to the presence of a bleeding diathesis.

Question 5: Are Abnormalities of Brain Function and Metabolism in Regions Not Shown to Be Damaged by Computed Tomography or Magnetic Resonance Imaging? Are Abnormalities of Blood Flow Not Detected by the Macro-Level Tests of Large Artery Vascular Imaging?

The tests described so far help localize and quantify morphologic structural abnormalities in the brain, larger blood vessels, and blood.

At times, especially during the acute ischemic period, brain tissue is ischemic but not irreversibly

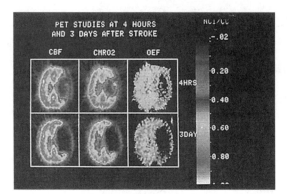

Figure 4-21. Positron emission tomography (PET) scans from a patient with a middle cerebral artery territory infarct (on right of scans); studies were taken at 4 hours (top row) and at 3 days (bottom row). (CBF = cerebral blood flow; CMRO$_2$ = cerebral metabolic rate for oxygen; OEF = oxygen extraction fraction.) (Courtesy of Robert Ackerman, Massachusetts General Hospital.)

damaged. Reduced regional cerebral blood flow (rCBF) in the range of 10 to 20 ml/100 g per minute can lead to stunning (not functioning normal but not irreversibly damaged), a state characterized by decreased electrical activity and reduced cerebral metabolism but increased extraction of oxygen. The stunned brain region has usually been called the *ischemic penumbra*, which borrows a term from astronomy to indicate the state of almost shadow that is characteristic of a partial solar eclipse.[171] Clinical and research techniques are available that can yield information about brain function, metabolism, and blood flow. In this section of the chapter, I first describe the tests available and then comment on their possible present and future use.

Positron Emission Tomography

PET is a functional imaging technique that makes it possible to measure in vivo chemical reactions in body organs. Only a small number of suitable positron-emitting radionuclides are available that are integral to most organic biological compounds. These radionuclides have short half-lives, and so a dedicated medical cyclotron is required on site for synthesis, thereby making the equipment and its maintenance quite expensive.

The positron-emitting radionuclides are tagged to physiologically active compounds and given to the patient at acceptably low radiation doses. CT or MRI studies of the distribution of these radionuclides allow for images of brain physiology and metabolism during life. PET scanning allows for quantification and imaging of CBF, the metabolic rate of oxygen, the metabolic rate of glucose, and the oxygen extraction fraction. These measurements give useful information about blood flow, the metabolic activity, and avidity for oxygen in the local regions studied.[172]

In the normal situation, blood flow and metabolism are coupled; however, flow and metabolism are often different in the core of infarcts, as compared with the peripheral zone (penumbra). When oxygen metabolism is markedly depressed, either in association with low rCBF or out of proportion to rCBF, the likelihood of useful return of function in the tissue is small. If oxygen metabolism is preserved and there is a relatively high oxygen extraction function, then the outlook for recovery is better.[173] Baron dubbed the situation of avidity of the local tissue for oxygen in the presence of poor perfusion the *misery perfusion syndrome*.[174] In chronic infarcts, CT regions of hypodensity and PET images of rCBF and the metabolic rate of oxygen are essentially congruous, showing dead tissue with little flow and little metabolism. During some phases of a stroke, rCBF may be increased relative to metabolism, a phenomenon that Lassen dubbed *luxury perfusion*.[175] Hyperperfusion in the early period after stroke onset correlates with open arteries by TCD and good clinical outcome.[176] The hyperperfusion is usually related to spontaneous recanalization of embolic occlusions.[176] Figure 4-21 illustrates the data generated from PET examinations.

Metabolic depression can also occur at sites distant from the zones of infarction. This finding has sometimes been called *diaschisis* and is most common in: (1) the thalamus ipsilateral to a cerebral infarct, (2) the cerebral cortex ipsilateral to a thalamic lesion, (3) the cerebral hemisphere contralateral to a supratentorial infarct of the opposite hemisphere, (4) the cerebellar hemisphere contralateral to a cerebral lesion, and (5) the cerebellar hemisphere ipsilateral to a pontine infarct. These distant effects provide insight into brain pathways and help guide physiologic approaches to rehabilitation. They also help in understanding previously confusing rCBF results associated with xenon inhalation.

Figure 4-22. Single-photon emission computed tomography scan shows lack of isotope uptake in the left posterior part of the brain (on the lower right of the picture).

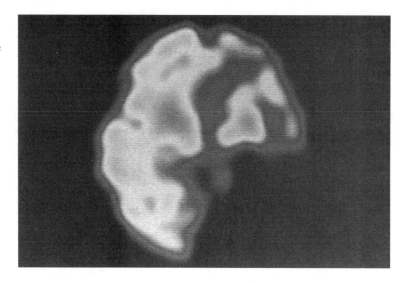

PET can also be used to study changes in flow and metabolism after various types of stimulation. Visual stimuli augment activity in the lateral geniculate body and striate regions. Auditory stimuli activate the medial geniculate body and various temporal and parietal regions, depending on whether music, language, or other auditory stimuli are used and the content of the sound. Speaking and right limb movement activate parasylvian and frontal regions, predominantly in the left cerebral hemisphere. These studies give important insights into how the brain functions. Also, in some circumstances, rCBF and metabolism might be adequate for baseline function but may not be able to augment satisfactorily after stimulation. These functional studies also have the potential of telling how the damaged brain functions with sensory stimuli and how patterns of metabolism and flow change with recovery. Insight into reparative and adaptive mechanisms could ensue.

Without question, PET has opened up large vistas with potential insights into brain function. The expense of the equipment, the length of time required for testing, and the importance of ancillary physicists and chemists limit the applicability of the PET technique to large research centers funded for their studies. Functional MRI studies have begun to develop the capability of demonstrating brain function and activity without the need for a cyclotron. Furthermore, functional MRI can be performed on the same equipment used for brain and vascular imaging.[177,178]

Single-Photon Emission Computed Tomography

SPECT uses ordinary radionuclear camera equipment and does not require a cyclotron to generate radionuclides. The equipment is thus less expensive than a CT or a PET scanner. The most common radioisotopes used now are technetium-99M–labeled hexamethylpropylene amineoxime and technetium-99m–labeled ethyl cysteinate dimer.[179,180] Regional radiotracer uptake can be imaged in three planes by the existing technology. The isotopes measure mostly rCBF rather than metabolic activity. A major advantage of SPECT scanning is that imaging does not have to be performed immediately after injection of the radionuclide. The findings on SPECT imaging represent those that were present at the time of injection. Acute treatment could be instituted immediately after injection even before imaging if so desired. SPECT is probably not as accurate or as definitive when compared to PET. The resolution of the SPECT images is much poorer than PET, but practical considerations favor the use of SPECT. SPECT images can be repeated at intervals. Like PET, it should be used in conjunction with standard neuroimaging (CT or MRI). The pattern of radiotracer uptake can suggest a stroke mechanism. Wedge-shaped regions of reduced uptake suggest embolism. Cortical regions of diminished uptake establish a non-lacunar type of stroke. Border-zone areas of decreased uptake suggest hemodynamically significant proximal arterial lesions.[180] Figures 4-22 and 4-23 show SPECT scans with different patterns

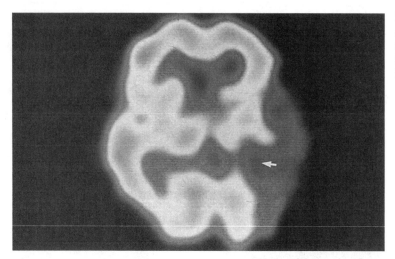

Figure 4-23. Single-photon emission computed tomography scan shows smaller areas of decreased isotope uptake in the left temporal-lobe region (*arrow*).

of abnormal uptake. Interpretation of both PET and SPECT are greatly enhanced if the vascular lesion is defined.[180] To date, there are insufficient data about the use of SPECT in the diagnosis and management of stroke patients, but the technique shows promise when the proper questions are asked.[181,182]

Xenon-Enhanced Computed Tomography

Inhalation of gases with calculation of total CBF and rCBF distribution of the gases has been used to quantify blood flow to the brain since 1944.[183-184] The inhalation technique for rCBF was performed on multiple occasions, thus allowing sequential determinations in individual patients. Technical problems limited the identification of some infarcts, imaging resolution was poor, and few well-designed studies considered the use of the technique in the diagnosis and management of individual stroke patients.

One of the major limitations of inhalation or injection rCBF techniques was the lack of anatomic definition. Because xenon, the most frequently used gas, was inert and was not metabolized by the brain, metabolic data were not obtained. The development of XeCT has allowed imaging of rCBF changes on sequential standard CT slices.[185,186] Xenon enhances or modifies the images, allowing visualization of relative rCBF in regions of interest. This technique facilitates comparison of the zone of infarction on CT with regions of reduced CBF. The technique, like SPECT but unlike PET, contains no metabolic information. XeCT and SPECT have

replaced and superseded all of the prior CBF measurement techniques that used inhalation or injection of labeled gases. Patients who show normal brain perfusion by XeCT in regions outside of the area of infarction usually have good outcomes and do not extend the infarcts.[187]

Newer Magnetic Resonance Techniques

Advances in the technology of MRI have now made it possible to safely and quickly acquire a great deal of information about brain ischemia and brain perfusion. Diffusion-weighted MRI shows regions of increased brain water content that usually represent regions that will become infarcted.[9,10,189] Brain perfusion can also be imaged using dynamic contrast-enhanced MR scans.[188-191] Ultrafast imaging after gadopentetate dimeglumine-diethylenetriaminepentaacetic acid injection is used to calculate regional cerebral blood volume, rCBF, and to produce so-called perfusion-weighted images.[188-191] Comparison of the region of probable infarction on diffusion-weighted scans with the region of reduced perfusion gives an indication of the part of the brain that is underperfused but not yet infarcted (the presumed ischemic penumbra). When the region of reduced perfusion matches the zone of infarction, progression of infarction and progression of neurologic signs are rare. When this information is supplemented by vascular imaging—usually MRA, which is acquired at the same time as the diffusion-weighted and perfusion MRI

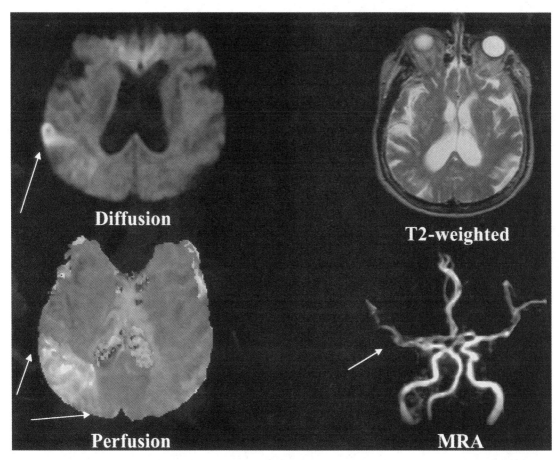

Figure 4-24. Magnetic resonance studies in a patient with atrial fibrillation who developed sudden aphasia. In these figures, which were taken 4 hours after symptom onset, the left side of the figures represents the left cerebral hemisphere. The upper left figure is a diffusion-weighted study that shows a small area of abnormality (*arrow*) in the left temporal lobe. The T2-weighted scan does not show a lesion in this region. A perfusion-weighted scanat the lower left shows a larger area of abnormality (*arrows*) than the diffusion-weighted scan above it. The magnetic resonance angiography (MRA) at the lower right shows a spontaneously partially recanalized left middle cerebral artery (*arrow*). After these acute scans, the patient rapidly improved. (Courtesy of Rafael Llinas, M.D.)

scans—the treating physician has all the useful information needed to assess brain perfusion and to allow a logical decision about the likely use of acute treatments such as thrombolysis. A patient with an occluded MCA shown by MRA, who has a large zone of reduced perfusion within the MCA territory, shown by perfusion MR—and a relatively small region of infarction shown by diffusion-weighted MR—represents the ideal candidate for thrombolysis. On the other hand, a large zone of infarction on diffusion-weighted MR, open ICA and MCA on MRA, and perfusion deficits that match or are less than the zone of infarction on dif-

fusion-weighted scans, are characteristics of candidates in whom thrombolysis has little likely use. All of this clinically relevant data can be acquired rapidly without risk on one machine, making modern MR imaging using the new technology the best method of studying acute stroke patients. Figures 4-24 and 4-25 illustrate acute modern MR studies.

Two other advances, MR spectroscopy (MRS) and functional MRI, have added new dimensions to the study of stroke and brain ischemia. During MRS, regions of interest as identified by MRI can be analyzed for the relative volumes and localization of various chemical constituents such as choline,

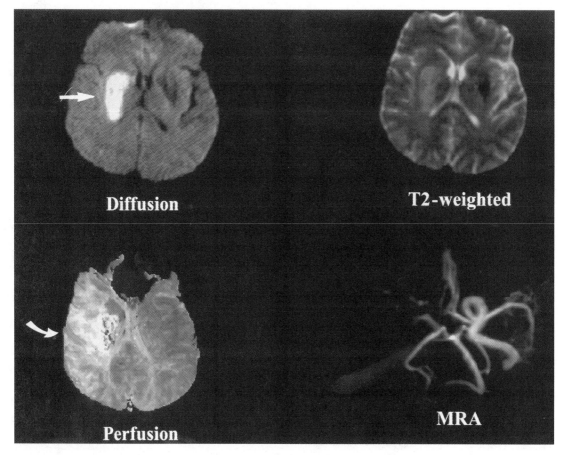

Figure 4-25. Magnetic resonance studies a few hours after symptom onset in a patient with a left internal carotid artery occlusion. The left cerebral hemisphere is on the left of these figures. The diffusion-weighted magnetic resonance imaging scan at the top left shows a large striatocapsular abnormality (*arrow*). The perfusion-weighted scan below shows a much larger area of decreased perfusion involving both the deep and superficial blood supply of the left middle cerebral artery (*curved arrow*). The T2-weighted MRI at the upper right shows the deep infarct but the abnormality is less intense than on the diffusion scan. The magnetic resonance angiography (MRA) scan shows no image of the left internal carotid and middle cerebral arteries. This patient worsened after these acute images were performed. (Courtesy of Rafael Llinas, M.D.)

creatine, *N*-acetyl aspartate, lactate, and glutamate.[192,193] Elevated lactate is found soon after infarction; decreased *N*-acetyl aspartate, creatine, and choline are characteristic of the MRS spectrum in the region of brain infarction. MRS analysis may be useful in the future in distinguishing tissue that is destined to become infarcted from tissue that is reversibly ischemic. MRS may also prove useful in studying patients with various stroke-related metabolic problems, such as mitochondrial disorders that alter brain metabolism.[194]

When certain MRI techniques are used during perceptual, cognitive, and motor tasks, small changes in signal intensity show alterations in local blood flow related to increased brain activity and function during these tasks.[195,196] Functional MRI can yield insights into which parts of the brain are being used to perform various brain functions. This information is probably most relevant to the study of recovery from stroke and may give important insights into spontaneous recovery and the potential of various rehabilitative therapies.

Electrical Tests of Brain Function

EEG is the oldest available noninvasive test of brain function. Experience has shown that the use of EEG in stroke diagnosis and management is limited. There are, however, occasional circumstances in which EEG is quite helpful. In some patients with stroke or other central nervous system lesions, worsening of a neurologic deficit is caused by clinically inapparent or subtle seizure activity, which is usually dramatically captured by EEG. Some patients with recent-onset strokes, especially those caused by subcortical ICHs or cerebral embolism, have seizures. In these patients, sequential EEGs can quantify seizure discharge and thereby guide anticonvulsant management. Because lacunar strokes are small and deep, they seldom influence the EEG, recorded primarily from superficial structures, whereas cortical lesions are usually more extensive, closer to the surface, and so produce more effect on the EEG.[197] In patients with a clinical deficit due to ischemia and normal CT, when other diagnostic tools such as MRI, SPECT, and XeCT are not available, EEG may help the clinician decide whether the lesion is subcortical or cortical. A normal or symmetric EEG suggests a deep subcortical or posterior fossa site of ischemia. An asymmetric EEG, with the abnormality located on the side appropriate to the neurologic symptoms and signs, suggests a cortical localization that has not produced enough irreversible damage to be visualized by CT. In patients with severe vascular insults causing coma, the EEG can provide valuable data about the viability and residual electrical function of the brain.

Modern computer technology has also been used to create topographical maps of the distribution of scalp-recorded electrical activity. Frequency analysis and topographical EEG mapping is superior to standard EEG in localizing electrical abnormalities.[198,199] The color-coded maps are easier to read, and the results are more quantified and consistent. This technology, however, has largely been superseded by functional MR imaging.

EEGs can also be recorded during somatosensory, visual, and auditory stimuli and while the patient is performing various cognitive tasks. Computers then subtract the baseline electrical activity and generate a printout of that part of the electrical activity directly attributable to the stimulus or the task—the evoked potentials.[198,199] Evoked potentials can also be studied via topographic mapping techniques to better localize the abnormalities. These techniques are particularly useful in unresponsive patients for whom it is impossible to clinically assess cognitive and sensory functions, and in patients under anesthesia. In patients with brain stem disease, both brain stem auditory evoked responses and quantified testing of the blink and masseter reflexes can help localize the functional abnormality to particular portions of the brain stem.[200]

These electrical tests are most helpful in answering the following questions: Is the patient having seizures? How much residual electrical activity is present in this comatose patient's cerebrum? Is this anesthetized patient now having cerebrovascular surgery undergoing damage during the procedure? Are there functional changes in the brain stem not shown by brain-imaging techniques?

In JH, I did not perform functional imaging or electrical testing. His clinical deficit was severe, and morphologic studies (CT) had shown an extensive infarct. Moreover, his vascular lesion was not treatable. Newer MR technologies were not available at the time he was treated.

Question 6: Are There Genetic Abnormalities That Might Clarify the Etiology of the Cerebrovascular Disease and Potentially Guide Treatment of the Patient and Prevention or Management of Relatives?

During the 1990s, there has been a revolution in molecular biology and genetics. Genetic influences clearly play a large influence in determining who will develop strokes and which subtypes of stroke they will have.[201,202] Genetic analysis of mutations has become instrumental in the diagnosis and understanding of some genetic and mitochondrial diseases.[201–204] A number of genetic disorders have been shown to cause abnormal bleeding and hypercoagulability.[151–153] The ensuing years will undoubtedly witness further advances. Pinpointing the genetic etiology and influences on cerebrovascular disease can help the patient's relatives and progeny as well as the patient. I have not included a discussion of molecular biology and genetics in this third edition because the field is still in its infancy. I discuss some specific genetic disorders in Chapter 9 on nonatherosclerotic causes of brain ischemia.

References

1. Caplan LR. Computed Tomography and Stroke. In F McDowell, L Caplan (eds), Cerebrovascular Survey Report for the National Institute of Neurological and Communicative Disorders and Stroke (NINCDS), Washington, D.C. revised. 1985;61–74.
2. von Kummer R, Nolte PN, Schnittger H, et al. Detectability of cerebral hemisphere ischaemic infarcts by CT within 6 hours of stroke. Neuroradiology 1996;38:31–33.
3. Norman D, Price D, Boyd D, et al. Quantitative aspects of computed tomography of the blood and cerebrospinal fluid. Radiology 1977;7:223–228.
4. Caplan LR, Flamm ES, Mohr JP, et al. Lumbar puncture and stroke: a statement for physicians by a committee of the Stroke Council of the American Heart Association. Stroke 1987;18:540A–544A.
5. Patel MR, Edelman RR, Warach S. Detection of hyperacute primary intraparenchymal hemorrhage by magnetic resonance imaging. Stroke 1996;27:2321–2324.
6. Beauchamp NJ, Bryan RN. Neuroimaging of Stroke. In KMA Welch, LR Caplan, DJ Reis, et al. (eds), Primer on Cerebrovascular Diseases. San Diego: Academic Press, 1997;599–611.
7. Meuli RA, Maeder P, Uske A. Magnetic Resonance Imaging. In MD Ginsberg, J Bogousslavsky (eds), Cerebrovascular Disease: Pathophysiology, Diagnosis, and Management. Boston: Blackwell Science, 1998;1265–1291.
8. Brant-Zawadski M, Atkinson D, Detrick M, et al. Fluid-attenuated inversion recovery (FLAIR) for assessment of cerebral infarction: initial clinical experience in 50 patients. Stroke 1996;27:1187–1191.
9. Warach S, Chien D, Li W, Ronthal M, Edelman RR. Fast magnetic resonance diffusion-weighted imaging of acute human stroke. Neurology 1992;42:1717–1723.
10. Warach S, Gaa J, Siewert B, Wielopolski P, Edelman RR. Acute human stroke studied by whole brain echo planar diffusion-weighted nagnetic resonance imaging. Ann Neurol 1995;37:231–141.
11. Dul K, Drayer BP. CT and MR Imaging of Intracerebral Hemorrhage. In CS Kase, LR Caplan. Intracerebral Hemorrhage. Boston: Butterworth-Heinemann, 1994;73–93.
12. Mohr JP, Biller J, Hilal SK, et al. Magnetic resonance versus computed tomographic imaging in acute stroke. Stroke 1995;26:807–812.
13. Bryan RN, Levy LM, Whitlow WD, et al. Diagnosis of acute cerebral infarction: comparison of CT and MR imaging. Am J Neuroradiol 1991;12:611–620.
14. Becker H, Desch H, Hacker H, et al. CT fogging effect with ischemic cerebral infarcts. Neuroradiol 1978;18:185–192.
15. Nicolaides AN, Papadakis K, Grigg M, et al. Amaurosis Fugax—Data from CT Scans. In E Bernstein (ed), Amaurosis Fugax. New York: Springer,1988:200–226.
16. Caplan LR. Significance of Unexpected (Silent) Brain Infarcts. In LR Caplan, EG Shifrin, AN Nicolaides, WS Moore (eds), Cerebrovascular Ischaemia, Investigation and Management. London: Med-Orion, 1996;423–433.
17. Brott T, Broderick J, Kothari R, et al. Early hemorrhage growth in patients with intracerebral hemorrhage. Stroke 1997;28:1–5.
18. Adams HP Jr, Kassell NF, Turner JC, et al. CT and clinical correlations in recent aneurysmal subarachnoid hemorrhage: a preliminary report of the Cooperative Aneurysm Study. Neurology 1983;33:981–988.
19. Fishman RA. Cerebrospinal Fluid in Cerebrovascular Disorders. In JH Barnett, JP Mohr, BM Stein, FJ Yatsu (eds), Stroke: Pathophysiology, Diagnosis, and Management. New York: Churchill Livingstone, 1986:109–117.
20. Van der Meulen JP. Cerebrospinal fluid xanthrochromia: an objective index. Neurology 1966;16:170–178.
21. Soderstrom CE. Diagnostic significance of CSF spectrophotometry and computer tomography in cerebrovascular disease: a comparative study in 231 cases. Stroke 1977;8:606–612.
22. Lee MC, Heaney LM, Jacobson RL, et al. Cerebrospinal fluid in cerebral hemorrhage and infarction. Stroke 1975;6:638–641.
23. Schluep M, Bogousslavsky J. Cerebrospinal Fluid in Cerebrovascular Disease. In MD Ginsberg, J Bogousslavsky (eds), Cerebrovascular Disease: Pathophysiology, Diagnosis, and Management. Boston: Blackwell Science, 1998;2:1221–1226.
24. Lovblad K-O, Laubach H-J, Baird AE, et al. Clinical experience with diffusion-weighted MR in patients with acute stroke. AJNR Am J Neuroradiol 1998;19:1061–1066.
25. Yamamoto H, Bogousslavsky J. Mechanisms of second and further strokes. J Neurol Neurosurg Psychiatry 1998;64:771–776.
26. Caplan LR. Reperfusion of Ischemic Brain: Why and Why Not? In W Hacke, G del Zoppo, M Hirschberg (eds), Thrombolytic Therapy in Acute Stroke. Berlin: Springer, 1991;36–45.
27. Ropper AH. Lateral displacement of the brain and level of consciousness in patients with an acute hemispheral mass. N Engl J Med 1986;314:953–958.
28. Ropper AH. A preliminary MRI study of the geometry of brain displacement and level of consciousness with acute intracranial masses. Neurology 1989;39:622–627.
29. Eckert B, Zeumer H. Brain Computed Tomography. In MD Ginsberg, J Bogousslavsky (eds), Cerebrovascular Disease: Pathophysiology, Diagnosis, and Management. Boston: Blackwell Science, 1998;2:1241–1264.
30. Weisberg LA, Stazio A, Shamsnia M, et al. Nontraumatic parenchymal brain hemorrhages. Medicine (Baltimore) 1990;69:277–295.
31. Kase CS. Cerebral Amyloid Angiopathy. In CS Kase, LR Caplan (eds), Intracerebral Hemorrhage. Boston: Butterworth–Heinemann, 1994;179–200.
32. Hauw J-J, Seilhean D, Duyckaerts CH. Cerebral Amyloid Angiopathy. In MD Ginsberg, J Bogousslavsky (eds), Cerebrovascular Disease: Pathophysiology, Diagnosis, and Management. Boston: Blackwell, 1998;1772–1794.
33. Kase C, Robinson R, Stein R, et al. Anticoagulant-related intracerebral hemorrhages. Neurology 1985;35:943–948.
34. Kase CS. Bleeding Disorders. In CS Kase, LR Caplan (eds), Intracerebral Hemorrhage. Boston: Butterworth–Heinemann, 1994;117–151.
35. Weisberg L. Computed tomography in aneurysmal subarachnoid hemorrhage. Neurology 1979;29:802–808.

36. Adams H, Kassell N, Torner J, et al. CT and clinical correlations in recent aneurysmal subarachnoid hemorrhage: a preliminary report of the cooperative aneurysm study. Neurology 1983;33:981–988.

37. van Gijn J, van Dongen K. Computerized tomography in subarachnoid hemorrhage: difference between patients with and without an aneurysm on angiography. Neurology 1980;30:538–539.

38. van Gijn J, van Dongen KJ, Vermeulen M, et al. Perimesencephalic hemorrhage: a non-aneurysmal and benign form of subarachnoid hemorrhage. Neurology 1985;35:493–497.

39. Rinkel GJ, Wijdicks EF, Vermeulen M, et al. Outcome in perimesencephalic (non-aneurysmal) subarachnoid hemorrhage: a follow-up study in 37 patients. Neurology 1990;40:1130–1132.

40. Kistler JP, Crowell R, Davis K, et al. The relation of cerebral vasospasm to the extent and location of subarachnoid blood visualized by CT scan: a prospective study. Neurology 1983;33:424–437.

41. Mohsen F, Pominis S, Illingworth R. Prediction of delayed cerebral ischemia after subarachnoid hemorrhage by computed tomography. J Neurol Neurosurg Psychiatry 1984;47:1197–1202.

42. O'Donnell TF, Erdoes L, Mackey W, et al. Correlation of B-mode ultrasound imaging and arteriography with pathologic findings at carotid endarterectomy. Arch Surg 1985;120:443–449.

43. Schenk EA, Bond G, Aretz T, et al. Multicenter validation study of real-time ultrasonography, arteriography and pathology: pathologic evaluation of carotid endarterectomy specimens. Stroke 1988;19:289–296.

44. Hennerici M, Freund H-J. Efficacy of CW-Doppler and duplex system examinations for the evaluation of extracranial carotid disease. J Clin Ultrasound 1984;12:155–161.

45. Gronholdt M-LM, Nordestgaard BG, Nielsen TG, Sillesen H. Echolucent carotid artery plaques are associated with elevated levels of fasting and postprandial triglyceride-rich lipoproteins. Stroke 1996;27:2166–2172.

46. Geroulakos G, Hobson RW, Nicolaides AW. Ultrasonic Carotid Plaque Morphology. In LR Caplan, EG Shifrin, AN Nicolaides, WS Moore (eds), Cerebrovascular Ischaemia, Investigation and Management. London: MedOrion, 1996;25–32.

47. von Reutern GM, von Budingen HJ. Ultrasound diagnosis of cerebrovascular disease, New York: Georg Thieme, 1993.

48. Bartels E. Color-coded Duplex ultrasonography of the cerebral vessels. Stuttgart: Schattauer, 1998

49. Steinke W, Kloetzsch C, Hennerici M. Carotid artery disease assessed by color Doppler flow imaging: correlation with standard Doppler sonography and angiography. AJNR Am J Neuroradiol 1990;11:259–266.

50. Tegeler CH, Kremkau FW, Hitchings LP. Color velocity imaging: introduction to a new ultrasound technology. J Neuroimaging 1991;1:85–90.

51. Steinke W, Kloetzsch CH, Hennerici M. Symptomatic and asymptomatic high-grade carotid stenosis in Doppler color-flow imaging. Neurology 1992;42:131–138.

52. Steinke W, Ries S, Artemis N, et al. Power Doppler imaging of carotid artery stenosis. Comparison with color Doppler flow imaging and angiography. Stroke 1997;28:1981–1987.

53. Griewing B, Doherty C, Kessler CH. Power Doppler ultrasound examination of the intracerebral and extracerebral vasculature. J Neuroimaging 1996;6:32–35.

54. Aaslid R. Transcranial Doppler Sonography. New York: Springer, 1986.

55. Babikian VL, Wechsler LR (eds). Transcranial Doppler Ultrasonography. St. Louis: CV Mosby, 1993.

56. Otis SM, Ringelstein EB. The Transcranial Doppler Examination: Principles and Applications of Transcranial Doppler Sonography. In CH Tegeler, VL Babikian, CR Gomez (eds), Neurosonology. St Louis: Mosby, 1996;113–128.

57. Caplan LR, Brass LM, DeWitt LD, et al. Transcranial Doppler ultrasound: present status. Neurology 1990;40:696–700.

58. Hennerici M, Rautenberg W, Sitzer G, et al. Transcranial Doppler ultrasound for the assessment of intracranial arterial flow velocity. Surg Neurol 1987;27:439–448.

59. Hennerici M, Rautenberg W, Schwartz A. Transcranial Doppler ultrasound for the assessment of intracranial arterial flow velocity: II. Evaluation of intracranial arterial disease. Surg Neurol 1987;27:523–532.

60. Burns PN. Overview of echo-enhanced vascular ultrasound imaging for clinical diagnosis in neurosonology. J Neuroimaging 1997;7(suppl 1):S2–S14.

61. Bogdahn U, Becker G, Schlief R, et al. Contrast-enhanced transcranial color-coded real-time sonography. Stroke 1993;24:676–684.

62. Delcker A, Turowski B. Diagnostic value of three-dimensional transcranial contrast duplex sonography. J Neuroimaging 1997;7:139–144.

63. Caplan LR. Posterior circulation disease. Clinical findings, diagnosis, and management. Boston: Blackwell, 1996.

64. Sliwka U, Rautenberg W. Multimodal ultrasound versus angiography for imaging the vertebrobasilar circulation. J Neuroimag 1998;8:182.

65. Piepgras A, Schmiedek P, Leinsinger G, et al. A simple test to assess cerebrovascular reserve capacity using transcranial Doppler sonography and acetazolamide. Stroke 1990;21:1306–1311.

66. Markus HS. Transcranial Doppler detection of circulating cerebral emboli, a review. Stroke 1993;24:1246–1250.

67. Markus HS, Harrison MJ. Microembolic signal detection using ultrasound. Stroke 1995;26:1517–1519.

68. Tong DC, Albers GW. Transcranial Doppler-detected microemboli in patients with acute stroke. Stroke 1995;26:1588–1592.

69. Sliwka U, Job F-P, Wissuwa D, et al. Occurrence of transcranial Doppler high-intensity transient signals in patients with potential cardiac sources of embolism, a prospective study. Stroke 1995;26:2067–2070.

70. Daffertshofer M, Ries S, Schminke U, Hennerici M. High-intensity transient signals in patients with cerebral ischemia. Stroke 1996;27:1844–1849.

71. Sliwka U, Lingnau A, Stohlmann W-D, et al. Prevalence and time course of microembolic signals in patients with acute strokes, a prospective study. Stroke 1997;28:358–363.

72. Teague SM, Sharma MK. Detection of paradoxical cerebral echo contrast embolization by transcranial Doppler ultrasound. Stroke 1991;22:740–745.

73. Chimowitz MI, Nemec JJ, Marwick TH, et al. Transcranial Doppler ultrasound identifies patients with right-to-

left cardiac or pulmonary shunts. Neurology 1991;41: 1902–1904.

74. Albert A, Muller HR, Hetzel A. Optimized transcranial Doppler technique for the diagnosis of cardiac right-to-left shunts. J Neuroimaging 1997;7:159–163.

75. Di Tullio M, Sacco RL, Venketasubramanian N, et al. Comparison of diagnostic techniques for the detection of a patent foramen ovale in stroke patients. Stroke 1993;24:1020–1024.

76. Klotzsch C, Janzen G, Berlit P. Transesophageal echocardiography and contrast-TCD in the detection of a patent foramen ovale. Experiences with 111 patients. Neurology 1994;44:1603–1606.

77. Culebras A, Leeson M, Cacayorin E, et al. Computed tomographic evaluation of cervical carotid plaque complications. Stroke 1985;16:425–431.

78. Essig M, von Kummer R, Egelhof T, Winter R, Sartor K. Vascular MR contrast enhancement in cerebrovascular disease. AJNR Am J Neuroradiol 1996;17:887–894.

79. Lazar EB, Russell EJ, Cohen BA, Brody B, Levy RM. Contrast-enhanced MR of cerebral arteritis: intravascular enhancement related to flow stasis within areas of focal arterial ectasia. AJNR Am J Neuroradiol 1992;13:271–276.

80. Edelman RR, Mattle HP, Atkinson DJ, et al. MR angiography. AJR Am J Roentgenol 1990;154:937–946.

81. Johnson BA, Heiserman JE, Drayer BP, Keller PJ. Intracranial MR angiography: its role in the integrated approach to brain infarction. AJNR Am J Neuroradiol 1994;15:901–908.

82. Gillard JH, Oliverio PJ, Barker PB, et al. MR angiography in acute cerebral ischemia of the anterior circulation: a preliminary report. AJNR Am J Neuroradiol 1997;18:343–350.

83. Yano T, Kodama T, Suzuki Y, Watanabe K. Gadolinium-enhanced 3D time-of-flight MR angiography. Acta Radiol 1997;38:47–54.

84. Leclerc X, Martinat P, Godefroy O et al. Contrast-enhanced three-dimensional fast imaging with steady-state precession (FISP) MR angiography of supraaortic vessels: preliminary results. AJNR Am J Neuroradiol 1998;19:1405–1413.

85. Levi CR, Mitchell A, Fitt G, Donnan GA. The accuracy of magnetic resonance angiography in the assessment of extracranial carotid artery occlusive disease. Cerebrovasc Dis 1996;6:231–236.

86. Mitti RL, Broderick M, Carpenter JP, et al. Blinded-reader comparison of magnetic resonance angiography and Duplex ultrasonography for carotid artery bifurcation stenosis. Stroke 1994;25:4–10.

87. Quereshi A, Isa A, Cinnamon J, et al. Magnetic resonance angiography in patients with brain infarction. J Neuroimaging 1998;8:65–70.

88. Caplan LR, Wolpert SM. Angiography in patients with occlusive cerebrovascular disease: a stroke neurologist and neuroradiologist's views. AJNR Am J Neuroradiol 1991;12:593–601.

89. Cumming MJ, Morrow IM. Carotid artery stenosis: a prospective comparison of CT angiography and conventional angiography. AJR Am J Roentgoenol 1994;163:517–523.

90. Dillon EH, van Leeuwen MS, Fernandez MA, et al. CT angiography: applications to the evaluation of carotid artery stenosis. Radiology 1993;189:211–219.

91. Leclerc X, Godefroy O, Pruvo JP, Leys D. Computed tomographic angiography for the evaluation of carotid artery stenosis. Stroke 1995;26:1577–1581.

92. Wong KS, Liang EY, Lam WWM, et al. Spiral computed tomography angiography in the assessment of middle cerebral artery occlusive disease. J Neurol Neurosurg Psychiatry 1995;59:537–539.

93. von Kummer R, Weber J. Brain and vascular imaging in acute ischemic stroke: the potential of computed tomography. Neurology 1997;49(suppl 4):S52–S55.

94. Na DG, Byun HS, Lee KH, et al. Acute occlusion of the middle cerebral artery:early evaluation with triphasic helical CT — preliminary results. Radiology 1998;207:113–122.

95. Caplan LR, Wolpert SM. Conventional Cerebral Angiography in Occlusive Cerebrovascular Disease. In JH Wood (ed), Cerebral Blood Flow: Physiological and Clinical Aspects. New York: McGraw-Hill, 1987;356–384.

96. Akers DL, Markowitz IA, Kerstein MD. The value of aortic arch study in the evaluation of cerebrovascular insufficiency. Am J Surg 1987;154:230–232.

97. DeRook FA, Comess KA, Albers GW, Popp RL. Transesophageal echocardiography in the evaluation of stroke. Ann Intern Med 1992;117:922-932.

98. Grullon C, Alam M, Rosman HS, et al. Transesophageal echocardiography in unselected patients with focal cerebral ischemia: when is it useful? Cerebrovasc Dis 1994;4:139–145.

99. Daniel WG, Mugge A. Transesophageal echocardiography. N Engl J Med 1995;332:1268–1279.

100. Horowitz DR, Tuhrim S, Weinberger J, et al. Transesophageal echocardiography: diagnostic and clinical applications in the evaluation of the stroke patient. J Stroke Cerebrovasc Dis 1997;6:332–336.

101. Caplan LR. Of birds and nests and cerebral emboli. Rev Neurol 1991;147:265–273.

102. Caplan LR, Brain Embolism. In LR Caplan, M Chimowitz, JW Hurst. Practical Clinical Neurocardiology. New York: Marcel Dekker, 1999;35–185.

103. Johnson LL, Pohost GM. Nuclear cardiology. In RC Schlant, RW Alexander (eds), Hurst's: The Heart (8th ed). New York: McGraw-Hill, 1994;2281–2323.

104. Weinberger J, Azhar S, Danisi F, et al. A new noninvasive technique for imaging atherosclerotic plaque in the aortic arch of stroke patients by transcutaneous real-time B-mode ultrasonography. Stroke 1998;29:673–676.

105. Lockwood K, Sherman D, Gerza C, et al. Detection of left atrial thrombi by cardiac CT. Neurology 1984;34(1):205.

106. Helgason C, Chomka E, Louie E, et al. The potential role for ultrafast cardiac computed tomography in patients with stroke. Stroke 1989;20:465–472.

107. Ezekowitz M, Wilson D, Smith E, et al. Comparison of indium 111 platelet scintigraphy and two-dimensional echocardiography in the diagnosis of left ventricular thrombi. N Engl J Med 1982;306:1509–1513.

108. Rokey R, Rolak LA, Harati Y, et al. Coronary artery disease in patients with cerebrovascular disease: a prospective study. Ann Neurol 1985;16:50–53.

109. Gibbons RJ, Zinsmeister AR, Miller TD. Supine exercise electrocardiography compared with exercise radionuclide angiography in non-invasive identification of severe coronary artery diseases. Ann Intern Med 1990;112:743–749.

110. Sirna S, Biller J, Skorton DJ, et al. Cardiac evaluation of the patient with stroke. Stroke 1990;21:14–23.

111. Verani M, Rokey R. Coronary Artery Disease: Diagnosis and Clinical Features. In: L Rolak, R Rokey (eds), Coronary and Cerebral Vascular Disease: a Practical Guide. Mt. Kisco, NY: Futura, 1990:19–49.

112. DiPasquale G, Andreoli A, Carini G, et al. Non-invasive screening for silent ischemic heart disease in patients with cerebral ischemia: use of dipyridamole-thallium myocardial imaging. Cerebrovasc Dis 1991;1:31–37.

113. Lieb WE, Flaharty PM, Sergott RC, et al. Color Doppler imaging provides accurate assessment of orbital blood flow in occlusive carotid artery disease. Opthalmology 1991;98:548–552.

114. Hedges TR. Ocular Ischemia. In Caplan LR (ed), Brain Ischemia. Basic Concepts and Clinical Relevance. London: Springer, 1995:61–73.

115. Levine SR, Brust JCM, Futrell N, et al. A comparative study of the cerebrovascular complications of cocaine—alkaloidal versus hydrochloride—a review. Neurology 1991;41:1173–1177.

116. Alberico RA, Patel M, Casey S, et al. Evaluation of the circle of Willis with three-dimensional CT angiography in patients with suspected intracranial aneurysms. AJNR Am J Neuroradiol 1995;16:1571–1578.

117. Sekhar L, Wechsler L, Yonas H, et al. Value of transcranial Doppler examination in the diagnosis of cerebral vasospasm after subarachnoid hemorrhage. Neurosurgery 1988;22:813–821.

118. Sloan MA, Haley EC, Kassell NF, et al. Sensitivity and specificity of transcranial Doppler ultrasonography in the diagnosis of vasospasm following subarachnoid hemorrhage. Neurology 1989;39:1514–1518.

119. Pollock S, Tsitsopoulas P, Harrison M. The effect of hematocrit on cerebral perfusion and clinical status following occlusion in the gerbil. Stroke 1982;13:167–170.

120. Harrison M, Pollock S, Kindoll B, et al. Effect of hematocrit on carotid stenosis and cerebral infarction. Lancet 1981;2:114–115.

121. Thomas D, duBoulay G, Marshall J, et al. Effect of hematocrit on cerebral blood flow in man. Lancet 1977;2:941–943.

122. Tohgi H, Yamanouchi H, Murakami M, et al. Importance of the hematocrit as a risk factor in cerebral infarction. Stroke 1978;9:369–374.

123. Grotta J, Ackerman R, Correia J, et al. Whole-blood viscosity parameters and cerebral blood flow. Stroke 1982;13:296-298.

124. Thomas D. Whole blood viscosity and cerebral blood flow. Stroke 1982;13:285–287.

125. Kee DB Jr, Wood JH. Influence of blood rheology on cerebral circulation. In: Wood JH, (ed). Cerebral Blood Flow: Physiological and Clinical Aspects. New York: McGraw-Hill, 1987;173–185.

126. Brass LM, Prohovnik I, Pavlakis SG, et al. Middle cerebral artery blood velocity and cerebral blood flow in sickle cell disease. Stroke 1991;22:27–30.

127. Adams RJ, Nichols FT, Figueroa R, et al. Transcranial Doppler correlation with cerebral angiography in sisckle cell disease. Stroke 1992;23:1073–1077.

128. Adams RJ, McVie V, Nichols FT, et al. The use of transcranial ultrasonography to predict stroke in sickle cell disease. N Engl J Med 1992;326:605–610.

129. Adams RJ, McKie V, Hsu L, et al. Prevention of a first stroke by transfusion in children with sickle cell anemia and abnormal results on transcranial Doppler ultrasonography. N Engl J Med 1998;339:5–11.

130. Mercuri M, Bond MG, Evans G, et al. Leukocyte count and carotid atherosclerosis. Stroke 1991;22:134.

131. Wu K. Platelet hyperaggregability and thrombosis in patients with thrombocythemia. Ann Intern Med 1978;88:7–11.

132. Coull BM, Goodnight SH. Antiphospholipid antibodies, prethrombotic states, and stroke. Stroke 1990;21:1370–1374.

133. Bailey DP, Coull BM, Goodnight SH. Neurological disease associated with antiphospholipid antibodies. Ann Neurol 1989;25:221–227.

134. Levine SR, Welch KMA. The spectrum of neurologic disease associated with antiphospholipid antibodies: lupus anticoagulants, and anticardiolipin antibodies. Arch Neurol 1987;44:876–883.

135. Atkinson JLD, Sundt TM, Kazmier FJ, et al. Heparin-induced thrombocytopenia and thrombosis in ischemic stroke. Mayo Clin Proc 1988;63:353–361.

136. Uchyama S, Takeuchi M, Osawa M, et al. Platelet function tests in thrombotic cerebrovascular disorders. Stroke 1983;14:511–517.

137. Helgason CH, Bolin KM, Hoff JA, et al. Development of aspirin resistance in persons with previous ischemic stroke. Stroke 1994;25:2331–2336.

138. Ludlam CA. Evidence for the platelet specificity of beta-thromboglobulin and studies on its plasma concentration in healthy individuals. Br J Haematol 1979;41:271–278.

139. Fisher M, Francis R. Altered coagulation in cerebral ischemia: platelet, thrombin, and plasmin activity. Arch Neurol 1990;47:1075–1079.

140. Qizilbash N, Duffy S, Prentice CRM, et al. Von Willebrand factor and risk of ischemic stroke. Neurology 1997;49:1552–1556.

141. Weiss EJ, Bray PF, Tayback M, et al. A polymorphism of a platelet glycoprotein receptor as an inherited risk factor for coronary thrombosis. N Engl J Med 1996;334:1090–1094.

142. Kannel WB, Wolf PA, Castelli WP, et al. Fibrinogen and risk of cardiovascular disease. JAMA 1987;258:1183–1186.

143. Coull BM, Beamer NB, deGarmo PL, et al. Chronic blood hyperviscosity in subjects with acute stroke, transient ischemic attack, and risk factors for stroke. Stroke 1991; 22:162–168.

144. Beamer N, Coull BM, Sexton G, et al. Fibrinogen and the albumin-globulin ratio in recurrent stroke. Stroke 1993;24:1133–1139.

145. Ernst E, Resch KL. Fibrinogen as a cardiovascular risk factor: a meta-analysis and review of the literature. Ann Intern Med 1993;118:956–963.

146. The Ancrod Stroke Study Investigators. Ancrod for the treatment of acute ischemic brain infarction. Stroke 1994;25:1755–1759.

147. Atkinson RP. Ancrod in the treatment of acute ischemic stroke. a review of clinical data. Cerebrovasc Dis 1998;8(suppl 1):23–28.

148. Radack K, Deck C, Huster G. Dietary supplementation with low-dose fish oils lowers fibrinogen levels: a randomized double-blind controlled study. Ann Intern Med 1989;111:757–758.

149. Lechner H, Walzl M, Walzl B, et al. H.E.L.P. Application in Cerebrovascular Disease. In E Ernst, W Koenig, GDO Lowe, TW Meade (eds), Fibrinogen: a New Cardiovascular Risk Factor. Vienna: Blackwell, 1992;408–412.

150. Dahlback B, Carlsson M, Svensson PJ. Familial thrombophilia due to a previously unrecognized mechanism characterized by poor anticoagulant response to activated protein C: prediction of a cofactor to activated protein C. Proc Natl Acad Sci U S A 1993;90:1004–1008.

151. Zoller B, Dahlback B. Linkage between inherited resistance to activated protein C and factor V gene mutation in venous thrombosis. Lancet 1994;343:1536–1538.

152. Ridker PM, Miletich JP, Stampfer MJ, et al. Factor V Leiden and risks of recurrent idiopathic venous thromboembolism. Circulation 1997;95:1777–1782.

153. Poort SR, Rosendaal FR, Reitsma PH, et al. A common genetic variation in the 3' untranslated region of the prothrombin gene is associated with elevated prothrombin levels and an increase in venous thrombosis. Blood 1996;88:3698–3703.

154. Martinelli I, Sacchi E, Landi G, et al. High risk of cerebral-vein thrombosis in carriers of a prothrombin-gene mutation and in users of oral contraceptives. N Engl J Med 1998;338:1793–1797.

155. Kosik KS, Furie B. Thrombotic stroke associated with elevated plasma Factor VIII. Arch Neurol 1980;8:435–437.

156. Estol C, Pessin MS, DeWitt LD, et al. Stroke and increased Factor VIII activity. Neurology 1989;39:225.

157. Markus HS, Hambley H. Neurology and the blood: haematological abnormalities in ischaemic stroke. J Neurol Neurosurg Psychiatry 1998;64:150–159.

158. Feinberg WM, Cornell ES, Nightingale SD, et al. Relationship between prothrombin activation fragment F1.2 and International Normalized Ratio in patients with atrial fibrillation. Stroke 1997;28:1101–1106.

159. Feinberg WM, Bruck DC, Ring ME, et al. Hemostatic markers in acute stroke. Stroke 1989;20:592–597.

160. Toghi H, Kawashima M, Tamura K, et al. Coagulation-fibrinolysis abnormalities in acute and chronic phases of cerebral thrombosis and embolism. Stroke 1990;21:1663–1667.

161. Jeppeson LL, Jorgensen HS, Nakayama H, et al. Tissue plasminogen activator is elevated in women with ischemic stroke. J Stroke Cerebrovasc Dis 1998;7:187–191.

162. Feinberg WM. Coagulation. In LR Caplan (ed), Brain Ischemia. Basic Concepts and Clinical Relevance. London: Springer, 1995;85–96.

163. Levine SR, Salowich-Palm L, Sawaya K, et al. IgG anticardiolipin antibody titer >40GPL and the risk of subsequent thrombo-occlusive events and death. A prospective cohort study. Stroke 1997;28:1660–1665.

164. Myers R, Yamaguchi S. Nervous system effects of cardiac arrest in monkeys. Arch Neurol 1977;34:65–74.

165. Pulsinelli W, Waldman S, Rawlinson D, et al. Hyperglycemia converts ischemic neuronal damage into brain infarction. Neurology 1982;32:1239–1246.

166. Plum F. What causes infarction in ischemic brain? Neurology 1983;33:222–233.

167. Pulsinelli W, Levy D, Sigsbel B, et al. Increased damage after ischemic stroke in patients with hyperglycemia with

168. Walker G, Williamson P, Ravich R, et al. Hypercalcemia associated with cerebral vasospasm causing infarction. J Neurol Neurosurg Psychiatry 1980;43:464–467.

169. Gorelick PB, Caplan LR. Calcium, hypercalcemia, and stroke. Current concepts of cerebrovascular disease. Stroke 1985;20:13–17.

170. Siesjo B, Kristian T. Cell Calcium Homeostasis and Calcium-Related Ischemic Damage. In KMA Welch, LR Caplan, DJ Reis, et al. (eds), Primer on Cerebrovascular Diseases. San Diego: Academic Press, 1997;172–178.

171. Lassen NA. Pathophysiology of brain ischemia as it relates to the therapy of acute ischemic stroke. Clin Neuropharmacol 1990;13:51–58.

172. Frackowiak R. PET CBF Investigations of Stroke. In KMA Welch, LR Caplan, DJ Reis, B Siesjo, B Weir (eds), Primer on Cerebrovascular Diseases. San Diego: Academic Press, 1997;636–640.

173. Phelps M, Mazziotta J, Huang S. Study of cerebral function with positron computed tomography. J Cereb Blood Flow Metab 1982;2:113–162.

174. Baron JC, Bousser M, Rey A, et al. Reversal of focal misery-perfusion syndrome by extra-intracranial arterial bypass in hemodynamic cerebral ischemia. Stroke 1981;12:454–459.

175. Lassen N. The luxury perfusion syndrome and its possible relation to acute metabolic acidosis localized within the lesion. Lancet 1966;2:1113–1115.

176. Marchal G, Furlan M, Beaudouin V, et al. Early spontaneous hyperperfusion after stroke: a marker of favorable tissue outcome. Brain 1996;119:409–419.

177. Cao Y. Functional Magnetic Resonance Imaging in the Investigation of Brain Recovery and Reorganization after Ischemic Infarct. In KMA Welch, LR Caplan, DJ Reis et al. (eds), Primer on Cerebrovascular Diseases. San Diego: Academic Press, 1997;640–644.

178. Belliveau JW, Kennedy DN, McKinstry RC, et al. Functional mapping of the human visual cortex by magnetic resonance imaging. Science 1991;254:716–719.

179. Therapeutics and Technology Subcommittee of the American Academy of Neurology. Assessment of brain SPECT. Neurology 1996;46:278–285.

180. Masdeu JC, Brass LM. SPECT imaging of stroke. J Neuroimaging 1995;5:514–522.

181. Caplan LR. Question-driven technology assessment: SPECT as an example. Neurology 1991;41:187–191.

182. Fayad P, Brass LM. Single photon emission computed tomography in cerebrovascular disease. Stroke 1991;22:950–954.

183. Lassen N, Ingvar D, Skinhoj E. Brain function and blood flow. Sci Am 1978;239:62–71.

184. Obrist W, Thompson H Jr, Wang H, et al. Regional cerebral blood flow estimated by ^{133}xenon inhalation. Stroke 1975;6:245–250.

185. Yonas H, Wolfson SK, Gur D, et al. Clinical experience with the use of xenon-enhanced CT blood flow mapping in cerebral vascular disease. Stroke 1984;15:443–450.

186. Yonas H, Darby JM, Marks EC, Durham SR, Maxwell C. CBF measured by Xe-CT: approach to analysis and normal values. J Cereb Blood Flow Metab 1991;11:716–725.

or without established diabetes mellitus. Am J Med 1983;74:540–544.

187. Firlik A, Rubin G, Yonas H, Wechsler LR. Relation between cerebral blood flow and neurologic deficit resolution in acute ischemic stroke. Neurology 1998;51:177–182.
188. Warach S, Li W, Ronthal M, Edelman RR. Acute cerebral ischemia: evaluation with dynamic contrast-enhanced MR imaging and MR angiography. Radiology 1992;182:41–47.
189. Fisher M, Prichard JW, Warach S. New magnetic resonance techniques for acute ischemic stroke. JAMA 1995;274:908–911.
190. Rother J, Guckel F, Neff W, et al. Assessment of regional cerebral blood flow volume in acute human stroke by use of a single-slice dynamic susceptibility contrast-enhanced magnetic resonance imaging. Stroke 1996;27:1088–1093.
191. Sorensen AG, Buonanno F, Gonzalez RG, et al. Hyperacute stroke: evaluation with combined multisection diffusion-weighted and hemodynamically weighted echoplanar MR imaging. Radiology 1996;199:391–401.
192. Duijn JH, Matson GB, Maudsley AA, et al. Human brain infarction: proton MR spectroscopy. Radiology 1992;183:711–718.
193. Castillo M, Kwock L, Mukherij SK. Clinical applications of Proton MR spectroscopy. AJNR Am J Neuroradiol 1996;17:1–15.
194. Pavlakis SG, Kingsley PB, Kaplan GP, et al. Magnetic resonance spectroscopy. Use in monitoring MELAS treatment. Arch Neurol 1998;55:849–852.
195. Belliveau JW, Cohen MS, Weisskoff R, et al. Functional studies of the human brain using high-speed magnetic resonance imaging. J Neuroimaging 1991;1:36–41.
196. Humberstone MR, Sawle GV. Functional magnetic resonance imaging in clinical neurology. Eur Neurol 1996;36:117–124.
197. Caplan LR, Young R. EEG findings in certain lacunar syndromes. Neurology 1972;22:403.
198. Nuwer MR, Jordan SE, Ahn SS. Evaluation of stroke using EEG frequency analysis and topographic mapping. Neurology 1987; 37:1153–1159.
199. Duffy FH. Clinical value of topographic mapping and quantified neurophysiology. Arch Neurol 1989;46:1133–1134.
200. Tettenborn B, Caplan LR, Krämer G, Hopf H. Electrophysiology in Posterior Circulation Disease. In R Berguer, LR Caplan (eds), Vertebrobasilar Arterial Disease. St. Louis: Quality Medical Publishing, 1991:124–129.
201. Natowicz M, Kelley RI. Mendelian etiologies of stroke. Ann Neurol 1987;22:175–192.
202. Massa SM. An update on genetic influences on stroke. J Neurovasc Dis 1998;3:109–116.
203. Joutel A, Corpechot C, Ducros, et al. Notch 3 mutations in CADASIL, a hereditary adult-onset condition causing stroke and dementia. Nature 1996;383:707–710.
204. Penn AMW, Lee JWK, Thuiller P, et al. MELAS syndrome with mitochondrial tRNA Leu(UUR) mutation: correlation of clinical state, nerve conduction, and muscle 31P magnetic resonance spectroscopy during treatment with nicotinamide and riboflavin. Neurology 1992;42: 2147–2152.

Chapter 5

Treatment

Some men see things as they are and say Why? I dream things that never were and say Why not?

—George Bernard Shaw

The 1990s can be legitimately thought of as the decade during which stroke theraputics seemed to finally get its just due. Advances in diagnostic technology made it possible to quickly and safely determine the cause of most strokes. The methodology of randomized therapeutic trials progressed as researchers and physicians began to systematically study various treatments. In this chapter, I introduce the general underlying principles of treatment and outline the types of therapy available. Factors that influence treatment and various therapeutic strategies are also discussed. More specific treatments for patients with individual vascular pathologies and mechanisms (e.g., stenosis of an internal carotid artery [ICA], cardiac-origin embolism, and cerebral venous sinus thrombosis) are considered in Part II of this book.

Past Failure to Generate Useful Therapeutic Data

Few therapies have been scientifically studied and thoroughly investigated in patients with particular stroke subtypes. However, lack of certainty of effectiveness is no excuse for therapeutic nihilism. As with other illnesses, physicians should select the best treatment available based on their own experience, the reported and shared advice and experience of others, and on their knowledge of basic pathophysiology. Stroke therapeutics have lagged far behind advances in the basic pathology,

pathophysiology, and diagnosis of stroke syndromes. The war against stroke has been impeded by bad strategy, insufficient ammunition and soldiers, and a militia with inadequate interest and training. Solid therapeutic information is now emerging from randomized trials of various medical and surgical therapeutic strategies.

Bad Strategy

Treatments have traditionally been evaluated in large groups of patients lumped together according to the tempo of the stroke and the presence or extent of brain damage. These groups include (1) transient ischemic attacks (TIAs), (2) minor stroke, (3) reversible ischemic neurologic deficit (RIND), (4) stroke in progress, and (5) completed stroke.[1]

Although these designations were perhaps of some use in the past, there is no rational reason to continue to rely heavily on them. After all, these terms concern only two factors—the time-sequenced course of the neurologic symptoms at that particular moment and the present, clinically detected degree of damage. The transient nature of a TIA may be the result of (1) relief of ischemia before significant neuronal damage, (2) small size of infarction, or (3) rapid compensation of function by other neuronal regions. In many patients with clinical TIAs and normal neurologic examinations, computed tomography (CT) and magnetic resonance imaging (MRI) show infarcts compatible with the clinical symptoms.[2] Classification of patients often changes with time; today's stroke is yesterday's TIA. To designate a stroke as completed implies an ability to infallibly predict the future. In fact, TIA, RIND, and completed stroke all share a high, relatively comparable risk of future stroke.[1–5] In other branches of medicine, physicians do not treat time courses. What would a gastroenterologist say when asked about treatment for transient or persistent abdominal pain? He or she would probably ask, "What is causing the stomach pain?" Physicians should not treat time courses but rather treat patients with particular pathologic and pathophysiologic problems. None of the time courses is specific for any single pathology or pathophysiology. In fact, most vascular pathologies and stroke mechanisms have the potential to produce most of the time course designations mentioned. Stenosis of the ICA, vasculopathy underlying lacunar infarction, and cardiogenic brain embolism can all cause TIAs, RIND, and progressive and completed strokes.

Investigators designate groups in an irrational manner and naively seek single remedies or cures for these groups. Even individual stroke mechanism groups, such as thrombosis and embolism, are heterogeneous designations that can join together fruits as divergent as grapes, watermelons, grapefruits, and mangoes. Does it make sense for divergent causes to respond the same way to a single treatment? If TIAs have many underlying causes, is it likely for one treatment to be effective for all or most underlying conditions? Despite the improbability of success, researchers continue to seek a panacea effective for all ischemic strokes. Hopes for omnipotence include vasodilators, aspirin, endarterectomy, and warfarin. These sorts of remedies have been hypothesized and enthusiastically endorsed before inevitable disenchantment.

Of course, physicians must consider the severity of the patient's condition: No profit comes from watering dead grass! The seriousness of the deficit is, however, not the only consideration. Grass that is now brown can turn green with proper nurturing. In the future, physicians clearly need studies of groups of patients with similar pathologies and stroke pathogenesis (e.g., studies of patients with severe ICA stenosis with various degrees of brain damage).[2,6] I do not discuss treatment of TIAs,

strokes in progress, RIND, or completed strokes in this volume. Clinicians should be discouraged from using these designations to determine treatment. Instead this book is organized by anatomy, pathology, and pathophysiology—the cornerstones of medicine. Clinicians must return to these foundations to successfully manage patients with cerebrovascular disease.

Inadequate Army and Equipment

Interest in stroke has lagged far behind interest in other areas, such as heart disease and cancer. Despite the fact that stroke is the third leading cause of death in the United States and an even more important cause of disability, stroke has been understudied and its research and treatment have been underfunded. Research funding for stroke and other diseases is compared in Figure 5-1.[7] In the past, there was no equipment capable of reliably separating stroke patients into meaningful etiologic subgroups. That circumstance has changed as a quick glance at Chapter 4 indicates. Modern technology needs wider dissemination and concentration in regional centers specially interested in stroke with trained personnel and the latest technology. Neurology has been an understaffed specialty but that too has dramatically changed. Many more neurologists are now in practice in communities and academic centers.

Insufficient Interest and Training

Nonstroke specialists frequently lack training, interest, and experience in caring for stroke patients. "A stroke is a stroke" is an all-too-prevalent feeling. Having brilliantly concluded that a stroke has occurred, many physicians attach a pseudoscientific set of meaningless initials, such as CVA (cerebrovascular accident), to the patient and rest on their laurels, not searching further along the diagnostic tree or suggesting anything but caregiver treatment. No wonder stroke treatment has been in such a bad fix! Practitioners must be encouraged to recognize different stroke mechanisms and pathophysiologies. Diagnosis of these subtypes can be made without sophisticated knowledge of neuroanatomy. Logical therapeutic

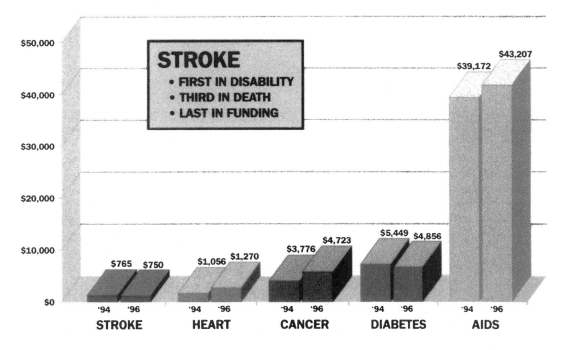

Figure 5-1. Funding statistics: research dollars per death in 1994 and 1996 (Department of Health and Human Services statistics). (Reprinted with permission from LR Caplan. Stroke 1989;29[3]:cover.)

strategies do exist. Centers and clinicians interested in and able to help nonspecialists with stroke diagnosis and management do exist. The brain is the most important organ in the body. The brain controls intelligence, behavior, personality, and character—traits that make us human. The brain is the Rolls Royce organ. Brain illness, especially stroke, deserves the best care and skills the medical system can offer.

Randomized Trials and Evidence-Based Medicine

Randomized trials are important but have limitations. Trials are expensive, timeconsuming, and require enormous resources. To provide statistically valid results, randomized trials must contain large numbers of patients with enough end points to analyze. Sufficient end points must be reached in a relatively short period. Many trials are unsuitable for the study of cerebrovascular conditions. The issue of numbers versus specificity limits trials. For randomized trials to yield statistically valid results, many patients must be included in the study. If the results are to be useful, the data must be specifically applicable to individual patients. To achieve an adequate number of patients, the condition studied must be common and a "lumping" strategy must predominate over "splitting." Patients who are too ill, old, young, and of childbearing age are often excluded from trials. Those incapable of giving informed consent, or who have too complex or multiple illnesses are also frequently left out of trials. These are just the type of stroke patients doctors care for every day.

The results of many randomized trials are impossible to apply directly to individual patients. The term *evidence-based* must be used cautiously when applied to a particular circumstance if that circumstance has not been specifically studied. Information from trials must be weighed according to the context of specific treatment decisions. Conducting trials is different from caring for sick patients. In trials, the same treatments are given to all eligible patients depending only on randomization. Departure from the specified treatment makes the results difficult to interpret. In the clinic, doctors treat individual patients. George Thibault said it well[8]:

We then need to decide which approach in our large therapeutic armamentarium will be most appropriate in a particular patient, with a particular stage of disease and particular coexisting conditions, and at a particular age. Even when randomized clinical trials have been performed (which is true for only a small number of clinical problems), they will often not answer this question specifically for the patient sitting in front of us in the office or lying in the hospital bed.

Factors Influencing Treatment

Enough has been said about what has gone wrong in the past. I turn to a discussion of what is known of treatment and some potentially useful strategies. First of all, what factors should the clinician consider when planning treatment for the individual stroke patient?

Socioeconomic and Psychological Factors

Socioeconomic and psychological factors may influence treatment for some patients and their families. A previously unreliable and noncompliant person cannot be depended on to take anticoagulants. Some patients do not have the economic resources for particular therapies. In other cases, lack of caring family members or friends limits subsequent follow-up and treatment. One person might be disabled by fear of impending disability when informed of the presence of carotid artery disease and a threat of stroke whereas another individual with a similar condition may weigh the alternatives more dispassionately.

Other Medical Conditions

Pre-existent or coexistent illness also limits or affects treatment. Physicians are more conservative when suggesting surgery for stroke patients who have severe heart disease or advanced cancer. Particular concomitant conditions contraindicate some treatments. An active peptic ulcer or severe arterial hypertension makes anticoagulation unwise. Other conditions, such as severe heart or lung disease, increase the risks of anesthesia and surgery. The patient's premorbid function and intellect are also critical. A hopelessly demented nursing home resident with a new stroke should be treated humanely but certainly not aggressively. An older widow depressed and lonely for many years after the death of her husband and friends would be managed differently from a happy and pleasant but slightly demented grandmother who draws joy from her family and surroundings. Age is never an absolute contraindication to stroke therapy. Elderly patients cannot tolerate medical and surgical treatments as well as younger patients, nor do they share the same ability to rebound from strokes. The eldery should be handled cautiously. The same diagnostic and therapeutic strategies that apply to younger individuals, however, should be considered for geriatric patients.

Nature of the Stroke

Arterial Lesion

Management of ICA occlusion is different from severe ICA stenosis or carotid plaque without stenosis. These extracranial large artery lesions differ greatly from lipohyalinosis of intracranial penetrating arteries caused by hypertension. These intrinsic vascular lesions differ from cardiogenic embolism and hypercoagulability as causes of vascular occlusion. The nature, location, and severity of the vascular lesions are key factors in selecting possible therapeutic strategies.

Blood That Courses through the Vessels

Does the patient have a high hematocrit (Hct) or platelet count? What is the blood viscosity? Are the platelets activated or sticky? Is there a bleeding diathesis? Abnormalities of blood constituents and coagulation functions might suggest some therapeutic strategies and contraindicate other treatments.

In a small number of patients, the hematologic disorder is the primary condition that leads to vascular thrombosis or hemorrhage. In many patients, the coagulation disorder contributes to vascular occlusion. Many acute medical conditions, including infections, systemic vascular occlusions (e.g., myocardial infarction), cancers, and inflammatory diseases such as regional enteritis and ulcerative colitis, are accompanied by platelet activation and an increase in acute phase reactants, which increase blood coagulability. In patients with pre-existing cardiac and vascular lesions (e.g., atrial fibrillation, congestive heart failure, and arterial stenosis or ulceration), the increase in coagulability and platelet activation incites the formation of white thrombi, red thrombi, or both at the site of the pre-existing condition.

Mechanisms and Pathophysiology of Stroke

Was the ischemia caused by local vascular thrombosis, embolism, or circulatory failure? (For example, was the brain ischemia caused by low cerebral blood flow or by embolism in patients with ICA stenosis?)

Extent and Reversibility of the Brain Lesions

If the entire middle cerebral artery (MCA) territory is destroyed, there is little point in reperfusing the MCA territory because only dead brain would be irrigated. Reperfusion might even be harmful.[9,10] If, however, the MCA territory ischemia is reversible and the neurons are stunned and dysfunctional but not completely knocked out, the argument for augmenting MCA blood flow is substantially greater. Functional tests, especially magnetic resonance (MR), diffusion and perfusion studies, and magnetic resonance angiography (MRA), are available as discussed in Chapter 4. These tests help determine if feeding arteries are still occluded and the potential reversibility of the ischemia. The cause of the ischemia and the severity and location of the cardio-cerebrovascular lesion is also important in determining the risk for further ischemia. Even if the entire MCA territory in one cerebral hemisphere is irreversibly damaged caused by cardiac-origin embolism, the opposite cerebral hemisphere and the territory supplied by the posterior circulation are still at risk for further damage.

The size of the lesion, degree of neurologic deficit, and length of time since the last worsening have traditionally been used to decide if a stroke is completed.[1] The term *completed stroke* is variously defined and applied and should be discarded. Short of an infallible crystal ball or direct guidance from a deity, doctors cannot predict the future. The fact that a patient is stable today does not tell whether he or she will worsen tomorrow. Patients with so-called completed stroke have as high a frequency of further brain ischemia as those with TIA or RIND.[2] If, however, the vascular mechanism and pathology are known, the tissue at risk can be estimated. In a patient with penetrating vessel disease, a 5 mm basal-ganglionic lacune may represent infarction of the entire territory of that artery. If the same patient with a small basal-ganglia infarct had severe stenosis of the MCA causing reduced flow in the lenticulostriate territory, the potential for further extensive damage is much greater.

Similarly, *stroke in evolution* is a nonspecific term. Almost 30% of stroke patients worsen after entry into the hospital. These worsening deficits are related to numerous factors, including (1) failure of collateral circulation, (2) systemic hypotension, (3) cardiac arrhythmias, (4) embolization or propagation of thrombus, (5) progressive occlusion of the vessel lumen, (6) psychological depression, (7) intercurrent infections, or (8) seizures. Knowledge that a patient is worsening should stimulate action. The nature of the therapeutic action, however, depends on the pathophysiology of the patient's particular problem.

Pace of the Stroke

I have already emphasized that tempo of the illness should not be used as the only criterion for treatment. This does not mean, however, that it should not be considered at all. In fact, the pace of progression dictates the urgency and speed of evaluation and treatment. Table 3-6 in Chapter 3 shows Harvard Stroke Registry data concerning timing of the first and last TIA before stroke in patients with severe ICA disease. A patient with a TIA this morning has a greater probability of stroke tomorrow than a patient with a single TIA 3 months ago. The patient with a single TIA a week ago differs from the patient with a flurry of 5 to 10 TIAs yesterday and today. Patients worsening under immediate supervision require more urgent management than patients stable for the past week. An improving patient makes the physician pause before deciding to tamper with natural forces that seem to be at least temporarily succeeding.

The goal of treatment is to prevent brain damage whenever possible. The major determinant of treatment is the nature of the causative cardiocerebrovascular lesion. Ideally, treatments indicated because of

Table 5-1. General Strategies of Stroke Treatment

Control stroke risk factors to prevent further strokes and
    vascular disease

Prevent stroke complications (e.g., decubitus ulcers, uri-
    nary infections, phlebothrombosis, and pulmonary
    embolism)

Treat specific pathologies and pathophysiologies (e.g.,
    draining a brain hematoma, reperfusion of an occlu-
    sive vascular lesion, managing increased intracranial
    pressure, reducing coagulability to prevent thrombus
    formation) in patients with atrial fibrillation

Facilitate recovery

Improve neurologic function

the nature of that lesion should begin before the
patient develops any neurologic worsening.

Personnel and Facilities Available for a Given Treatment or Evaluation

Complications and success rates vary widely
between different hospitals and even within the
same medical center depending on the personnel
involved. Figures from Springfield, Illinois,[11] Cincinnati, Ohio,[12] and elsewhere[13,14] document striking variability in morbidity and mortality for the
same surgical procedure—carotid endarterectomy.
The risk to benefit ratio of carotid endarterectomy
when the complication rate is 2% is quite different
from the situation when it is 20%. The use and complication rate for diagnostic tests, such as cerebral
angiography, also vary with the skill, training, and
experience of the angiographer and the equipment
available. Especially in this era of limited resources,
not all medical centers are economically able to specialize equally in all fields. Physicians owe patients
the best possible care. Responsibility to the patient
must exceed loyalty to one's colleagues and institution if physicians are to continue to deserve the
respect of the community. If a physician or hospital
has limited interest and capability in stroke management and the patient's condition and socioeconomic
status make it feasible for the patient to go elsewhere, then the physician should send the patient to
where the best care is available. The Golden Rule is
the most important guide to treatment.

Some therapeutic strategies are general and
apply to all stroke patients[15] whereas other strate-

gies depend on the specific problems in the individual patient. Examples of specific problems
include (1) focal brain ischemia caused by low
flow in a patient with a documented occlusive vascular lesion, (2) increased intracranial pressure
(ICP) caused by the mass effect of a hematoma and
its surrounding cerebral edema, (3) a threatened
second embolism in a patient with a known cardiac
source of embolism, and (4) a threatened recurrence of subarachnoid hemorrhage in a patient with
a cerebral aneurysm. General treatment strategies
are listed in Table 5-1.

General Care

Important general care goals for physicians are to
limit suffering, give comfort, and prevent complications. Patients deserve excellent nursing and
general care even when no specific therapy seems
warranted because of the severity of the deficit,
type of stroke, or severe comorbidities. Stroke
patients are often at least partially immobilized
and may not be able to care for their bodily needs.
Key goals are (1) maintenance of adequate nutrition; (2) prevention of contractures or painful,
stiff, or frozen joints; (3) prevention of decubiti
and of pressure-related peripheral nerve palsies;
and (4) prevention of thromboembolic, pulmonary,
genitourinary, and skin complications. Table 5-2
lists some stroke complications and general types
of treatment for prevention. Perhaps just as important as these physical problems is maintenance of a
positive but realistic outlook for patients, their
families, and significant others. Depression is common after stroke, so measures should be instituted
early to prevent discouragement.[16] Depression
should be recognized and treated when it occurs.

Patients' visits to doctors and hospitals give
physicians important opportunities to view the
whole person and his or her environment. In the
hurry to diagnose and treat acute stroke problems,
preventive measures are often overlooked. The
stroke patient of today, irrespective of cause, is at
risk for future strokes and vascular disease in other
important organs. Prevention strategies should
begin as early as possible. Patients receive wrong
messages when some factors are neglected (e.g.,
food trays rich in red meats, cheese, and ice cream
tell the patient with hypercholesterolemia that diet

Table 5-2. General Problems and Treatments in Patients with Stroke

Problems	Treatments
Nutritional maintenance (especially if dysphagia is present)	Balanced diet that conforms to suggested calories and content (e.g., low cholesterol and low salt), vitamins when indicated, intravenous feeding, nasogastric tubes, gastronomy
Pulmonary complications (aspiration, pneumonia atelectasis, pulmonary emboli)	Care or avoidance in oral feeding; in dysphagics, study of swallowing before oral feeding; respiratory therapy; early antibiotic treatment of infection; no smoking; anticoagulants (miniheparin or heparinoids); use of special leg boots to prevent phlebothrombosis
Immobility (body or one or more limbs)	Frequent full range-of-motion exercises, frequent turning, prevention of pressure palsies and joint dislocations by slings, and careful limb positioning
Urinary tract complications (bladder distension, urinary retention, infection)	Catheterization using sterile technique when needed; avoidance when possible of indwelling catheters; early antibiotic treatment; urinary acidification
Skin (decubiti)	Careful, frequent turning; pillows and pads to protect pressure areas; water beds; skin surveillance
Psychological (apathy and depression)	Positive outlook; entire medical care personnel functioning as a team; antidepressants

Source: Modified with permission from LR Caplan. A General Therapeutic Perspective on Stroke Treatment. In R Dunkel, J Schmidley (eds). Stroke in the Elderly: New Issues in Diagnosis; Treatment and Rehabilitation. New York: Springer, 1987;60–69.

is not important). Nurses or aides who help the patient smoke also convey approbation. While the specific stroke mechanism is investigated and treated, explore general health practices and stroke risk factors and deal with them early in the course. Table 5-3 lists some of these risk factors. These factors are explored in more detail in Chapter 17.

While exploring diagnosis and treatment of acute stroke, begin to develop rehabilitation strategies. Restorative or rehabilitation therapy depends on the type of handicap and disability, not on the stroke etiology or mechanism. Limb weakness, gait abnormalities, language disturbances, dysphagia, neglect of the left side of space, and hemianopia are different problems that require different rehabilitation and therapy strategies. To be maximally effective, rehabilitation should focus on the individual patient, taking past capabilities, activities, and future needs into consideration.

Rehabilitation involves an educational process, training patients to understand their handicaps, and devising strategies to overcome them. Recall that the word *doctor* is derived from the Latin word *docere*, which means "to teach" or "to lead." Sometimes well-learned routine tasks, such as walking, eating, or getting on and off a toilet seat, must be performed in a different way. Patients must be instructed and trained to use new

approaches. To be successful, the rehabilitation and education process must be shared with the family and others who live with and help the patient. They must carry on and amplify the gains made in the hospital after the patient returns home. If friends and family know the nature of the patient's disabilities, they understand when the patient cannot perform particular tasks and thus modify the patient's environment to make things easier. A kind, understanding, and unhurried approach by all personnel involved is needed. Rehabilitation, like prevention, should start early during the acute stroke period. Passive range-of-movement exercises, speech therapy, and explanation of the neurologic dysfunction can begin during the first days after the stroke.

In many medical centers and physician practices, the locations and personnel involved in stroke prevention, acute treatment, and rehabilitation are different. Primary care physicians have the most opportunity to encourage stroke prevention practices when they see patients in their offices. Neurologists and other acute-care specialists treat acute strokes in acute-care facilities, sometimes in special stroke or intensive care units. Neurologists do not usually see patients until they already have had a stroke or other cerebrovascular event. Other specialists, such as physiatrists, often manage the

Table 5-3. Risk Factors and Potentially
Unhealthy Practices

Smoking
Heart disease
Hypertension
Illicit drug use (especially cocaine and amphetamines)
Prescription drugs and their overuse
Overuse of alcohol
Abnormal blood lipids
Oral contraceptives
Sedentary lifestyle
Diabetes
Highly stressful work and home situations
Being overweight

patient during the recuperative period in rehabilitation hospitals. All phases of care should be a continuum. Ideally, the three types of practitioners should be involved during the acute-care phase. Rehabilitation personnel must be aware of the preventive and acute treatment strategies used during rehabilitation. After being urged to refrain from smoking and watch their diet in the acute-care hospital, what message do patients receive if they are allowed to smoke and eat as they please in the rehabilitation hospital?

Ischemic Stroke

Although mechanisms of ischemia vary, particular themes are applicable to all patients with brain ischemia. *Ischemia* means inadequate delivery of blood containing required nutrients. Maximizing blood flow to ischemic zones is clearly important. Can areas of vascular blockage in large arteries be opened or circumvented by medical or surgical treatments? Can local perfusion through the microcirculation supplying the ischemic zone be improved? Occlusive thrombosis and thromboembolism are important in most patients with ischemic stroke. Can the coagulation system be altered to diminish the development of so-called white platelet-fibrin clots and red thrombin-dependent clots? Metabolic changes within the ischemic zone are important in causing cell death. Can the brain be made more resistant to ischemia by manipulating its chemical environment? Edema

and raised ICP can potentiate nerve cell damage. Can they be controlled? I discuss these different issues separately.

Maximizing Blood Flow

Different medical and surgical strategies are available to try to improve circulation to an ischemic region distal to a vascular occlusive lesion.

Controlling Position and Activity

In some patients, sitting, standing, and even elevating the head of the bed increase ischemic symptoms.[17] The minor reduction in cephalad flow accompanying postural change decreases blood flow through the stenotic vessel or collateral channels just enough to decompensate a fragile equilibrium.[17,18] Physicians should note if patients are sensitive to postural changes. Initially after the acute stroke, patients should be observed when first sitting or standing, to ensure that blood pressure does not drop excessively or postural symptoms appear. Patients with progressive symptoms caused by ischemia should be nursed supine, sometimes with the feet slightly or moderately elevated.

Managing Blood Pressure, Blood Volume, and Cardiac Output

Cerebral blood flow (CBF) increases with rising blood pressure until the pressure becomes high, approaching the malignant range. For this reason, surgeons often administer intravenous agents, such as phenylephrine, to raise blood pressure just before clamping the ICA during an endarterectomy. During the acute period of ischemic stroke, it is unwise to lower the systemic pressure unless it is extremely high (e.g., above 200/120 mm Hg). In some emergency rooms or intensive care units, however, exposing physicians to an elevated blood pressure is like waving a red flag before a bull; they want to move all of the patient's numbers into the normal range, including blood pressure. Remember that physicians treat patients, not numbers. The patient's symptoms, signs, and neurologic function are better guides for the appropriateness of a treatment than the measured blood pressure. Blood volume also affects perfusion pressure and blood flow.

Some patients who are not able to eat normally become dehydrated and relatively hemoconcentrated. Other factors (i.e., vomiting, eating restrictions because of concern for aspiration, or simply the rush of diagnostic testing occupying patients at mealtimes) contribute to reduced fluid intake during the early hours and days after stroke onset. In general, it is wise to keep blood volume, especially plasma volume, high. Fluids must often be given intravenously or by nasogastric tube. Care, however, must be taken to avoid fluid overload and the complications of cardiac failure and brain edema. Careful monitoring of cardiac and cerebral function should accompany any therapeutic attempt to augment fluid volume.

Some patients have anoxic-ischemic brain damage caused by cardiac malfunction; in others, a strong pump helps maximize CBF. Attention to cardiac rhythm and pump function is important, especially during the acute, fragile period of cerebral ischemia. Cardiac output can sometimes be improved by (1) use of digitalis, vasodilators, pacemakers, or medications to treat slow rhythms and heart block; (2) adjustment of already prescribed drugs such as digitalis and diuretics; (3) correction of abnormal serum K^+ and Ca^{++} levels; and (4) control of tachyrhythmias. Cardiac-ejection fractions and output can be monitored noninvasively by echocardiography.

Relieving Vascular Obstructions

Surgical Endarterectomy or Local Reconstruction

Endarectomy is the most common method of unblocking a vessel by direct surgery. This strategy differs from other techniques that augment flow because endarterectomy of a tightly stenotic vessel produces a suddenly large increase in flow. Capillaries, small arterioles, and neurons are often damaged during ischemia. When flooded with blood under high pressure, these abnormal vessels can then bleed. The carotid sinus is also damaged during endarterectomy, leading to failure of the carotid sinus reflex and accelerated hypertension in the hours and days after carotid endarterectomy.[19–21] Elevated blood pressure and flooding of damaged vessels can lead to brain edema and ICH after carotid endarterectomy.[21,22] Care must be taken in the timing of endarterectomy. Blood pressure of patients undergoing carotid endarterectomy must be carefully monitored during the postoperative period. Usually, completely occluded vessels do not lend themselves to direct repair because clots form and propagate distally beyond the site of surgical access in the presence of low flow.

Carotid endarterectomy has been shown to be clearly more effective than medical therapy in patients with neurologically symptomatic, severe (70% luminal narrowing) carotid artery stenosis.[23–25] Endarterectomy not only removes the obstructing lesion dramatically augmenting flow but also removes the source of intra-arterial emboli. Endarterectomy has also been shown to be somewhat effective in selected patients with luminal stenosis in the 50–69% range.[26,27] However, patients must be carefully chosen because neurologic and cardiac morbidity and mortality are significant risks. Vertebral artery surgery can also be performed successfully with low morbidity and mortality when performed by surgeons with extensive experience with the procedure.[28,29] The most common method of vertebral artery reconstruction is to anastamose the vertebral artery to the carotid artery. Vertebral artery endarterectomy can also be performed. In one study, the Asymptomatic Carotid Atherosclerosis Surgery trial, endarterectomy was more effective than medical treatment in preventing strokes in selected patients who had no symptoms of retinal or brain ischemia, severe cardiac disease, or other serious comorbidities when operated on by selected surgeons who had low surgical complication rates.[30] Endarterectomy has also occasionally been performed successfully in stenosing lesions of the intracranial vertebral arteries.[31,32] Insufficient cases have been studied to determine the indications and effectiveness of surgery versus medical therapy in patients with vertebral artery lesions. Emboli have also been removed directly from the MCA but the procedure did not lessen stroke severity.[33]

Angioplasty

Since the 1980s, interventional radiology techniques have become an important therapeutic alternative for many cerebrovascular conditions. At first, interventional techniques using coils, catheters, balloons, glues, and other devices were applied mostly to treatment of patients with intracranial aneurysms and vascular malformations.

Transluminal angioplasty, sometimes with insertion of vascular stents, is often performed in patients with coronary artery and peripheral vascular occlusive disease of the limbs. Radiologists and other trained interventionalists use catheters and balloons to mechanically split plaques and dilate vessels. Mechanical vascular dilation has also been used to treat fibromuscular dysplasia. Carotid and vertebral artery angioplasty for stenotic disease of the neck arteries was first performed in patients considered poor candidates for surgical endarterectomy. Carotid artery angioplasty is now being performed more widely. Trials are planned to study the relative effectiveness and complication rate of angioplasty versus carotid artery surgery in patients with severe carotid artery stenosis.

Intracranial angioplasty is effective in dilating vasoconstricted intracranial arteries after subarachnoid hemorrhage (SAH).[34] Percutaneous transluminal angioplasty using intra-arterial balloons has also occasionally been performed for stenosis of intracranial arteries the size of the MCA, and the vertebral and basilar arteries.[35–37] Dissections, vasospasm, and blockage of penetrating arteries during balloon insufflation are important complications of intracranial angioplasty.[36] Angioplasty of intracranial arteries at sites of the origins of important penetrating arteries carries a risk of infarction in the territorial supply of these penetrators. For this reason, angioplasty of the mainstem MCA at the site of the lenticulostriate arterial origins and the basilar artery have the highest risk for complications. Thrombosis can also complicate intracranial angioplasty.[37] The technology used to treat extracranial and intracranial stenoses by interventional techniques is improving rapidly. Stents are used more widely. In the future, angioplasty will undoubtedly prove to be a more commonly used strategy to treat occlusive cerebrovascular disease.

Thrombolysis

Clots can also be lysed chemically. In the body, thrombus formation stimulates an endogenous fibrinolytic mechanism for thrombolysis. Factor XII, the release of tissue plasminogen activator, and other substances promote conversion of plasminogen to plasmin, the active fibrinolytic enzyme.[38,39] Plasmin activity is concentrated at the sites of fibrin deposition. Endogenous formation of plasmin is probably responsible for some examples of spontaneous recanalization of thrombosed arteries.

Beginning in the late 1950s, clinicians have given stroke patients thrombolytic agents in an attempt to open thrombosed arteries. Early attempts used bovine or human thrombolysins or streptokinase.[39] During the early 1960s, Meyer and colleagues randomized 73 patients with worsening strokes to receive streptokinase intravenously or anticoagulants (or both) within 3 days of stroke onset.[40–42] Clots were lysed in some patients. Ten patients treated with streptokinase died, however, and some patients had brain hemorrhages. After these studies, streptokinase was thought to be too dangerous to use. In fact, the use of streptokinase for systemic and cardiac thromboembolism was considered contraindicated in the presence of brain lesions or past strokes.

During the 1980s, stimulated by the successful use of thrombolytic agents for the treatment of coronary artery thrombosis, clinicians turned again to these "clot busters" to treat cerebrovascular thromboembolism.[39,42,43] Streptokinase, urokinase, and recombinant tissue plasminogen activator (rt-PA) were the most common substances used. These agents were given intravenously or intra-arterially by catheter into the thrombosed artery. Anterior and posterior circulation thromboembolism was treated. Arteries, especially MCA branches and the basilar artery, were recanalized in many patients.[42,43] Some treated patients developed hemorrhagic transformation of infarcts and frank intracerebral hematomas.[43] As in coronary artery disease, after occlusive thrombi were lysed, stenosing plaques remain and rethrombosis is an imminent threat in the hours and days after thrombolytic treatment. Concomitant use of heparin, aspirin, or warfarin after thrombolytic agents might prevent rethrombosis but clearly increase the risk of hemorrhage.

Thrombolytic treatment of stroke patients is one of the most controversial topics in clinical medicine. The release of a report from investigators sponsored by the National Institute of Neurological Diseases and Stroke (NINDS) gave momentum to a movement to quickly introduce intravenous thrombolysis into the treatment of patients with acute ischemic strokes. During the summer of 1996, approximately one-half year after the publication of the NINDS rt-PA Study Group,[44] the U.S. Food and Drug Administration approved the use of rt-PA for the treatment of stroke patients if the drug was given within the first 3 hours of stroke onset. Subsequent published treatment protocols adopted by committees of the American Heart Association (AHA)[45] and the American Academy of Neurology (AAN)[46] recommend intravenous administration of rt-PA (0.9 mg/kg—maximum of 90 mg) given in a 10% bolus followed by an infusion lasting 60 minutes to patients within 3 hours of onset of ischemic stroke. The recommendations stipulate that a CT scan done before the infusion should not show major infarction, mass effect, edema, or hemorrhage. Neither the NINDS rt-PA Study Group, AHA, nor the AAN committees require or suggest vascular tests before treatment of thrombolysis.

To place the NINDS study results within the context of past studies and knowledge of the effectiveness and risks of thrombolytic drugs, I review those studies in which the arterial lesions have been shown by angiography before intra-arterial and intravenous thrombolysis. These studies contain important data about the effectiveness of the drug in producing recanalization and the relation of recanalization to clinical outcome. They also indicate the risks of intracranial bleeding in patients with known occlusive lesions. I also review studies that involved thrombolytic drug use without prior clarification of the vascular occlusive lesions, including the NINDS study.

Intra-arterial studies, by definition, are performed under angiographic control. After a diagnostic angiogram shows an acute vascular occlusion, a physician trained and experienced in interventional endovascular therapy positions a catheter into the thrombus and introduces the thrombolytic drug at or near the proximal end of the clot. At times, physicians use the catheter to physically manipulate the clot to facilitate clot fragmentation and lysis. Table 5-4 lists data including drugs used, occluded vessels, frequency of successful reperfusion, presence of hemorrhagic complications, and outcomes from published studies of intra-arterial therapy.[47–64] The timing of treatment varied considerably in these studies, but the agent was always given within 24 hours. In one study that included only patients treated with urokinase after MCA occlusions related to angiographic or endovascular procedures, the patients were all treated within 3 hours.[58]

The presence and extent of reperfusion depended greatly on the pathophysiology of the stroke and the location of the occluded artery.[65] Among the 449 patients treated in these 17 studies, 64% had effective recanalization after therapy. In general, mainstem and MCA occlusions responded best, whereas ICA occlusions responded least well. Distal MCA branch occlusions did not respond as well as more proximal MCA lesions. Sixty-nine percent of patients with basilar artery occlusion showed recanalization. Thrombolytic treatment of patients with occlusion of the ICA bifurcation (the carotid "T" portion) was almost invariably unsuccessful. Embolic occlusions were generally more successfully recanalized than thrombosis engrafted on in situ atherosclerosis. In some patients, transluminal angioplasty was needed after thrombolysis to keep the occluded artery open.[66] Recanalization was helped by mechanical clot disruption. This was especially important in patients with carotid artery thromboses when emboli originating from the carotid thrombus had occluded the MCA. Penetration of the catheter through the clot in the neck allowed placement of the catheter at the MCA clot with subsequent successful recanalization. Intracranial hemorrhagic complications occurred in 18.5% of patients. Forty-two percent of the treated patients had a good outcome as judged by the authors of the reports (see Table 5-4).

The results of two randomized therapeutic trials of intra-arterial therapy have been reported.[67,68] Each compared intra-arterial Prolyse (recombinant pro-urokinase [r-proUK]) and heparin versus heparin delivered intra-arterially to patients with angiographically confirmed MCA occlusions who were treated within 6 hours of stroke onset. In each trial, interventional radiologists were instructed to deliver the agent by infusion using a catheter placed at the proximal end of the thrombus; mechanical manipulation of the clot was not permitted. In the first Prolyse in Acute Cerebral Thromboembolism Trial (PROACT I), within 2 hours after the start of the intra-arterial infusion, 15 of 26 (57.7%) patients treated with r-proUK had successful recanalization of the MCA compared with two of 14 (14.3%) of controls.[67] In PROACT II, 40% of patients treated with r-proUK followed by heparin had modified Rankin scores of two or less compared with 25% of 59 patients treated with heparin alone. The recanalization rate was 66% in the r-proUK group compared with 18% in controls given heparin alone.[68]

Table 5-4. Intra-Arterial Thrombolytic Studies

Author	Drug	Total	Reperfusion of Arteries			Hem	"Good Outcome"
			ICA	MCA	Basilar		
del Zoppo[47]	U/S	19	7/8	9/11	—	4	17 (89%)
Hacke[48]	U/S	43	—	—	19/43	4	13 (30%)
Zeumer[49]	U/t-PA	59	129/3	—	28/28	8	17 (29%)
Mori[50]	U	22	—	8/22	—	4	11 (50%)
Mori[51]	UPA	44	1/8	13/31	2/5	10	16 (36%)
Mobius[52]	U/S	18	—	—	14/18	—	10 (56%)
Matsumoto[53]	U/t-PA	93	21/36	28/41	9/16	25	30 (32%)
Theron[54]	S/U	12	3/3	9/9	—	3	11 (92%)
Zeumer[55]	S	5	—	—	4/5	—	3 (60%)
Casto[56]	U	12	—	8/8	3/4	3	5 (42%)
Barnwell[57]	U	12	2/2	5/8	2/2	3	9 (75%)
*Berg-Dammer[58]	S/U	14	—	13/14	—	—	9 (64%)
Mitchell[59]	U	16	—	—	13/16	2	7 (44%)
Jansen[60]	U/t-PA	16	2/16	—	—	3	1 (6%)
Becker[61]	U	12	—	—	10/13*	2	3 (25%)
Cross[63]	U	20	—	—	11/20	7	4 (20%)
Wijdicks[62]	U	9	—	—	7/9	1	5 (56%)
Gonner[64]	U	43	1/9	13/23	5/10	8	26 (60%)
Total	—	469	37/82	106/167	127/189	87	197 (42%)
Recanalized	—	299 (64%)	45%	62%	67%	18.5%	—

Hem = hemorrhagic changes; ICA = internal carotid artery; MCA = middle cerebral artery; S = streptokinase; t-PA = tissue plasminogen activator; U = urokinase.
*13 occlusions/12 patients; 2 basilar, 10 vertebral artery.

In seven clinical studies, the vascular lesions were also defined by angiography but the thrombolytic drug was delivered intravenously.[60,69–75] In these studies, the angiographic catheters were left in situ so that angiography could be performed before and after intravenous delivery of the drug. Table 5-5 outlines the results of these studies. Only two of these studies had control patients whom were not given a thrombolytic drug. In all of the series except one,[74] rt-PA was given within 6 hours whereas in the other study there was an 8-hour limit. Among the total 370 patients treated with rt-PA, one-third of the arteries treated showed significant recanalization as compared to only 5% of 58 control arteries. MCA branch occlusions recanalized best followed by occlusions of the superior and inferior divisions of the MCA. Mainstem MCA occlusions recanalized less often than branch and division MCA lesions. ICA occlusions recanalized seldom. There were no recanalizations when the ICA and MCA were occluded. Few patients with documented basilar artery occlusions were given intravenous rt-PA and only one out of six recanalized. In one study, Grond et al. reported favorable results of treatment in 10 of 12 patients with acute vertebrobasilar territory ischemia given intravenous rt-PA followed by heparin. The occlusive vascular lesions, however, were not documented before treatment.[76] Embolic occlusions recanalized more often than in situ thrombosis of atherostenotic arteries. Recanalization was better when there was angiographic evidence of good collateral circulation before administration of rt-PA. Hemorrhagic infarction and parenchymatous hematomas were slightly more common after intravenous, as compared with intra-arterial, delivery of the thrombolytic agents.

The first large, multicenter, randomized trial of intravenous thrombolysis without definition of

Table 5-5. Intravenous Angiographic Thrombolytic Studies

Author	Time	# Pts	Arteries ICA	Canalized MCA	Total BA	Hem	Outcome
Yamaguchi[69]	<6 h	51 t-PA 47 c	10/47 t-PA	2/46 c	0	24 HI, 4 PH 22 HI, 5 PH	37 good; good
Yamaguchi[70,a]	<6 h	121 t-PA	28/121	—	0	11 HI & PH	MCA >ICA
Mori[71]	<6 h	19 t-PA 12 c	1/6 0/4 c	7/13 1/8 c	0	8 HI, 1 PH 4 HI, 1 PH	t-PA >c
von Kummer[72]	<6 h	32 t-PA	1/11	10/21	0	9 HI, 3 PH	44% good
von Kummer[73]	<6 h	27 t-PA	3/10	9/17	1/5	6 HI, 0 PH	44% good
Jansen[60,b]	<6 h	8 t-PA	2/16	0	0	1 PH	19% good
del Zoppo[74,75]	<8 h	104 (93c) t-PA	2/23	12/34 m 14/26 m2 29/44 br	0/1	21 HI, 11 PH	—
Totals	—	370 thromb 59 c	33% t-PA	5% c	16%	58HI, 20PH 26HI, 6PH	—

BA = basilar artery; br = branch; c = control; Hem = hemorrhage; HI = hemorrhagic infarct; ICA = internal carotid artery; m = mainstem middle cerebral artery; MCA = middle cerebral artery; m2 = MCA divisions; PH = parenchymatous hemorrhage; thromb = thrombosis; t-PA = tissue plasminogen activator.
[a]Only patients with ICA/MCA emboli included.
[b]Only intracranial ICA occlusions.
[c]Ninety-three of the 104 completed rt-PA therapy according to protocol; recanalization data presented as arteries not as patients.

the vascular occlusive lesions to be reported was the European Cooperative Acute Stroke Study (ECASS).[77,78] In this study, 620 patients with acute hemispheral strokes were recruited in 75 hospitals in 14 European countries. A total of 313 patients were randomized to receive rt-PA (1.1 mg/kg), and 307 patients were randomized to the placebo group. Treatment was given within 6 hours of the onset of symptoms of brain ischemia. Patients with hemorrhage or major early infarct signs (e.g., diffuse hemispheral swelling, parenchymal hypodensity, and effacement of cerebral sulci in more than one-third of the MCA territory) on the initial CT scans were excluded. CT scans were initially read on site. An independent, blinded, CT scan–reading panel then retrospectively reviewed the CT scans and determined protocol violations of the CT scan entry criteria. A large number of protocol deviations were found in this study, mostly because of failure at the local centers to recognize CT abnormalities that should have excluded patients. One hundred nine patients were excluded after review at the coordinating center, including 66 patients in the rt-PA group and 43 in the placebo-treated group.

The results were calculated through an intention-to-treat analysis and by analyzing only those patients in the "target population" (i.e., those patients who did not have protocol violations). In the target population, the rt-PA–treated patients had significantly better outcome as measured by combined Barthel Index and modified Rankin Scale scores at 90 days. Stay in the hospital was significantly shorter in rt-PA–treated patients. Intracerebral hemorrhages and mortality were higher in the rt-PA–treated patients, but these differences were not statistically significant. Large parenchymal hematomas were more often found in patients treated with rt-PA. Patients treated within 3 hours did better after rt-PA than controls and those treated with rt-PA between 3 and 6 hours.[79]

The ECASS study showed that treatment of patients with early infarct signs on CT scan was particularly dangerous. Initial analysis of the CT scans at local hospitals was often unreliable. Some hemorrhages and many early infarcts were missed by local physicians. The mortality and brain hemorrhage rates among patients with protocol violations randomized to the rt-PA group were extremely high; 33.3% and 40%, respectively. Among 52 patients included in the study, despite major early infarct signs, 40% died. Among the 31 patients with major early infarct signs on CT treated with rt-PA, 15 (48.4%) died mostly during the first week. An editorial commenting on the results of the ECASS study pointed out the trade-off between improvement and hemorrhage.[78] Comparing the target population with the placebo group, for every 1,000 patients treated, 117 more than the number expected by chance recovered essentially normal neurologic function. One hundred twenty-six more than expected had an ICH, however.

The next study reported was the NINDS study.[44] The major differences in this study compared with ECASS were (1) more rapid entry into the study, (2) lower dose of rt-PA, (3) earlier treatment (302 patients were treated within 90 minutes and 322 between 90 and 180 minutes after ischemic symptom onset), and (4) the absence of exclusion of patients because of brain ischemia found on entry CT scans. The NINDS study consisted of two parts. In Part I, 291 patients were enrolled to test whether treatment with rt-PA given intravenously would result in an improvement of 4 points or more in the National Institutes of Health Stroke Scale or be associated with resolution of the neurologic deficit within 24 hours of stroke onset. Part II studied the results of thrombolytic treatment versus placebo using a number of clinical outcome scales measured at 3 months after stroke onset.[44] Although in Part I no major differences were found between the placebo and treatment groups in the percentages of patients with neurologic improvement at 24 hours, there was a statistically significant benefit for rt-PA over placebo for all outcome measures at 3 months. In Part II patients, there was a 1.7 (95% confidence interval, 1.2–2.6) global odds ratio for a favorable outcome at 3 months when compared with the placebo group. Patients receiving intravenous rt-PA were at least 30% more likely to have minor or no disability at 3 months. No significant difference in effectiveness was found in the patients treated within 90 minutes versus those treated between 90 and 180 minutes. Symptomatic ICHs were more common in the patients treated with rt-PA (6.4% vs 0.6%) and

were especially more common in patients with more severe neurologic deficits at entry and in patients older than 75 years. The mortality at 3 months was 17% in the rt-PA group versus 21% in the placebo group.

In the NINDS study, few patients had recognized important CT abnormalities (18 had edema and 12 had mass effect).[44] No important difference in outcome was found in the groups with varying etiologies. Quick entry and absence of vascular and cardiac imaging, however, made the clinical diagnosis of stroke etiology tentative at best.

In the ECASS II trial, investigators treated 800 patients from Europe, Australia, and New Zealand with rt-PA or placebo within 6 hours of stroke onset.[80] Stroke patients were treated with the same dose used in the NINDS trial rather than the higher dose used in ECASS I. Patients with major infarcts on CT scan were excluded, but vascular imaging was not performed before treatment. Guidelines for control of hypertension were more explicit than in ECASS I. In ECASS II, 36.6% of patients in the placebo-treated group had favorable outcomes—a much better result than in the ECASS I and NINDS trials. Among the rt-PA–treated group, 40.3% had favorable outcomes; this was not significantly different from the placebo-treated group.[80] Treatment results and frequency of hemorrhages were similar in the 0–3 hour and 3–6 hour treatment groups. Symptomatic hemorrhages developed in 8.8% of the rt-PA–treated patients.[80]

Three therapeutic trials have been performed of intravenous streptokinase in patients without identification of the vascular lesions—the Australian Streptokinase Trial,[81] Multicenter Acute Stroke Trial in Italy,[82] and Multicenter Acute Stroke Trial in Europe.[83] All were stopped prematurely because of the high rate of brain hemorrhages in patients treated with intravenous streptokinase. Lyden and his colleagues in the NINDS study group reviewed the results of intravenous thrombolysis trials for stroke and their implications for stroke care.[84]

Since the planning of the NINDS and ECASS I trials in the early 1990s, major advances have been made in vascular imaging. I have already discussed MRA, CT angiography (CTA), ultrasound, and echocardiography in Chapter 4. These tests can be performed quickly and safely. Information about vascular occlusions can be obtained at the same time as brain imaging. CTA can be performed immediately after CT brain imaging. MRA can be performed with MRI. In some centers, MR diffusion and perfusion studies can also be performed at the same time. Neck and transcranial ultrasound is an effective method of screening for extracranial and intracranial large artery occlusions and can be performed quickly. These vascular imaging procedures are all sensitive and specific for complete occlusions of large arteries.

Therapeutic decisions regarding whether to use thrombolytics are complex and depend on more than simply the time that has expired since stroke symptom onset and findings on CT scan. Much has been learned, but there is still much more to be understood.[85,86]

Issues Related to the Occluded Artery

Angiographically controlled studies show:

1. Intravenous thrombolysis is most likely successful when the occluded arteries are intracranial and relatively small. MCA branch occlusions are much more likely to lyse than ICA siphon lesions. ICA siphon and mainstem MCA lesions are more likely to lyse than ICA origin occlusions in the neck. Neck lesions rarely recanalize. Occlusions of the extracranial and intracranial vertebral arteries have not been well studied.

2. The more recent the thrombosis, the more likely thrombolysis will be successful.

3. Thrombolysis leads to clinical improvement only when recanalization occurs.

4. Emboli are more easily lysed than thrombi that form in situ in regions of atherostenosis. Thrombolysis is less successful when there is severe underlying atherostenosis and when the thrombus is organized and adherent. In the presence of severe atherostenosis, lysis of small occlusive thrombi is usually only temporary. Thrombi often recur if the stenosis is not treated.

5. Intra-arterial thrombolysis is often effective in patients with basilar artery, mainstem, and divisional MCA occlusions. Manipulation of the clot by the intra-arterial catheter contributes to the success of intra-arterial therapy. Angioplasty is sometimes needed after thrombolysis to keep the recanalized artery open.

6. Long thrombi in large arteries are difficult to lyse successfully.

7. Soft, red, fresh clots are more readily lysed than older clots. Some embolic substances (e.g., calcific valves, cholesterol-rich plaques, myxomatous material, and white platelet-fibrin thrombi) are probably not susceptible to thrombolysis.

Issues Related to the Ischemic Brain and Blood Flow

Preliminary results show:

1. The longer the brain ischemia, the less likely reversibility. The most common window of opportunity is probably less than 3–6 hours, but some patients with much longer duration ischemia may gain from reperfusion. MR studies show that some patients retain regions of stunned brain for many hours.

2. The longer the duration of ischemia and vascular occlusion, the more likely that reperfusion will be complicated by hemorrhage. Systemic hypertension also increases the likelihood of reperfusion hemorrhage.

3. Collateral blood flow is an important determinant of recanalization.[87] Poor collaterals usually mean less adequate delivery of thrombolytic agent to the brain.

4. Large areas of infarction and severe neurologic deficits present at the time of thrombolysis greatly increase the risk of brain hemorrhage and poor outcome.

Although not well studied, it is likely that blood composition and function (e.g., Hct, platelet count, viscosity, fibrinogen levels, and coagulability) have important effects on thrombolysis. The amount of plasminogen and plasminogen inhibitor present and available are also important, especially if rt-PA is used, but has not been studied. Plasminogen activators are ineffective if inadequate plasminogen is present. Coagulation factors undoubtedly affect the success of thrombolytics and the likelihood of hemorrhagic complications.

Issues Related to the Thrombolytic Agent and its Delivery

Fewer data exist about thrombolytic agent factors than those discussed so far. Streptokinase, in the doses used in trials, causes more hemorrhage than either rt-PA or urokinase. Newer fibrin-selective agents are being developed. Unlike the situation in coronary artery disease, there has been little comparison of different agents using the same protocols. Intravenous therapy is more rapidly and widely applicable because interventional neuroradiologists are not required. Angiography and an experienced, trained interventionalist are needed for intra-arterial delivery. Intra-arterial treatment allows for local delivery of the drug that might be safer and more effective. Mechanical disruption of the clot is feasible at the time of intervention, and angioplasty can also be performed at the same time as thrombolysis. No trials that directly compare intravenous and intra-arterial treatment using the same agent and a uniform protocol have been performed. The safety and effectiveness of adding other drugs concurrently or after thrombolysis have not been well studied in patients with cerebrovascular disease. Dosage and delivery factors relating to effectiveness and risk of various agents are still unsettled. Thrombolysis has not been compared with other treatments (e.g., low-molecular-weight or standard heparin, or antiplatelet agents).

The factors that predict hemorrhagic complications have not been thoroughly characterized. In some studies, length of time after symptom onset did not predict intracranial bleeding.[80] Although most serious hemorrhages are intracranial, bleeding can occur at puncture sites and has been described in the pericardium in patients with myocardial ischemia given rt-PA for acute strokes.[88]

I believe that the decision regarding whether to use thrombolytic agents should be based on thorough evaluation of the individual patient by a physician with great experience in treating stroke patients. The evaluation must include a thorough history and general and neurologic examinations. Brain imaging should always precede thrombolysis. Patients with large infarcts and severe neurologic deficits have a higher risk of hemorrhage and edema after thrombolysis. These patients have less likelihood of a good outcome than patients with small or no infarcts. Vascular imaging should also be performed whenever possible. I do not use thrombolytic agents if vascular imaging studies do not show an occluded artery at the time treatment is considered. Some patients with acute onset of neurologic deficits do not have cerebrovascular disease. Among those patients that do have brain ischemia, some have preocclusive vascular lesions, vasoconstriction, and nonthrombotic emboli. Some patients have had thromboemboli that have already recanalized. In each individual stroke patient, evaluation of the stroke pathophysiology and vascular lesions should precede consideration of thrombolytic treatment.[86] The use of intravenous thrombolytic drugs as suggested in the published protocols[45,46] exposes patients who do not have the condition that thrombolytic drugs treat to needless risk of brain hemorrhage. Physicians have always been admonished that above all else they should do no harm—primum non nocere. Even if a majority of patients benefit from a treatment that has significant serious risks, it is wrong to expose patients who cannot benefit to the risks of that treatment. Some patients with certain vascular lesions do benefit from thrombolytic treatment. More clinical research, however, is needed.

Surgically Bypassing Regions of Blockage

A surgical bypass can be created connecting one vessel to another beyond an obstruction (e.g., a common carotid artery to verterbral artery connection) or intracranially creating an artificial conduit between extracranial branches and intracranial vessels. One artery can be directly sewn to another, or a venous conduit can be interposed. When the vessel to be bypassed is stenotic but still patent, creation of a distal shunt has been shown to further reduce flow through the region of stenosis and promote thrombotic occlusion of the previously stenotic artery.[89,90] Clots that form at the site of occlusion might embolize distally, causing new ischemic damage.

Many anecdotal reports noted the effectiveness of extracranial to intracranial artery bypass using the superficial temporal artery as the donor artery and an MCA branch as the recipient artery. A large, randomized study of the effectiveness of such extracranial–intracranial bypasses, however, proved beyond reasonable doubt that the surgery as it was customarily performed had no benefit. In some circumstances, operated patients fared worse than patients treated medically.[91] The patients in this series had surgery approximately 6 weeks after stroke to prevent reperfusion hemorrhage in regions where the capillaries and arterioles might be ischemic and vulnerable to leakage. Several questions remain:

1. Might bypass procedures earlier in the course (although more risky) be more effective?
2. Might a different recipient artery (e.g., the mainstem MCA or a large conduit such as an interposed vein or larger artery) improve results?
3. Is posterior circulation bypass surgery effective?
4. Might there be some small groups of patients (e.g., those with severe persistent hypoperfusion confirmed by positron emission tomography scanning) who could benefit?[92]

Bypass operations are still performed in patients with critical flow, reducing intracranial occlusive disease in the vertebrobasilar system. Most often, the occipital artery is anastomosed to the posterior inferior cerebellar artery or to the anterior inferior cerebellar artery.[31,93] Occasionally, the superficial temporal artery is used as the donor vessel and the superior cerebellar or posterior cerebral artery as the recipient.[31] Most bypass procedures performed, however, involve the branches of the aortic arch and are conducted by vascular surgeons. These iatrogenic shunts are created to augment blood flow in the recipient arteries. During the procedure, the proximal portion of the occluded or stenotic artery is at times ligated to prevent embolic material from traveling to the brain.

Increasing Collateral Circulation and Perfusion in the Ischemic-Zone Capillary Bed

Vasodilating agents have long been prescribed to increase blood flow. Carbon dioxide (CO_2) is the oldest known vasodilator. Physicians have attempted to dilate brain arteries by asking patients to breathe air with high CO_2 content. Other agents include cyclandelate, isoxsuprine, hydergine, papaverine, and nicotinic acid. A woeful lack of information exists regarding the effect and use of vasodilating agents on CBF in patients with TIAs or ischemic strokes.[94] Abnormal or even paradoxical responses of the cerebral circulation in stroke patients might theoretically render vasodilator treatment ineffective or even harmful.[94] Cerebral arteries have relatively few medial elastic fibers and are less responsive than systemic vessels to vasodilator stimuli. Vasodilator agents produce more systemic than cerebral vasodilation and could thus lead to hypotension or globally decreased CBF. Arteries within nonischemic regions should retain the ability to vasodilate, whereas arteries within ischemic zones could be sufficiently damaged by ischemia losing their ability to dilate. In that circumstance, vasodilating drugs could result in an increased flow into nonischemic areas creating a type of "steal away" from the ischemic areas.

Some pharmaceutical agents have vasoconstrictive effects in some arteries and vasodilator effects in others. Even individual drugs sometimes have different effects on the same circulation depending on dose and other factors. Serotonin has been shown to dilate normal coronary arteries but constrict coronary arteries when the endothelium is diseased.[95] None of the available agents have been thoroughly studied in individuals with cerebrovascular disease. Technology to study regional cerebral blood flow (rCBF) and flow in the brain arteries is available (e.g., xenon-enhanced CT, positron emission tomography scans, perfusion MR, transcranial Doppler, and single-photon emission CT scans).

Headache and faintness have been described after inhalation of glyceryl trinitrate, a known vasodilator. In situations such as SAH or migraine, in which there is known vasospasm, agents that decrease vasoconstriction may have beneficial effects. Acetazolamide (Diamox) has been used as a provocative agent to acutely dilate brain arteries to test the brain's vascular reserve capability to further augment blood flow. Flow is measured in basal intracranial arteries by transcranial Doppler before and after 1 g of acetazolamide is given intravenously.[96] In one study of patients with occlusive disease of intracranial or extracranial arteries, intravenous acetazolamide did increase rCBF but mostly on the nonobstructed side.[97] Acetazolamide has not been extensively tried as a treatment in ischemic stroke patients.

Calcium channel–blocking agents have been tested since 1987 to determine if they improve function in patients with ischemic stroke and SAH. Calcium has a number of actions that can influence the outcome of ischemia.[98] These include promoting vasoconstriction by effects on vascular smooth muscle, altering coagulation (some of the coagulation reactions require Ca^{++}), killing cells when extracellular Ca^{++} passes through cell membranes into the intracellular compartment, and lowering systemic blood pressure.[98,99] Calcium channel–blocking agents may ameliorate migraine.[100]

A preliminary study of nimodipine in patients with SAH suggested some beneficial effects on cerebral vasospasm.[101] Later studies also showed some beneficial effects on morbidity, mortality, and on prevention of delayed ischemic infarction in patients with SAH. It was not clear in these studies whether nimodipine successfully increased blood flow or decreased the arterial vasoconstriction.[102–104] A Dutch trial of oral nimodipine in ischemic stroke patients found that the drug reduced mortality in men and had a beneficial effect in reducing the clinical deficits in patients with moderate and severe neurologic abnormalities.[105] Trials of the effectiveness of nimodipine in patients with ischemic stroke, however, have had disappointing results,[106] although nimodipine may help in the most severe cases if given early enough.[107] Therapeutic benefits probably result more from blockage of extracellular-to-intracellular movement of Ca^{++} than from reversal of vasoconstriction.

Newer calcium channel blockers might have more selective cerebral vasodilating effects. Newer technology allows monitoring of blood flow acutely, chronically, focally, and globally. Newer drugs and some untested, older agents can be studied in the laboratory and clinic.

Volume expansion is another method used to attempt to augment cerebral blood flow and increase perfusion within the microcirculation of the brain. Physicians have attempted to increase blood volume by simply increasing fluid intake or by using various volume expanders. Albumin, plasma, and solutions of colloids and crystalloids have been used.[108] Mannitol, most often used to treat brain edema in patients with edematous brain infarcts and brain hemorrhages, may also temporarily expand intravascular volume and increase microcirculatory blood flow. Most often, the expansion of blood volume related to use of these agents is in serum volume, thus effec-

tively diluting the more viscous erythrocyte portion of the blood. This is referred to as *hemodilution*. The two major determinants of blood viscosity within brain vessels are fibrinogen and Hct. Lowering the Hct by hemodilution may reduce whole blood viscosity and increase blood flow.[109,110] The optimal Hct for blood flow and preservation of oxygen transport is approximately 33%.[111] Rapid hemodilution with reduction of the Hct theoretically could significantly improve blood flow to ischemic zones. Hemodilution may be isovolemic (i.e., blood replaced with equivalent fluid volume) or replacement may be more (hypervolemic) or less (hypovolemic) than the original blood volume. Plasma, Ringer's lactate solution, or colloid solutions such as dextran 40 or hydroxyethyl starch are often used for fluid replacement. Volume is important to maintain during hemodilution because either hypovolemia with excessively reduced volume, hypervolemia with potential cardiac overload, and brain edema can be harmful. Centers using hemodilution therapy must have experience in this technique.

The most frequently used colloidal solutions are dextrans and starches. Dextrans are polysaccharide molecules made by the action of bacteria on sucrose. The most commonly used solution (10% dextran solution in normal saline or 5% dextrose) is called *dextran 40* and contains molecules ranging from 10,000 to 80,000 molecular weight (average 40,000). Infusion causes rapid volume expansion but rapid urinary excretion of the dextran molecules of less than 50,000 molecular weight leads to an osmotic diuresis with reduction in plasma volume. Dextran also coats red blood cells, platelets, and endothelium which are posited to decrease blood viscosity and prevent cellular aggregation to improve microcirculatory flow. Dextran has a potential antithrombotic action by its hemodiluting effect, erythrocyte coating, and decreased platelet aggregation. Another frequently used colloidal solution is hydroxyethyl starch. Dextran and hydroxyethyl starch solutions have been used to treat stroke, usually as part of hemodilution protocols,[108,111–115] but these agents have not been shown to improve outcome. Plasma and Ringer's lactate solution have also been used but have not been well studied in therapeutic trials.

Another means of reducing viscosity and also potentially altering blood coagulability is the use of substances that reduce fibrinogen levels. Fibrinogen contributes significantly to viscosity[116] and high fibrinogen levels have been noted to predict stroke recurrence in high-risk patients.[117] Ancrod, a substance derived from the purified protein fraction of venom from the Malayan pit viper, has a thrombin-like enzymatic effect. Ancrod selectively acts on fibrinogen and inhibits formation of cross-linked fibrin.[118] Ancrod can reduce fibrinogen levels to approximately 100 mg/dl and is being studied for its use in patients with brain ischemia.[118–120] In one study at onset, the mean plasma fibrinogen level was 385 mg/dl.[118] After intravenous infusions of ancrod, D-dimer levels rose, indicating clot lysis. Fibrinogen levels fell to a mean of 116 mg/dl at 6 hours and 52 mg/dl at 24 hours after start of treatment.[118]

Another method of rapidly reducing blood fibrinogen levels and whole blood viscosity is to use plasmaphoresis techniques. Investigators in Austria have developed a technique that they call *Heparin-Induced Extracorporeal Low Density Lipoprotein Precipitation* (HELP).[121,122] In this system, blood is removed from a cubital vein and passed through a filter that separates the cellular components from the plasma. Isovolemic acetate buffer and heparin are added to the plasma. Fibrinogen, low-density lipoprotein cholesterol, and triglycerides are removed by this process. The blood is then reinfused into the cubital vein on the opposite side. HELP treatment reduces fibrinogen levels, lowers whole blood viscosity at high and low shear rates, lowers plasma viscosity, and reduces red cell transit time.[121,122] This treatment has been used acutely to augment cerebral blood flow and can also be used repeatedly in patients with microvascular occlusive disease with vascular dementia who have high fibrinogen levels.

Omega-3 fatty acids, especially eicosopentanoic acid, can also lower blood fibrinogen levels.[123] In a preliminary study, eicosopentanoic acid also reduced blood viscosity, especially in those patients with high baseline viscosities.[124] Eicosopentanoic acid and omega-3 fatty acids, plentiful in various fish oils, have the potential to reduce platelet aggregability in addition to their effects on fibrinogen and viscosity. Reduced incidence of atherosclerosis in Eskimos has been attributed by some to diets rich in fish and omega-3 fatty acids. These substances have not been tested in stroke

prevention or treatment. Atromid, ticlopidine, and pentoxyfylline also have some fibrinogen-lowering effects.

Another strategy that has been used experimentally to improve microcirculatory flow and oxygen delivery is the use of perfluorochemicals. Perfluorochemicals are relatively small molecules, much smaller than erythrocytes. They can carry and release oxygen yet are not metabolized, remain chemically inert, and have low surface tension.[125] When patients or laboratory animals breathe 100% oxygen, these small molecules become saturated with oxygen. Animal experiments have shown promise that perfluorochemicals (e.g., Fluosol-DA) might be useful in ameliorating the extent of infarction in cats with transorbital ligation of an MCA.[126]

In humans, perfluorochemicals have been used mostly as so-called white blood given to patients who are severely anemic but refuse blood transfusions for religious reasons.[127] Theoretically, small molecules can squeeze through vascular passages that block erythrocytes and thereby succeed in delivering needed oxygen to the ischemic stunned penumbral brain tissue. In clinical studies, however, investigators have not been able to attain concentrations of perfluorochemicals ("fluocrits") high enough to provide useful oxygen-carrying capabilities.[128] In cat stroke models, perfusion of the ventricular and subarachnoid fluid spaces with highly oxygenated fluorocarbons decreases the extent of brain infarction.[129,130] The concept of delivering oxygen to tissues by using fluorocarbon emulsions shows promise.

In patients with low flow, stagnation causes clot formation and embolization. Measures to prevent embolization, discussed in the following section, are also applicable to many low-flow situations.

Prevention of Clot Formation, Propagation, and Embolism

The formation of a thrombus depends on a number of interrelated factors that include local vascular injury or roughening, the number of platelets and their activation, and the presence of serum coagulant and anticoagulant substances. In general, so-called red clots, erythrocyte-fibrin thrombi, tend to form in regions where there is low flow or stagnation, whereas smaller, so-called white platelet clots adhere to roughened places in faster-moving streams of blood.[131,132] Standard anticoagulants, such as heparin (and low-molecular-weight heparin and heparinoids) and warfarin, theoretically should be more useful in preventing red clots whereas antiplatelet agglutinating agents should be better at preventing white platelet plugs.[131,132] Heparin and warfarin should work best in occlusive disease of veins and large arteries and in cardiac disorders that predispose to cardiac-origin thromboembolism, whereas agents that decrease platelet aggregation might have an advantage in arterial plaque disease without severe stenosis. Some evidence documents the failure of aspirin, an antiplatelet agglutinating agent, in patients with severe carotid artery disease.[133]

Polycythemia and thrombocytosis increase the probability of clot formation. Frequent blood donations, removal of causes of secondary erythremia such as cigarette smoking, and specific antineoplastic treatment of polycythemia vera are therapeutic alternatives for reduction of Hct. In the acute situation, hemodilution decreases the Hct reducing viscosity and thrombotic tendencies. Thrombocytosis can also cause a clotting tendency and usually accompanies hematologic proliferative disorders that require specific therapy.

Heparin

Heparin, a biological substance derived from tissues of various animals (most often bovine lungs and porcine intestines), has been used clinically since the 1940s. It decreases hyperlipemia and has a variety of different anticoagulant effects. The major anticoagulant activity occurs when heparin binds to and activates antithrombin III, a naturally occurring plasma inhibitor of coagulation. Activated antithrombin III slowly binds to thrombin and the other serum protease coagulation factors and neutralizes these compounds. Heparin also antagonizes thromboplastin and prevents thrombi from reacting with fibrinogen to form fibrin. Heparin is a heterogeneous mixture of sulfated mucopolysaccharides containing at least 21 compounds ranging in size from 3,000 to 37,500 daltons.[134–135] Heparin has been used most often during the acute phase of thrombosis or embolism. The necessity of giving the drug parenterally has limited its long-term use. Heparin has also been used during pregnancy in patients who require anti-coagulation because of the potential adverse effects of warfarin on the fetus. Heparin can be given as an intravenous bolus, a continuous-drip infusion, or, less effectively, subcutaneously. Dosage is usually adjusted to keep the partial thromboplastin time (PTT) at 1.5–2.0 times the normal control values.[136,137] Heparin is usually given acutely to maintain anticoagulation until warfarin therapy produces therapeutic prolongation of the prothrombin time (PT). Some patients treated with heparin develop a drop in their platelet count (thrombocytopenia) and new ischemic events.[138,139] There are two varieties of heparin-induced thrombocytopenia. The most common variety involves a slight degree of thrombocytopenia usually beginning 1–5 days after the start of heparin as a result of heparin-induced platelet aggregation. Ischemia does not result and platelet counts return to normal despite continued heparin use. In the more severe form of heparin-induced thrombocytopenia, antibodies of the IgG and IgM groups become bound to platelets and platelet counts fall, usually during the second week of treatment. Often, thrombocytopenia is severe (10,000 mm^3) and thromboembolic and hemorrhagic complications rarely occur, presumably owing to consumption of coagulation factors and platelets.[138,139] Blockage of small arteries by white platelet-fibrin clots can cause regions of skin and visceral organ necrosis, termed the *white clot syndrome*. Occasionally, thrombosis seems to be precipitated by heparin without thrombocytopenia.[140]

The anticoagulant activities of various commercial preparations of heparin vary among sources and even within batches from the same source.[134,135] These variations lead to variability in clinical effectiveness and unexpected bleeding. Unfractionated heparin has begun to be replaced by low-molecular-weight heparins and heparinoids. Crude commercial preparations of heparin can be separated into low- and high-molecular-weight fractions. Low-molecular-weight heparins are fragments of standard heparin with molecular weights of 4,000–6,000.[141,142] Heparinoids are heparin analogues, natural or semisynthetic sulfated glycosaminoglycans, prepared by tissue extraction or by blending various components.[142,143] They are related structurally to heparin and have similar biological functions, especially anticoagulant effects. Heparins, low-molecular-weight heparins, and heparinoids act as anticoagulants by binding to plasma antithrombin III. This interaction induces a conformational change in anti-thrombin III that increases its ability to inactivate coagulation enzymes, including thrombin and activated factor X (factor Xa).

Low-molecular-weight heparins are thought to have more favorable bioavailability and pharmacokinetics than standard heparin. Their plasma half-lives are two to four times that of heparin.[141] Low-molecular weight heparins cause fewer hemorrhagic complications than standard heparin because they have less pronounced effect on platelet function and vascular permeability.[141,142] Some evidence suggests that low-molecular-weight heparin has more anticoagulant effect than unfractionated heparin and does not activate platelets.[135,143] Studies support the probability that heparin's bleeding complications relate to effects on platelets, especially inhibition of platelet aggregation which is mostly an action of the high-molecular-weight components in heparin.[143] Low-molecular-weight heparins also cause less heparin-related thrombocytopenia, heparin-related skin necrosis, and white clot syndromes. While heparin is monitored closely using the PTT, low-molecular-weight heparins and heparinoids can be monitored by measuring anti–factor Xa activity. Heparinoids and low-molecular-weight heparins are more convenient to use than standard heparin and are often used in patients outside of acute-care hospital settings.

The effectiveness of heparin in ischemic stroke has not been well studied. Ramirez-Lassepas and colleagues found good to excellent recovery in 81% of 136 patients treated with heparin and believe the drug might reduce fluctuations and late deteriorations.[144] However, Duke and colleagues found no benefit regarding stroke progression among patients with "partial stable strokes."[145] Neither study was controlled, and the arterial pathology and stroke mechanisms underlying the ischemia were not investigated or reported. Newer studies suggest that heparin is effective in patients with cerebral dural sinus thrombosis and in selected patients with large artery occlusive disease. Heparin might also be useful in preventing recurrence of cardiac-origin embolism in patients at high risk for early re-embolization.

Beginning in the 1960s, a number of single case reports and retrospective reviews suggested that heparin was a safe and effective treatment for patients with intracranial dural venous sinus thrombosis. Patients given heparin did not worsen or have new hemorrhages. Bousser et al. noted that among 82 patients treated with heparin, 77% of patients had a complete recovery and no deaths occurred.[146] In a retrospective review of several other series of patients with dural sinus thrombosis, among 79 patients given anticoagulants, 94% improved and survived whereas only approximately half of the 157 patients not given anticoagulants survived.[147]

A randomized, double-blinded, prospective trial of heparin use in patients with intracranial venous thrombosis was reported by Einhaupl and colleagues.[148] Ten of their 20 patients with angiographically proven venous sinus thrombosis were given heparin by intravenous bolus of 3,000 IU and then 25,000–65,000 IU each day by continuous intravenous infusion. The dose of heparin was adjusted to double the initial prothrombin time but not exceed 120 seconds (target, 80–100 seconds). The other 10 patients were given placebo. At the start of treatment, three patients in the heparin treated group and two in the placebo group had hemorrhages on CT scans. The authors used the results of a specially designed severity score and the development of ICH on treatment as outcome measures. To evaluate the occurrence of brain hemorrhage, each patient had at least two CT scans. CT was performed when hemorrhage was clinically suspected. The investigators planned to admit 60 patients with an interim analysis after the first 20 patients. The interim analysis was considered so favorable for heparin that the study was terminated after the first 20 patients were entered. The severity scores in the heparin-treated group were much improved over the placebo group. No patient in the heparin-treated group had a new brain hematoma. In the placebo group, there were three new brain hemorrhages; two of the new hematomas were in patients who did not have hemorrhages at onset. In the three patients with brain hemorrhages present before heparin treatment, two had complete recovery.

Einhaupl and colleagues also retrospectively analyzed their data from 102 patients with angiographically proven intracranial dural sinus and venous occlusions studied between 1977 and 1991.[148,149] Among the 102 patients, 43 had ICHs. Two patients had their first ICH after heparin treatment. One patient who had an ICH before treatment had another on heparin. Altogether six patients had ICH after heparin and 33 not treated with heparin had new hemorrhages. They also analyzed data from 40 patients who had known ICH before heparin treatment (27 patients) and before no heparin treatment (13 patients). Among those treated with heparin, 14 out of 27 had full recovery and 4 died; among those not treated with heparin, only 3 out of 13 recovered fully and 9 out of 13 died. The patients not treated with heparin clearly fared worse and had a higher mortality. In a randomized trial of Dutch patients with dural sinus thromboses treated with low-molecular-weight heparin vs placebo, there was a trend for better outcomes in the anticoagulant-treated group, but the difference was not statistically significant.[150] The data are quite convincing that heparin does not worsen or predispose to ICH. Heparin leads to a better outcome. The available data support the use of heparin in patients with intracranial dural and venous thrombosis unless there is a strong contraindication.

The results of two trials also suggest heparin might be effective in patients with acute ischemic stroke caused by large artery thromboembolism. In a trial performed in Hong Kong among 312 patients with acute ischemic stroke, low-molecular-weight heparin was more effective than placebo.[151] There was a significant dose-dependent reduction in the risk of death or dependency among patients treated with low-molecular-weight heparin (χ^2 for trend = 8.066, p = .005). Although vascular studies were not mandated in this study, most patients with ischemic stroke in Hong Kong have intracranial artery occlusive disease. Patients with cardiac lesions that required anticoagulation were not included in this study.

In the Trial of ORG 10172 in Acute Stroke Treatment (TOAST), a heparinoid showed some effectiveness in a subgroup of patients with large artery occlusive disease.[152] In this study, the low-molecular-weight heparinoid ORG 10172 (Danaparoid) was given within 24 hours of the onset of symptoms of an acute ischemic stroke.[152] This heparinoid was given by continuous intravenous infusion for 7 days with the dose adjusted after 24 hours to maintain the anti–factor Xa activity at 0.6–0.8 anti–factor Xa units/ml. ORG 10172 is a mixture of glycosaminoglycans isolated from porcine intestinal mucosa with a mean molecular weight of 5,500. The anti–factor Xa activity of ORG 10172 is attributed to its heparin sulfate component that has a high affinity for antithrombin III.

Although ORG 10172 treatment was not effective in the entire group of patients with ischemic stroke, overall, there was effectiveness for the group of patients that were diagnosed as having large artery atherosclerosis.[152] In the TOAST trial in patients classified as having large artery atherosclerosis, heparinoid reduced the number of recurrences of stroke during the 7 days of infusion. The rates of favorable outcomes were significantly higher in patients given heparinoid when compared with placebo. Sixty-eight percent of patients with large artery atherosclerosis treated with ORG 10172 had favorable outcome versus 54.7% treated with placebo (p = .04); 43% of patients with large artery atherosclerosis treated with ORG 10172 had very favorable outcomes versus 29.1% treated with placebo (p = .02). Recurrent strokes developed in 6% of ORG 10172-treated patients with large artery atherosclerosis versus 11% of those treated with placebo. Recurrent strokes also developed in 7.3% of patients with cardioembolism treated with placebo versus 2.8% of patients treated with ORG 10172. Because of the small numbers the figures for recurrent strokes did not meet statistical significance.[152] ORG 10172 was effective among the group of patients with large artery atherosclerosis who had severe internal carotid artery stenosis in the neck (>50% luminal narrowing or occlusion).[153] This was the only subgroup of patients in the TOAST study who had vascular tests that defined large artery lesions. Significantly, more patients with severe carotid artery disease had favorable outcomes among patients treated with heparinoid. The results of the TOAST trial for patients with carotid artery disease are shown in Table 5-6.

Although heparin would be predicted to prevent acute recurrence of embolism in patients with cardiac-origin embolism, there are explanations why these studies did not show an effect in this group. Patients with high-risk embolic sources thought to require anticoagulation were excluded from the Hong Kong study, and many such patients were probably not entered into the TOAST study. Among all patients with cardioembolism, a task force that studied embolism recurrence showed that most recurrences do not occur during the first week after a first embolus.[154] Results in the TOAST trial among patients with cardioembolism suggested that

Table 5-6. Outcomes in Patients with Carotid Artery Stenosis (>50%) or Occlusion Treated with Danaparoid versus Placebo in the Trial of ORG 10172 in Acute Stroke Treatment Trial

Outcome	Danaparoid	Placebo	*p* Value
Outcome at 7 days			
Favorable	64/119 (53.8%)	41/108 (38.0%)	.023
Very favorable	33/119 (27.7%)	19/108 (17.6%)	.082
Outcome at 3 months			
Favorable	82/120 (68.3%)	58/109 (53.2%)	.021
Very favorable	53/120 (44.2%)	35/109 (32.1%)	.077

Source: Submitted by BH Bendixen from a slide presented at the 1998 meeting of the American Academy of Neurology. Reprinted with permission from BH Bendixen, HP Adams, EC Leira, et al. Responses to treatment with a low molecular weight heparinoid or placebo among patients with acute ischemic stroke secondary to large artery atherosclerosis. Neurology 1998;50:A345.

fewer recurrences developed among patients treated with ORG 10172. The numbers were too small, however, for statistical significance.[152]

A study of acute anticoagulation with heparin in patients with documented large artery atherostenosis and cardiac origin embolism showed that the treatment could be performed safely with a minimum of hemorrhagic complications.[155] Theoretical and practical arguments support the use of heparin to prevent red clot formation in selected individuals. I continue to use heparin in patients with fresh thrombi in large arteries, presumed cardiac thrombi at high risk of brain embolism, and severe stenosis impeding flow in large arteries.

Warfarin

Warfarin is a water-soluble derivative of coumaric acid that is absorbed by the small intestine and transported in the blood loosely bound to albumin. Its therapeutic effect is to inhibit the action of vitamin K necessary for the biological synthesis of factors II (prothrombin), VII, IX, and X.[156] By depressing these procoagulant factors, warfarin affects the so-called intrinsic cascade and the extrinsic coagulation pathway.[156,157] Warfarin works quite differently from heparin. In some patients who have continued transient spells or progressive ischemic symptoms despite warfarin anticoagulation, symptoms may almost miraculously stop when heparin is substituted for warfarin. Heparin should be given before beginning warfarin anticoagulation, because initiation of therapy with warfarin alone can be associated with an initial period of hypercoagulability.

In the past, PTs were usually maintained at 2.0–2.5 times the control value. This therapeutic range was selected as that level slightly below that at which bleeding occurred.[156,157] Wessler and Gitel provide data that persuasively show that the dosage at which warfarin protects against thrombosis is probably far below that needed to cause bleeding.[156] In one study of 96 patients with venous thromboses treated with various intensities of oral anticoagulation, higher intensity therapy (i.e., more prolonged PTs) caused more bleeding. Less intense therapy was equally effective in preventing recurrent thromboembolism.[158] Others have also corroborated the safety and effectiveness of less intense warfarin anticoagulation.[159,160] Because of the wide variation in thromboplastin reagents used, the World Health Organization designated a single batch of human brain thromboplastin as an international standard.[161] Manufacturers calibrate their reagent against the international standard and calculate an International Sensitivity Index that relates their reagent to the international standard. Using the International Sensitivity Index and the PT, the international normalized ratio (INR) can be readily calculated. Various expert groups have published recommendations for intensity of anticoagulation based on the international system.[161,162] Generally, two intensities of anticoagulation have been recommended: a less intense range (INR 2.0–3.0, approximately equivalent to a PT of 1.3–1.5) and a more intense range (INR 3.0–4.5, approximately equivalent to a PT of 1.5–2.0 times control).[161] The higher intensity range clearly has more risk of bleeding. Stroke Prevention in Reversible Ischemia Trial (SPIRIT), a large Dutch trial that compared the effectiveness of aspirin versus oral anticoagulation (INR target range, 3.0–4.5) was prematurely stopped after an interim analysis showed an unacceptable rate of hemorrhage in the anticoagulant-treated group.[163] The frequency of bleeding increased by a factor of 1.43 for each 0.5 unit increase in the INR.[163] The Atrial Fibrillation Investigators analyzed the results of five trials of anticoagulation in patients with atrial fibrillation (INR target range, 1.4–4.2) and recommended a target range of 2.0–3.0 as having the best benefit and risk results.[164,165] Hylek and colleagues also analyzed the results of anticoagulation in atrial fibrillation trials and found that the rate of stroke increased when the INR fell below 2.0. Optimal protection occurred in patients with INRs between 2.0 and 3.0.[166] No further protection was attributable to INRs above 3.0.[166] In most patients, I follow the recommendations of these studies and aim at an INR between 2.0 and 3.0, which translates to a PT of approximately 1.3–1.5 times control value. In patients older than 75 years, I use an INR target of 2.0–2.5.

Until the 1990s, the effectiveness of warfarin administration had not been tested in modern randomized trials in patients with known pathologies. Early observational studies showed the effectiveness of warfarin in patients with rheumatic mitral stenosis who had brain embolism.[167–169] Trials of stroke prophylaxis in patients with atrial fibrillation who did not have valvular heart disease have now documented a dramatic benefit of warfarin treatment.[170–178] Table 5-7 reviews the six major randomized trials that studied this issue.[179] All trials showed a consistent and considerable risk reduction for stroke in patients treated with warfarin. Warfarin is approximately 50% more effective than aspirin in reducing the rate of stroke in patients with atrial fibrillation who do not have valvular disease.[180] The rate of intracranial hemorrhages and major bleeding episodes was low in all groups in all trials except in warfarin-treated patients older than 75 years in the Stroke Prevention in Atrial Fibrillation (SPAF II) study. In that study, 7 of 197 warfarin-treated older patients had intracranial hemorrhages that were most often fatal. Caution must be used in prescribing warfarin to patients older than 75 years. INR targets of 2.0–2.5 may be advisable.

Although there have been no published results to date of trials of warfarin in patients with docu-mented cerebrovascular occlusive lesions, a retrospective review of patients with intracranial occlusive lesions suggests a probable benefit of warfarin over aspirin.[181,182] In the Warfarin-Aspirin Symptomatic Intracranial Study, 151 patients had angiographically documented greater than 50% stenosis of intracranial anterior circulation (55% of patients) or posterior circulation (45%) arteries and were treated with either aspirin or oral warfarin anticoagulants.[181] Among 63 patients treated with aspirin (median duration, 19.3 months), 15 patients (24%) had a stroke and 11 (17%) had a myocardial infarct or sudden death. The overall rate of major vascular events in the aspirin-treated group was 18.1 per 100 patient-years of follow-up. Among 88 patients treated with warfarin (median time, 14.7 months), 6 patients (7%) had an ischemic stroke and 8 (9%) had a myocardial infarct or sudden death. The overall rate of major vascular events in the warfarin group was 8.4 per 100 patient-years of follow-up.[181] The Kaplan-Meier curves showing the proportion of patients in each treatment group who survived without a major vascular event are shown in Figure 5-2.

Clearly, more trials are needed in patients with documented cardiac and cardiovascular lesions. Until the results of such trials are available, I use and recommend the use of warfarin anticoagulation in patients who have or are at risk of developing red clots. In some, after preliminary use of heparin, warfarin is given for a period of 3–6 weeks until clots become organized and adhere to the vascular wall. In other patients, mostly those with cardiac thrombi, arrhythmias, cardiac lesions promoting thrombus formation, or severe stenosis of large arteries, warfarin is given indefinitely until the risk of thrombosis diminishes or anticoagulants become contraindicated. My present practice is to monitor vascular occlusive lesions by ultrasound or vascular imaging (CTA or MRA). I stop warfarin approximately 1 month after stenotic lesions are shown to have become occluded or after arteries recanalize. Warfarin is also used for some patients with congenital or acquired hypercoagulable states.

Drugs That Modify Platelet Functions

Agents that modify platelet adhesion and aggregation have been of great clinical interest in thrombotic disorders, particularly ischemic stroke.

Table 5-7. Trials of Prophylactic Therapy in Patients with Atrial Fibrillation without Valvular Disease

Trial	Design	Results
Copenhagen AFASAK[173]	1,007 patients; mean age 73; coumadin (INR 2.8–4.2) vs aspirin (75mg/day) vs placebo	Thromboemboli (stroke, TIA, systemic embolism); coumadin 2%/yr; aspirin 5.5%/yr; placebo 5.5%/yr
BAATAF[170]	628 patients; mean age 68; coumadin (INR 1.5–2.7) vs other medical Rx (could include aspirin)	Coumadin 2 strokes (0.4%/year); control 13 (3%/yr); no benefit of aspirin (8 of 13 strokes in controls on aspirin); 2 hemorrhages–1 each group
SPAF[174]	1,330 patients; mean age 67; warfarin-eligible patients randomized to warfarin (INR 2–3.5), aspirin (325 mg/day), or placebo; warfarin-ineligible patients randomized to aspirin or placebo	Warfarin 2.3%/yr vs 7.4%/yr placebo; stroke in warfarin-ineligible aspirin group 3.6%/yr vs 6.3% in placebo group; major bleeding 1.5%, 1.4%, 1.6% in warfarin, aspirin, placebo groups
EAFT[171]	1,007 patients, mean age 73; warfarin-eligible patients randomized to warfarin (INR 2.54), aspirin (300 mg), or placebo; warfarin-ineligible to aspirin or placebo	Strokes in 8% of 225 in warfarin group,15% of 404 in aspirin group, 19% of 378 in placebo group; major bleeding 2.8%/yr warfarin group and 0.9%/yr aspirin group
SPAF II[176]	1,100 patients; mean age 69.6; warfarin (INR 2–4.5) vs ASA (325 mg/day) compared in patients <75 yrs and patients >75 yrs	715 patients <75; ischemic stroke & systemic embolism 1.3%/year warfarin vs 1.9%/yr ASA; major hemorrhage 0.9%/yr; ASA 1.7%/yr warfarin; 385 >75; ischemic stroke & systemic embolism 3.6%/yr warfarin, 4.8%/yr ASA; major bleeds 4.2% warfarin,* 1.6% ASA
SPAF III[177]	1,044 patients with 1 or more risk factors; mean age 72; low-intensity fixed dose warfarin (INR 1.2–1.5) plus ASA (325 mg/day) vs adjusted dose warfarin (INR 2–3)	INR 1.3 fixed dose warfarin vs INR target 2.4 adjusted group; ischemic stroke and systemic embolism in 7.9% of fixed dose and ASA vs 1.9% in adjusted dose group
SPAF III[178]	892 patients with posited low risk were given 325 mg ASA	The rate of ischemic stroke was low (2%/yr) and disabling ischemic stroke only 0.8%/yr; the rate of major bleeding was 0.5%/yr

AFASAK = Copenhagen Atrial Fibrillation Aspirin Anticoagulation Study; ASA = aspirin; BAATAF = Boston Area Anticoagulation Trial for Atrial Fibrillation; EAFT = European Atrial Fibrillation Trial; INR = international normalized ratio; SPAF = Stroke Prevention in Atrial Fibrillation Study.
*71% of intracranial hemorrhages fatal; 29% had residual deficit.

Perhaps the first clinical observations on aspirin as an anticoagulant were made by a practitioner named Craven.[183] Craven, observing that dental patients bled more if they had used aspirin, urged friends and patients to take one or two aspirin tablets a day. He later published the effectiveness of this strategy in preventing coronary and cerebral thrombosis among 8,000 men in articles in the *Mississippi Valley Medical Journal*, not a periodical on every neurologist's bookshelf.[183–185] Twenty years later, case reports from the United States and Britain on the effectiveness of aspirin in preventing attacks of transient monocular blindness brought more attention to the subject.[186,187] The American[188] and Canadian[189] aspirin trials soon ensued in the late 1970s. Aspirin and other nonsteroidal anti-inflammatory drugs, such as indomethacin, phenylbutazone, and ibuprofen, inhibit platelet release reactions secondary to adenosine diphosphate–induced platelet aggregation and platelet adhesion to collagen when tested in vitro.[190] Aspirin probably inhibits platelet aggregation and secretion by preventing the synthesis of prostaglandins and thromboxane A_2. This action is achieved by inhibiting the cyclo-oxygenase enzyme that converts arachidonic acid to prostaglandin G_2, the precursor of thromboxane A_2.[191] Aspirin, however, also inhibits the production of prostacyclin by endothelial cells. Prostacyclin has a potent platelet antiaggregant and vasodilator effect.[192]

The optimal therapeutic dosage of aspirin is still controversial. The American[188] and Canadian[189] therapeutic trials used four 5-grain aspirin tablets each day. Some investigators posit that smaller doses produce the desired inhibition of platelet

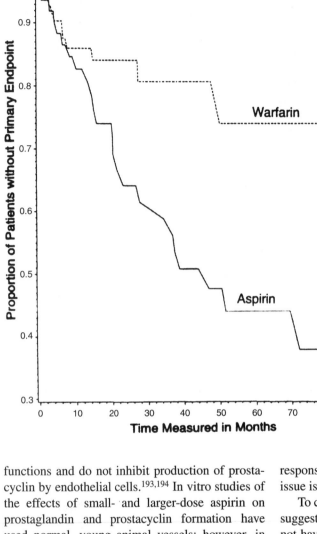

Figure 5-2. Graph shows Kaplan-Meier estimates of the proportion of patients in the Warfarin-Aspirin Symptomatic Intracranial Disease Study remaining free of ischemic stroke, myocardial infarction, or sudden death in those treated with warfarin or aspirin. (Reprinted with permission from MI Chimowitz, J Kokkinos, J Strong, et al. The Warfarin-Aspirin Symptomatic Intracranial Disease Study. Neurology 1995;45:1488–1493.)

functions and do not inhibit production of prostacyclin by endothelial cells.[193,194] In vitro studies of the effects of small- and larger-dose aspirin on prostaglandin and prostacyclin formation have used normal, young animal vessels; however, in patients with extracranial vascular disease, the endothelium is frequently damaged and might no longer be able to synthesize prostacyclin. In the British UK-TIA Trial, one 300-mg aspirin a day was as effective as higher doses.[195] In the Swedish Aspirin Low-Dose Trial, 75 mg of aspirin a day resulted in a statistically significant 18% reduction in stroke and death,[196] whereas in the Dutch TIA trial, even 30 mg was as effective and better tolerated than 300 mg of aspirin a day.[197] In the Canadian trial, relatively few women were tested, so the benefits of aspirin for women could not be shown.[189] In subsequent trials, sex differences in

responsiveness have not been prominent, but the issue is still often raised.[198]

To complicate matters, preliminary observations suggest that some patients who are given aspirin do not have significant effects on platelet functions as measured in vitro.[199,200] Helgason and colleagues studied the effectiveness of aspirin on platelet function measured in vitro.[200] Among 107 patients who received 325 mg of aspirin per day, inhibition of platelet aggregation was complete in 85 (79%) and partial in 22 (20.5%). Among nine patients who did not respond to 325 mg of aspirin, escalating the dose to 650 mg a day resulted in complete platelet inhibition in five (56%). An increase to 975 mg caused complete inhibition in one of the four patients who did not respond to 650 mg. The three patients who did not respond to 975 mg had only partial inhibition at a 1,300-mg aspirin dose.[200]

Genetic factors clearly play a role. Some patients require more aspirin than others. Platelets interact with the endothelium and arterial wall, so platelet function is only one of the factors that relates to the deposition of platelet-fibrin and erythrocyte-fibrin thrombi. Aspirin dosage should be decided by future clinical trials ideally in homogeneous subtypes of patients[6] and by anatomic and functional tests of platelet vascular function in animals and humans. Gastrointestinal bleeding and gastritis are important and common side effects of aspirin. The frequency of these side effects is dose related.

A variety of other agents that decrease platelet aggregation are in clinical use. Dipyridamole (Persantine) is a pyramidopyrimidine compound quite different chemically from the nonsteroidal anti-inflammatory drugs. Acting as a phosphodiesterase inhibitor, it also reduces platelet function. Dipyridamole reduces platelet function by raising the levels of cyclic adenosine monophosphate and of cyclic guanosine monophosphate.[201] These raised levels of cyclic adenosine monophosphate and cyclic guanosine monophosphate have platelet anti-aggregating effects.[201,202] In rabbits, a combination of aspirin and dipyridamole protected against thrombosis induced by combined chemical and electrical stimuli when neither drug did so separately.[203] The optimal dosage of dipyridamole is uncertain, but 400 mg per day was used with warfarin to effectively inhibit embolization from prosthetic heart valves.[204] Even when combined with aspirin, doses below 200 mg per day are probably ineffective.[205] Two trials reported in the early 1980s showed no benefit of dipyridamole even when added to aspirin.[206,207] In the Canadian-American randomized trial, dipyridamole in doses of 300 mg per day had no demonstrable therapeutic effect when added to 1,300 mg per day aspirin in patients with TIA or minor stroke.[206] In the Accidents Ischemiques Cerebraux Lies a l'Atherosclerose trial, 225 mg dipyridamole used with 1,000 mg aspirin was not better than aspirin alone.[207]

Two European Stroke Prevention Studies (ESPS 1 and ESPS 2) reported an effect on stroke prevention of dipyridamole when used with aspirin. In ESPS 1, dipyridamole, 75 mg 3 times a day, and aspirin, 330 mg 3 times a day for 2 years, showed a 38% reduction in stroke compared with placebo in patients with prior ischemic strokes or TIAs.[208] In the ESPS 2 trial, 6,602 patients took placebo, aspirin (25 mg twice a day), dipyridamole in a modified-release form (200 mg twice a day), or aspirin and dipyridamole (25 mg aspirin and 200 mg modified-release dipyridamole twice a day).[201] The relative risk reduction for the combined end points of stroke and death were 13.2% for aspirin, 15.4% for dipyridamole, and 24.4% for the combination of aspirin and dipyridamole. The combined therapy reduced the stroke risk 23.1% over aspirin alone and 24.7% over dipyridamole alone.[201] Note that the ESPS 2 trial used a much lower dose of aspirin and a new form of delayed-release dipyridamole when compared with the earlier French[207] and Canadian-American trials.[206] Headache and gastrointestinal symptoms (e.g., nausea, indigestion, abdominal pain, and diarrrhea) are common side effects of dipyridamole treatment, but headache is less of a problem if low doses of dipyridamole are used initially.

Ticlopidine hydrochloride, a thienopyridine derivate, is an effective platelet antiaggregant that has also been widely used in patients with occlusive vascular disease.[209,210] Ticlopidine functions mostly as an inhibitor of the adenosine diphosphate pathway of platelet aggregation. The drug inhibits most known stimuli to platelet aggregation but, unlike aspirin, does not inhibit the cyclooxygenase pathway.[209,210] Ticlopidine may also have the capability of reducing fibrinogen levels and increasing erythrocyte deformability.[209,211] Clopidogrel, a thienopyridine analogue of ticlopidine that differs from ticlopidine by the addition of a carboxymethyl side group, has been introduced as another effective platelet antiaggregant.[210,212] Clopidogrel and ticlopidine have similar effects on platelets, but clopidogrel has fewer serious hematologic side effects compared with ticlopidine.[209,210,212] In a large, randomized trial, the Ticlopidine-Aspirin Stroke Study, ticlopidine showed a relative risk reduction of approximately 30% in minimizing the rate of stroke, myocardial infarction, and vascular death in men and women who had a previous minor stroke.[213] In the Canadian-American Ticlopidine Study, ticlopidine (500 mg daily) was slightly more effective than aspirin (1,300 mg daily) in reducing the rate of stroke in patients with TIAs or minor strokes.[214] Ticlopidine has also been shown to be effective when used with aspirin in preventing thrombosis in coronary artery stents.[210,215] Ticlopidine had a relatively high rate of side effects, especially diarrhea and skin rash.

Neutropenia, sometimes severe, also was a serious but infrequent complication of ticlopidine (approximately 1% of patients).[213,214] Patients taking ticlopidine had a slightly elevated cholesterol level.[213] Bennett et al. reported 60 patients with thrombotic thrombocytopenic purpura after using ticlopidine,[216] and thrombocytopenia has been noted by others as a ticlopidine side effect.[210] Clearly, ticlopidine is an effective drug but side effects, especially neutropenia and thrombocytopenia, require careful monitoring. In most circumstances, neutropenia develops within the first 3 months of drug use, and white blood cell counts return to normal within days to weeks of ticlopidine termination. Thrombotic thrombocytopenic purpura usually develops within the first month of ticlopidine use.[216] During a consensus conference in 1995, a committee of the American College of Chest physicians reviewed the data on platelet antiaggregants in patients with TIAs and minor strokes. These physicians recommended that ticlopidine only be used in aspirin-intolerant patients and only when close hematologic monitoring was feasible.[217]

The Clopidogrel versus Aspirin in Patients at Risk of Ischemic Events (CAPRIE) trial was a randomized, double-blinded trial of clopidogrel (75 mg per day) versus aspirin (325 mg per day) in preventing ischemic events (e.g., ischemic stroke, myocardial infarction, and vascular death).[212] During 3 years, 19,185 patients were entered, including 6,421 ischemic stroke patients, 6,302 patients with myocardial infarcts, and 6,452 patients with atherosclerotic peripheral vascular occlusive disease. Clopidogrel had a relative risk reduction over aspirin of 8.7%, considering all end points. The frequency of stroke was 405 out of 17,636 (2.30%) for clopidogrel versus 430 out of 17,519 (2.45%) for aspirin. The frequency of myocardial infarction was more effectively reduced by clopidogrel than the frequency of stroke.[212] Clopidogrel had an excellent safety record in this large trial; the frequency of neutropenia and thrombocytopenia in patients using clopidogrel were no different than for aspirin.[212] Although clopidogrel has not been directly compared with ticlopidine, the results of the CAPRIE study suggest that clopidogrel is probably at least equally effective as ticlopidine and has a much better safety profile. I use clopidogrel rather than ticlopidine in patients when I believe an antiplatelet aggregant therapy is warranted and aspirin is prob-

lematic. Because the majority of serious adverse hematologic complications of ticlopidine occurs during the first 3 months, it is probably safe to continue ticlopidine in patients who have been using this drug for longer than 3 months. Because the antiplatelet aggregants discussed (aspirin, dipyridamole, ticlopidine, clopidogrel) have different modes of action and produce partial inhibition of platelet functions, some clinicians have begun to treat patients with less than full-dose combinations of two agents, positing more platelet inhibition with this strategy than that obtained with any of the drugs individually.

Interest is also growing in the potential effects of natural substances, such as eicosopentanoic acid[218] and omega-3 oils, substances found in high concentration in fish, and black-tree fungus, a substance found in most Chinese restaurant foods. Eicosopentanoic acid reduces fibrinogen levels[123] and inhibits platelet functions. It is an excellent substance to use in aspirin-sensitive or intolerant patients.

The advent of newer drugs that are antagonists of the glycoprotein platelet IIb/IIIa complex gives promise of even more effective inhibition of platelet functions. The platelet glycoprotein IIb/IIIa complex is the site of binding to adhesive proteins including fibrinogen. Binding to fibrinogen activates platelet aggregation and adhesion to blood vessels. Glycoprotein platelet IIb/IIIa inhibitors have been used acutely and intravenously, [219,220] but agents that can be used orally and chronically are being tested.[221] Because these glycoprotein platelet IIb/IIIa inhibitors are antagonists of the final common pathway of platelet adhesion with fibrinogen, they give promise of being the most effective agents to prevent white clot formation.

The Antiplatelet Trialists Collaboration[222] and others[217,223] reviewed the relative effects of antiplatelet drugs on stroke prevention and other vascular events in detail. None of the published studies mandated rigorous evaluation of the heart, aorta, and craniocerebral arteries or technology-assisted diagnosis of stroke mechanisms. None of the studies showed which drugs were effective for which vascular lesions. More studies are needed comparing antiplatelet drugs with other strategies in patients with well-defined vascular lesions.

Some investigators have used a combination of warfarin anticoagulants and platelet antiaggregants, usually aspirin, in patients with severe atherosclerosis who did not respond to more conventional treatments.[224] This combination was effective but resulted in a higher bleeding-complication rate.[224,225] I have also used this strategy in patients in whom warfarin was indicated but was ineffective when used alone.

A useful strategy may be to use platelet antiaggregants when there is no obstruction to flow and ischemia is most likely due to the process of platelet plugs and small white (or white and red) clots. Heparin (or low-molecular-weight heparin or heparinoids) and warfarin are reserved for situations of tight stenosis or clots within the heart. These standard anticoagulants are also used for 3–4 weeks in patients with a recent in situ occlusion within a large artery. This method is strictly hypothetical. Results to date are anecdotal and have not been tested scientifically. Table 5-8 reviews my present recommendations for the use of platelet antiaggregants and anticoagulants.

Increasing the Brain's Resistance to Ischemia

I have discussed ways of improving the circulation. In this section, I turn to means of helping the brain survive despite poor perfusion. Neuronal death probably depends on multiple factors,[226] including (1) level of activity[227] (the more work that goes on, the more fuel is needed), (2) presence of local metabolites such as lactic acid[226,228,229] and oxygen-free radicals,[230–233] (3) temperature of the system (at low temperatures there is less metabolism and less need for fuel),[234,235] (4) integrity of the neuronal cell membranes,[226,236] and (5) influx of calcium into cells and the extracellular-to-intracellular gradient for calcium.[237–239] Preliminary evidence from experimental whole-brain ischemia in young animals indicates that hyperglycemia makes the brain more vulnerable to ischemia. Sugar increases metabolism and leads to the production of lactic acid. Acidosis can be destructive to brain tissue.[240] In experimental animals, work can lead to increased vulnerability to ischemia when compared with the resting state.[227] A high concentration of extracellular calcium can also contribute to final neuronal death.[237–239] Neurotransmitters, especially glutamate, released at sites of ischemia might overexcite neurons and cause toxic damage increasing the effects of the initial ischemia.[241,242] This theory, often referred to as the *excitotoxin hypothesis*, has

Table 5-8. Present Recommended Use of Platelet Aggregants and Anticoagulants

---

Heparin (standard intravenous dose) (short-term, 2–4 weeks)

Usually given by constant intravenous infusion keeping aPTT between 60 and 100 seconds (1.5–2 × control aPTT)

1. Immediate therapy of definite cardiac-origin brain embolism (large cerebral infarct, hypertension, bacterial endocarditis, or sepsis would delay or contraindicate this use)
2. For patients with severe stenosis or occlusion of the ICA origin, ICA siphon, MCA, VA, or basilar artery, with less than a severe clinical deficit—treatment then could be shifted to warfarin or surgery

Heparin (subcutaneous mini dose)

For prophylaxis of deep-vein occlusion in patients immobilized by stroke (unless contraindicated)

Warfarin

Usually overlapped with heparin, keeping INR between 2.0 and 3.0

1. Long-term (greater than 3 months) in patients with cardiogenic brain embolization and rheumatic heart disease, atrial fibrillation with large atria or prior cerebral embolism, prosthetic valves, and some hypercoagulable states
2. Long-term (greater than 3 months) in patients with severe stenosis of the ICA origin, ICA siphon, MCA stem, VA, basilar artery—used until studies show artery has been occluded for at least 3 weeks
3. Shorter-term (3–6 weeks) in patients with recent occlusion of the ICA, MCA, VA, or basilar arteries

Platelet antiaggregants (aspirin, clopidogrel, combined aspirin-dipyridamole)

1. For patients with plaque disease of the extracranial and intracranial arteries without severe stenosis
2. For patients with polycythemia or thrombocytosis and related ischemic attacks

---

aPTT = activated partial thromboplastin time; ICA = internal carotid artery; INR = international normalized ratio; MCA = middle cerebral artery; VA = vertebral artery.

stimulated much research concerning neurotransmitters and ischemia.

These observations on factors that influence brain vulnerability to anoxic and ischemic insults have stimulated interest in many possible therapeutic regimens. Treatments aimed at reducing cell damage are usually referred to as *neuroprotective* or *cytoprotective* therapies. Although a variety of neuroprotective strategies have shown some effectiveness in laboratory animals, none has shown definite benefits in randomized trials of human patients with strokes.

Although early studies suggested that hyperglycemia, with or without diabetes mellitus, might aggravate ischemic brain damage,[228,243] some reviews indicate that the issues are complex.[244] Studies of glycosylated hemoglobin allow an estimation of the adequacy of blood-glucose control in diabetics. Elevated fasting blood sugar levels,[244,245] especially when accompanied by high levels of glycosylated hemoglobin,[244] do predict poor outcome. Others have related high glucose levels in stroke patients to a stress response[246,247]; large hemorrhages and infarcts induce catecholamine secretion, which in turn increases the white blood cell count and the blood sugar levels. Reduction of elevated blood sugar levels by insulin might decrease brain lactate production in ischemic zones and thereby reduce necrosis. This idea, however, remains an unproven hypothesis. It seems prudent to avoid hyperglycemia and treat high blood sugar levels with insulin. Insufficient data exist to warrant reducing normal blood sugars to hypoglycemic levels.

Hypothermia[248] and barbiturate anesthesia[249,250] are nonspecific strategies that reduce cerebral energy and metabolism and thereby reduce the brain's requirements for fuel, oxygen, and blood. Each can lead to circulatory changes and can complicate the examination and management of stroke patients. Some have hypothesized that ischemia and spinal injury can result in release of endogenous opiates (endorphins) that cause further injury.[251,252] Early reports suggested that naloxone, an opiate receptor antagonist, was effective in reducing stroke severity in gerbils[253] and humans,[254] but later studies showed an equivocal or lack of naloxone effect. In high doses, naloxone may be effective in reversing some clinical signs,[255] but this probably occurs mostly in patients with stunned brain regions and not in patients with established infarcts. At present, naloxone is not being used in patients with ischemia.

Another strategy being tested for effectiveness in protecting neurons from the effects of ischemia is the use of gangliosides.[256] The ganglioside compounds used are monogangliosides (GM1) that are composed of glycosphingolipids, normal components of plasma membranes that are particularly abundant in the cells of the central nervous system. Exogenous gangliosides are important chemical constituents of neurons. Monosialoganglioside GM1 enters neural plasma membranes and might protect membranes from injury. Early studies showed promise,[257,258] but larger trials showed no benefit from GM1 treatment.[256,259,260]

Some investigators posit that free radicals found during hypoxic injury may lead to further neuronal damage.[230–233] A free radical is an atom, group of atoms, or molecule having one or more unpaired electrons in its outermost orbit. Covalent chemical bonds usually have paired electrons; free radicals are molecules with an open bond, which accounts for their extreme reactivity. The free radicals of importance in brain ischemia are superoxide and hydroxyl radicals.[230] Hydrogen peroxide can generate hydroxyl radicals in reaction with superoxide. Xanthine oxidase is the major enzyme that generates superoxide radicals. Free radicals can react with and damage proteins, nucleic acids, lipids, and other molecules and can initiate destructive chain reactions.[231,232] Oxygen radicals can also damage blood vessels and cause vasodilation, increased permeability, endothelial and smooth muscle injury, and increased platelet aggregation.[261]

Strategies to prevent and neutralize oxygen free radicals have been attempted mostly in experimental animals. The agents used are often referred to as *free radical scavengers*. Allopurinol inhibits xanthine oxidase but does not penetrate well into the brain. Inhibition has not proved effective. Superoxide dismutase is an enzymatic scavenger that could alter the oxygen radicals as they are formed. Mice that overexpress superoxide dismutase have reduced ischemic damage when exposed to glutamate neurotoxicity.[262] Other putative antioxidants include vitamin E, glutathiones, and a new class of compounds called *lazaroids* that are usually 21-aminosteroids.[263,264] One of these 21-aminosteroids, tirilizad mesylate, is being studied for its effect in brain ischemia.[265] These compounds and strategies have been tried in experimental animals, but there are fewer data on their safety and effectiveness in humans. A large trial that included 1,023 patients with aneurysmal subarachnoid hemorrhage showed some benefit from 6 mg/kg of tirilizad mesylate when used with nimodipine in men.[265,266] Some of the benefit from tirilizad was attributed to a decrease in the frequency and severity of vasoconstriction.[265,266] Two trials of tirilizad mesylate (6 mg/kg) given within 6 hours of stroke onset and continued for 3 days in patients with acute ischemic stroke showed good tolerability and safety, but tirilizad conveyed no improvement in recovery after 3 months in either trial.[265,267,268]

The most compelling theory of nerve cell damage has undoubtedly been the excitotoxin hypothesis.[241,242] The concept was introduced by Olney and colleagues to describe the mechanism by which glutamate and some other acidic amino acids caused neuronal lesions in periventricular structures when given systemically to mice.[241,269,270] Electrophysiologic studies showed that these compounds functioned as neuronal excitants and damaged the periventricular structures studied. Hypothetically, hypoxia and ischemia caused energy depletion and release of glutamate into the tissues. Glutamate then was taken up by receptors and excited the cells already depleted of blood supply, ultimately leading to neuronal death. Putative neurotoxins include glutamate, kainic acid, N-methyl-D-aspartate (NMDA), and homocysteic acid. By far, glutamate has been the most studied. These compounds have various receptor types, usually referred to as *NMDA* and *non-NMDA* receptors, including quisqualate and kainate receptors.

Experimental evidence supports the role of excitotoxins in potentiating ischemia. When kainic acid is injected into the hippocampus of experimental animals it causes a pattern of cell death similar to hypoxic-ischemic damage.[270] The concentration of glutamate in the extracellular compartment in ischemic brain is increased. Deafferentation of specific intrahippocampal excitatory pathways seems to protect against ischemic damage. Finally, drugs that block excitatory neurotransmission are sometimes protective when given to animals early after experimentally induced ischemia.

Glutamate opens membrane sodium conductance allowing a large influx of sodium to enter cells. Chloride ion and water follow the sodium causing cytotoxic edema. Transmembrane influx of calcium into cells leads to a toxic increase in cytosolic free calcium that can kill cells.[236–239] Experimentally, a number of competitive and noncompetitive NMDA receptor antagonists have been used, including MK 801, dextrorphan, dextromethorphan, ketamine, magnesium, memantine, selfotel, aptiganel, felbamate, and phencyclidine.[256,271–273] Adenosine, its agonists, and propentofylline, an adenosine transport inhibitor, also reduce glutamate release.[256,274,275] Although the vast bulk of the work on excitatory neurotransmitters has been in laboratory animals, preliminary studies

have been carried out in human stroke patients.[256,271,272] Many of the agents used have had prominent central nervous system or cardiovascular toxicity. Agitation, confusion, sedation, hallucinations, catatonia, and psychotic behavior occur during therapy with many of the NMDA channel antagonists.[256,272] Aptinogel (Cerestat) and some other NMDA antagonists cause a significant rise in blood pressure.[273,276] These side effects have limited the tolerability of these compounds, and preliminary studies have not showed convincing benefit.

Lubelazole, a benzathiazole compound, showed promise as an effective neuroprotective agent in animal stroke models, but two large, randomized trials did not show clear-cut benefit in humans.[277,278] Another cytoprotective strategy has been to give animal stroke models and humans cytidine-5-diphosphocholine (citicoline), an intermediary in the biosynthesis of the membrane phospholipid phosphatidylcholine, to enhance the synthesis of this lipid in the brain. Preliminary human studies seemed to show some beneficial effects of citicoline in human stroke patients.[279] In animals, citicoline seemed to have a beneficial synergistic effect with MK 801, an NMDA antagonist.[280]

The final common pathway of neuronal death in ischemia may well be calcium influx into cells. Excitotoxins, free radicals, acidosis, and other substances may ultimately kill cells by injuring membranes and allowing Ca^{++} into the cells.[237–239] Calcium has been shown to accumulate in the interstitial space and inside cells during ischemia.[281,282] A number of calcium channel blockers have been used to attempt to block or alter the entry of calcium into cells. Trials have shown inconsistent effects of nimodipine.[105–107] Perhaps newer pharmacological agents given early after the onset of brain ischemia might provide more effective calcium channel blockade within brain tissue in ischemic zones. I list in Table 5-9 some of the tested neuroprotective strategies.[283] Armchair ideas and theories abound and far outweigh the data, but this field of investigation may prove fruitful in the future. Trials in human stroke patients have not always been well designed to show an effect of the various therapies. Ideally, neuroprotective agents would be posited to work when given early to patients who had stunned brain at risk for infarction. Patients with lacunar infarcts and those that already have important

Table 5-9. Neuroprotective Therapies
for Ischemic Stroke

Voltage-sensitive calcium channel antagonists (e.g., nimodipine, darodipine, flunarazine)

Noncompetitive *N*-methyl-D-aspartate (NMDA) receptor
antagonists (e.g., dextromethorphan, eliprodil, aptinagel,
remacemide)

Competitive NMDA antagonists (e.g., selfotel)

Calcium channel modulators (e.g., eliprodil, ACEA-1021)

Antioxidants (e.g., tirilazad a 21-aminosteroid, superoxide
dysmutase)

Alpha-amino-3-hydroxy-5-methyl-4-isoxazole propionic
acid (AMPA) and kainate receptor antagonists (e.g.,
NBQX, YM90K)

Presynaptic gamma-aminobutyric acid inhibitors (e.g., fos-
phenytoin)

Gamma-aminobutyric acid receptor agonists (e.g., chlome-
thiazole)

Presynaptic modulation of glutamate release (e.g., riluzole)

Adenosine analogs (e.g., propentofylline)

Calpain antagonists (e.g., AK 275)

Polypeptide growth factors (e.g., basic fibroblast growth
factor)

Antiadhesion molecules (e.g., antibodies against ICAM-I,
CD11b/18)

Phosphatidylcholine synthesis (e.g., citicoline)

Apoptosis inhibitors (e.g., cycloheximide)

Source: Reprinted with permission from LR Caplan. New
stroke therapies. Arch Neurol 1997;54:1222–1224. Copyright ©
American Medical Association.

brain infarction are unlikely to respond. Most of
the trials have given therapeutic agents too late
and have not required sufficient brain and vascular
imaging to limit treatment to those expected to
respond.

Statins (HMG-CoA Reductase Inhibitors)

The 3-hydroxy-3-methylglutaryl coenzyme A reductase inhibitors (statins), were initially prescribed
because of their potent affect in lowering serum cholesterol, especially the low-density lipoprotein component. Early trials showed that statin drugs not only
reduced cholesterol levels but also were effective in
reducing coronary artery disease–related events and
mortality, even in patients with average levels of cholesterol.[284–286] Analysis of randomized trials of

statins also shows a clear and rather dramatic reduction in the incidence of stroke.[287–289] Use of statin
drugs slows progression of carotid artery atherosclerotic plaques.[290–292] The beneficial effects of the
statins on nearly all aspects of atherosclerotic disease
morbidity and mortality are not entirely explained by
reduction in serum lipid levels. Basic research indicates some other important salutory effects of the
statins including (1) normalization of the vascular
endothelium, (2) anti-inflammatory effects, (3)
depletion and stabilization of the lipid core content
of plaques, (4) strengthening of the fibrous cap of
plaques, (5) decrease in formation of platelet-fibrin
thrombi and decreased deposition of white clots on
endothelial surfaces, and (6) reduction in the thrombogenicity of plaque elements.[293]

Neurotransmitter Replacement and the Effect
of Pharmacological Agents on Recovery

The previous sections discussed prevention and
minimization of ischemic brain damage. What if
damage has already occurred and an infarct or
hemorrhage is already present? Are there agents or
strategies that might improve function or acceler-
ate and promote maximum recovery? Injury to
nerve cells affects their ability to secrete or
respond to neurotransmitters. One strategy that has
become popular since 1980 is to attempt to restore
function by replacing neurotransmitters known to
be active in damaged regions. L-Dopa is given to
patients with Parkinson's disease to replace
depleted dopamine because of nigrostriatal degeneration. Acetylcholine-like drugs have been tried in
an attempt to treat the hypothesized cholinergic
deficit in Alzheimer's disease. After this lead, a few
clinicians have tried neurotransmitters in stroke
patients. In one patient with bilateral paramedian
thalamic infarcts who was apathetic and habitually
assumed sleeping postures, bromocriptine, a
dopamine agonist, led to improvement in spontaneity and less time in bed.[294] In a patient who had
been aphasic since a left frontal-lobe hemorrhage
3.5 years before study, bromocriptine led to an
improvement in speech fluency and a reduction in
hesitancy when talking.[295] Bromocriptine was also
effective in a patient with neglect of the left side of
space caused by a right frontoparietal and striatal
infarct.[296] Neglect and lack of attention were

improved while taking bromocriptine and worsened after the drug was withdrawn. Bromocriptine and lisuride have been used effectively to treat abulia in four patients with degenerative diseases and strokes.[297] In all of these circumstances, bromocriptine presumably had no healing effect on the damaged tissues; it merely improved functional capacity.

Amphetamines have also been given to promote recovery and enhance function. After the animal experiments of Feeney and colleagues,[298,299] who found that amphetamines coupled with motor activity accelerated recovery of beam-walking ability in rats, some investigators began to try amphetamines in stroke patients.[300,301] In rats, neither saline (if the rats had low blood volumes, also used as a control) nor amphetamine alone facilitated recovery after sensorimotor-cortex lesions. A single 2-mg/kg injection of amphetamines and continued experience walking on the beam were needed.[300,301] In contrast, animals given haloperidol performed far worse than controls.[299] Amphetamines were also effective in promoting recovery of function in animals with experimental sensorimotor-cortex lesions.[302] In a preliminary human study, 10 mg of D-amphetamine sulfate and physical therapy led to accelerated recovery when compared with patients given placebo and therapy.[300] Amphetamine had to be given early to be effective. From the available studies, it is not clear whether amphetamine has a specific effect in promoting recovery or merely a generally pepped-up function when combined with physical activity. Amphetamine administration might lead to long-term potentiation of cell function[303] or merely a nonspecific stimulation of less-than-normal cells.

Some pharmacological agents have the potential of retarding recovery. Haloperidol has a definite negative effect on recovery.[298–300] Similarly, drugs that enhance gamma-aminobutyric acid transmission, such as diazepam, might increase inhibition of function and also delay recovery.[304] Stroke patients are often exposed to polypharmacy.[305,306] Some drugs have been prescribed before the stroke and others are given after the stroke to treat various symptoms and general medical conditions. In general, the acute and chronic effects of concurrent drugs on recovery have been poorly studied but are clearly important.[306,307] Table 5-10 reviews available information on the effect of various drugs on recov-

ery as studied in the laboratory or clinically.[306] Sedatives, anticonvulsants, haloperidol, and opiates should be avoided when possible.

Increased Intracranial Pressure and Brain Edema and Their Control

Large ischemic and hemorrhagic strokes often increase the volume and pressure inside the cranium. Herniations, shifts in intracranial contents, and generalized increase in ICP are all common causes of death in patients with large strokes. Treatment of these patients often involve strategies to control changes in ICP. Subarachnoid hemorrhage is also accompanied by increased blood within the cranium, often complicated by decreased drainage of cerebrospinal fluid. Patients with subarachnoid hemorrhage almost always have increased ICP.

The cranium can be thought of as an almost completely closed structure within a rigid container. The brain and its interstitial fluid account for approximately 80% of the intracranial volume, whereas cerebrospinal fluid (CSF) and blood within vessels each account for approximately 10% of the volume.[308] When ICP rises, adaptation occurs mostly by altering the CSF and vascular compartments. Less CSF can be produced or more can be absorbed. Blood volume inside the cranium can also be reduced. Most blood is contained in the low-pressure venous system, and this volume can be reduced.[308] ICP has a major effect on pressure and flow in brain blood vessels. To maintain viability of brain tissue, there must be adequate cerebral perfusion pressure. In supine patients, cerebral perfusion pressure is approximately equal to the mean systemic arterial blood pressure minus the mean ICP.[308] Either an increase in ICP or a decrease in systemic blood pressure can further compromise rCBF to already ischemic brain regions. For practical purposes, there are only a few mechanisms of ICP elevation in stroke patients. These include (1) introduction of new contents into the cranium, such as a hematoma within the brain or subarachnoid hemorrhage; (2) edema in and around infarcts and hemorrhages; (3) obstruction of the ventricular system leading to hydrocephalus; and (4) decreased absorption of CSF caused by subarachnoid bleeding. Each of these problems dictates different treatment strategies.

Table 5-10. Results of Laboratory and Clinical Studies of Recovery After Focal Brain Injuries

Transmitter, Substance, or Class	Action	Lab Effect	Clinical Effect
Norepinephrine		+	
Amphetamine sulfate	Sympathomimetic	+	+/Neutral
Phenteramine	Sympathomimetic	+	
Phenylpropanolamine	Sympathomimetic	+	
Methylphenidate	Sympathomimetic	+	?
Yohimbine	Alpha$_2$-AR antagonist	+	
Idazoxan	Alpha$_2$-AR antagonist	+	
Clonidine	Alpha$_2$-AR antagonist	−	(−)
Haloperidol	Alpha$_1$-AR antagonist	−	(−)
Prazosin	Alpha$_1$-AR antagonist	−	(−)
Propanolol	Beta-AR antagonist	Neutral	
GABA		−	
Diazepam	GABA agonist	−	
Muscimol	GABA agonist	−	
Anticonvulsants			
Phenytoin		−	(−)
Phenobarbital		−	
Carbamazepine		Neutral	
Vigabatrin		Neutral	
Antidepressants			
Trazodone	5-HT reuptake blocker	−	+
Fluoxetine	5-HT reuptake blocker	Neutral	+
Desipramine	NE reuptake blocker	+	
Amitryptiline	Mixed 5-HT NE reuptake blocker	−/Neutral	
Dopamine			
Haloperidol	Butyrophenone	−	(−)
Fluanisone	Butyrophenone	−	
Droperidol	Butyrophenone	−	
Spiroperidol	Antagonist	−	
Apomorphine	Agonist	+	

AR = adrenergic receptor; GABA = gamma-aminobutyric acid; NE = norepinephrine; 5-HT = 5 hydroxytryptamine (serotonin); + = beneficial effect; − = detrimental effect; ? = insufficient testing; (−) = drugs included in lists of potentially harmful agents in two retrospective studies but have not been examined sufficiently separately.
Source: Modified from LB Goldstein. Potential effects of common drugs on stroke recovery. Arch Neurol 1998;55:454–456.

Reducing or Limiting the Size of an Intracerebral Hemorrhage

Unlike brain infarction, a hemorrhage always introduces extra volume into the closed cranial cavity. The larger the hemorrhage, the more the intracranial volume is expanded. In addition, the local blood collection induces surrounding edema, which further increases the volume of extra matter within the brain. ICP is generally elevated, especially in the region of the hematoma; the pressure changes can lead to a shift of midline structures and herniation into other dural compartments. The aim of therapy is to limit the size of the hemorrhage. This can be accomplished by limiting the bleeding, treating the accompanying edema, or draining the hematoma. In the case of hemorrhage caused by a vascular malformation or aneurysm, removing the offending vascular lesion also prevents recurrent hemorrhage.

The most important method to stop the bleeding is to reduce arterial tension. Overzealous blood pressure reduction, however, can be harmful because the elevated blood pressure helps perfuse brain tissue remote from the hemorrhage to some degree. Venous and dural sinus pressures are also raised pari passu when ICP is elevated. The arterial pressure must rise to produce an effective arteriovenous pressure differential to perfuse the brain. Excessive reduction in blood pressure may decrease perfusion. The patient's alertness and neurologic findings must be carefully monitored as the blood pressure is lowered. When hemorrhage is caused by a bleeding diathesis, correction of the coagulopathy is critical in containing the hemorrhage. Use of antihemophilic globulin in hemophiliacs and reversal of warfarin-induced hypoprothrombinemia by fresh frozen plasma or vitamin K are examples of such therapeutic interventions.

Drainage of hematomas can provide rapid decompression. Some patients may decompress their own lesions through spontaneous dissection of the clot that drains into the ventricle or the subarachnoid space. Ease of surgical drainage will depend on the location of the lesion and its proximity to the surface. Lobar, putaminal, and cerebellar hemorrhages are easiest to drain surgically; thalamic and pontine hemorrhages are difficult to drain effectively.[309,310] The purpose of drainage is to reduce critical volume expansion that threatens life. Drainage of the hematoma leaves a residual cavity that disconnects brain pathways. Although allowing survival, drainage probably does not reduce the neurologic deficit. In comparable-sized infarcts, the cortex is invariably destroyed, whereas hematomas usually spare the cortex. For this reason, recovery from hemorrhages is usually better than from infarcts of equal size. Surgical drainage should be performed if life is threatened by the volume of the lesion and if the hematoma is accessible. The decision to operate must take into consideration the severity of the residual deficit and the wishes of the patient and family after they have been fully informed of the alternatives.

Hematomas are easiest to drain early in the course when the hemorrhage is liquid. Surgeons have begun to drain hematomas stereotactically through a burr hole.[309–312] Some surgeons use fibrinolytic agents to liquify hematomas and then aspirate the contents.[309–312] Brain edema surrounding the lesion can be treated with agents discussed in the next section.

Treatment of Brain Swelling

Brain infarcts, hemorrhages, and subarachnoid bleeding can cause secondary effects that lead to swelling of the brain. The resulting increase in ICP contributes to reduction in consciousness and increases the likelihood of a bad outcome. The three major processes that swell the brain are vascular congestion, so-called vasogenic brain edema, and cytotoxic edema. The potential volume of distended brain capillaries is great. When consciousness is reduced, patients may hypoventilate, thus raising the partial pressure of arterial carbon dioxide. Carbon dioxide is a potent vasodilator. The potential importance of vascular congestion can be shown by the use of mechanical hyperventilation in rapidly reducing elevated ICP.[308,313] Hyperventilation causes an almost immediate decrease in ICP but the peak decrement occurs approximately 30 minutes after the carbon dioxide partial pressure (PCO_2) is reduced.[308,314] The initial acute reduction in PCO_2 of 5–10 mm Hg often reduces ICP by 25–30%.[308] The PCO_2 should be kept between 25 and 35 mm Hg.[308,314] Blood gases should be monitored using capillary oximetry in patients with reduced consciousness. The ICP-reducing effect of hyperventilation is temporary and lasts only 1–2 days.[314] In many patients, it may be necessary to use sedation and a curare-like drug to adequately control mechanical hyperventilation. Reducing the volume of blood in the head reduces ICP irrespective of the cause. Even when there is no important vascular dilation or congestion, decreasing the amount of venous blood volume in the cranium allows acute decompression of intracranial contents.

Infarcts and hematomas are often accompanied by considerable edema during the acute period. The two basic types of brain edema are vasogenic and cytotoxic.[315] Water in the interstitial or extracellular compartment has been traditionally called *vasogenic edema* after Klatzo.[316] This type of edema responds to osmotic diuretics, such as mannitol and glycerol. Glycerol is an effective osmotic dehydrating agent that reduces ICP and can be given either orally or intravenously.[317–319] When given intravenously, glycerol should be infused every 2 hours but can be given every 4–6 hours orally.[308] A 20–25% solution of mannitol has become the most common osmotic agent used to reduce ICP. Although dosage varies, the typical initial dose of mannitol is 0.75 to 1 g/kg followed by 0.25–0.5 g/kg every 3 to 5 hours depending on the ICP.[308] Small doses of 0.25g/kg may decrease ICP as well as higher doses, but the effect of small doses lasts a shorter time.[308,320] Mannitol may also improve microcirculatory perfusion in the regions directly surrounding hematomas. Elevated head position and barbiturate sedation also reduce ICP. The effect of corticosteroids is controversial, but most studies show no benefit of steroids in patients with brain hemorrhages and infarcts.[308] Vasogenic edema commonly surrounds hematomas. Many clinicians use mannitol in patients with large hematomas. There is theoretical concern, however, that hypertonic agents could diffuse into the hematoma during continued bleeding and increase the volume of the hematoma.

The second type, so-called cytotoxic edema,[315] is caused by swelling of the cells so that the water is intracellular. Most of the edema in patients with ischemia is intracellular and does not respond to corticosteroids. Ischemia can also produce some vasogenic edema. This develops later, however, when brain cell necrosis has released substances that compromise the blood–brain barrier and lead to extracellular edema. Both vasogenic and cytotoxic edema may be potentiated by reperfusion of brain tissue.[315,321] When the arterial supply to a brain region is blocked, the capillaries and small blood vessels may be damaged by the resulting ischemia. When this region is reperfused, the damaged capillaries leak fluid because of injury to the endothelium and basement membranes. The reperfused blood may also carry or promote circulation of substances to the region, such as excitotoxins and Ca^{++} ions, which might enhance cell damage leading to more cytotoxic edema.[9,239] Clinical trials have not shown a general beneficial effect from corticosteroids in ischemic stroke.[308,322] Most authorities do not recommend their use in patients with brain infarcts. In most infarct patients, edema is not clinically important except when there is massive infarction and the prognosis is already poor. Dramatic edema does develop in certain younger patients, however, despite seemingly limited infarction. In this circumstance, osmotic agents and steroids are probably helpful.

Occasionally, surgical decompression with removal of infarcted and edematous brain has been performed in patients with herniations or increased ICP. Most often, the infarction has involved the cerebellum with resultant compression of the brain stem and fourth ventricle.[323–325] The infarcted cerebellum acts much like a hematoma causing critical mass effect in the posterior cranial fossa, a relatively small, enclosed compartment. Hemicraniectomy has been increasingly used to treat patients with large cerebral infarcts.[326–328] Decompressive hemicraniectomy involves removing a large bone flap of approximately 12 cm that usually includes the frontal, parietal, and temporal bones and part of the occipital squama.[328] The dura mater is opened and a dural patch is used for closure. At first, the surgery was limited to patients with large right cerebral hemisphere infarcts because it was thought that survivors with large left hemisphere infarcts would remain hopelessly disabled by aphasia and right hemiplegia.[326] Initially, surgery was only performed after a major shift in brain contents had occurred and the patient became stuporous. Some studies, however, show surprisingly good results even in patients with large left hemisphere infarcts.[327,328] The prognosis of patients with large middle cerebral artery territory infarcts is so poor[329] that aggressive therapy is warranted, especially in young, previously healthy individuals. Occasional patients, even those with uncal herniation, do respond and survive after the use of acute hyperventilation followed by mannitol.[330] Survival from massive cerebral infarction is better when hemicraniectomy is performed early before herniation occurs.[327,328]

Hydrocephalus can be caused by ventricular drainage system blockage, most commonly the aqueduct or fourth ventricle, or by failure of CSF absorption caused by plugging of the meninges by blood and blood products. In SAH, the ventricles may enlarge early in the course, and some patients develop persistent hydrocephalus.[331] Ventricular shunting is needed in only a minority of patients with SAH because, in many patients, the hydrocephalus is temporary. Most other patients respond to repeated LPs and the use of acetazolamide to decrease CSF production. Large cerebellar infarcts and hemorrhages distort the fourth ventricle, leading to obstructive hydrocephalus.[323,332] Insertion of a ventricular drain or shunt can be lifesaving in that situation and can allow recovery in some patients, without the need for direct surgery on the posterior fossa lesion.[333] The decision whether to treat patients with large cerebellar infarcts with ventricular drainage or removal of a large portion of the infarct depends on the clinical and neuroimaging findings in the individual patient.[323,334]

Stroke Units and the Role of Multiple Treatments and Strategies

During the 1990s, many general and specialty hospitals have begun to designate units that are dedicated to the care of stroke patients. These units vary in their makeup and emphasis. Some are administered by internal medicine specialists, some by neurologists, and others by specialists in physical medicine and rehabilitation. Some emphasize acute stroke care and monitoring of acute stroke patients. These units are excellent resources for clinical research and clinical stroke trials that study acute phase treatments and practices. Others emphasize early rehabilitation. Some units have access to the most advanced diagnostic technology. All stroke units have specialized nursing care, protocols and practices to prevent the complications of stroke, and education for stroke patients, their families, and significant others. Treatment in stroke units reduces mortality, decreases stroke morbidity, and allows more patients to remain independent and to return to their homes.[335–339] Randomized trials and systematic reviews and meta-analyses of trials all have shown a considerable benefit for acute stroke units.

Stroke is a complex disease. Care should include (1) stroke and atherosclerosis risk assessment and stroke prevention strategies, (2) rapid clinical evaluation and diagnosis, (3) rapid complete brain and vascular imaging studies and blood tests, (4) management of blood pressure and fluid balance, (5) medical or surgical treatment (or both) of the process causing the acute stroke, (6) early use of rehabilitation techniques, (7) surveillance and treatment to prevent the common stroke complications (e.g., aspiration, phlebothrombosis, urinary and pulmonary infections, and bed sores), and (8) education for patients and their families regarding their specific problems and stroke in general.

In the foregoing discussions, I have mostly discussed individual treatments. Because most stroke patients have more than one pathophysiologic problem, combinations of treatment are often indicated. Neuroprotective agents could be used with throm-

bolytics; theoretically, neuroprotective agents could delay brain infarction until thrombolytics were able to recanalize clots and reperfuse ischemic zones.[340,341] Patients with brain ischemia and increased ICP have been treated with volume expanders (e.g., hypertonic saline hydroxyethyl starch) and mannitol, a combination aimed at reducing brain edema while maintaining perfusion.[342] Because patients with strokes often develop second and third strokes that are different in etiology from the initial stroke,[343] all patients should be fully investigated for conditions that may cause future strokes. Consideration should be given to prophylaxis of all of the risks found.[344]

Summary and Rules

The field of stroke treatment is changing so quickly that I have included much armchair theorizing and investigational strategies. I suggest the following rules clinicians should use when approaching treatment in their patients with strokes and cerebrovascular disease:

1. Begin preventive strategies early. Educate patients and families about stroke risk factors and their control early during hospitalization.
2. Treatment of the acute stroke, prevention of the next stroke, and rehabilitation should be concurrent themes throughout hospitalization and recovery.
3. Avoid common stroke complications, such as deep-vein thrombosis, aspiration, hypovolemia, pressure sores, contractures, and urinary tract infections. These problems are easier to prevent than treat.
4. Plan treatment of the acute stroke by analyzing the mechanism and pathophysiology in the individual patient. The time course of the symptoms should never be the sole guide to treatment.
5. The clinician should determine the location and severity of the vascular lesion, the blood constituents and coagulation functions, and the state of the brain (e.g., normal, stunned, or irreversibly damaged).
6. Determine precisely what is wrong with every stroke patient. Stroke is a cerebrovascular disease and diagnosis involves finding the cardiac-cere-

brovascular-hematologic cause. Precise diagnosis has great intrinsic value. It allows better estimates of prognosis and guides logical treatment.

7. Unblocking occlusive arterial lesions with endarterectomy or thrombolysis should be considered when there is no brain damage or when ischemia is recent and possibly reversible.

8. Prevention of thrombus formation, propagation, and embolization is often possible by using drugs that modify platelet aggregation and adhesion and by using anticoagulants of the heparin, heparinoid, and warfarin groups. I suggest using antiplatelet aggregants (e.g., aspirin) to prevent white clots and heparin and warfarin to counteract red clots.

9. When an artery is acutely occluded, anticoagulants are used for 3–6 weeks until the occlusive thrombus has organized and become adherent to the artery. In contrast, longer-term anticoagulants are warranted for severe stenosis in large arteries and for continued potential for embolism (e.g., in chronic cardiac lesions that represent a risk for cardiogenic embolism).

10. Try to maximize blood flow to ischemic regions during the acute stroke. Avoid excessive reduction of blood pressure and hypovolemia during the acute stage of infarction.

11. Cardiac disease and mortality are high in most stroke patients. Always consider the heart and its blood supply in addition to the brain.

Discussion of these general treatments and strategies is expanded in Part II (Stroke Syndromes) and III (Prevention, Complications, and Rehabilitation) of this book.

References

1. Caplan LR. Are terms such as *completed stroke* or *RIND* of continued usefulness? Stroke 1983;14:431–433.
2. Caplan LR. TIAs—we need to return to the question, what is wrong with Mr. Jones? Neurology 1988;38:791–793.
3. Matsumoto N, Whisnant J, Kurland L, et al. Natural history of stroke in Rochester, Minnesota, 1955–1969. Stroke 1973;4:20–29.
4. Whisnant J, Goldner J, Taylor W. Natural History of Transient Ischemic Attacks. In J Moosy, R Janeway (eds), Cerebral Vascular Disease: Proceedings of the Seventh Princeton Conference. New York: Grune & Stratton, 1971;161–169.
5. Wiebers D, Whisnant J, O'Fallon W. Reversible ischemic neurologic deficit (RIND) in a community: Rochester, Minnesota, 1955–1974. Neurology 1982;32:459–465.
6. Caplan LR. Treatment of cerebral ischemia: where are we headed? Stroke 1984;15:571–574.
7. Stroke 1998;29(3):(cover).
8. Thibault GE. Clinical problem solving: too old for what? N Engl J Med 1993;328:946–950.
9. Caplan LR. Reperfusion of Ischemic Brain: Why and Why Not? In W Hacke, G Del Zoppo, M Hirschberg (eds), Thrombolytic Therapy in Acute Ischemic Stroke. Berlin: Springer, 1991;36–45.
10. Babbs C. Reperfusion injury of post ischemic tissue. Ann Emerg Med 1988;17:1148–1157.
11. Easton JD, Sherman D. Stroke and morbidity rate in carotid endarterectomy: 228 consecutive operations. Stroke 1977;8:565–568.
12. Brott T, Thalinger K. Carotid endarterectomy in Cincinnati 1980: indications and morbidity in 431 cases. Neurology 1983;33(Suppl 2):93.
13. Cebul RD, Snow RJ, Pine R, et al. Indications, outcomes, and provider volumes for carotid endarterectomy. JAMA 1998;279:1282–1287.
14. Wennberg DE, Lucas FL, Birkmeyer JD, et al. Variation in carotid endarterectomy mortality in the Medicare population. Trial hospitals, volume, and patient characteristics. JAMA 1998;279:1278–1281.
15. Caplan LR. A General Therapeutic Perspective on Stroke Treatment. In R Dunkel, J Schmidley (eds), Stroke in the Elderly: New Issues in Diagnosis, Treatment and Rehabilitation. New York: Springer, 1987;60–69.
16. Robinson RG, Lipsey JR, Price TR. Diagnosis and clinical management of post-stroke depression. Psychosomatics 1985;26:769–778.
17. Caplan LR, Sergay S. Positional cerebral ischemia. J Neurol Neurosurg Psychiatry 1976;39:385–391.
18. Toole J. Effects of change of head, limb, and body position on cephalic circulation. N Engl J Med 1968;279: 307–311.
19. Lehv M, Salzman E, Silen W. Hypertension complicating carotid endarterectomy. Stroke 1970;1:307–313.
20. Holton P, Wood J. The effects of bilateral removal of the carotid bodies and denervation of the carotid sinus in two human subjects. J Physiol 1965;181:365–378.
21. Breen JC, Caplan LR, DeWitt LD, et al. Brain edema after carotid surgery. Neurology 1996;46:175–181.
22. Caplan LR, Skillman J, Ojemann R, et al. Intracerebral hemorrhage following carotid endarterectomy: a hypertensive complication. Stroke 1978;9:457–460.
23. North American Symptomatic Carotid Endarterectomy Trial Collaborators. Beneficial effect of carotid endarterectomy in symptomatic patients with high-grade carotid stenosis. N Engl J Med 1991;325:445–453.
24. MRC European Carotid Surgery Trial. Interim results for symptomatic patients with severe (70-99%) or with mild (0–29%) carotid stenosis. Lancet 1991;337:1235–1243.
25. Biller J, Feinberg WM, Castaldo JE et al. Guidelines for carotid endarterectomy. A statement for healthcare professionals from a special writing group of the Stroke Council, American Heart Association. Stroke 1998;29:554–562.

26. Barnett HJM, Taylor DW, Eliasziw M, et al. for the North American Symptomatic Carotid Endarterectomy Trial Collaborators. Benefit of carotid endarterectomy in patients with symptomatic moderate or severe stenosis. N Engl J Med 1998;339:1415–1425.

27. European Carotid Surgery Trialists' Collaborative Group. Randomised trial of endarterectomy for recently symptomatic carotid stenosis: final results of the MRC European Carotid Surgery Trial (ECST). Lancet 1998;351: 1379–1387.

28. Spetzler RF, Hadley MN, Martin NA, et al. Vertebrobasilar insufficiency: I. Microsurgical treatment of extracranial vertebrobasilar disease. J Neurosurg 1987;66:648–661.

29. Kieffer E, Koskas F, Bahnini A, et al. Long-term Results after Reconstruction of the Cervical Vertebral Artery. In LR Caplan, EG Shifrin, AN Nicolaides, WS Moore (eds), Cerebrovascular Ischaemia—Investigation and Management. London: Med-Orion, 1996;617–625.

30. Executive Committee for the Asymptomatic Carotid Atherosclerosis Study. Endarterectomy for symptomatic carotid artery stenosis. JAMA 1995;273:1421–1428.

31. Hopkins LN, Martin NA, Hadley MN, et al. Vertebrobasilar insufficiency: II. Microsurgical treatment of intracranial vertebrobasilar disease. J Neurosurg 1987;66:662–674.

32. Ausman JI, Diaz FG, Pearce JE, et al. Endarterectomy of the vertebral artery from C2 to posterior inferior cerebellar artery intracranially. Surg Neurol 1982;18:400–404.

33. Meyer FB, Piepgras DG, Sundt TM, et al. Emergency embolectomy for acute occlusion of the middle cerebral artery. J Neurosurg 1985;62:639–647.

34. Higashida RT, Hieshima GB, Tsai FY, et al. Transluminal angioplasty of the vertebral and basilar artery. AJNR Am J Neuroradiol 1987;8:745–749.

35. Higashida RT, Halbach W, Tsai FY, et al. Interventional neurovascular techniques for cerebral revascularization in the treatment of stroke. AJR Am J Roentgenol 1994;163: 793–800.

36. Takis C, Kwan ES, Pessin MS, et al. Intracranial angioplasty: experience and complications. AJNR Am J Neuroradiol 1997;18:1661–1668.

37. Nakano S, Yokogami K, Ohta H, et al. Direct percutaneous transluminal angioplasty for acute middle cerebral artery occlusion. AJNR Am J Neuroradiol 1998;19:767–772.

38. Collen D. On the regulation and control of fibrinolysis: Edward Kowalsky Memorial Lecture. Throm Haemost 1980;43:77–89.

39. Sloan MA. Thrombolysis and stroke, past and future. Arch Neurol 1987;44:748–768.

40. Meyer JS, Gilroy J, Barnhart ME, et al. Anticoagulants plus streptokinase therapy in progressive stroke. JAMA 1964;189:373.

41. Meyer JS, Gilroy J, Barnhart ME, Johnson JF. Therapeutic Thrombolysis, in Cerebral Thromboembolism: Randomized Evaluation of Streptokinase. In C Millikan, R Siekert, JP Whisnant (eds), Cerebral Vascular Disease, 4th Princeton Conference. New York: Grune & Stratton, 1965;200–213.

42. del Zoppo GJ. Thrombolytic therapy in cerebrovascular disease. Stroke 1988;19:1174–1179.

43. Pessin MS, del Zoppo GJ, Furlan AJ. Thrombolytic Treatment in Acute Stroke: Review and Update of Selected Topics. In M Moskowitz, LR Caplan (eds). Cerebrovascular Diseases, 19th Princeton Conference, 1994. Boston: Butterworth–Heinemann, 1995;409–418.

44. The National Institute of Neurological Disorders and Stroke rt-PA Study Group. Tissue plasminogen activator for acute ischemic stroke. N Engl J Med 1995;333:1581–1587.

45. Adams HP, Brott TG, Furlan AJ, et al. Use of thrombolytic drugs. A suppement to the guidelines for the management of patients with acute ischemic stroke. A statement for Health Care Professionals from a special writing group of the Stroke Council American Heart Association. Stroke 1996;27:1711–1718.

46. Quality Standards Subcommittee of the American Academy of Neurology. Practice advisory: Thrombolytic therapy for acute ischemic stroke—summary statement. Neurology 1996;47:835–839.

47. del Zoppo G, Ferbert A, Otis S, et al. Local intra-arterial fibrinolytic therapy in acute carotid territory stroke. A pilot study. Stroke 1988;19:307–313.

48. Hacke W, Zeumer H, Ferbert A, et al. Intra-arterial thrombolytic therapy improves outcome in patients with acute vertebrobasilar occlusive disease. Stroke 1988;19:1216–1222.

49. Zeumer H, Freitag H-J, Zanella F, et al. Local intra-arterial fibrinolytic therapy in patients with stroke: urokinase versus recombinant tissue plasminogen activator (r-tPA). Neuroradiology 1993;35:159–162.

50. Mori E, Tabuchi M, Yoshida T, Yamadori A. Intracarotid urokinase with thromboembolic occlusion of the middle cerebral artery. Stroke 1988;19:808–812.

51. Mori E. Fibrinolytic Recanalization Therapy in Acute Cerebrovascular Thromboembolism. In W Hacke, GJ del Zoppo, M Hirschberg (eds), Thrombolytic Therapy in Acute Ischemic Stroke. Heidelberg: Springer, 1991;137–145.

52. Mobius E, Berg-Dammer E, Kuhne D, Nahser HC. Local thrombolytic therapy in acute basilar artery occlusion. Experience with 18 patients. In W Hacke, GJ del Zoppo, M Hirschberg (eds), Thrombolytic Therapy in Acute Ischemic Stroke. Heidelberg: Springer, 1991;213–215.

53. Matsumoto K, Satoh K. Topical Intraarterial Urokinase Infusion for Acute Stroke. In W Hacke, GJ del Zoppo, M Hirshberg (eds), Thrombolytic Therapy in Acute Ischemic Stroke. Heidelberg: Springer, 1991;207–212.

54. Theron J, Courtheoux P, Casasco A, et al. Local intraarterial fibrinolysis in the carotid territory. AJNR Am J Neuroradiol 1989;10:753–765.

55. Zeumer H, Hacke W, Ringelstein EB. Local intra-arterial thrombolysis in vertebrobasilar thromboembolic disease. AJNR Am J Neuroradiol 1983;4:401–404.

56. Casto L, Caverni L, Canerlingo M, et al. Intra-arterial thrombolysis in acute ischaemic stroke: experience with a superselective catheter embedded in the clot. J Neurol Neurosurg Psychiatry 1996;60:667–670.

57. Barnwell SL, Clark WM, Nguyen TT, et al. Safety and efficacy of delayed intraarterial urokinase therapy with mechanical clot disruption for thromboembolic stroke. AJNR Am J Neuroradiol 1994;15:1817–1822.

58. Berg-Dammer E, Henkes H, Nahser HC, Kuhne D. Thromboembolic occlusion of the middle cerebral artery due to angiography and endovascular procedures: safety and efficacy of local intra-arterial fibrinolysis. Cerebrovasc Dis 1996;6:222–230.

59. Mitchell PJ, Gerraty RP, Donnan GA, et al. Thrombolysis in the vertebrobasilar circulation: the Australian Urokinase Stroke Trial. Cerebrovasc Dis 1997;7:94–99.

60. Jansen O, von Kummer R, Forsting M, et al. Thrombolytic therapy in acute occlusion of the intracranial internal carotid artery bifurcation. AJNR Am J Neuroradiol 1995;16:1977–1986.

61. Becker KJ, Monsein LH, Ulatowski J, et al. Intraarterial thrombolysis in vertebrobasilar occlusion. AJNR Am J Neuroradiol 1996;17:255–262.

62. Wijdicks EFM, Nichols DA, Thielen KR, et al. Intra-arterial thrombolysis in acute basilar artery thromboembolism: the initial Mayo Clinic experience. Mayo Clin Proc 1997;72:1005–1013.

63. Cross DT III, Moran CJ, Akins PT, et al. Relationship between clot location and outcome after basilar artery thrombosis. AJNR Am J Neuroradiol 1997;18:1221–1228.

64. Gonner F, Remonda L, Mattle H, et al. Local intra-arterial thrombolysis in acute ischemic stroke. Stroke 1998;29:1894–1900.

65. Brandt T, von Kummer R, Muller-Kuppers M, Hacke W. Thrombolytic therapy of acute basilar artery occlusion, variables affecting recanalization and outcome. Stroke 1996;27:875–881.

66. Tsai FY, Berberian B, Matovich V, et al. Percutaneous transluminal angioplasty adjunct to thrombolysis for acute middle cerebral artery rethrombosis. AJNR Am J Neuroradiol 1994;15:1823–1829.

67. del Zoppo GJ, Higashida RT, Furlan AJ, et al. PROACT: A phase II randomized trial of recombinant pro-urokinase by direct arterial delivery in acute middle cerebral artery stroke. PROACT Investigators. Prolyse in Acute Cerebral Thromboembolism. Stroke 1998;29:4–11.

68. Furlan AJ, Higashida RT, Wechsler L, et al. for the PROACT investigators. Intra-arterial prourokinase for acute ischemic stroke. The PROACT II study: A randomized controlled trial. JAMA 1999;282:2003–2011.

69. Yamaguchi T, Hayakawa T, Kikuchi H, for the Japanese Thrombolysis Study Group. Intravenous Tissue Plasminogen Activator in Acute Thromboembolic Stroke: a Placebo-controlled Double-blind Trial. In GJ del Zoppo, E Mori, W Hacke (eds), Thrombolytic Therapy in Acute Ischemic Stroke II. Berlin: Springer, 1993;59–65.

70. Yamaguchi T, Kikuchi H, Hayakawa T, for the Japanese Thrombolysis Study Group. Clinical Efficacy and Safety of Intravenous Tissue Plasminogen Activator in Acute Embolic Stroke: a Randomized Double-blind, Dose-comparison Study of Duteplase. In T Yamaguchi, E Mori, K Minematsu, GJ del Zoppo (eds), Thrombolytic Therapy in Acute Ischemic Stroke III. Tokyo: Springer, 1995;223–229.

71. Mori E, Yoneda Y, Tabuchi M, et al. Intravenous recombinant tissue plasminogen activator in acute carotid artery territory stroke. Neurology 1992;42:976–982.

72. von Kummer R, Hacke W. Safety and efficacy of intravenous tissue plasminogen activator and heparin in acute middle cerebral artery stroke. Stroke 1992;23:646–652.

73. von Kummer R, Forsting M, Sartor K, Hacke W. Intravenous Plasminogen Activator in Acute Stroke. In W Hacke, GJ del Zoppo, M Hirschberg (eds), Thrombolytic Therapy in Acute Ischemic Stroke. Heidelberg: Springer, 1991; 161–167.

74. del Zoppo GJ, Poeck K, Pessin MS, et al. Recombinant tissue plasminogen activator in acute thrombotic and embolic stroke. Ann Neurol 1992;32:78–86.

75. Wolpert SM, Bruckmann H, Greenlee R, et al. The rt-PA Acute Stroke Study Group. Neuroradiologic evaluation of patients with acute stroke treated with recombinant tissue plasminogen activator. AJNR Am J Neuroradiol 1993;14:3–13.

76. Grond M, Rudolf J, Schmulling S, et al. Early intravenous thrombolysis with rt-PA in vertebrobasilar stroke. Arch Neurol 1998;55:466–469.

77. Hacke W, Kaste M, Fieschi C, et al. Intravenous thrombolysis with recombinant tissue plasminogen activator for acute hemispheric stroke. The European Cooperative Acute Stroke Study (ECASS). JAMA 1995;274:1017–1025.

78. Fisher M, Pessin MS, Furlan AJ. ECASS: lessons for future thrombolytic stroke trials. JAMA 1995;274:1058–1059.

79. Steiner T, Bluhmki E, Kaste M, et al. The ECASS 3-hour cohort. Secondary analysis of ECASS data by time stratification. Cerebrovasc Dis 1998;8:198–203.

80. Hacke W, Kaste M, Fieschi C, et al. Randomised double-blind placebo-controlled trial of thrombolytic therapy with intravenous alteplase in acute ischaemic stroke (ECASS ll). Lancet 1998;352:1245–1251.

81. Donnan GA, Davis SM, Chambers BR, et al. Trials of streptokinase in severe acute ischemic stroke. Lancet 1995;345:578–579.

82. Multicenter Acute Stroke Trial-Italy (MAST-I) Group. Randomised controlled trial of streptokinase, aspirin, and combination of both in treatment of acute ischaemic stroke. Lancet 1995;346:1509–1514.

83. The Multicenter Acute Stroke Trial-Europe Study Group. Thrombolytic therapy with streptokinase in acute ischemic stroke. N Engl J Med 1996;335:145–150.

84. Lyden PD, Grotta JC, Levine SR, et al. Intravenous thrombolysis for acute stroke. Neurology 1997;49:14–29

85. Easton JD, Hacke W, Caplan LR, et al. Thrombolysis for stroke. Cerebrovasc Dis 1998;8:191–197.

86. Caplan LR, Mohr JP, Kistler JP, Koroshetz W. Thrombolysis—not a panacea for ischemic stroke. N Engl J Med 1997;337:1309–1310, 1313.

87. Brandt T, von Kummer R, Muller-Kuypers M, Hacke W. Thrombolytic therapy of acute basilar artery occlusion. Variables affecting recanalization and outcome. Stroke 1996;27:875–881.

88. Kasner SE, Villar-Cordova C, Tong D, Grotta JC. Hemopericardium and cardiac tamponade after thrombolysis for acute ischemic stroke. Neurology 1998;50:1857–1859.

89. Furlan A, Little J, Dohn D. Arterial occlusion following anastomosis of the superficial temporal artery to middle cerebral artery. Stroke 1980;11:91–95.

90. Gumerlock M, Ono H, Neurvelt E. Can a patent extracranial-intracranial bypass provoke the conversion of an

intracranial arterial stenosis to a symptomatic occlusion? Neurosurgery 1983;12:391–400.

91. The EC-IC Bypass Study Group. Failure of the extracranial-intracranial arterial bypass to reduce the risk of ischemic stroke. N Engl J Med 1985;313:1191–1200.

92. Przybylski GJ, Yonas H, Smith HA. Reduced stroke risk in patients with compromised cerebral blood flow reactivity treated with superficial temporal artery to distal middle cerebral artery bypass surgery. J Stroke Cerebrovasc Dis 1998;7:302–309.

93. Roski RA, Spetzler RF, Hopkins LN. Occipital artery to posterior inferior cerebellar artery bypass for vertebrobasilar ischemia. Neurosurgery 1982;10:44–49.

94. Caplan LR. Use of Vasodilating Drugs for Cerebral Symptomatology. In R Miller, D Greenblatt (eds), Drug Therapy Reviews. Amsterdam: Elsevier, 1979;305–317.

95. Golino P, Pisclone F, Willerson JT, et al. Divergent effects of serotonin in coronary-artery dimensions and blood flow in patients with coronary atherosclerosis and control patients. N Engl J Med 1991;324:641–648.

96. Piepgras A, Schmiedek P, Leinsinger G, et al. A simple test to assess cerebrovascular reserve capacity using transcranial Doppler sonography and acetazolamide. Stroke 1990;21:1306–1311.

97. Hojer-Pedusen E. Effect of acetazolamide on cerebral blood flow in subacute and chronic cerebrovascular disease. Stroke 1987;18:887–891.

98. Braunwald E. Mechanism of action of calcium-channel blocking agents. N Engl J Med 1982;307:1618–1627.

99. Gorelick PB, Caplan LR. Calcium, hypercalcemia and stroke. Current concepts of cerebrovascular disease. Stroke 1985;20:13–17.

100. Solomon G, Steel J, Spaccevento L. Verapamil prophylaxis of migraine. JAMA 1983;250:2500–2502.

101. Allen G, Ahn H, Preziosi T, et al. Cerebral arterial spasm: a controlled trial of nimodipine in patients with subarachnoid hemorrhage. N Engl J Med 1983;308:619–624.

102. Phillipon J, Grob R, Dagreou F, et al. Prevention of vasospasm in subarachnoid hemorrhage: a controlled study with nimodipine. Acta Neurochir (Wien) 1986;82:110–114.

103. Jan M, Buchheit F, Tremoulet M. Therapeutic trial of intravenous nimodipine in patients with established cerebral vasospasm after rupture of intracranial aneurysms. Neurosurg 1988;23:154–157.

104. Pickard JD, Murray GD, Illingworth R, et al. Effect of oral nimodipine on cerebral infarction and outcome after subarachnoid hemorrhage: British Aneurysm Nimodipine Trial. BMJ 1989;298:636–642.

105. Gelmers HJ, Gorter K, deWeerdt C, et al. A controlled trial of nimodipine in acute ischemic stroke. N Engl J Med 1988;318:203–207.

106. TRUST study group. Randomized, double-blind placebo-controlled trial of nimodipine in acute stroke. Lancet 1990;336:1205–1209.

107. The American Nimodipine Study Group. Clinical trial of nimodipine in acute ischemic stroke. Stroke 1992;23:3–8.

108. Heros RC, Korosue K. Hemodilution for cerebral ischemia. Stroke 1989;20:423–427.

109. Thomas DJ. Hemodilution in acute stroke. Stroke 1985;16:763–764.

110. Thomas DJ, duBoulay GH, Marshall J, et al. Effect of haematocrit on cerebral blood flow in man. Lancet 1977;2:941–943.

111. Wood JH, Kee DB. Hemorrheology of the cerebral circulation in Stroke. Stroke 1985;16:765–772.

112. Strand T, Asplund K, Eriksson S, et al. A randomized controlled trial of hemodilution therapy in acute stroke. Stroke 1984;15:980–989.

113. Staedt U, Schlierf G, Oster P, et al. Hypervolemic Hemodilution with 10% HES 200/0.5 and 10% Dextran 40 in Patients with Ischemic Stroke. In A Hartmann, E Kuschinsky (eds), Cerebral Ischemia and Hemorrheology. New York: Springer, 1987;429–435.

114. Scandinavian Stroke Study Group. Multicenter trial of hemodilution in acute ischemic stroke: results of subgroup analyses. Stroke 1988;19:464–471.

115. Aichner FT, Fazekas F, Brainin M, et al. Hypervolemic hemodilution in acute ischemic stroke. The Multicenter Austrian Hemodilution Stroke Trial (MAHST). Stroke 1998;29:743–749.

116. Grotta J, Ackerman R, Correia J, et al. Whole-blood viscosity parameters and cerebral blood flow. Stroke 1982;13:296–298.

117. Coull BM, Beamer NB, deGarmo PL, et al. Chronic blood hyperviscosity in subjects with acute stroke, transient ischemic attacks, and risk factors for stroke. Stroke 1991;22:162–168.

118. Olinger CP, Brott TG, Barsan TG, et al. Use of ancrod in acute or progressing ischemic cerebral infarction. Ann Emerg Med 1988;17:1208–1209.

119. Hossmann V, Dieter-Heiss W, Bewermeyer H, et al. Controlled trial of ancrod in ischemic stroke. Arch Neurol 1983;40:803–808.

120. Liu M, Counsell C, Wardlaw J, Sandercock P. A systematic review of randomized evidence for fibrinogen-depleting agents in acute ischemic stroke. J Stroke Cerebrovasc Dis 1998;7:63–69.

121. Schuff-Werner P, Schutz E, Seyde WC, et al. Improved haemorheology associated with a reduction in plasma fibrinogen and LDL in patients being treated by heparin-induced extracorporeal LDL precipitation (HELP). Eur J Clin Invest 1989;19:30–37.

122. Walzl M, Lechner H, Walzl B, Schied G. Improved neurological recovery of cerebral infarctions after plasmapheretic reduction of lipids and fibrinogen. Stroke 1993;24: 1447–1451.

123. Radack K, Deck C, Huster G. Dietary supplementation with low-dose fish oils lowers fibrinogen levels: a randomized double-blind controlled study. Ann Intern Med 1989;111:757–758.

124. Kobayashi S, Hirai A, Terano T, et al. Reduction in blood viscosity by eicosopentaenoic acid. Lancet 1981;2:197.

125. Geyer RP. Oxygen transport in vivo by means of perfluorochemical preparations. N Engl J Med 1982;307:304–306.

126. Peerless SJ, Nakamura R, Rodriguez-Salazar A, et al. Modification of cerebral ischemia with fluosol. Stroke 1985;16:38–43.

127. Tremper KK, Friedman AE, Levine EM, et al. The preoperative treatment of severely anemic patients with a perfluorochemical oxygen-transport fluid, Fluosol-DA. N Engl J Med 1982;307:277–283.

128. Gould SA, Rosen AL, Sehgal L, et al. Fluosol-DA as a red-cell substitute in acute anemia. N Engl J Med 1986;314:1653–1656.

129. Bose B, Osterholm JL, Triolo A. Focal cerebral ischemia: reduction in size of infarcts by ventriculo-subarachnoid perfusion with fluorocarbon emulsions. Brain Research 1985;328:223–231.

130. Bell RD, Frazer GD, Osterholm JL, Duckett SW. A novel treatment for ischemic intracranial hypertension in cats. Stroke 1991;22:80–83.

131. Weksler B. Antithrombotic Therapies in the Management of Cerebral Ischemia. In F Plum, W Pulsinelli (eds), Cerebrovascular Diseases: Proceedings of the Fourteenth Princeton Conference. New York: Raven Press, 1985: 211–223.

132. Deykin D. Thrombogenesis. N Engl J Med 1967;276: 622–628.

133. Carson S, Demling R, Esquivel C. Aspirin failure in symptomatic atherosclerotic carotid artery disease. Surgery 1981;90:1084–1092.

134. Wu K. New pharmacologic approaches to thromboembolic disorders. Hosp Pract 1985;20:101–120.

135. Caplan LR. Anticoagulation for cerebral ischemia. Clin Neuropharmacol 1986;9:399–414.

136. Hirsh J. Heparin. N Engl J Med 1991;324:1565–1574.

137. Salzman E, Deykin D, Shapiro R, et al. Management of heparin therapy. N Engl J Med 1975;292:1046–1050.

138. Warkentin TE, Levine MN, Hirsh J, et al. Heparin-induced thrombocytopenia in patients treated with low-molecular-weight heparin or unfractionated heparin. N Engl J Med 1995;332:1330–1335.

139. Becker PS, Miller VT. Heparin-induced thrombocytopenia. Stroke 1989;20:1449–1459.

140. Phelan BK. Heparin-associated thrombosis without thrombocytopenia. Ann Intern Med 1983;99:637–638.

141. Weitz JI. Low-molecular-weight heparins. N Engl J Med 1997;337:688–698.

142. Gordon DL, Linhardt R, Adams HP. Low-molecular-weight heparins and heparinoids and their use in acute or progressing ischemic stroke. Clin Neuropharmacol 1990;13:522–543.

143. Rosenberg R, Lam L. Correlation between structure and function of heparin. Proc Natl Acad Sci U S A 1979; 76:3198–3202.

144. Ramirez-Lassepas M, Quinones MR, Nino HH. Treatment of acute ischemic stroke: open trial with continuous intravenous heparinization. Arch Neurol 1986;42:386–390.

145. Duke RJ, Bloch RF, Alexander GG, et al. Intravenous heparin for the prevention of stroke progression in acute partial stable stroke: a randomized controlled trial. Ann Intern Med 1986;105:825–828.

146. Ameri A, Bousser M-G. Cerebral venous thrombosis. Neurol Clin 1992;10:87–111.

147. Jacewicz M, Plum F. Aseptic Cerebral Venous Thrombosis. In K Einhaupl, O Kempski, A Baethmann (eds), Cerebral Sinus Thrombosis. Experimental and Clinical Aspects. New York: Plenum, 1990;157–170.

148. Einhaupl KM, Villringer A, Meister W, et al. Heparin treatment in sinus venous thrombosis. Lancet 1991;338: 597–600.

149. Meister W, Einhaupl K, Villringer A, et al. Treatment of Patients with Cerebral Sinus and Vein Thrombosis with Heparin. In K Einhaupl, O Kempski, A Baethmann (eds), Cerebral Sinus Thrombosis. Experimental and Clinical Aspects. New York: Plenum, 1990;225–230.

150. De Bruijn SF, Stam J. Randomized, placebo-controlled trial of anticoagulant treatment with low-molecular-weight heparin for cerebral spinal thrombosis. Stroke 1999;30:484–488.

151. Kay R, Wong KS, Yu YL, et al. Low-molecular-weight heparin for the treatment of acute schemic stroke. N Engl J Med 1995;333:1588–1593.

152. The Publications Committee for the Trial of ORG 10172 in Acute Stroke Treatment (TOAST) Investigators. Low molecular weight heparinoid, ORG 10172 (Danaparoid), and outcome after acute ischemic stroke. A randomized controlled trial. JAMA 1998;279:1265–1272.

153. Adams HP Jr, Bendixen BH, Leira E, et al. Antithrombotic treatment of ischemic stroke among patients with occlusion or severe stenosis of the internal carotid artery: a report of the Trial of Org 10172 in Acute Stroke Treatment (TOAST). Neurology 1999;53:122–125.

154. Cerebral embolism task force. Cardiogenic brain embolism. Arch Neurol 1986;43:71–84.

155. Camerlingo M, Casto L, Censori B, et al. Immediate anticoagulation with heparin for first-ever ischemic stroke in the carotid artery territories observed within 5 hours of onset. Arch Neurol 1994;51:462–467.

156. Wessler S, Gitel S. Warfarin: from bedside to bench. N Engl J Med 1984;311:645–652.

157. Deykin D. Warfarin therapy. N Engl J Med 1970;283: 691–694.

158. Hull R, Hirsch J, Jay R, et al. Different intensities of oral anticoagulant therapy in the treatment of proximal-vein thrombosis. N Engl J Med 1982;307:1676–1681.

159. Taberner D, Poller L, Burslem R, et al. Oral anticoagulants controlled by the British cooperative: thromboplastin versus low dose heparin in prophylaxis of deep vein thromboses. BMJ 1977;1:272–274.

160. Frances CW, Marder VJ, Evan CM, et al. Two-step warfarin therapy: prevention of post-operative venous thrombosis without excessive bleeding. JAMA 1983;249:374–378.

161. Hirsh J, Poller L, Deykin D, et al. Optimal therapeutic range for oral anticoagulants. Chest 1989;95(Suppl):S5–S11.

162. Poller L. The effect of low-dose warfarin on the risk of stroke in patients with nonrheumatic atrial fibrillation. N Engl J Med 1991;325:129–130.

163. The Stroke Prevention in Reversible Ischemia Trial (SPIRIT) Study Group. A randomized trial of anticoagulants versus aspirin after cerebral ischemia of presumed arterial origin. Ann Neurol 1997;42:857–865.

164. Atrial Fibrillation Investigators: Risk factors for stroke and efficacy of antithrombotic therapy in atrial fibrillation: analysis of pooled data from 5 randomized clinical trials. Arch Intern Med 1994;154:1949–1957.

165. Hart RG. Oral anticoagulation for secondary prevention of stroke. Cerebrovasc Dis 1997;7(Suppl 6):24–29.

166. Hylek EM, Skates SJ, Sheehan MA, Singer DE. An analysis of the lowest effective intensity of prophylactic antico-

agulation for patients with nonrheumatic atrial fibrillation. N Engl J Med 1996;335:540–546.
167. Fleming HA, Bailey SM. Mitral valve disease, systemic embolism and anticoagulants. Postgrad Med J 1971;47: 599–604.
168. Adams GF, Merrett JD, Hutchinson WM, Pollock AM. Cerebral embolism and mitral stenosis: survival with and without anticoagulants. J Neurol Neurosurg Psychiatry 1974;37:378–383.
169. Carter AB. Prognosis of cerebral embolism. Lancet 1965; 2:514–519.
170. The Boston Area Anticoagulation Trial for Atrial Fibrillation Investigators. The effect of low-dose warfarin on the risk of stroke in patients with nonrheumatic atrial fibrillation. N Engl J Med 1990;323:1505–1511.
171. EAFT Study Group. Silent brain infarction in nonrheumatic atrial fibrillation. Neurology 1996;46:159–165.
172. Bogousslavsky J, Van Melle G, Regli F, Kappenberger L. Pathogenesis of anterior circulation stroke in patients with nonvalvular atrial fibrillation: The Lausanne Stroke Registry. Neurology 1990;40:1046–1050.
173. Petersen P, Godtfredsen J, Boysen G, et al. Placebo-controlled, randomized trial of warfarin and aspirin for prevention of thromboembolic complications in chronic atrial fibrillation: The Copenhagen AFASAK study. Lancet 1989;1:175–179.
174. The Stroke prevention in Atrial Fibrillation Investigators. The stroke prevention in atrial fibrillation study: final results. Circulation 1991;84:527–539.
175. EAFT (European Atrial Fibrillation Trial) Study Group. Secondary prevention in non-rheumatic atrial fibrillation after transient ischaemic attack or minor stroke. Lancet 1993;342:1255–1262.
176. Stroke Prevention in Atrial Fibrillation Investigators. Warfarin versus aspirin for prevention of thromboembolism in atrial fibrillation: Stroke Prevention in Atrial Fibrillation II Study. Lancet 1994;343:687–691.
177. Stroke Prevention in Atrial Fibrillation Investigators. Adjusted-dose warfarin versus low-intensity, fixed-dose warfarin plus aspirin for high-risk patients with atrial fibrillation: Stroke Prevention in Atrial Fibrillation III randomised clinical trial. Lancet 1996;348:633–638.
178. Stroke Prevention in Atrial Fibrillation Investigators. Prospective identification of patients with nonvalvular atrial fibrillation at low risk of stroke during treatment with aspirin: Stroke Prevention in Atrial Fibrillation III Study. Circulation 1997;96(Suppl 1):281(abst).
179. Caplan LR. Brain Embolism. In LR Caplan, MI Chimowitz, JW Hurst (eds), Clinical Neurocardiology. New York: Marcel Dekker, 1999;35–185.
180. Albers G. Atrial fibrillation and stroke. Three new studies, three remaining questions. Arch Intern Med 1994;154: 1443–1448.
181. Chimowitz MI, Kokkinos J, Strong J, et al. The Warfarin-Aspirin Symptomatic Intracranial Disease Study. Neurology 1995;45:1488–1493.
182. The Warfarin-Aspirin Symptomatic Intracranial Disease Study Group. Prognosis of patients with symptomatic vertebral or basilar artery stenosis. Stroke 1998;29: 1389–1392.
183. Fields WS, Lemak NA. A History of Stroke: Its Recognition and Treatment. New York: Oxford University Press, 1989;115–119.
184. Craven LL. Experiences with aspirin (acetylsalicylic acid) in the nonspecific prophylaxis of coronary thrombosis. Mississippi Valley Med J 1953;75:38–44.
185. Craven LL. Prevention of coronary and cerebral thrombosis. Mississippi Valley Med J 1956;78:213–215.
186. Mundall J, Quintero P, von Kaulla K, et al. Transient monocular blindness and increased platelet aggregability treated with aspirin—a case report. Neurology 1971; 21:402.
187. Harrison MJG, Marshall J, Meadows JC, et al. Effect of aspirin in amaurosis fugax. Lancet 1971;2:743–744.
188. Fields WS, Lemak N, Frankowski R, et al. Controlled trial of aspirin in cerebral ischemia. Stroke 1977;8:301–306.
189. Barnett HJM. The Canadian Cooperative Study: a randomized trial of aspirin and sulfinpyrazone in threatened stroke. N Engl J Med 1978;299:53–59.
190. Moncada S, Vane J. Arachidonic acid metabolites and the interactions between platelets and blood vessel walls. N Engl J Med 1979;300:1142–1147.
191. Nurden AT. Platelet function and pharmacology of antiplatelet drugs. Cerebrovasc Dis 1997;7(Suppl 6):2–9.
192. Moncada C. Biologic and therapeutic potential of prostacyclin. Stroke 1983;14:157–168.
193. Preston F, Whipps S, Jackson C, et al. Inhibition of prostacyclin and platelet thromboxane A_2 after low dose aspirin. N Engl J Med 1981;304:76–79.
194. Weksler B, Pelt S, Alonso D, et al. Differential inhibition by aspirin of vascular and platelet prostaglandin synthesis in atherosclerotic patients. N Engl J Med 1983;308:800–805.
195. UK-TIA Study Group. The UK-TIA Aspirin Trial: the interim results. BMJ1988;296:316–320.
196. The SALT Collaborative Group. Swedish Aspirin Low-Dose Trial (SALT) of 75 mg aspirin as secondary prophylaxis after cerebrovascular ischemic events. Lancet 1991; 338:1345–1349.
197. The Dutch TIA Trial Study Group. A comparison of two doses of aspirin (30 mg vs 283 mg a day) in patients after a transient ischemic attack or minor stroke. N Engl J Med 1991;325:1261–1266.
198. Dyken M. Aspirin with and without dipyridamole. Cerebrovasc Dis 1997;7(Suppl 6):10–16.
199. Helgason CM, Hoff JA, Kondos GT, Brace LD. Platelet aggregation in patients with atrial fibrillation taking aspirin or warfarin. Stroke 1993;24:1458–1461.
200. Helgason CM, Tortorice L, Winkler S, et al. Aspirin response and failure in cerebral infarction. Stroke 1993;24:345–350.
201. Diener HC, Cunha L, Forbes C, et al. European Stroke Prevention Study 2. Dipyridamole and acetylsalicylic acid in the secondary prevention of stroke. J Neurol Sci 1996;143:1–13.
202. Alheid U, Reichwehr I, Foerstermann U. Human endothelial cells inhibit platelet aggregation by separately stimulating platelet cyclic AMP and cyclic GMP. Eur J Pharmacol 1989;164:103–110.
203. Honour A, Hochaday T, Mann J. The synergistic effect of aspirin and dipyridamole upon platelet thrombi in living blood vessels. Br J Exp Pathol 1977;58:268–272.
204. Sullivan J, Harken D, Gorlin R. Pharmacologic control of thromboembolic complications of aortic valve replacement. N Engl J Med 1971;284:1391–1394.
205. Fitzgerald GA. Dipyridamole. N Engl J Med 1987;316: 1247–1257.

206. Fields WS, Yatsu F, Conomy J, et al. Persantine-aspirin trial in cerebral ischemia: the American-Canadian Cooperative Study group. Stroke 1983;14:97–103.

207. Bousser MG, Eschwege E, Hagenah M, et al. "AICLA" controlled trial of aspirin and dipyridamole in the secondary prevention of athero-thrombotic cerebral ischemia. Stroke 1983;14:5–14.

208. ESPS Group. European Stroke Prevention Study (ESPS): principal endpoints. Lancet 1987;2:1351–1354.

209. Bousser M-G, Roberts RS, Gent M. Ticlopidine and Clopidogrel in secondary stroke prevention. Cerebrovasc Dis 1997;7(Suppl 6):17–23.

210. Sharis PJ, Cannon CP, Loscalzo J. The antiplatelet effects of ticlopidine and clopidogrel. Ann Intern Med 1998; 129:394–405.

211. Ono S, Ashida S, Abiko Y. Hemorheological effect of ticlopidine in the rat. Thromb Res 1983;31:549–556.

212. CAPRIE Steering Committee. A randomised, blinded, trial of clopidogrel versus aspirin in patients at risk of ischaemic events. Lancet 1996;348:1329–1339.

213. Hass WK, Easton JD, Adams HP, et al. A randomized trial comparing ticlopidine hydrochloride with aspirin for the prevention of stroke in high-risk patients. N Engl J Med 1989;321:501–507.

214. Gent M, Easton JD, Hachinski V, et al. The Canadian American Ticlopinine Study (CATS) in thromboembolic stroke. Lancet 1989;1:1215–1220.

215. Hall P, Nakamura S, Maiello I, et al. A randomized comparison of combined ticlopidine and aspirin therapy versus aspirin therapy alone after successful intravascular ultrasound-guided stent implantation. Circulation 1996; 93:215–222.

216. Bennett CL, Weinberg PD, Rozenberg-Ben-Dror K, et al. Thrombotic thrombocytopenic purpura associated with ticlopidine. A report of 60 cases. Ann Intern Med 1998; 128:541–544.

217. Sherman DG, Dyken ML. Gent M, et al. Antithrombotic therapy for cerebrovascular disorders: an update. Chest 1995;108:S444–S456.

218. Dyerberg J, Bang H, Stofferson E, et al. Eicosopentanoic acid and prevention of thrombosis and atherosclerosis. Lancet 1978;2:117–119.

219. Lefkovits J, Plow EF, Topol EJ. Platelet glycoprotein IIb/IIIa receptors in cardiovascular medicine. N Engl J Med 1995;332:1553–1559.

220. Wallace RC, Furlan AJ, Moliterno DJ, et al. Basilar artery rethrombosis: successful treatment with platelet glycoprotein IIb/IIIa receptor inhibitor. AJNR Am J Neuroradiol 1997;18:1257–1260.

221. Mousa SA, Mu D-X, Lucchesi BR. Prevention of carotid artery thrombosis by oral platelet GP IIb/IIIa antagonists in dogs. Stroke 1997;28:830–836.

222. Antiplatelet Trialists' Collaboration. Collaborative overview of randomised trials of antiplatelet therapy. 1. Prevention of death, myocardial infarction, and stroke by prolonged antiplatelet therapy in various categories of patients. BMJ 1994;308:81–106.

223. Sivenius J, Puranen J. Antiplatelet therapy in secondary prevention of stroke. A review of efficacy and tolerability. CNS Drugs 1997;8:38–50.

224. Miller A, Lees R. Simultaneous therapy with antiplatelet and anticoagulant drugs in symptomatic cardiovascular disease. Stroke 1985;16:668–675.

225. Chesebro J, Fuster V, Elveback L, et al. Trial of combined warfarin plus dipyridamole or aspirin therapy in prosthetic heart valve replacement: danger of aspirin combined with warfarin. Am J Cardiol 1983;51:1537–1541.

226. Garcia J. Mechanisms of Cell Death in Ischemia. In LR Caplan (ed), Brain Ischemia, Basic Concepts and Clinical Relevance. London: Springer, 1995;7–18.

227. Dietrich W, Busto R, Ginsberg M, et al. Influence of functional activity on metabolic recovery following experimental ischemia. Neurology 1984;34(1):261.

228. Plum F. What causes infarction in ischemic brain? Neurology 1983;33:222–233.

229. Myers R. Lactic Acid Accumulation as a Cause of Brain Edema and Cerebral Necrosis Resulting from Oxygen Deprivation. In R Korobkin, C Guilleminault (eds), Advances in Perinatal Neurology. New York: Spectrum, 1979;88–114.

230. Schmidley JW. Free radicals in central nervous system ischemia. Stroke 1990;21:1086–1090.

231. McCord JM. Oxygen-derived free radicals in post ischemic tissue injury. N Engl J Med 1985;312:159–163.

232. Floyd RA. Production of Free Radicals. In KMA Welch, LR Caplan, DJ Reis, BK Siesjo, B Weir (eds), Primer on Cerebrovascular Diseases. San Diego: Academic, 1997;165–169.

233. Siesjo BK, Agardh CD, Bengtsson F. Free radicals and brain damage. Cerebrovasc Brain Metab Rev 1989;1: 165–211.

234. Busto R, Dietrich WD, Globus MYT, et al. The importance of brain temperature in cerebral ischemic injury. Stroke 1989;20:1113–1114.

235. Dietrich WD, Busto R. Hyperthermia and Brain Ischemia. In KMA Welch, LR Caplan, DJ Reis, BK Siesjo, B Weir (eds), Primer on Cerebrovascular Diseases. San Diego: Academic, 1997;165–169.

236. Siesjo BK. Brain Energy Metabolism. New York: Wiley, 1978.

237. Siesjo BK, Bengtsson F. Calcium fluxes, calcium antagonists, and calcium-related pathology in brain ischemia, hypoglycemia and spreading depression: a unifying hypothesis. J Cereb Blood Flow Metab 1989;9:127–140.

238. Tymianski M, Sattler RG. Is calcium involved in excitotoxic or ischemic neuronal damage? In KMA Welch, LR Caplan, DJ Reis, BK Siesjo, B Weir (eds), Primer on Cerebrovascular Diseases. San Diego: Academic, 1997; 190–192.

239. Siesjo B. Historical overview: calcium, ischemia and death of brain cells. Ann N Y Acad Sci 1988;522:638–661.

240. Siesjo B, Smith M-L. Mechanism of Acidosis-related Damage. In KMA Welch, LR Caplan, DJ Reis, BK Siesjo, B Weir (eds), Primer on Cerebrovascular Diseases. San Diego: Academic, 1997;223–226.

241. Choi DW. The Excitotoxic Concept. In KMA Welch, LR Caplan, DJ Reis, BK Siesjo, B Weir (eds), Primer on Cerebrovascular Diseases. San Diego: Academic, 1997;187–190.

242. Choi DW. Excitotoxicity and Stroke. In LR Caplan (ed), Brain ischemia, Basic Concepts and Clinical Relevance. London: Springer, 1995;29–36.

243. Pulsinelli WA, Levy DE, Sigsbee B, et al. Increased damage after ischemic stroke in patients with hyperglycemia

with or without established diabetes mellitus. Am J Med 1983;74:540–544.

244. Helgason C. Blood glucose and stroke. Stroke 1988;19:1049–1053.

245. Adams HP, Olinger CP, Marler JR, et al. Comparison of admission serum glucose concentration with neurologic outcome in cerebral infarction. Stroke 1988;19:455–458.

246. Woo E, Ma JTC, Robinson JD, et al. Hyperglycemia is a stress response in acute stroke. Stroke 1988;19:1359–1364.

247. Woo E, Lam CWK, Kay R, et al. The influence of hyperglycemia and diabetes mellitus on immediate and 3-month morbidity and mortality after acute stroke. Arch Neurol 1990;47:1174–1177.

248. Ginsberg MD. Hypothermic Neuroprotection in Cerebral Ischemia. In KMA Welch, LR Caplan, DJ Reis, BK Siesjo, B Weir (eds), Primer on Cerebrovascular Diseases. San Diego: Academic, 1997;272–275.

249. Safar P. Amelioration of post ischemic brain damage with barbiturates. Current concepts in cerebrovascular disease. Stroke 1980;15:1–5.

250. Black K, Weidler J, Jallad N, et al. Delayed pentobarbital therapy of acute focal cerebral ischemia. Stroke 1978;9:245–251.

251. Faden AI, Jacobs TP, Holaday JW. Opiate antagonist improves neurologic recovery after spinal injury. Science 1981;211:493–494.

252. Faden AI, Hallenbeck JM, Brown CQ. Treatment of experimental stroke: comparison of naloxone and thyrotropin releasing hormone. Neurology 1982;32:1083–1087.

253. Hosobuchi Y, Baskins DS, Woo SK. Reversal of induced ischemic neurologic deficit in gerbils by the opiate antagonist naloxone. Science 1982;215:69–71.

254. Baskin DS, Hosobuchi Y. Naloxone reversal of ischemic neurological deficits in man. Lancet 1981;2:272–275.

255. Faden AI. Opiate antagonists in the treatment of stroke. Stroke 1984;15:575–578.

256. Wahlgren NG. Cytoprotective Therapy for Acute Ischemic Stroke. In M Fisher (ed), Stroke Therapy. Boston: Butterworth–Heinemann, 1955;315–350.

257. Argentino C, Sacchetti ML, Toni D, et al. GM1 ganglioside therapy in acute ischemic stroke. Stroke 1989;20:1 143–1149.

258. Leon A, Lipartiti M, Seren MS, et al. Hypoxic-ischemic damage and the neuroprotective effects of GM1 ganglioside. Stroke 1990;21(Suppl 3);95–97.

259. Sygen Acute Stroke Study (SASS) investigators. Ganglioside GM1 in acute ischemic stroke; the SASS trial. Stroke 1994;25:1141–1148.

260. Lenzi GL, Grigoletto F, Gent M, et al. Early treatment of stroke with monoganglioside GM1. Efficacy and safety results of the Early Stroke Trial. Stroke 1994;25:1552–1558.

261. Kontos HA. Oxygen Radicals in Cerebral Ischemia. In MD Ginsberg, WD Dietrich (eds), Cerebrovascular Disease. New York: Raven Press, 1989;365–371.

262. Chan PH, Chu L, Chen SF, et al. Reduced neurotoxicity in transgenic mice overexpressing human copper-zinc-superoxide dismutage. Stroke 1990;21(Suppl 3):80–82.

263. Hall E, Pazara KE, Braughler JM, et al. Nonsteroidal lazaroid U78517F in models of focal and global ischemia. Stroke 1990;21(Suppl 3):83–87.

264. Hall ED, Pazara KE. Effects of Novel 21-amino Steroid Antioxidants on Post Ischemic Neuronal Degeneration. In MD Ginsberg, WD Dietrich (eds), Cerebrovascular Disease. New York: Raven Press, 1989;387–391.

265. Hall ED. 21-Aminosteroids. In KMA Welch, LR Caplan, DJ Reis, BK Siesjo, B Weir (eds), Primer on Cerebrovascular Diseases. San Diego: Academic, 1997;257–261.

266. Kassell N, Haley EC, Appersen-Hansen C, Alves WM. A randomized, double-blind, vehicle-controlled trial of tirilizad mesylate in patients with aneurysmal subarachnoid hemorrhage: a cooperative study in Europe/Australia/New Zealand. J Neurosurg 1996;84:221–228.

267. Peters GR, Hwang L-J, Musch D, et al. Safety and efficacy of 6 mg/kg/day tirilizad mesylate in patients with acute ischemic stropke (TESS Study). Stroke 1996; 27:195.

268. Randomized Trial of Tirilizad in Acute Stroke (RANITAS) Investigators. Randomized trial of tirilizad in acute stroke. Stroke 1996;27:195.

269. Olney JW. Brain lesion, obesity, and other disturbances in mice treated with monsodium glutamate. Science 1969;164:719–721.

270. Meldrum B. Excitotoxicity in Ischemia: an Overview. In MD Ginsberg, WD Dietrich (eds). Cerebrovascular Diseases. New York: Raven Press, 1989;47–60.

271. Small DL, Buchan AM. NMDA and AMPA Receptor Antagonists in Global and Focal Ischemia. In KMA Welch, LR Caplan, DJ Reis, BK Siesjo, B Weir (eds), Primer on Cerebrovascular Diseases. San Diego: Academic, 1997;244–247.

272. Onai MZ, Fisher M. Thrombolytic and cytoprotective therapies for acute ischemic stoke: a clinical overview. Drugs Today 1996;32:573–592.

273. Lees KR. Cerestat and other NMDA antagonists in ischemic stroke. Neurology 1997;49(Suppl 4);S66–S69.

274. Dux E, Fastborn J, Umgerstedt U, et al. Protective effect of adenosine and a novel xanthine derivative propentofylline on the cell damage after bilateral carotid occlusion in the gerbil hippocampus. Brain Res 1990;516:248–256.

275. Huber M, Kittner B, Hojer C, et al. Effect of propentofylline on regional cerebral glucose metabolism in acute ischemic stroke. J Cereb Blood Flow Metab 1993;13:526–530.

276. Muir KW, Lees KR. Clinical experience with excitatory amino acid antagonist drugs. Stroke 1995;26:503–513.

277. Grotta J. Lubelazole treatment of acute ischemic stroke. The U.S. and Canadian Lubelazole Ischemic Stroke Study Group. Stroke 1997;28:2338–2346.

278. Diener HC. Multinational randomised controlled trial of lubelazole in acute ischaemic stroke. The European and Australian Lubelazole Ischaemic Stroke Study Group. Cerebrovasc Dis 1998;8:172–181.

279. Clark WM, Warach SJ, Pettigrew LC, et al. A randomized dose-response trial of citicoline in acute ischemic stroke patients. Citicoline Stroke Study Group. Neurology 1997;49:671–678.

280. Onal MZ, Li F, Tatlisumak T, et al. Synergistic effects of citicoline and MK-801 in temporary experimental focal ischemia in rats. Stroke 1997;28:1060–1065.

281. Marcoux FW, Probert AW, Weber ML. Hypoxic neuronal injury in tissue culture is associated with delayed calcium accumulation. Stroke 1990;21(Suppl 3):71–74.

282. Goldberg M, Choi DW. Intracellular free calcium increases in cultured cortical neurons deprived of oxygen and glucose. Stroke 1990;21(Suppl 3):75–77.

283. Caplan LR. New stroke therapies. Arch Neurol 1997;54: 1222–1224.

284. Shepherd J, Cobbe SM, Ford I, et al. Prevention of coronary heart disease with pravastatin in men with hypercholesterolemia. N Engl J Med 1995;333:1301–1307.

285. Scandinavian Simvastatin Survival Study Group. Randomised trial of cholesterol lowering of 444 patients with coronary heart disease: the Scandinavian Simvastatin Survival Study (4S). Lancet 1994;344:1383–1389.

286. Sacks FM, Pfeffer MA, Moye LA, et al. The effect of pravastatin on coronary events after myocardial infarction in patients with average cholesterol levels. N Engl J Med 1996;335:1001–1009.

287. Hebert P, Gaziano JM, Chan KS, Hennekens CH. Cholesterol lowering with statin drugs, risk of stroke, and total mortality. An overview of randomized trials. JAMA 1997;278:313–321.

288. Blauw GJ, Lagaay AM, Smelt AHM, et al. Stroke, statins, and cholesterol. A meta-analysis of randomized placebo-controlled double-blind trials with HMG-CoA reductase inhibitors. Stroke 1997;28:946–950.

289. Bucher HC, Griffith LE, Guyatt GH. Effect of HMGcoA reductase inhibitors on stroke. A meta-analysis of randomized controlled trials. Ann Intern Med 1998;128:89–95.

290. Furberg CD, Adams HP, Applegate WB, et al. Effect of lovostatin on early carotid atherosclerosis and cardiovascular events. The Asymptomatic Carotid Artery Progression Study (ACAPS) Research Group. Circulation 1994;90:1679–1687.

291. Crouse JR, Byington RP, Bond MG, et al. Pravastatin, lipids, and atherosclerosis in the carotid arteries (PLAC ll). Am J Cardiol 1995;75:455–459.

292. Hodis HN, Mack WJ, LaBree L et al. Reduction in carotid arterial wall thickness using lovastatin and dietary therapy. A randomized controlled clinical trial. Ann Intern Med 1996;124:548–556.

293. Rosenson RS, Tangney CC. Antiatherothrombotic properties of statins. Implications for cardiovascular event reduction. JAMA 1996;279:1643–1650.

294. Catsman-Beirevoets C, Harskamp F. Compulsive presleep behavior and apathy due to bilateral thalamic stroke: response to bromocriptine. Neurology 1988;38:647–648.

295. Albert ML, Bachman D, Morgan A, et al. Pharmacotherapy for aphasia. Neurology 1988;38:877–879.

296. Fleet WS, Watson RT, Valenstein E, et al. Dopamine agonist therapy for neglect in humans. Neurology 1986; 36(Suppl):347.

297. Barrett K. Treating organic abulia with bromocriptine and lisuride: four case studies. J Neurol Neurosurg Psychiatry 1991;54:718–721.

298. Feeney DM, Gonzalez A, Law WA. Amphetamine, haloperidol and experience interact to affect the rate of recovery after motor cortex injury. Science 1982;217:855–857.

299. Houda DA, Feeney DM. Haldoperidol blocks amphetamine induced recovery of binocular depth perception after bilateral visual cortex abilities in the cat. Proc West Pharmacol Soc 1985;28:209–211.

300. Davis JN, Crisostomo EA, Duncan P, et al. Amphetamine and Physical Therapy Facilitate Recovery of Function From Stroke: Correlative Animal and Human Studies. In ME Raichle, W Powers (eds), Cerebrovascular Diseases. New York: Raven Press, 1987;297–304.

301. Goldstein LB. Amphetamine-Facilitated Functional Recovery After Stroke. In MD Ginsberg, WD Dietrich (eds), Cerebrovascular Diseases. New York: Raven Press, 1989:303–308.

302. Hurwitz BE, Dietrich D, McCabe PM, et al. Amphetamine promotes recovery from sensory-motor integration deficit after thrombotic infarction of the primary somatosensory rat cortex. Stroke 1991;22:648–654.

303. Goldstein LB. Pharmacology of recovery after stroke. Stroke 1990;21(Suppl 3):139–142.

304. Hernandez TC, Kiefel J, Barth TM, et al. Disruption and Facilitation of Recovery of Behavioral Function: Implication of the Gamma-aminobutyric Acid/benzodiazepine Receptor Complex. In MD Ginsberg, WD Dietrich (eds), Cerebrovascular Diseases. New York: Raven Press, 1989:327–334.

305. Goldstein LB, Davis JN. Physician prescribing patterns following hospital admission for ischemic cerebrovascular disease. Neurology 1988;38:1806–1809.

306. Goldstein LB. Potential effects of common drugs on stroke recovery. Arch Neurol 1998;55:454–456.

307. Goldstein LB. Common drugs may influence motor recovery after stroke. The Sygen in Acute Stroke Study Investigators. Neurology 1995;45:865–871.

308. Ropper AH. Neurological and Neurosurgical Intensive Care (3rd ed). New York: Raven Press, 1993.

309. Kase CS, Crowell RM. Prognosis and Treatment of Patients with Intracerebral Hemorrhage. In CS Kase, LR Caplan (eds), Intracerebral Hemorrhage. Boston: Butterworth–Heinemann, 1994;467–489.

310. Kase CS, Caplan LR. Therapy of Intracerebral Hemorrhage. In T Brandt, LR Caplan, J Dichgans, HC Diener, C Kennard (eds), Neurological Disorders, Course and Treatment. San Diego: Academic,1996;277–288.

311. Shields CB, Friedman WA. The role of stereotactic technology in the management of intracerebral hemorrhage. Neurosurg Clin North Am 1992;3:685–702.

312. Kopitnik TA, Kaufman HH. The future: prospects of innovative treatment of intracerebral hemorrhage. Neurosurg Clin North Am 1992;3:703–707.

313. Zervas N, Hedley-White J. Successful treatment of cerebral herniation in five patients. N Engl J Med 1973;286: 1075–1077.

314. Krieger D, Hacke W. The intensive care of the stroke patient. Stroke pathophysiology, diagnosis, and management (3rd ed). New York: Churchill Livingstone, 1998;1133–1154.

315. O'Brien MD. Ischemic Cerebral Edema. In LR Caplan (ed), Brain Ischemia, Basic Concepts and Clinical Relevance. London: Springer, 1995;43–50.

316. Klatzo I. Neuropathological aspects of brain edema. J Neuropathol Exp Neurol 1967;26:1–14.

317. Newkirk T, Tourtellotte W, Reinglass J. Prolonged control of increased intracranial pressure with glycerin. Arch Neurol 1972;27:95–96.

318. Buckell M, Walsh L. Effect of glycerol by mouth on raised intracranial pressure in man. Lancet 1964;1:1151–1152.

319. Frank MS, Nahata MC, Hilty MD. Glycerol: a review of its pharmacology, pharmacokinetics, adverse reactions and clinical use. Pharmacotherapy 1981;1:147–160.

320. Marshall LF, Smith RW, Rauscher LA, et al. Mannitol dose requirements in brain-injured patients. J Neurosurg 1978;48:169–172.

321. Kuroiwa M, Shibutani M, Okeda R. Blood-brain barrier disruption and exacerbation of ischemic brain edema after restoration of blood flow in experimental focal cerebral ischemia. Acta Neuropathol 1988;76:62–70.

322. Mulley G, Wilcox R, Mitchell J. Dexamethasone in acute stroke. BMJ 1978;2:994–996.

323. Caplan LR. Posterior Circulation Disease: Clinical Findings, Diagnosis, and Management. Boston: Blackwell Science, 1996.

324. Lehrich J, Winkler G, Ojemann R. Cerebellar infarction with brainstem compression: diagnosis and surgical treatment. Arch Neurol 1970;22:490–498.

325. Feeley MP. Cerebellar infarction. Neurosurg 1979;4:7–11.

326. Delashaw JB, Broaddus WC, Kassell NF, et al. Treatment of right hemispheric cerebral infarction by hemicraniotomy. Stroke 1990;21:874–881.

327. Schwab S, Rieke K, Aschoff A, et al. Hemicraniotomy in space-occupying hemispheric infarction: useful early intervention or desperate activism. Cerebrovasc Dis 1996; 6:325–329.

328. Schwab S, Steiner T, Aschoff A, et al. Early hemicraniectomy in patients with complete middle cerebral artery infarction. Stroke 1998;29:1888–1893.

329. Heinsius T, Bogousslavsky J, Van Melle G. Large infarcts in the middle cerebral artery territory. Etiology and outcome patterns. Neurology 1998;50:341–350.

330. Wijdicks E, Schievink W, McGough PF. Dramatic reversal of the uncal syndrome and brain edema from infarction in the middle cerebral artery territory. Cerebrovasc Dis 1997;7:349–352.

331. Fujita K, Kusonoki T, Noda M, et al. Normal pressure hydrocephalus (NPH) following subarachnoid hemorrhage (SAH): clinical considerations of CT and development of hydrocephalus after SAH. Brain Nerve 1981; 33:845–851.

332. Greenberg J, Shubick D, Shenkin H. Acute hydrocephalus in cerebellar infarct and hemorrhage. Neurology 1961;11: 697–700.

333. Khan M, Polyzoidis K, Adegbite A, et al. Massive cerebellar infarction: "conservative" management. Stroke 1983;14:745–751.

334. Rieke K, Krieger D, Adams H-P, et al. Therapeutic strategies in space-occupying cerebellar infarction based on clinical, neuroradiological,and neurophysiological data. Cerebrovasc Dis 1993;3:45–55.

335. Kaste M, Palmomaki H, Sarna S. Where and how should elderly stroke patients be treated? A randomized trial. Stroke 1995;26:249–253.

336. Indredavik B, Slordahl SA, Bakke F, Rokseth R, Haheim LL. Stroke unit treatment. Long term effects. Stroke 1997;28:1861–1866.

337. Stroke Unit Trialists' Collaboration. Collaborative systematic review of the randomized trials of organised inpatient (stroke unit) care after stroke. BMJ 1997;314: 1151–1159.

338. Stroke Unit Trialists' Collaboration. How do stroke units improve patient outcomes? A collaborative systematic review of the randomized trials. Stroke 1997;28:2139–2144.

339. Ronning OM, Gulvog B. Outcome of subacute stroke rehabilitation. A randomized controlled trial. Stroke 1998;29:779–784.

340. Steiner T, Hacke W. Combination therapy with neuroprotectants and thrombolytics in acurte ischaemic stroke. Eur Neurol 1998;40:1–8.

341. Zivin JA, Mazzarella V. Tissue plasminogen activator plus glutamate antagonists improves outcome after embolic stroke. Arch Neurol 1991;48:1235–1240.

342. Schwarz S, Schwab S, Bertram M, et al. Effects of hypertonic saline hydroxyethyl starch solution and mannitol in patients with increased intracranial pressure after stroke. Stroke 1998;29:1550–1555.

343. Yamamoto H, Bogousslavsky J. Mechanisms of second and further strokes. J Neurol Neurosurg Psychiatry 1998; 64:771–776.

344. Caplan LR. Prevention of strokes and recurrent strokes. J Neurol Neurosurg Psychiatry 1998;64:716.

Part II
Stroke Syndromes

Chapter 6

Large Artery Occlusive Disease
of the Anterior Circulation

Specific clinical and laboratory aspects of occlusive disease of the commonly involved arteries are analyzed in this chapter. Examples of typical patients are included to discuss management and illustrate the common clinical and imaging findings. The general epidemiologic, etiologic, and pathologic features that relate to large artery occlusive lesions are discussed in Part I of this book.

Occlusive Disease of the Internal Carotid Artery

Internal Carotid Artery Disease at Its Origin

The modern era in ischemic cerebrovascular disease began in 1951 with Miller Fisher's key report, which called attention to the clinical findings associated with occlusion of the internal carotid artery (ICA) in the neck.[1,2] Previously, ischemic strokes in the anterior circulation were invariably attributed to middle cerebral artery (MCA) disease. Fisher called attention to warning episodes in patients with carotid artery disease that preceded strokes. He dubbed these episodes *transient ischemic attacks* (TIAs).[1–3] Fisher commented, "It is even conceivable that some day surgery will find a way to bypass the occluded portion of the artery during the period of ominous fleeting symptoms." At that time, angiography required a surgical cutdown and only single-frame, hand-pulled films were available. During the next decades, the advent of safer and more widespread angiography led to increased recognition of the frequency and importance of ICA disease in the neck. Newer, noninva-

sive techniques now make possible reliable detection of carotid artery lesions in outpatients.

The first carotid surgical procedures were performed in the early 1950s.[1,4] During the 1960s and 1970s, improved diagnostic capability, safer anesthesia, advanced surgical techniques, and an increase in the number of vascular surgeons caused an explosion in the amount of operative procedures performed on the carotid arteries. In 1985, more than 107,000 endarterectomies were performed in the United States, making it one of the three most common surgical procedures.[4] After 1987, the number of endarterectomies began to decrease in response to widespread concern about the indications, use, and complications of the procedure.[5,6] In 1991, the North American and European controlled trial results[7,8] showed an important therapeutic benefit of endarterectomy in symptomatic patients with high-grade stenosis. These reports gave the procedure more credibility and was an impetus for more vascular surgery. The frequency of complications, morbidity, and mortality figures still vary widely among surgeons and medical centers, even within the same city.[9,10] I return to the important question of treatment after reviewing the epidemiologic, clinical, and laboratory features of ICA occlusive disease in the neck.

A 58-year-old man, HL, awakened with a numb and weak left hand. He had a myocardial infarction 6 years earlier and continued to have angina pectoris on moderate exertion. He developed pain in the left calf that abated when he stopped to rest or walked more than two blocks.

The major cause of ICA occlusive disease in the neck is atherosclerotic narrowing of the vessel. The lesion usually begins in the distal common carotid artery (CCA) and extends to the few proximal centimeters of the ICA and external carotid artery (ECA), almost always more severely narrowing the ICA. This lesion is found more often in whites than in African-Americans or Asians, and in men more than women.[11,12] Occlusive disease of the large systemic vessels, especially the coronary, iliac, and femoral arteries, often accompanies carotid atherosclerosis. Coexisting angina pectoris, myocardial infarction, and limb claudication are common.[13] Risk factors for the development of proximal ICA disease are similar to those for coronary artery disease and include hypertension, smoking, diabetes, and hypercholesterolemia. Mortality in patients with ICA disease is usually cardiac. Attention is appropriately focused on the heart and brain, and the brain's circulation.

> Although HL did not volunteer other symptoms, direct questioning revealed several important warning signs. In the months before presentation, he had two brief episodes of transient obscuration of vision in his right eye. A dark shade descended from above, rather quickly blocking vision completely on one occasion, and obscuring only the upper half of vision during the other episode. The attacks were brief and lasted less than a minute each. He also had three episodes of transient neurologic dysfunction. These episodes consisted of stumbling after his left leg gave way, slurred speech, and numbness of the left arm and hand and left face. The initial episode was 3 months earlier, the most recent 3 days earlier. He noted unaccustomed, frequent headaches in the weeks before presentation.

Atherosclerotic plaques gradually narrow the ICA lumen. Ulceration, attachment of platelet nidi and clot to crevices in plaques, and hemorrhage into plaques become more common as the artery becomes increasingly stenosed. Plaques usually contain a lipid core and fibrous cap. When there is a break in the fibrous cap, contact of the lipid core with the contents of the lumen activates platelets

and can activate the coagulation cascade, promoting the deposition of white and red thrombi onto the plaque surface. Plugs of platelets and thrombi may detach from the arterial wall and embolize to distal vessels, causing transient or prolonged neurologic dysfunction. Reduction in blood flow can also lead to periodic insufficiency in distal perfusion. For these reasons, TIAs often occur as the vessel narrows to warn of an impending stroke. Many times when an artery occludes, adequate collateral circulation develops and no permanent neurologic damage ensues.

The most important clue to an ICA localization of the occlusive process is an attack of transient monocular blindness. Often, the vision loss is described as a dimming, darkening, or obscuration. An apparent shade or curtain usually falls from above, but may move from the side like a theater curtain. After a brief period of seconds or a few minutes, the curtain lifts or recedes. This usually leaves no permanent vision loss. These attacks of transient visual obscuration are caused by decreased blood flow through the ophthalmic artery, the first branch of the ICA. Amaurosis fugax occurs when the lesion affects the ICA proximal to the ophthalmic artery (in the neck or proximal carotid siphon) or involves the ophthalmic artery itself. Diminished flow or pressure in the ophthalmic artery is a clue to the presence of carotid artery disease. In migraine, the most common differential diagnostic consideration, patients usually describe brightness, glittering, flickering, and movement within the visual field, which lasts 15–30 minutes and is seldom monocular. Occasionally, patients with severe ICA occlusive disease report unilateral spells of reduced vision after exposure to bright light, a type of retinal claudication.[14] In some patients with bilateral ICA disease, the transient vision loss can be bilateral. As with HL, individuals may not volunteer information about temporary vision loss because they think it is completely unrelated to the present problem. The physician must directly and repeatedly ask about specific symptoms of ocular and brain ischemia.

Episodes of hemispheral ischemia are also usually brief. Attacks may be quite varied and include different deficits in different limbs during individual attacks. Sometimes, however, the spells are stereotyped. In some patients with critical stenosis, the attacks are frequent and may be precipitated by sud-

Table 6-1. Symptoms of Internal Carotid
Artery Disease

Attacks of transient monocular blindness
Transient ischemic attacks, sometimes variegated, and
    occurring during a span of weeks or months
Frequent, unaccustomed headache
Commonly associated history of coronary or peripheral
    vascular disease

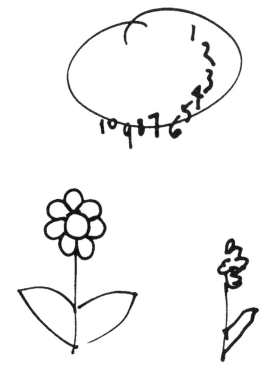

Figure 6-1. At the top is a clock drawn by the patient who
had a right parietal lobe lesion. At the bottom is the patient's
copy (*right*) of a daisy drawn by the examiner (*left*).

denly standing or a drop in blood pressure.[15] Frequent, brief, machine-gun–like attacks usually mean low flow caused by proximal severe stenosis. Emboli generally produce longer, less frequent attacks. In disease of larger vessels, such as the ICA, TIAs may occur during a period of months, as compared with a briefer span of hours, days, or a week in patients with lacunar infarction caused by disease of smaller blood vessels. As the ICA narrows, collateral circulation develops, leading to dilation of arteries and the onset of unaccustomed headache. It is unusual, however, for headache to be the only symptom; in my experience, headache is usually accompanied by TIAs. The common symptoms of ICA disease in the neck are listed in Table 6-1.

On examination, HL had moderate weakness of the left arm, slight weakness of the left psoas muscle, and severe weakness of the left hand. Position sense was decreased in the left hand and HL could not accurately localize left-limb touch stimuli, nor recognize objects in the left hand. He drew a clock poorly (Figure 6-1, top) and also copied inaccurately (Figure 6-1, bottom). A soft, high-pitched bruit was audible at the right carotid bifurcation in the neck. A right Horner's syndrome was noted.

Physical examination of the blood vessels and eyes may yield important clues to an ICA location of the lesion (Table 6-2). Palpation of the neck is not helpful unless the CCA is occluded, in which case there is no palpable carotid pulse on that side. Even when the ICA is occluded, the CCA pulse is usually transmitted to the ICA in the neck. The presence of a typical bruit (i.e., a high-pitched, long, focal sound heard loudest over the carotid bifurcation) is virtually diagnostic of localized ICA dis-

ease. In some patients with severe ICA occlusive disease, however, flow is so severely diminished that no bruit is audible. When a bruit at the bifurcation is also audible over the ipsilateral eye, the physician can be confident that the bruit is of ICA

Table 6-2. Signs of Internal Carotid Artery Disease

Neck
    High-pitched, focal, long bruit at bifurcation
Face
    Increased angular, brow, cheek[17] pulses
    Frontal artery sign[18]
    Increase in superficial temporal artery
Retina
    Cholesterol crystals[19]
    Platelet plugs[20]
    Retinal infarcts
    Reduced caliber of arteries
    Less severe hypertensive changes
    Venous stasis retinopathy[21,22]
    Reduced retinal artery pressure

origin and that the artery is patent. A bruit also can arise from the proximal ECA. In this case, the bruit usually radiates toward the jaw and can be diminished by pressure on ECA branches.[16] When the ICA is occluded or severely stenosed, ECA collaterals may feed into the orbit and may be palpable at the angular, brow, and cheek (ABC) regions (see Figure 3-2).[17,18]

Ischemia to the iris or retina on the side of the carotid occlusive lesion is another helpful clue. Retinal arteries on the side of the carotid lesion may be reduced in caliber or show fewer hypertensive changes than their counterparts in the opposite retina. White, fluffy exudates or focal retinal atrophy can represent infarction. Small cholesterol crystal emboli are highly refractile bodies that usually lodge at bifurcations of retinal arteries.[19] White platelet plugs can also be transiently seen within retinal arteries.[20] *Venous stasis retinopathy* is a descriptive term for the ophthalmoscopic appearance found in patients with ICA occlusion, and is characterized by microaneurysms, small-dot retinal hemorrhages, and dilatated, dark retinal veins, sometimes of irregular caliber.[21,22] This disorder resembles diabetic retinopathy but can usually be distinguished by unilaterality, location in the midportion of the retina, and its association with low retinal arterial pressure as measured by diminished ophthalmic blood-flow velocities by transcranial Doppler (TCD). The presence of venous stasis retinopathy always means that flow reduction in the ophthalmic artery is severe and longstanding.

Neurologic findings are caused by infarction of brain regions within the ICA circulation. Signs in patients with ICA disease are difficult to separate clinically from those in patients with intrinsic lesions of the MCA.[23,24] The most common loci of infarction are within the MCA territory. Weakness is common and usually affects the contralateral hand and face more than the leg. When sensory loss is present, it usually is of the cortical type with loss of position sense, point localization, and stereognosis on the opposite side of the body. Again, the hand and face often show more sensory abnormalities than the trunk and lower extremity. When bilateral simultaneous tactile stimuli are presented to the arms, the stimulus contralateral to the lesion is often not reported by the patient. Neglect of the opposite side of visual space and an attentional hemianopia are also common findings, especially

when the infarct is in the right cerebral hemisphere. Poor drawing and copying, impersistence with tasks, diminished emotional responsiveness, and anosognosia (lack of awareness of the deficit) also frequently accompany right ICA-territory infarction.[25,26] Aphasia is a common sequel to left-sided infarction. Occasionally, the infarct is located predominantly in the territory of the anterior cerebral artery (ACA); foot, leg, and shoulder weakness predominate. Rarely, when the posterior cerebral artery (PCA) is supplied directly by the ICA, an infarct caused by ICA occlusion can lie solely within the PCA territory and can manifest as a hemianopia without other signs.[27,28]

A duplex scan was performed. B-mode showed some flat plaques within the distal right CCA and severe atherosclerotic disease at the right ICA origin with near occlusion (Figure 6-2A). The Doppler frequencies also suggested high-grade stenosis of the right ICA (Figure 6-2B, C). The left carotid artery showed only minor disease. TCD examination revealed lower flow velocities in the right ICA siphon, and the right MCA and ACA. Computed tomography (CT) showed a hypodensity in the cortical parietal lobe affecting the postcentral gyrus and superior parietal lobule (Figure 6-3). Cerebral angiography by femoral artery catheterization using the Seldinger technique demonstrated severe, irregular narrowing of the ICA at its origin with a residual lumen of approximately 1 mm (95% luminal narrowing) (Figure 6-4). The carotid siphon and MCA were normal, but there was a branch occlusion of one of the parietal branches of the superior trunk of the MCA. Echocardiography and Holter monitoring were normal.

Noninvasive diagnostic tests are discussed in Chapter 4. In this patient, ultrasonography suggested a severe flow-reducing lesion at the ICA origin. Because of the likelihood that the lesion would require surgery, and the necessity of opacifying the intracranial vessels, it was decided to proceed with standard angiography. Alternatively, magnetic resonance angiography (MRA) or computed tomography angiography (CTA) might have adequately

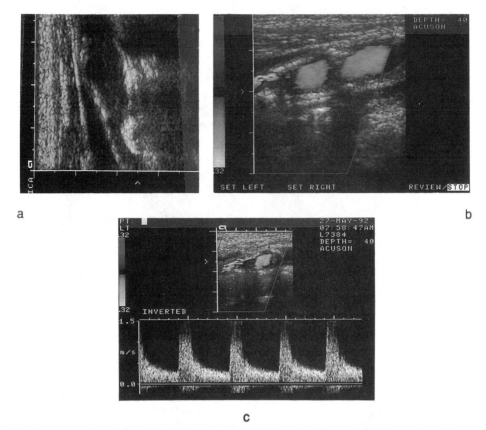

Figure 6-2. Ultrasound studies. (**a**) B-mode from duplex scan. Hard plaque is seen narrowing the internal carotid artery; in this view, the artery is narrowed approximately 60%; in other views, the narrowing is more severe. (**b**) Color Doppler flow imaging shows the stenosis and change in flow. (**c**) Doppler spectrum from duplex scan corresponds to (**a**). High blood-flow velocities through area of stenosis. (Courtesy of Professor Michael Hennerici.)

shown the lesion. Angiography confirmed and further quantified the nature of the stenotic lesion.

In patients with ICA atherosclerotic occlusive disease, there are several frequent patterns of disease that are diagrammed in Figure 6-5. When the ICA is occluded, the vessel may be angiographically absent or show a pointed, tapering, or rounded stump.[29] Barnett and colleagues called attention to embolization from the stump of previously occluded carotid arteries.[30] Stenotic lesions can be ulcerated, smooth, or irregular. The lesions may be long and tapered or may slope abruptly like a shelf. B-mode scans and color Doppler flow ultrasound imaging (CDFI) studies of the carotid origin can help define the nature of plaques, presence of ulceration, and dynamics of flow. Calcific, smooth plaques are less often the source of intra-arterial emboli and usually do not show rapid enlargement, whereas irregular, heterogeneous,

ulcerated, soft plaques often progress and are frequently the source of emboli. When angiography is complete, it is often possible to detect embolic occlusion of the MCA or its branches, so-called occlusio supra occlusionem.[31]

Imaging Findings in Patients with Internal Carotid Artery Disease

CT scans of patients with carotid artery occlusion or severe stenosis show several common patterns of distribution of infarction (Figure 6-6). These patterns include (1) watershed or border-zone infarction between the territories of the ACA and MCA, and between the MCA and PCA; (2) subcortical white matter infarcts; (3) wedge-shaped, pial artery–territory infarcts; and (4) infarction of the basal ganglia and lentiform nucleus.[31] The bor-

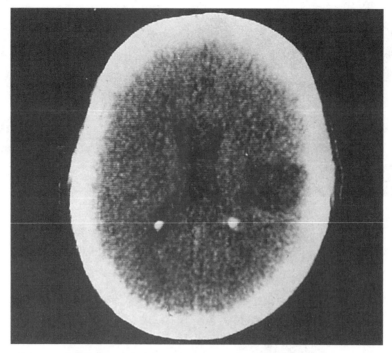

Figure 6-3. Computed tomography shows an infarct in the right parietal lobe (on right side of figure).

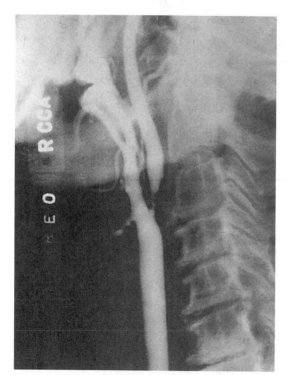

Figure 6-4. Right carotid angiogram: lateral view shows severe stenosis of the proximal internal carotid artery.

der zone and subcortical white matter lesions are probably caused by reduced flow, whereas the pial and basal ganglia infarcts are caused by emboli to the mainstem MCA, its superior or inferior division trunks, or penetrating artery branches. In my experience, watershed infarction and large, superficial infarcts in the MCA territory are the most common lesions found on CT in patients with severe ICA obstructive disease.[23] The mechanism of stroke in patient HL was a small superior parietal-lobe infarct caused by an embolus from the ICA stenosis in the neck. Cardiac testing did not show an alternative embologenic donor source in the heart.

HL was placed on heparin therapy for 1 week of treatment and was then switched to warfarin. The international normalized ratio (INR) was maintained between 2.0 and 3.0. At 4 weeks, an uncomplicated carotid endarterectomy was performed. Blood pressure was carefully monitored postoperatively, but did not elevate. The patient had minimal residual neurologic signs of clumsiness and slight numbness

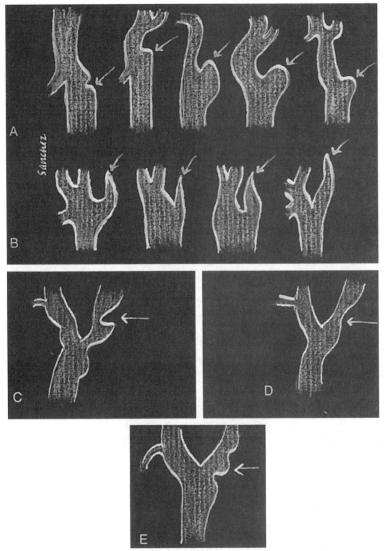

Figure 6-5. Examples of appearance on angiography of carotid artery lesions: (**A**) rounded stump; (**B**) pointed stump; (**C**) shelf plaque; (**D**) regular plaque; and (**E**) ulcerated plaque. (Adapted from MS Pessin, G Duncan, K Davis, et al. Angiographic appearance of carotid occlusion in acute stroke. Stroke 1980;11:485–487.)

of his left hand, but was able to return to his former work.

In my present practice, choice of treatment for patients with ICA disease in the neck depends on the following:

1. Severity of the stenosis.
2. Anatomy of the carotid artery and stenosing plaque: A high carotid artery bifurcation and a long stenotic lesion increase the difficulty of surgery.
3. Presence of a recent cerebral infarct as determined by a persistent clinical deficit, an appropriate CT, or magnetic resonance imaging (MRI) lesion.
4. General health of the patient, especially any contraindication to surgery, warfarin anticoagulation, or agents that decrease platelet agglutination.

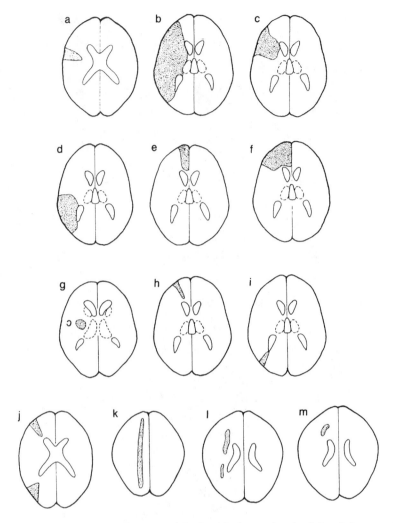

Figure 6-6. Most common computed tomography locations of infarcts in the anterior circulation. Infarcts are shown by hatched gray: **(a)** wedge-shaped middle cerebral artery infarct, **(b)** entire middle cerebral artery territory, **(c)** superior-division middle cerebral artery, **(d)** inferior-division middle cerebral artery, **(e)** anterior cerebral artery, **(f)** anterior cerebral artery and middle cerebral artery, **(g)** striatocapsular infarct, **(h)** wedge-shaped anterior watershed infarct, **(i)** wedge-shaped posterior watershed infarct, **(j)** anterior and posterior watershed infarcts, **(k)** linear watershed infarct, **(l)** ovular deep watershed infarct, and **(m)** small white matter watershed infarct. (Reprinted with permission from LR Caplan. Cerebrovascular Disease: Larger Artery Occlusive Disease. In S Appel (ed), Current Neurology, Vol 8. Chicago: Yearbook Medical, 1988;179–226.)

5. Morbidity and mortality record of the surgeon who would undertake surgery and of the hospital where the surgery would take place.
6. Attitude of the patient and family toward the situation after the alternative courses of action have been discussed.

Physicians and surgeons at the Mayo clinic carefully analyzed the neurologic, medical, and angiographic risks of carotid surgery. I rely heavily on their analysis.[32] I consider symptomatic patients with TIAs or small, nondisabling strokes who have various ICA lesions in the following section.

Complete Occlusion of the Internal Carotid Artery in the Neck

I do not recommend surgery for complete occlusion of the ICA in the neck. When the ICA occludes, clot quickly propagates high into the neck, often to the carotid siphon and beyond. Because there are no ICA branches in the neck, collateral flow patterns promote extension of clot toward the first branch, the ophthalmic artery. It is technically difficult to open completely occluded ICAs, and attempts to suction clots can lead to distal embolization. If it were known that an occlusion had become complete minutes or a few hours before, as might happen after angiography, exploration of the neck would be reasonable. That circumstance is rare in my experience. Angiography can yield clues as to the extent of the occlusive thrombosis. If opacification of the contralateral ICA shows retrograde filling of the occluded ICA down into the neck, it is more likely that the surgeon might be able to open the ICA surgically.

When the patient arrives at the hospital soon after the onset of stroke symptoms, and CT or MRI does not show a large region of infarction, thrombolytic therapy can be considered. Intravenous recombinant tissue plasminogen activator has seldom been effective in recanalizing occlusions of the ICA in the neck or intracranially.[33] Some interventionists have been able to physically manipulate the ICA clot with a catheter and inject urokinase directly into the thrombus. This lyses the clot and allows recanalization.[34,35] When an embolus arising from the ICA has blocked the MCA, the interventionist can manipulate the catheter to the MCA clot and affect thrombolysis by injecting urokinase or another thrombolytic agent into the intracranial thrombus.[34,35] When neck or intracranial thrombi are superimposed on severe atherostenotic lesions, however, thrombi almost always reoccur, unless the stenosis is removed by angioplasty shortly after successful thrombolysis. The use of thrombolysis in the setting of ICA thrombosis has never been compared with anticoagulant therapy. I have not had occasion to use this aggressive approach in patients with acute ICA thrombosis.

I treat patients with acute ICA thrombosis with bed rest, keeping the head flat or slightly lower than the feet, to augment blood flow to the head. I try to avoid hypotension and have used agents, such as ephedrine, which raise blood pressure in some patients. I avoid antihypertensive drugs during the first 1–2 weeks unless the blood pressure is in the malignant range (e.g., greater than 225/125 mm Hg). If the patient is normotensive and there is no contraindication to the use of anticoagulants, I use intravenous heparin, followed by warfarin for a short period (2–6 weeks), to attempt to prevent embolization of fresh clots and discourage clot propagation. After this period, I do not use anticoagulants, but do use aspirin in doses of one 325-mg tablet per day. I use 75 mg of clopidogrel in patients who are aspirin-intolerant or have peptic ulcer disease.

Caution must be exercised in the diagnosis of complete ICA occlusion because a severe reduction in flow can lead to collapse of the artery above the high-grade block. Angiography produces a picture that closely resembles occlusion, so called pseudo-occlusion,[36] but late films usually show a trickle of dye ascending anterograde toward the siphon. CDFI also sometimes visualizes flow through a pseudo-occlusion not seen with standard angiography.[37] CT in cross section of the high neck after contrast can show blood in the ICA, documenting preserved anterograde flow.[38] In pseudo-occlusion, the residual flow, albeit small, makes it possible for the surgeon to open the vessel. Patients with pseudo-occlusion are considered to have severe stenosis. Analysis of the data from the North American Symptomatic Carotid Endarterectomy Trial (NASCET) showed that patients with near occlusion do not have an increased risk of acute stroke compared with those with lesser degrees of severe stenosis (70–94%), nor do they have a higher rate of surgical complications.[39]

In patients with ICA occlusion, the deficit usually develops at, or shortly after, the time of occlusion when embolization and low flow are maximal. A chronic low-flow state, so-called misery perfusion,[40] may occur but only rarely persists. Occasionally, patients with known ICA occlusion develop transient symptoms, especially if they become hypotensive from overzealous antihypertensive treatment, or from dehydration or hypovolemia. The most common symptoms are transient obscurations of vision in the ipsilateral eye and/or weakness or numbness of the contralateral limbs.

An unusual, but characteristic, sign of hypoperfusion is a so-called limb-shaking TIA.[41,42] Usually when standing or active, the patient develops a tremor with impressive shaking and oscillation of the arm and hand contralateral to the occluded ICA. Occasionally, the lower extremity is involved. The shaking stops when the patient sits or lies down and is caused by ischemia rather than a seizure. I have not referred patients with ICA occlusion for ECA-ICA bypass, but would consider doing so if there were persistent, recurrent ischemic attacks or if positron emission tomography (PET), single-photon emission computed tomography (SPECT), or other new technology documented persistent misery perfusion. Sequential TCD studies of blood-flow velocity in the MCA and ACA, especially after acetazolamide infusion, also yield information about distal flow and the reserve capacity of the carotid tributaries to dilate. These laboratory techniques are discussed in Chapter 4.

Severe Stenosis of the Internal Carotid Artery in the Neck

In my opinion, severe stenosis of the ICA in the neck, when symptomatic, requires surgery unless there is a severe, disabling distal infarction. The reported results of the North American[7,43] and European trials[8,44] support this strategy. What constitutes a severe stenosis? The two principal criteria are (1) the degree of anatomic narrowing of the artery and presence of significant reduction in flow velocity and (2) pressure in tributary vessels shown by TCD.[45] A residual lumen of less than 1.5 mm (70–99% stenosis) invariably represents severe stenosis and nearly always impedes distal flow. When the severely stenotic ICA is examined histologically, compound ulcers are often found.[46] Although these lesions may also be found in nonstenosed vessels, they become more frequent as the artery narrows.

When patients have TIAs, but no persistent neurologic deficit, and severe stenosis of the ICA with a residual lumen of less than 1.5 mm (70–99% stenosis), I believe that carotid endarterectomy should be performed urgently. If there is evidence of infarction, persistent abnormal neurologic signs or symptoms, or a new infarct on CT, I prefer to wait 3–6 weeks before surgery because of the possibility of intracerebral hemorrhage (ICH) after endarterectomy.[47,48] Many instances of postendarterectomy ICH are explained by hypertension after manipulation of the carotid receptors in the neck.[49,50] Careful postoperative monitoring of blood pressure and effective treatment of hypertension (if it develops) should prevent ICH. Endarterectomy on patients with severe stenosis can also be followed by a "hyperperfusion syndrome."[51,52] Sudden flooding of the previously underperfused brain with blood can overwhelm the autoregulatory capacity of the region and lead to headache, seizures, focal neurologic signs, brain edema, and brain hemorrhage.[52] Hypertension, often acute and severe, is also usually present in patients with severe effects of the hyperperfusion syndrome. Recognition of the syndrome and rapid, effective treatment of hypertension usually prevents serious brain edema and hemorrhage.

When there is a persistent neurologic deficit, I prefer to use heparin, then warfarin, to keep the INR between 2.0 and 3.0. As long as the patient remains stable or improves, I wait 6 weeks. If, however, there are further attacks or worsening during this waiting interval, I suggest endarterectomy without further delay, because in my experience, severe deficits commonly develop if surgery is not performed in these patients. Also, if patients worsen during observation in the hospital and continue to progress despite heparin therapy, I urge emergency correction of a critical ICA stenosis. Some patients improve dramatically immediately after surgery.

In patients with severe ICA stenosis, if surgery cannot be performed or if the patient refuses operation, I choose to anticoagulate with warfarin. The duration of anticoagulation is uncertain and should be individualized. I use the results of sequential duplex scans to guide the duration of treatment. Arteries with tight stenosis often occlude on follow-up scans, often without new symptoms.[53,54] During the 4–6 weeks after occlusion, thrombi become organized and adherent, after which embolization is rare. I switch from warfarin to one aspirin, per day, 4–6 weeks after vascular studies show complete occlusion. While the lumen remains narrowed but patent, I continue warfarin. In some patients, plaques seem to regress and the lumen may become less narrowed. In these individuals, a switch to aspirin also seems logical. No studies have been undertaken to test the strategy I have outlined.

*Plaque Disease of the Internal Carotid Artery
in the Neck with Slight or Moderate Stenosis*

I suggest prophylactic treatment with 3-hydroxy-3-methylglutaryl coenzyme A reductase inhibitors (statins) and an agent that decreases platelet aggregation for ICA plaque disease in the neck. I do not recommend warfarin anticoagulation or surgery. Although it is true that ulceration can occur in nonstenotic lesions, and that ulcers can be the source of artery-to-artery embolization, this occurs less frequently in patients without severe stenosis. In the presence of a severe stenosing lesion, the physician can be more confident that this is the responsible lesion rather than another plaque. Furthermore, the natural history of plaques has not been well studied. They may reendothelialize and heal. Plaques are ubiquitous in individuals older than 40 years, and current angiographic and noninvasive techniques do not infallibly predict the presence of ulceration on histologic examination. Agents that decrease platelet aggregation are posited to be most effective when there are nonstenosing plaques and high-velocity flow continues.

I prefer aspirin over surgery because aspirin is likely to be safer and, perhaps, as effective for these lesions. Aspirin also has theoretical advantages over warfarin, an agent that probably works best in slow-moving vascular streams to prevent red thrombi. At present, I prefer aspirin to other agents. The dose of aspirin is uncertain. I usually prescribe one 325-mg tablet per day. An accurate, reproducible in vitro test of the effectiveness of the platelet antiaggregants might lead clinicians to titrate the dose in individual patients, and so monitor effectiveness of the drug. Clopidogrel, 75 mg a day, and dipyridamole, preferably in a modified-release form (200 mg with 25 mg aspirin), given twice each day are alternative antiplatelet aggregants.

When plaques are shallow, the decision to use platelet antiaggregant agents is clear. As plaques become larger, more irregular, or clearly ulcerated, and luminal narrowing approaches 50–70%, however, the therapeutic decision becomes more difficult and should be individualized. NASCET and the European Carotid Surgery Trials showed modest benefit from surgery in patients with this severity of stenosis. The risk to benefit ratio, however, depends much on the individual patient and surgeon characteristics.[43,44] In a young patient with a lesion in this gray zone of near-critical stenosis, who has several TIAs and is a good surgical candidate, I probably would choose surgery.

Carotid Artery Clots

Some patients with atherosclerotic plaques in the neck, with or without severe stenosis, have thrombi that are grossly visible on angiography.[55–57] In some of these patients, free-floating thrombi are attached to plaques and coagulation functions are normal, whereas in others, a hypercoagulable state has promoted the formation of carotid thrombi. These patients should be treated urgently. In a review of prior cases of patients with intraluminal clot, both surgery and warfarin anticoagulation were effective in preventing further stroke.[55] Clot recurred after surgery, however, in patients with coagulopathy[56] The blood coagulation profiles of these patients should be carefully studied before treatment. In the NASCET study, the presence of ICA thrombi increased the surgical risk.[43]

*Asymptomatic Patients with Internal
Carotid Artery Disease in the Neck*

The preceding discussion of treatment concerned symptomatic patients with TIA or stroke. It now has become commonplace to document ICA disease in the neck in patients who have no apparent central nervous system symptoms. The most common circumstances provoking carotid artery investigation are an audible neck bruit or imminent surgical procedures on the aorta, coronary, or peripheral-limb vessels. Some cases are discovered at angiography for indications other than vascular disease, or when an angiogram shows ICA disease on the asymptomatic side. Should these lesions be repaired before symptoms develop?

I seldom recommend carotid endarterectomy in asymptomatic patients. These patients do not have an unusual risk of stroke during surgery on other major vessels. Furthermore, stroke is unusual without preceding TIAs. In most medical centers, the risk of surgery and angiography (approximately 6% combined morbidity and mortality)[58–60] is probably as great as, if not greater than, the risk of stroke without prior TIA.

Results of several studies of asymptomatic lesions are important to consider. In one series of 168 prospectively studied patients with known ICA stenosis, 26 patients (15%) had TIAs only; three patients had TIAs but refused surgery and had subsequent strokes; and just one patient developed sudden stroke without warning.[61] In another series of patients with carotid stenosis followed for 2 years among 318 patients, 5% developed TIAs, but only two patients had a stroke without a preceding TIA.[62] Sequential studies show that stenotic arteries often occlude without symptoms.[54] In patients undergoing endarterectomy who have bilateral carotid artery stenosis, subsequent stroke on the unoperated side is uncommon.[62] Even when a bruit is detected before elective surgery, the incidence of postoperative stroke is not increased.[63] Postoperative strokes are usually caused by cardiogenic emboli.

Treatment of asymptomatic patients must be individualized.[64] I do not think surgery on asymptomatic patients should be seriously considered unless the stenosis is severe (>80% luminal narrowing). When made aware of a definite risk of stroke, some patients become quite anxious and psychologically tolerate the risk poorly. They prefer the small gamble of an intraoperative complication to the sword that they sense hangs perpetually over them. The situation must be fully discussed with the patient, and the benefits and risks of medical and surgical therapy explained. In patients who do not elect surgery, I teach them about TIAs and urge them to immediately report any attacks. I prescribe statin drugs and antiplatelet aggregants and follow the carotid artery disease with sequential duplex ultrasound examinations. Significant increase in severity of the stenosis does increase the risk of a stroke and is some evidence favoring surgery.[65] The occurrence of TIAs puts patients in the symptomatic category and makes them surgical candidates.

The Asymptomatic Carotid Artery Study showed a modest benefit for carotid endarterectomy in men who had more than 60% carotid stenosis, and did not have important cardiac or other comorbidity.[66] Surgeons who participated in this study were carefully selected, and the perioperative surgical morbidity and mortality was low (2.3%). The risk of stroke after angiography was 1.2%. The results of this study and the topic of treatment of patients who have carotid artery stenosis with no symptoms have aroused considerable controversy.[67–69] Many neurologists and vascular surgeons question the need for catheter angiography in these patients and rely on duplex ultrasound and vascular imaging with MRA or CTA. The decision remains an individual one for each patient. The anatomic aspects of the plaque (e.g., location, extent, degree of stenosis, heterogeneity, and echodensity); change during conservative medical treatment with statins and platelet antiaggregants; comorbidity, especially the presence of hypertension and coronary artery disease; the experience and results of the surgeon chosen; and the biases and wishes of the well-informed patient should be considered when deciding between medical or surgical treatment.[64]

Extracranial Carotid Artery Dissections

After atherosclerosis, dissection is the next most common lesion that affects the carotid artery in the neck. Dissections usually involve the pharyngeal portion of the artery above the origin but below entry into the skull. Dissections are tears in arteries, almost always involving the medial coat. Dissections are customarily referred to as *traumatic* or *spontaneous* in origin. The great majority of dissections, however, probably involves some trauma or mechanical stress. Sudden neck movements and stretching are likely to cause dissection. Some inciting events are trivial, such as lunging for a tennis shot or turning the neck while driving to see other cars to the side and rear. Many patients forget such events or believe them to be too inconsequential to mention. Congenital and acquired abnormalities of the arterial media and elastic tissue, especially fibromuscular dysplasia, make patients more vulnerable to dissection. Most patients with dissection, however, do not have concurrent disorders. Migraine is more common in patients with dissection. The posited explanation for the relationship between migraine and dissection is that edema of the vessel wall during a migraine attack makes the involved artery more vulnerable to tearing.

Dissections probably begin with a tear in the media, that then leads to bleeding within the arterial wall. Intramural blood then dissects longitudinally, spreading along the vessel proximally and distally. Dissections can tear through the intima, allowing the partially coagulated intramural blood to enter the lumen of the artery. The arterial wall, expanded by intramural blood, also compresses the lumen. Dissections probably begin at the intimal surface in some patients and dissect into the media. Intimal flaps are often present on the intimal surface. At times, the major dissection plane is between the media and the adventitia, causing an aneurysmal outpouching of the arterial wall.

Extracranial dissections cause symptoms primarily by the presence of luminal compromise and luminal clot. Dissections through the adventitia lead to rupture into the surrounding neck, muscles and fascia, a process that causes neck pain and formation of a pseudoaneurysm, but usually does not further compromise blood flow. Thrombus is present within the lumen because of rupture of intramural clot into the lumen or thrombus formation in situ within the lumen. Narrowing of the lumen by the intramural blood, with alteration in blood flow and irritation of the endothelium, causing release of endothelins and tissue factors, and activation of platelets and the coagulation cascade, each contributes to formation of intraluminal thrombus. Brain ischemia can result from hypoperfusion, usually from acute luminal compromise, embolism, or both. Hypoperfusion usually causes transient ischemia, but seldom is prolonged enough to cause infarction. Infarction is more often caused by embolization or propagation of luminal thrombus.

The major symptoms of extracranial carotid artery dissection are (1) neck, head, and face pain; (2) Horner's syndrome; (3) pulsatile tinnitus; (4) transient ipsilateral monocular vision loss; (5) transient hemispheral attacks with contralateral limb numbness or weakness; (6) sudden-onset strokes; and (7) palsy of lower cranial nerves (IX-XII).[70-72] Many patients present pain and headache as their only symptoms and do not have neurologic findings. The pain is often in the neck, face, or jaw. Headaches may be generalized but are most common on the side of the dissection. Features of Horner's syndrome are caused by involvement of the sympathetic fibers along the dilated carotid artery segments. Pulsatile tinnitus is another common symptom because the carotid artery courses near the tympanic membrane. Neurologic symptoms related to hypoperfusion are usually multiple, brief TIAs, referred to as *carotid allegro* by Miller Fisher because of their rapidity. Sudden-onset strokes are usually caused by embolism of clot from the region of dissection. The dis-

tended, dilated carotid artery at the skull base can compress the lower cranial nerves (IX–XII) that exit this region. The diagnosis of carotid artery dissection can be suggested by ultrasound when the ultrasonographer explores the neck with the probe from above the carotid bifurcation to the skull base.[73] MRA, CTA, and standard angiography are helpful. Cut MRI sections of the neck often show the lesion. The best treatment is anticoagulation for as long as severe stenosis persists. When the ICA is occluded and remains occluded, 2–3 months of anticoagulation is sufficient.

Intracranial Internal Carotid Artery Occlusive Disease

Narrowing and thrombotic occlusion of the ICA occur at the siphon far less frequently than at the ICA origin. The siphon includes the S-shaped portion of the carotid artery from its entry through the carotid foramen into the petrous bone to its exit from the cavernous sinus above the petrous clinoid. The ophthalmic artery originates from the ICA within the siphon. Less is known about the pathology of the artery in its entirely intraosseous course because the bone is seldom removed for study. Calcification of the ICA in the siphon is common.[74] Studies of groups of patients with ICA siphon disease document a high incidence of strokes, frequent coexistent extracranial vascular disease, and a high death rate from coronary artery disease.[75-78]

> RY, a 70-year-old man, had an attack of transient weakness of his right leg 1 week before he awakened with weakness of the right foot and face. This was accompanied by an unaccustomed reluctance to speak. He repeated spoken language normally and comprehension of written and spoken language was good. There was a history of angina pectoris, and a high-pitched focal bruit was audible over the right neck.

The epidemiology of carotid siphon disease is probably similar to ICA-origin disease. African-Americans, however, have an unexpectedly high incidence of this lesion.[11] Accompanying disease at the ICA and vertebral artery origins is common. Tandem ICA origin and siphon disease occurred in

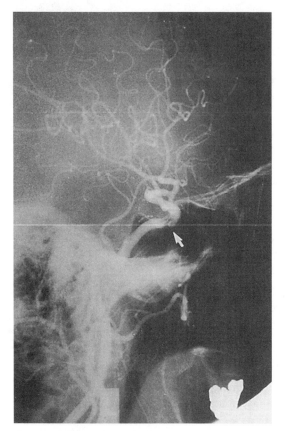

Figure 6-7. Carotid artergram: lateral view shows stenosis of the left internal carotid artery in the siphon (*arrow*).

62% of the series of patients with siphon disease, as reported by Marzewski and colleagues.[75] TIAs are less frequent and fewer in number in patients with siphon disease when compared with ICA-origin disease. The ratio of strokes to TIAs and of asymptomatic patients is higher in carotid-siphon disease.

The presence of amaurosis fugax depends on the level of the lesion in the siphon. In my experience, the occlusive lesion is most often distal to the ophthalmic artery origin, so that ICA siphon disease is an infrequent cause of transient monocular blindness. On examination, there are usually no signs of collateral circulation through the ECA vessels of the face. The ocular and retinal pathologies discussed in ICA-origin disease are uncommon. I have, however, seen a number of patients with angiographically verified thrombotic occlusion of the carotid siphon, who days later developed signs of decreased ophthalmic flow and reduced central retinal artery pressure. The mechanism of delayed

ophthalmic ischemia is retrograde extension of the clot below the ophthalmic artery branch, a phenomenon documented postmortem in patients with stenosis and thrombosis of the ICA siphon.[79] Retrograde extension of clot is, however, rare if the siphon occlusion is caused by embolism.[79]

Too few patients have been well studied to allow a comparison of the topography and distribution of cerebral infarcts in patients with ICA-siphon disease, as compared with disease of the ICA origin or the MCA. My impression is that separate infarcts in portions of the ACA and MCA territories are more common in siphon disease. The leg is more often paretic in siphon disease, indicating ACA-territory damage. Sometimes, the lesions affect the center of the ACA and MCA territories, causing weakness of the foot and face with relative sparing of the hand, whereas in ICA-origin disease, upper-extremity weakness is most common.

> In RY, a carotid duplex scan showed moderate stenosis (50%) of the right ICA origin. TCD showed increased blood-flow velocities through the orbital window at the left carotid siphon, and normal velocities in the MCA and ACA. Velocities in the right intracranial arteries were normal. Angiography by femoral catheterization revealed severe irregularity and stenosis of the left ICA siphon, the lesion beginning above the ophthalmic-artery origin (Figure 6-7). The left ICA origin had a shallow plaque without stenosis. No definite distal-branch artery occlusion was seen. CT showed a small infarct in the paramedian frontal lobe.

Ultrasound studies confirmed severe carotid siphon disease on the side, appropriate to the symptoms and the CT lesion. TCD is an effective diagnostic technology for detecting and quantifying stenotic lesions of the intracranial ICA.[80] MRAs of the carotid siphon are often difficult to interpret. Tortuosity makes this a common area for artefacts. CTAs are more useful than MRAs in this region. The contralateral ICA-origin lesion was asymptomatic and not severe enough to reduce flow. The clinical signs of leg and foot weakness and transcortical motor aphasia were caused by ACA-territory ischemia. The infarct was caused by either low flow with good MCA collaterals or embolism originating from the irregular siphon stenosis.

> RY was given intravenous heparin. After a slight increase in leg weakness during the first day, he stabilized. Warfarin was begun on day 5. On day 7, heparin was discontinued. The patient was maintained on warfarin therapy for 1 year, at which time he developed a fatal myocardial infarction.

Reviews in the 1980s confirm that ICA-siphon disease has a worse prognosis than ICA-origin disease.[75–78] Late strokes and cardiac death are common. Stenosis of the ICA in the siphon seems to be more stable than other intracranial lesions. Follow-up angiography shows a low rate of progression or regression of stenotic carotid siphon atherosclerotic lesions.[81] Lesions within the siphon cannot be treated surgically. Therapeutic alternatives include antiplatelet agglutinating agents, warfarin, angioplasty, and ECA-ICA bypass to MCA branches. There have been no prospective controlled studies to fully document the effectiveness, or lack thereof, of any medical treatment in patients with disease of the carotid siphon. In some series, white men with TIAs relating to siphon disease had a relatively good outcome after warfarin therapy.[77,78] The tortuous, windy course and calcification within the siphon makes angioplasty of stenotic lesions difficult and risky. Some balloon angioplasties, however, have been performed without subsequent insertion of stents.[82,83] In the ECA-ICA bypass study, there was no difference in outcome in patients with severe intracranial carotid artery occlusive disease who were treated medically or by bypass.[84] ECA-ICA bypass should not be considered in patients with severe stenosis of surgically inaccessible vessels that still retain luminal patency. A patent shunt distal to an artery with low flow can further discourage flow through the stenosis, promoting thrombosis. Occlusion of stenotic vessels after a shunt has been documented in eight patients.[85,86] The thrombus could embolize distally, leading to cerebral infarction, despite the presence of a shunt that delivers adequate flow. Since the results of the ECA-ICA bypass study have been published, I have not suggested bypass in patients with occlusion of the ICA siphon. There may rarely be patients with ICA siphon or MCA occlu-

sion with chronic low perfusion, and with stunned but not infarcted brain, who might benefit from revascularization. Such could only be detected by sophisticated blood flow and metabolic studies using PET, MRI, SPECT, and TCD.

I suggest warfarin for those patients with tight ICA siphon stenosis, and preserved anterograde flow who have no contraindication to anticoagulation. I reserve antiplatelet agglutinating agents, such as aspirin, clopidogrel, and combined low-dose aspirin and dipyridamole for patients who have minor irregularity of the artery without severe impediment to flow. As with disease of the ICA origin, attention should also be directed to the heart because of the high incidence of associated cardiac morbidity (as in the case of RY).

In some patients, there is associated severe disease of the ICA origin in addition to the siphon stenosis. In these patients with tandem lesions, operation on the ICA in the neck is sometimes followed by opening of the siphon lesion on follow-up angiography.[87] This occurrence is explained by preoperative distal collapse or narrowing of the vessel as a result of diminished flow. In the face of complete occlusion of the ICA siphon, there is no gain in opening an ICA-origin stenosis. If, however, the ICA stenosis at the siphon is not critical, carotid endarterectomy of the more proximal ICA-origin lesion might greatly augment flow. In the presence of severe critical stenosis at both sites, often accompanied by stenosis of other vessels, I usually choose a trial of warfarin therapy before considering surgery.

Top of the Carotid Artery Occlusions

Occlusions of the intracranial carotid artery bifurcation are predominantly embolic.[88,89] This portion of the ICA is often called the *T portion* because of its shape. When an embolus blocks the distal intracranial ICA, the result is usually a large infarct that includes the anterior and MCA territory. Death or severe disability results. Occlusions of the distal intracranial carotid artery seldom recanalize with either intravenous or intra-arterial thrombolytic treatment.[89–91] Severe stenosis and thrombotic occlusion of the supraclinoid carotid artery before its intracranial bifurcation into MCA and ACA branches (top of the carotid) rarely occurs. In my experience, an unusual number of patients with a lesion at this site have had coagulation abnormalities, such as sickle cell disease or circulating lupus anticoagulant.

Occlusion or Severe Stenosis of the Middle Cerebral Artery Stem or Its Major Upper and Lower Trunks

Occlusion of the MCA was a common diagnosis in the era before cerebral angiography. After Fisher and others called attention to the high incidence of extracranial ICA disease[1–3] and angiography became prevalent, most patients formerly diagnosed with MCA occlusion were found instead to have extracranial ICA disease. The vast majority of

MCA occlusions was embolic, arising from a proximal ICA plaque or from the heart.[13,79] These observations on the rarity of occlusive lesions in the intracranial anterior circulation were generated at hospitals with a predominance of white patients. Studies of African-American[11,12,92,93] and Asian[94–99] patients, however, show a higher frequency of intracranial occlusive disease of the MCA and its major trunk branches than is found in white patients. Figure 6-8 shows the most common patterns of infarction in patients with MCA occlusions.

A 48-year-old African-American woman, AC, awakened with weakness of the right face and was unable to speak. These symptoms cleared during the day. During the next morning, however, she noted

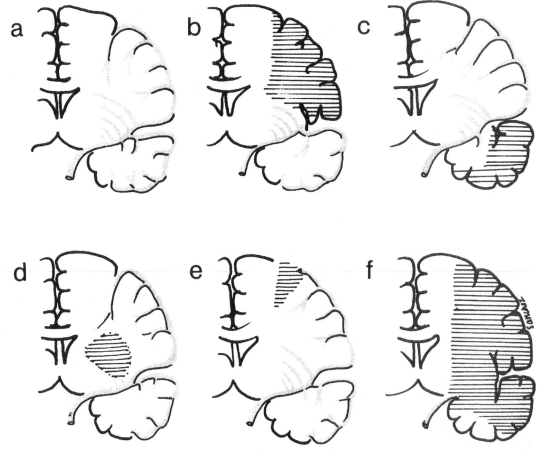

Figure 6-8. Common patterns of infarction with middle cerebral artery occlusion: (**a**) diagram of the middle cerebral artery in coronal section, (**b**) occlusion of the upper trunk of the middle cerebral artery, (**c**) occlusion of the lower trunk of the middle cerebral artery, (**d**) infarct of the deep basal ganglia, (**e**) wedge infarct in the pial territory, and (**f**) whole middle cerebral artery occlusion.

aphasia and weakness of her right limbs. She had a history of slight hypertension but had no history of coronary or peripheral vascular disease.

In my experience, patients with MCA occlusive disease, when compared with patients with ICA disease, are more often African-American or Asian, young, female, hypertensive, and diabetic.[12,23,97,99] They also have had a lower incidence of hypercholesterolemia and associated coronary and peripheral vascular disease. Patients of Japanese, Chinese, and Thai descent, as well as diabetics and women taking contraceptive pills, share a propensity for MCA pathology with African-Americans. Although TIAs do occur in patients with MCA disease, they are probably less frequent with ICA disease and occur during a shorter time span.[23,99] The frequency of TIAs in patients with MCA disease also seems to vary with race. In four series of predominantly white patients with MCA occlusive disease, TIAs were a more frequent presentation than stroke.[78,100–103] The TIA to stroke ratios in these studies were 15 to 1,[100] 15 to 6,[101] 13 to 11,[102] and 9 to 4.[103] In contrast, the TIA to stroke ratio in a predominantly African-American patient series was 4 to 16.[23] It was 3 to 20 in a series of mostly Chinese patients,[99] and 8 to 28 in a series of Japanese patients.[104] Smoking was an important risk factor in a large study that reported its frequency. Eighty percent of patients with MCA occlusion and 72% of patients with MCA stenosis had a history of cigarette smoking.[98] Because the vascular lesion is intracranial and, of course, beyond the ophthalmic artery supply, transient monocular blindness does not occur.

During the first 3 days in the hospital, AC progressively worsened, gradually developing a complete right hemiplegia, minor tingling of the right limbs, and mutism. Examination revealed no bruits, facial, or limb-pulse abnormalities.

Patients with MCA disease often develop their deficits more gradually than comparable series of patients with ICA disease.[23,99] Patients with MCA disease often note their abnormalities on awakening in the morning or from a nap and have a high incidence of subsequent fluctuation or progression during the next 1–7 days. This gradual onset and progressive course support a low-flow mechanism for the ischemia. Deficits begin when flow is most sluggish, and collateral circulation takes time to develop and equilibrate. In contrast, patients with ICA disease more commonly have sudden-onset deficits while awake and thereafter remain stable—a course better explained by distal embolism from their ICA lesion than by low flow.

Because the occlusive process is intracranial, there are no important associated signs of extracranial disease. Neurologic findings vary, depending on the location of the vascular occlusion and the brain ischemia. The following sections discuss the most common patterns of neurologic deficits seen in patients with MCA disease. Although these syndromes are discussed under the heading of intrinsic MCA-occlusive disease, the patterns are more commonly caused by embolism to the MCA territory. Figure 6-9 shows the common patterns of MCA occlusion and their anatomic and clinical correlates.

Occlusion or Stenosis of the Upper Trunk of the Middle Cerebral Artery

The superior trunk of the MCA supplies the frontal and superior parietal lobes. Occasionally, when the mainstem MCA is short, the lenticulostriate vessels arise from the proximal portion of the superior trunk.[23,105,106] In that case, the internal capsule and lateral basal ganglia are also nourished by the superior trunk.

The findings include (1) hemiplegia, more severe in the face, hand, and upper extremity, with relative sparing of the lower extremity; (2) hemisensory loss, usually including decreased pinprick and position sense, sometimes sparing the leg; (3) conjugate eye deviation, with the eyes resting toward the side of the brain lesion; and (4) neglect of the contralateral side of space, especially to visual stimuli. Visual neglect is usually more severe in patients with right hemisphere lesions.

When the lesion is in the left dominant hemisphere, there invariably is an accompanying aphasia. Verbal output is sparse and patients do not do what they are asked with either hand. They may follow whole-body commands, however, such as turn over, sit, and stand. They may be able to nod appropriately to yes and no questions, but comprehension of written material is poor. With time, a pattern of Broca's aphasia evolves with sparse, effortful speech, poor pronunciation of syllables, and omission of filler words. Comprehension of spoken language, however, is preserved.

In superior-division MCA infarcts in the right hemisphere, patients frequently seem unaware of their deficit (anosognosia) and may not admit they are hemiplegic or impaired in any way.[25,26,107] Some patients are also impersistent, performing requested tasks quickly, but cannot persevere and terminate tasks prematurely.[85,107,108] When asked to read, patients with right superior-trunk occlusions often omit the left of the page or paragraph, and cannot see people or objects to their left.

Occlusion of the Inferior Trunk of the Middle Cerebral Artery

The inferior division of the MCA usually supplies the lateral surface of the temporal lobe and inferior parietal lobule (Figure 6-9). The anterior, medial, and inferior portions of the temporal lobes are supplied by other arteries.

In contrast to patients with lesions of the superior division, patients with occlusion of the MCA inferior trunk usually have no elementary motor or sensory abnormalities. They often have a visual field defect, either a hemianopia or an upper quadrantanopia, affecting the contralateral visual field.

When the left hemisphere is involved, patients have a Wernicke-type aphasia. Speech is fluent, and syllables are well pronounced. Patients use wrong or nonexistent words, however, and what is said makes little sense. Comprehension and repetition of spoken language are poor. There may be relative sparing of written comprehension, with the patient preferring that words be written.[109,110] When the right hemisphere is affected, patients draw and copy poorly and may have difficulty finding their way about or reading a map.

Behavioral abnormalities also frequently accompany temporal-lobe infarctions. Patients with Wernicke's aphasia are often irascible, paranoid, and may become violent. Patients with right temporal infarcts often have an agitated hyperactive state resembling delirium tremens.[111–113] Diagnosis of right inferior-trunk occlusion is sometimes difficult. The key findings are a left visual-field defect and poor drawing and copying in an agitated person.[113]

Deep Infarction of the Middle Cerebral Artery Territory

Basal ganglia and internal-capsule infarction (Figure 6-9) is usually explained by occlusion of the mainstem MCA before its lenticulostriate branches. Excellent potential exists for collateral circulation over the convexities but poor collateral circulation in the deep basal gray nuclei and the internal capsule. For this reason, some patients with MCA occlusion have selective ischemia of the deep lenticulostriate territory. Collateral circulation, however, is adequate to prevent cortical infarction. On CT, the lesions can be confused with lacunes but are larger and often extend to the inferior brain surface. Some have called these lesions *giant lacunes*.[23,114] The preferred term for these deep MCA lenticulostriate-territory lesions, however, is *striatocapsular infarcts.*[88,115,116]

Patients with striatocapsular infarcts are invariably hemiparetic, but the distribution of weakness in face, arm, and leg is variable. Sensory loss is usually minor because the posterior portion of the internal capsule is spared. When the lesion is in the left hemisphere after a short period of temporary mutism, speech is sparse and dysarthric, but repetition of spoken language is preserved. Comprehension of spoken and written language depends on the size and anteroposterior extent of the lesion.[117,118] When the right hemisphere is involved, there often is neglect of contralateral visual and tactile stimuli, but this is usually more transient than with parietal cortical infarction.

Mainstem Occlusion with Total Infarction of the Middle Cerebral Artery Territory

Mainstem occlusion with total infarction of the MCA territory is most common in patients with

Figure 6-9. ➤Patterns of occlusion of the middle cerebral artery and their anatomic correlates. (Reprinted with permission from The Netter Collection of Medical Illustrations, illustrated by Frank H. Netter, M.D. Copyright © Novartis. All rights reserved.)

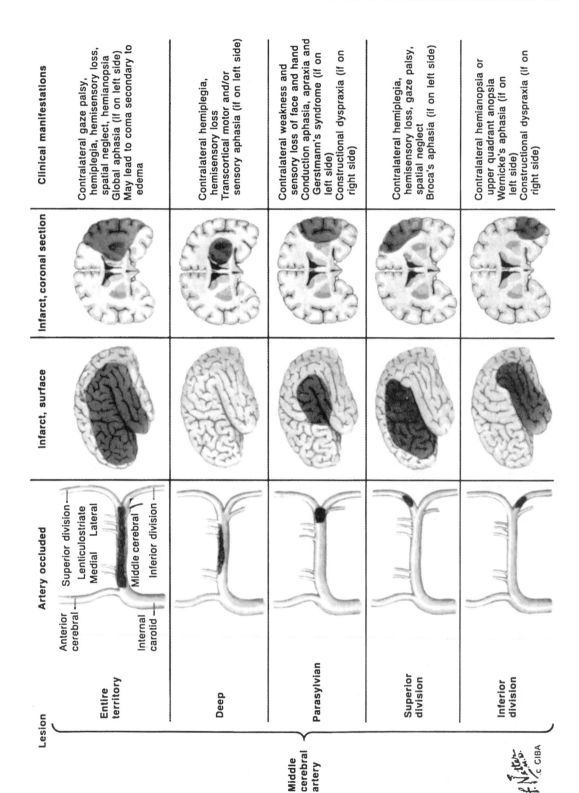

Lesion	Artery occluded	Infarct, surface	Infarct, coronal section	Clinical manifestations
Middle cerebral artery — Entire territory	Anterior cerebral, Superior division, Lenticulostriate (Medial, Lateral), Internal carotid, Middle cerebral, Inferior division			Contralateral gaze palsy, hemiplegia, hemisensory loss, spatial neglect, hemianopsia. Global aphasia (if on left side). May lead to coma secondary to edema
Deep				Contralateral hemiplegia, hemisensory loss. Transcortical motor and/or sensory aphasia (if on left side)
Parasylvian				Contralateral weakness and sensory loss of face and hand. Conduction aphasia, apraxia and Gerstmann's syndrome (if on left side). Constructional dyspraxia (if on right side)
Superior division				Contralateral hemiplegia, hemisensory loss, gaze palsy, spatial neglect. Broca's aphasia (if on left side)
Inferior division				Contralateral hemianopsia or upper quadrant anopsia. Wernicke's aphasia (if on left side). Constructional dyspraxia (if on right side)

embolism to the proximal MCA (see Figure 6-9). In most patients with intrinsic occlusive disease of the MCA, there is sufficient collateral circulation to spare at least the outer borders of the territory.

These patients are usually devastated. Among 208 patients with large MCA-territory infarcts in one series, the mortality rate was 17%. Fifty percent of patients had severe disability.[119] Severe paralysis, hemisensory loss, attentional hemianopia, and conjugate eye deviation to the opposite side were found. When the left hemisphere is involved, there is a global aphasia. Right hemisphere lesions produce severe neglect, anosognosia, disinterest or poor motivation, apathy, and severe constructional apraxia. Recovery to useful function is unusual.[120]

Brain edema with swelling of the infarcted hemisphere, causing a midline shift and brain herniations, is an important complication in patients with large MCA-territory infarction.[119,121,122] This complication is especially apt to develop in young patients with large embolic MCA-territory infarcts. Coma usually heralds a fatal outcome. Some patients with large MCA-territory infarcts and severe brain edema have been treated with hemicraniectomy with favorable outcomes.[121,122]

Segmental Infarction in the Middle Cerebral Artery Territory

Segmental infarctions in the MCA territory are caused by occlusion of the distal cortical branches of the upper or lower division of the MCA (see Figure 6-9). They are almost invariably embolic and are seldom caused by intrinsic atheromatous occlusion of a convexity branch. The syndromes are quite variable and depend on the branch affected.

> Neck ultrasound in patient AC was normal. Bloodsugar levels were 240 on admission and remained elevated until insulin was begun. CT revealed a deep striatocapsular infarct. TCD showed an absence of flow velocities in the left MCA with normal ACA and right-sided values. Angiography showed occlusion of the left mainstem MCA after a tapered, irregular origin.

CT patterns of MCA-territory infarction have already been described. The most common patterns are wedge-shaped, pial-territory infarcts, and subcortical, deep basal ganglia and internal-capsule infarcts.[99] Hyperdensity of the MCA in noncontrast-enhanced CT scans is an important and relatively common finding in patients with acute-onset MCA-territory infarcts. In one series among 55 patients, one-third had the hyperdense MCA sign.[123] TCD is a useful technique for demonstrating MCA disease.[80,124,125] Stenosis often causes high velocities when insonating at the depth of the lesion. When the MCA is occluded, flow and velocities decline, and often no signal can be obtained. TCD can be used to rapidly diagnose embolic MCA occlusion and monitor recanalization during and after thrombolysis.[125] TCD monitoring sometimes shows micro-embolic signals in patients with MCA stenosis.[126] This indicates embolism from the MCA lesion, a situation also documented to occur at necropsy in patients with thrombi engrafted on MCA stenotic lesions.[127]

MRA and CTA, with concentration on intracranial views, can also usually document severe MCA occlusive lesions.[128] Using standard angiography, MCA occlusion is best seen on the anteroposterior view of a selective ICA injection. At times, the occlusion is near the MCA trifurcation, so oblique views are needed. The area of poorest supply of MCA tributaries is best identified on lateral views. At times, poor opacification of inferior and superior trunk arteries is seen, and it is difficult to identify the precise point of narrowing or occlusion.

> AC was treated with heparin. The stroke, however, progressed. She remained on warfarin for 2 months. Repeat angiography showed good collateral filling of the MCA from ACA and PCA branches. The infarct on a T2-weighted MRI scan at 2 months matched the perfusion defect on perfusion-weighted MRI.

Therapy of intrinsic MCA disease is uncertain because there have been few series of patients studied, and none has been studied in large, randomized, controlled trials. In patients with acute thrombotic or embolic MCA occlusion, thrombolytic treatment is sometimes effective if given early enough. Thrombolytic therapy is more likely to lead to recanalization in patients with MCA emboli than in those with in situ thrombosis engrafted on atherostenosis. Intravenous[129–131] and intra-arterial[90,91,132] thrombolysis have been effective in recanalizing MCA embolic occlusions. In patients with thrombotic disease within the MCA, thrombi usually reform within the MCA after thrombolysis unless angioplasty is performed after the clot is lysed.

Angioplasty has occasionally been performed to dilate occlusive MCA-stenotic lesions.[82,83,133] Angioplasty can be complicated by occlusion of lenticulostriate branches with resultant striatocapsular infarction.[83] Dissection and vasoconstriction are other complications of angioplasty on the mainstem MCA.[83] The success of angioplasty depends greatly on the location, length, angulation, and morphology of the MCA-occlusive lesion.[133]

Heparin, low-molecular-weight heparin, and heparinoids are often given to patients with acute-thrombotic and embolic-MCA occlusions. Warfarin is then used to attempt to prevent propagation and embolization from the MCA thrombus during a period of 6 weeks to 3 months. During this time, the clot becomes organized and adherent, and collateral circulation maximizes.

Warfarin is also used to prevent total occlusion of a stenosed MCA. In the series of Hinton et al., patients frequently stabilized while taking warfarin.[100] In the Warfarin-Aspirin Symptomatic Intracranial Disease Study, which retrospectively compared outcome in patients with intracranial occlusive disease treated with aspirin or warfarin, warfarin was more effective.[134] In this study, MCA-stenotic lesions were the most common intracranial stenotic lesions studied.[134] I use warfarin anticoagulation in patients with severe MCA stenosis, keeping the INR between 2.0 and 3.0. If ischemic symptoms are not controlled, I pursue angioplasty in selected patients with lesions amenable to this treatment.

Occlusion or Severe Stenosis of the Anterior Cerebral Artery

Intrinsic occlusive disease of the ACA is unusual. Most ACA-territory infarcts are caused by embolism from the heart or ICA. Many patients with intrinsic disease of the ACA also have extensive ICA and MCA disease, often with multiple infarcts, making clinicopathologic correlation of the ACA lesions difficult.[135] Some ACA-territory infarcts are caused by occlusive disease of the ICA. Others are caused by vasospasm-related ischemia in patients with SAH who have aneurysms of the anterior communicating artery.[136] In one study of cerebral infarcts documented by CT, 13 of 413 (3%) were in the ACA territory.[137] Eight of the 13 patients with ACA-territory ischemia had angiography that showed five ACA occlusions. In three other patients, angiography showed ACA occlusion, but the CT showed no infarction in this territory. Nearly all patients in this series with occlusion of the ACA had severe occlusive disease at the origin of the ICA in the neck or in the carotid siphon on the side of the ACA lesion.[137] The most likely mechanism of ACA-territory infarction in this group of patients was intra-arterial embolism arising from the more proximal ICA lesions. In one patient, the authors postulated that intra-arterial embolic material traveled from an occluded ICA origin to the contralateral ACA, through a widely patent anterior communicating artery. In the Lausanne Stroke Registry, 27 of 1,490 patients (1.8%) with first-ever strokes had infarcts limited to the ACA territory.[138] Ten of the 27 patients had ICA-occlusive lesions and seven had cardiac-origin embolism. Only one patient, a Vietnamese man, had intrinsic ACA-occlusive disease. In the remainder of the patients, the cause of the ACA-territory infarcts was not discovered.[138]

My experience and that of others[137–139] lead me to the following opinions about the mechanisms of ACA-territory infarction: (1) ACA-territory infarction is most often embolic; (2) embolism is most often intra-arterial, arising from proximal ICA occlusive disease; (3) when intrinsic atherostenosis affects the ACA, patients usually have widespread extracranial and intracranial occlusive disease with multiple brain infarcts; (4) patients of Asian extraction often have predominantly intracranial occlusive disease, sometimes involving the ACA; and (5) stenotic lesions of the ACA are not always in the horizontal first portion of the artery, but can involve the pericallosal artery and other branches. Figure 6-10 depicts patterns of ACA occlusion and their anatomic correlates.

The ACA, after its brief horizontal A1 segment, gives off the artery of Heubner and medial striate

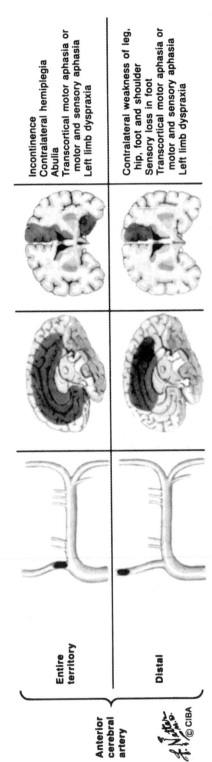

Anterior cerebral artery				
Entire territory				Incontinence Contralateral hemiplegia Abulia Transcortical motor aphasia or motor and sensory aphasia Left limb dyspraxia
Distal				Contralateral weakness of leg, hip, foot and shoulder Sensory loss in foot Transcortical motor aphasia or motor and sensory aphasia Left limb dyspraxia

Figure 6-10. Patterns of occlusion of the anterior cerebral artery and their anatomic correlates. (Reprinted with permission from The Netter Collection of Medical Illustrations, illustrated by Frank H. Netter, M.D. Copyright © Novartis. All rights reserved.)

arteries, which supply anteromedial portions of the caudate nucleus, anterior limb of the internal capsule, and anterior perforated substance.[140–144] After reaching the midline, the ACA swings posteriorly and divides to form the pericallosal and callosomarginal arteries that supply the paramedian frontal lobe above the corpus callosum. Figures 2-6, 2-8, and 2-10 show the ACA and its usual region of supply. At times, the A1 segment of the ACA on one side may be absent or hypoplastic, so that both ACAs are supplied by one ICA. The extent of the infarction depends on the location of the obstruction and the pattern of the anterior circle of Willis.

> A 75-year-old man, CF, awakened from a nap with paralysis of his left leg and foot. He also had slight tingling in his left toes. Examination showed complete paralysis of the left lower extremity. When asked to salute, wave goodbye, or pretend to throw a ball, he performed these functions normally with the right arm but used incorrect movements with the left arm. His arms, however, were not weak or clumsy. The patient was surprised to find that, on occasion, the left hand would grasp the right hand in the midst of an activity and seemed to do things without his will.

The single most important clue to an ACA-territory infarct is the distribution of motor weakness. Paralysis is usually greatest in the foot, but is also severe in the proximal thigh. Shoulder shrug is weak on the involved side, but the hand and face are usually normal if the deep ACA territory is spared. Some patients with anterior or large ACA-territory infarcts have a hemiplegia.[138–140] Some patients with medial frontal infarcts in the ACA territory have prominent motor neglect.[145] These individuals have little voluntary movement on the hemiparetic side. Despite the lack of spontaneous movement, strong prodding induces slow, clumsy arm movements. In these patients, the lower-extremity paralysis is explained by involvement of the precentral gyrus motor cortex. The upper limb motor dysfunction, however, is related to infarction of the premotor cortex anterior to the precentral gyrus.[145] Cortical sensory loss is also present in the weak limbs but is usually slight. The patient may

have difficulty touching the spot on his or her lower extremity touched by the examiner, be unable to identify numbers written on his or her foot with a blunt pencil, or extinguish bilateral tactile stimuli on the paralyzed foot and leg. A grasp reflex is often present in the hand contralateral to the infarct.

Another helpful sign is apraxia of the left arm. Normally, speech is received in the left posterior hemisphere. To communicate language to regions of the right hemisphere that control the left limbs, the information goes forward toward the left frontal region and then across the corpus callosum to the right frontal region. In ACA-territory infarcts, the callosum or its adjacent white matter is often infarcted. This interrupts the pathway, regardless of whether the right or left ACA territory is infarcted.[146] This disconnection can be detected by simple bedside tests:

1. Ask the patient to perform spoken commands with the right and left arms. Patients with ACA infarction are usually unable to perform with the left hand. The fact that they follow the commands normally with the right hand proves they understand the commands.

2. Ask the patient to write or print first with the right hand, then with the left hand. Some patients with ACA infarction write aphasically with the left hand.

3. Ask the patient to name objects placed first in the left hand, then in the right hand. Patients with an ACA infarct may be unable to name objects in their left hand, but can select the same objects by vision or touch and can name them correctly when placed in the right hand.

This topic of left limb apraxia was reviewed by Geschwind and Kaplan,[146,147] and has often been referred to as an *anterior disconnection syndrome*.

When the infarct involves the left ACA territory and supplementary motor cortex, a transcortical motor and sensory aphasia often results.[138,139,148–150] Despite reduced spontaneous speech, the patient can repeat spoken language well. Incontinence—characterized by inability to control micturition although the urge to urinate is preserved—may occur, especially in patients with bilateral lesions. Patients with unilateral ACA infarcts or bilateral frontal infarcts are usually abulic. They are apathetic with decreased spontaneity, slow in responding to queries or commands, and use terse speech that is limited in amount.[138,140,151,152] These patients have difficulty counting backwards quickly from 20 to 1, or in persevering with any protracted task, such as crossing off all the letter As in a paragraph or telling the examiner without prodding each time their finger is moved or touched. In some patients, the decreased activity is intermittent. At one moment patients speak. The next moment they stare blankly and pay no heed to queries or conversation, as if the machine were temporarily shut off.[153]

Another phenomenon found in some patients with frontal-lobe infarction related to ACA disease has been called the *alien hand sign*.[154–156] CF had noticed that his left hand had a mind of its own, often doing things he did not will it to do. This sign is most common in the right hand that interferes with willed movements of the left hand. One hand acts against the other or acts involuntarily. Similar findings occur in patients with epilepsy after surgical cutting of the corpus callosum, making it likely that the phenomenon is caused by defective interhemispheric connections. Forced grasping and a heightened grasp reflex found often contralateral to frontal-lobe lesions may also play a role in causing this sign.

> CT showed a moderate-sized right medial frontal infarct in CF (Figure 6-11A, B), and angiography documented severe stenosis of the right ACA before it formed the callosomarginal artery (Figure 6-11C). After physical therapy, he was able to walk with a brace.

MRI is able to show the topography of ACA-territory infarction quite well. Figure 6-12 shows a typical paramedian frontal ACA-territory infarct on MRI in a patient who had paralysis of the contralateral foot, leg, and thigh. Little is known about treatment for intrinsic ACA disease. I elected not to expose this older gentleman with an already sizable infarct to the risk of anticoagulation because little additional damage would ensue, even if the remainder of the right ACA territory were infarcted.

Occasionally, patients have the sudden development of bilateral ACA-territory infarction.[151,157–159] Figure 6-13 is a CT scan that shows a large, bilateral ACA-territory infarct. Figure 6-14 is a necropsy specimen of a patient with asymmetric large right and left ACA-territory infarcts. Bilateral ACA-territory infarction is most often explained by hypoplasia or absence of the A1 segment of the ACA on one side. In that circumstance, the territories of the ACA on both sides are supplied by one ACA. On angiography, dye instillation into one ICA produces bilateral ACA opacification. Occlusion of the ICA or ACA supplying both sides leads to bilateral frontal-lobe infarction. The resulting clinical picture is sudden apathy, abulia, and incontinence.[151,157–159] When the paracentral lobule is involved, weakness on one or both sides occurs. This predominantly affects the lower extremities. The sudden onset of dementia presents a striking clinical picture, especially to those unfamiliar with this rare syndrome.

Caudate Infarcts

One of the major branches of the ACA is the recurrent artery of Heubner, which supplies the head of the caudate nucleus and the anterior limb of the internal capsule.[141–144] Although older descriptions spoke of a single vessel, newer dissections show there usually are multiple, parallel penetrating arteries arising from the ACA near the anterior communicating artery junction. In approximately 25% of individuals, there is a single Heubner's artery; often, there are two, three, or even four recurrent arteries.[142] Occlusion of one of these penetrating arteries, or of the parent ACA before the origin of the perforators, leads to infarcts in the head of the caudate nucleus. Frequently, the infarction also involves the anterior limb of the internal capsule and the most anterior part of the putamen. Medial and lateral lenticulostriate artery branches of the MCA also supply the caudate nucleus, anterior limb of the internal capsule, and the putamen. Figure 6-15 shows a montage of the findings from CT scans from a series of patients with caudate infarcts.[143]

The clinical signs of caudate infarction are quite variable. Motor weakness is not prominent, although many patients have slight, but usually transient, hemiparesis. Among 18 patients in one series, 13 patients (78%) had some weakness in the limbs contralateral to the infarct. In most patients, however, the motor dysfunction was minor and recovered quickly.[143] Dysarthria is a more common finding and was present in 11 of 18 patients (61%)

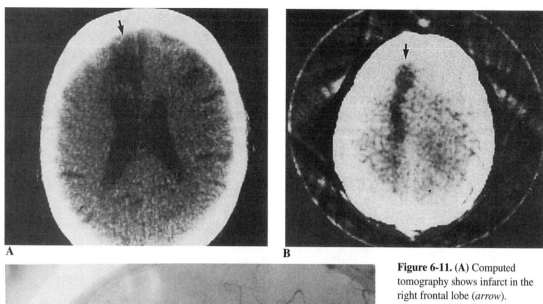

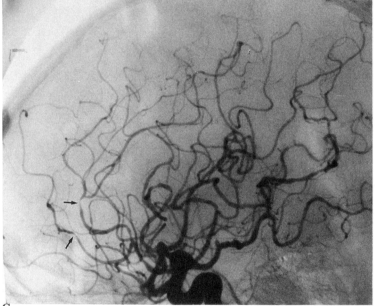

Figure 6-11. (A) Computed tomography shows infarct in the right frontal lobe (*arrow*). (B) Computed tomography shows linear infarct in the right anterior cerebral artery territory (*arrow*). (C) Carotid arteriogram, lateral intracranial view, shows stenosis of branches of the right anterior cerebral artery (*arrows*).

with caudate infarcts in one series,[143] and in 18 of 21 patients (86%) in another series.[160] Occasionally, patients with caudate infarcts have a movement disorder, usually choreoathetosis in the contralateral limbs, as the major clinical manifestation of caudate nucleus infarction.[161]

Most important are changes in behavior. The most common behavioral change, in my experience, has been abulia.[143,151,160] Families describe the patients as more apathetic, uninterested, inert, laconic, and inactive than they were before the stroke. Slowness is a frequent theme; each activity takes longer and requires more concentration and effort. Another frequent abnormality, especially in patients with right caudate infarcts, is restlessness and hyperactivity. Some patients speak incessantly, call out, and appear agitated, confused, and delirious, closely resembling patients with right temporal-lobe infarcts.[113,143] In some patients with caudate infarction, restlessness and agitation alternate with apathy and inertia. Slight aphasia can be found in left caudate infarcts. Some patients with right caudate lesions have left visual field neglect.[143,160]

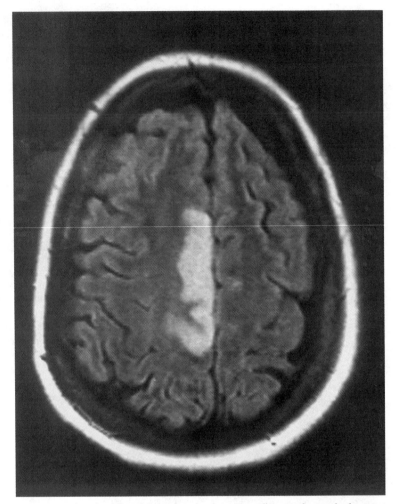

Figure 6-12. Magnetic resonance imaging T2-weighted scan shows a paramedian anterior cerebral artery territory infarct.

The cognitive and behavioral changes found in patients with caudate infarcts closely resemble the clinical signs found in patients with lesions in the medial thalamus and the frontal and temporal lobes. Anatomic and physiologic studies have shown strong interconnections between the caudate nucleus and various cortical regions, and between the caudate nucleus and the thalamus, globus pallidus, and substantia nigra.[162,163] Caudato-nigro-thalamo-cortical circuits are intimately related to planning, thinking, acting, and other higher cortical functions.[143,162]

The causes of caudate infarction are diverse. The most lateral portion is supplied by the medial and lateral striate penetrators of the MCA. Occlusion of these branches, or of the parent proximal MCA, can lead to striatocapsular infarction, including the caudate nucleus. Occlusion of the ACA, by intrinsic atherosclerosis or more often by embolism, is another important mechanism of caudate infarction. In most patients, the lesions are probably caused by atheromatous branch disease at the origins of these penetrating arteries.[143,164] In a 1990 series of patients with caudate infarcts, risk factors for small artery disease were prevalent.[143] Among the 18 patients, hypertension (77%) and diabetes (33%) were common; five patients had both diabetes and hypertension; and only 3 of 18 patients had neither hypertension nor diabetes. Only 1 of the 18 patients had confirmed large artery disease (ICA siphon stenosis). One patient had a cardiac source of embolism (mitral stenosis).[143] These data sug-

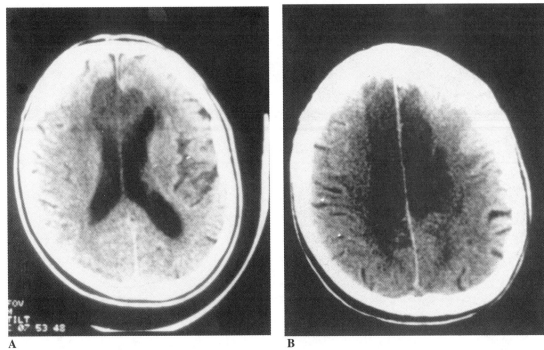

A   B

Figure 6-13. Computed tomography scan shows large bilateral paramedian anterior cerebral artery territory infarcts in a patient who suddenly developed bilateral, lower-limb paralysis and mutism. **(A)** Computed tomography shows bilateral infarction involving the corpus callosum and cingulate gyri just anterior to the lateral ventricles. **(B)** Higher computed tomography section shows extensive bilateral paramedian anterior cerebral artery territory infarction. (Courtesy of Noble David, M.D.)

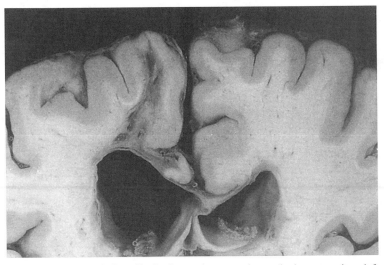

Figure 6-14. Postmortem necropsy coronal slice of brain shows a large anterior cerebral artery territory infarct above the enlarged left lateral ventricle. The corpus callosum is necrotic and the infarct extends toward the right cingulate gyrus.

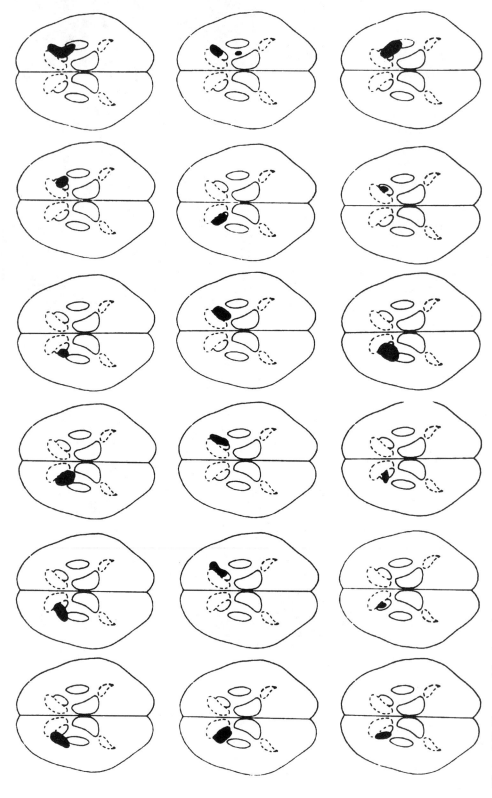

Figure 6-15. Montage of drawings of computed tomography shows caudate-nucleus infarcts. (Reprinted with permission from LR Caplan, JD Schmohmann, CS Kare, et al. Arch Neurol 1990;47:134. Copyright © American Medical Association.)

gest that most caudate infarcts are caused by atheromatous branch disease. This conclusion, however, must be tentative without more clinical and necropsy data. At present, I suggest screening patients with caudate infarcts with cardiac testing, ultrasound, or MRA before diagnosing a small artery etiology.

Occlusion of the Anterior Choroidal Artery

Neuroimaging (CT and MRI) often shows infarction limited to the territory of the anterior choroidal artery (AChA). This vessel originates from the ICA after its ophthalmic and posterior communicating branches, and courses posteriorly and laterally to supply the globus pallidus, lateral geniculate body, posterior limb of the internal capsule, and medial temporal lobe.[165,166] Figure 2-7 shows the AChA and its supply regions. Occasionally, there are anomalies of the AChA.[167] The artery can occasionally arise from the MCA or from the posterior communicating artery. Sometimes, the AChA is a larger-than-normal vessel that supplies the temporo-occipital lobes, the usual territory of the posterior cerebral artery.[167] Before CT, occlusion of the anterior choroidal artery had seldom been diagnosed during life. Cooper, at first inadvertently and later purposefully, tied this vessel in parkinsonian patients to stop tremor. The results were variable.[168]

Analyses of various series of patients[169–173] shows that the syndrome of the anterior choroidal artery includes:

1. Hemiparesis affecting the face, arm, and leg
2. Prominent hemisensory loss that is often temporary
3. Homonymous hemianopia
4. When the lateral geniculate body is infarcted, an unusual hemianopia, with sparing of a beak-shaped tongue of vision, within the center of the hemianopic visual field[174]
5. Absence of persistent neglect, aphasia, or other higher cortical-function abnormalities

Hemiparesis is the most consistent finding. Dysarthria and hemisensory abnormalities are present less often and usually do not persist. Hemianopia is the least common sign. Some patients with bilateral AChA-territory capsular infarcts have severe dysarthria and may even become mute.[175] The diagnosis is verified by CT (Figure 6-16) or MRI, which shows infarction in the pallidum and lateral geniculate body adjacent to the temporal horn,[169,173,176] and by occlusion of the AChA demonstrated angiographically. Many of the patients with AChA-territory infarcts have been diabetic or hypertensive.[169,173,177] Most often, infarction in AChA territory is caused by occlusion of the AChA. The pathology is probably that of intracranial branch atheromatous disease.[164] Carotid artery occlusion, vasospasm in patients with carotid artery aneurysms, and cardiac-origin embolism are occasionally responsible for AChA-territory infarction, often coupled with MCA-territory infarcts.[178,179]

The PCA is occasionally supplied directly through the posterior communicating branch of the ICA. This vessel is considered in Chapter 7 because it usually arises from the basilar artery.

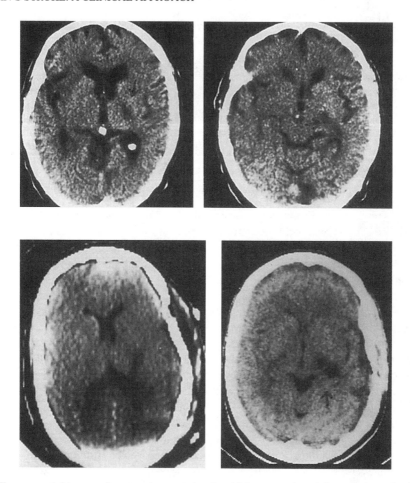

Figure 6-16. Four computed tomography scans show anterior choroidal artery territory infarcts in the region just above the temporal horn, in the region of the posterior limb of the internal capsule, and the globus pallidus. All of the infarcts are on the right of the figures.

References

1. Estol CJ. Dr. C. Miller Fisher and the history of carotid artery disease. Stroke 1996;27:559–566.
2. Fisher CM. Occlusion of the internal carotid artery. Arch Neurol Psychiatry 1951;65:346–377.
3. Fisher M. Occlusion of the carotid arteries. Arch Neurol Psychiatry 1954;72:187–204.
4. Thompson JE. The evolution of surgery for the treatment and prevention of stroke: the Willis lecture. Stroke 1996;27:1427–1434.
5. Dyken M. Carotid endarterectomy studies: a glimmering of science. Stroke 1986;17:355–358.
6. Barnett HJ, Plum F, Walton J. Carotid endarterectomy—an expression of concern. Stroke 1984;15:941–943.
7. NASCET Collaborators. Beneficial effect of carotid endarterectomy in symptomatic patients with high-grade carotid stenosis. N Engl J Med 1991;325:445–453.
8. European Carotid Surgery Trialists Collaborative Group. Interim results for symptomatic patients with severe (70-99%) or with mild (0-19%) carotid stenosis. Lancet 1991;337:1235–1243.
9. Wennberg DE, Lucas FL, Birkmeyer JD, et al. Variation in carotid endarterectomy mortality in the Medicare population. JAMA 1998;279:1278–1281.
10. Kempczinski RF, Brott TG, Labutta RJ. The influence of surgical specialist and caseload on the results of carotid endarterectomy. J Vasc Surg 1986;3:911–916.
11. Gorelick PB, Caplan LR, Hier DB, et al. Racial differences in the distribution of anterior circulation occlusive disease. Neurology 1984;34:54–59.
12. Caplan LR, Gorelick PB, Hier DB. Race, sex, and occlusive cerebrovascular disease: a review. Stroke 1986;17:648–655.
13. Mohr JP, Caplan LR, Melski J, et al. The Harvard Cooperative Stroke Registry: a prospective registry. Neurology 1978;28:752–754.

14. Furlan A, Whisnant J, Kearns T. Unilateral visual loss in bright light. Arch Neurol 1979;36:675–676.

15. Caplan LR, Sergay S. Positional cerebral ischemia. J Neurol Neurosurg Psychiatry 1976;39:385–391.

16. Reed C, Toole J. Clinical technique for identification of external carotid bruits. Neurology 1981;31:744–746.

17. Fisher CM. Facial pulses in internal carotid artery occlusion. Neurology 1970;20:476–478.

18. Caplan LR. The frontal artery sign. N Engl J Med 1973;288: 1008–1009.

19. Hollenhorst R. Ocular manifestations of insufficiency or thrombosis of the internal carotid artery. Am J Ophthalmol 1959;47:753–767.

20. Fisher CM. Observations of the fundus oculi in transient monocular blindness. Neurology 1959;9:333–347.

21. Kearns T, Hollenhorst R. Venous stasis retinopathy of occlusive disease of the carotid artery. Mayo Clin Proc 1963;38: 304–312.

22. Carter JE. Chronic Ocular Ischemia and Carotid Vascular Disease. In EF Bernstein (ed), Amaurosis Fugax. New York: Springer, 1988:118–134.

23. Caplan LR, Babikian V, Helgason C, et al. Occlusive disease of the middle cerebral artery. Neurology 1985;35:975–982.

24. Saver JL, Biller J. Superficial Middle Cerebral Artery. In J Bogousslavsky, LR Caplan (eds), Stroke Syndromes. Cambridge: Cambridge University Press, 1995;247–258.

25. Caplan LR, Bogousslavsky J. Abnormalities of the Right Cerebral Hemisphere. In J Bogousslavsky, LR Caplan (eds), Stroke Syndromes. Cambridge: Cambridge University Press, 1995;162–168.

26. Hier DB, Mondlock J, Caplan LR. Behavioral abnormalities after right hemisphere stroke. Neurology 1983;33:337–344.

27. Pessin MS, Kwan E, Scott RM, Hedges TR. Occipital infarction with hemianopsia from carotid occlusive disease. Stroke 1989;20:409–411.

28. Linn FH, Chang H-M, Caplan LR. Carotid artery disease: a rare cause of posterior cerebral artery territory infarction. J Neurovasc Dis 1997;2:31–34.

29. Pessin M, Duncan G, Davis K, et al. Angiographic appearance of carotid occlusion in acute stroke. Stroke 1980;11:485–487.

30. Barnett HJM, Peerless S, Kaufmann J. "Stump" of internal carotid artery: a source for further cerebral embolic ischemia. Stroke 1978;9:448–452.

31. Ringelstein E, Zeumer H, Angelou D. The pathogenesis of strokes from internal carotid artery occlusion: diagnostic and therapeutic implications. Stroke 1983;14:867–875.

32. Sundt T, Sandok BA, Whisnant JP. Carotid endarterectomy: complications and preoperative assessment. Mayo Clin Proc 1975;50:301–306.

33. del Zoppo GJ, Poeck K, Pessin MS, et al. Recombinant tissue plasminogen activator in acute thrombotic and embolic stroke. Ann Neurol 1992;32:78–86.

34. Casto L, Caverni L, Canerlingo M, et al. Intra-arterial thrombolysis in acute ischaemic stroke: experience with a superselective catheter embedded in the clot. J Neurol Neurosurg Psychiatry 1996;60:667–670.

35. Barnwell SL, Clark WM, Nguyen, et al. Safety and efficacy of delayed intra-arterial urokinase therapy with mechanical clot disruption for thromboembolic stroke. AJNR Am J Neuroradiol 1994;15:1817–1822.

36. Sekhar L, Heros R. Atheromatous pseudo-occlusion of the internal carotid artery. J Neurosurg 1980;52:782–789.

37. Steinke W, Kloetzsch C, Hennerici M. Symptomatic and asymptomatic high-grade carotid stenosis in Doppler color-flow imaging. Neurology 1992;42:131–138.

38. Riles T, Posner M, Cohen W, et al. Rapid sequential CT scanning of the occluded internal carotid artery. Stroke 1982;13:124.

39. Morganstern LB, Fox AJ, Sharpe BL, et al. The risks and benefits of carotid endarterectomy in patients with near occlusion of the carotid artery. Neurology 1997;48:911–915.

40. Baron JC, Bousser M, Comar D, et al. Human Hemispheric Infarction Studied by Positron Emission Tomography and the ^{15}O Continuous Inhalation Technique. In J Caille, C Salamon (eds), Computerized Tomography. Berlin: Springer, 1980;231–237.

41. Baquis GD, Pessin MS, Scott RM. Limb shaking—a carotid TIA. Stroke 1985;16:444–448.

42. Yanigahara T, Piepgras DG, Klass DW. Repetitive involuntary movement associated with episodic cerebral ischemia. Ann Neurol 1985;18:244–250.

43. Barnett HJM, Taylor DW, Eliasziw M, et al. Benefit of carotid endarterectomy in patients with symptomatic moderate or severe stenosis. North American Symptomatic Carotid Endarterectomy Trial Collaborators. N Engl J Med 1998;339:1415–1425.

44. European Carotid Surgery Trialists Collaborative Group. Randomised trial of endarterectomy for recently symptomatic carotid stenosis: final results of the MRC European Carotid Surgery Trial (ECST). Lancet 1998;351:1379–1387.

45. Can U, Furie K, Suwanwela N, et al. Transcranial Doppler ultrasound criteria for hemodynamically significant internal carotid artery stenosis based on residual lumen diameter calculated from en bloc endarterectomy specimens. Stroke 1997;28:1966–1971.

46. Fisher CM, Ojemann RG. A clinico-pathological study of carotid endarterectomy plaques. Rev Neurol (Paris) 1986;39: 273–299.

47. Caplan LR, Skillman J, Ojemann R, et al. Intracerebral hemorrhage following carotid endarterectomy: a hypertensive complication. Stroke 1978;9:457–460.

48. Piepgras DG, Morgan MK, Sundt TM, et al. Intracerebral hemorrhage after carotid endarterectomy. J Neurosurg 1988; 68:532–536.

49. Wade J, Larson C, Hickey R, et al. Effect of carotid endarterectomy on carotid chemoreceptor and baroreceptor function in man. N Engl J Med 1970;282:823–829.

50. Countee R, Sapru H, Vijayanathan T, et al. "Other Syndromes" of the Carotid Bifurcation. In RR Smith (ed), Stroke and the Extracranial Vessels. New York: Raven Press, 1984;345–357.

51. Reigel MM, Hollier LH, Sundt TM, et al. Cerebral hyperperfusion syndrome: a cause of neurologic dysfunction after carotid endarterectomy. J Vasc Surg 1987;5:628–634.

52. Breen JC, Caplan LR, DeWitt LD, et al. Brain edema after carotid surgery. Neurology 1996;46:175–181.

53. Hennerici M, Rautenberg W, Struck R. Spontaneous clinical course of asymptomatic vascular processes of the extracranial cerebral arteries. Klin Wochenschr 1984;62: 570–576.

54. Hennerici M, Hulsbower HB, Hefter K, et al. Natural history of asymptomatic extracranial disease: results of a long term prospective study. Brain 1987;110:777–791.

55. Caplan LR, Stein R, Patel D, et al. Intraluminal clot of the carotid artery detected angiographically. Neurology 1984; 34:1175–1181.

56. Pessin MS, Abbott BF, Prager R, et al. Clinical and angiographic features of carotid circulation thrombus. Neurology 1986;36:518–523.

57. Buchan A, Gates P, Pelz D, Barnett HJM. Intraluminal thrombus in the cerebral circulation. Implications for surgical management. Stroke 1988;19:681–687.

58. Toronto Cerebrovascular Study Group. Risks of carotid endarterectomy. Stroke 1986;17:848–852.

59. Fode NC, Sundt T, Robertson J, et al. Multicenter retrospective review of results and complications of carotid endarterectomy. Stroke 1986;17:370–376.

60. Caplan LR, Pessin MS. Symptomatic carotid artery disease and carotid endarterectomy. Annu Rev Med 1988;39:273–299.

61. Humphries A, Young J, Santilli P, et al. Unoperated asymptomatic significant carotid artery stenosis: a review of 182 instances. Surgery 1976;80:694–698.

62. Durward Q, Ferguson G, Barr H. The natural history of asymptomatic carotid bifurcation plaques. Stroke 1982;13:459–464.

63. Ropper A, Wechsler L, Wilson L. Carotid bruits and the risk of stroke in elective surgery. N Engl J Med 1982;307:1387–1390.

64. Caplan LR. A 79-year-old musician with asmptomatic carotid artery disease. JAMA 1995;274:1383–1389.

65. Chambers BR, Norris JW. Outcome in patients with asymptomatic neck bruits. N Engl J Med 1986;315:860–865.

66. Executive Committee for the Asymptomatic Carotid Atherosclerosis Study (ACAS). Endarterectomy for asymptomatic carotid artery stenosis. JAMA 1995;273:1421–1428.

67. Brott T, Toole J. Medical compared with surgical treatment of asymptomatic carotid artery stenosis. Ann Intern Med 1995;123:720–722.

68. Warlow C. Surgical treatment of asymptomatic carotid stenosis. Cerebrovasc Dis 1996;6(Suppl 1):7–14.

69. Perry JR, Szalai JP, Norris JW for the Canadian Stroke Consortium. Consensus against both endarterectomy and routine screening for asymptomatic carotid artery stenosis. Arch Neurol 1997;54:25–28.

70. Ojemann RG, Fisher CM, Rich JC. Spontaneous dissecting aneurysms of the internal carotid artery. Stroke 1972;3:434–440.

71. Ehrenfeld WK, Wylie EG. Spontaneous dissection of the internal carotid artery. Arch Surg 1976;111:294–330.

72. Bogousslavsky J, Despland PA, Regli F. Spontaneous carotid dissection with acute stroke. Arch Neurol 1987;44:137–140.

73. Sturznegger M. Ultrasound findings in spontaneous carotid artery dissection: the value of Duplex sonography. Arch Neurol 1991;48:1057–1063.

74. Fisher CM, Gore I, Okabe N, et al. Calcification of the carotid siphon. Circulation 1965;32:538–548.

75. Marzewski D, Furlan A, St Louis P, et al. Intracranial internal carotid artery stenosis: long-term prognosis. Stroke 1982;13:821–824.

76. Craig D, Meguro K, Watridge G, et al. Intracranial internal carotid artery stenosis. Stroke 1982;13:825–828.

77. Wechsler LR, Kistler JP, Davis KR, et al. The prognosis of carotid siphon stenosis. Stroke 1986;17:714–718.

78. Caplan LR. Cerebrovascular Disease: Larger Artery Occlusive Disease. In S Appel (ed), Current Neurology, Vol 8. Chicago Yearbook Medical, 1988;179–226.

79. Castaigne P, Lhermitte F, Gautier JC, et al. Internal carotid artery occlusion: a study of 61 instances in 50 patients with postmortem data. Brain 1970;93:231–258.

80. Ley-Pozo J, Ringelstein EB. Noninvasive detection of occlusive disease of the carotid siphon and middle cerebral artery. Ann Neurol 1990;28:640–647.

81. Akins PT, Pilgram TK, Cross DT, Moran CJ. Natural history of stenosis from intracranial atherosclerosis by serial angiography. Stroke 1998;29:433–438.

82. Callahan AS III, Berger BL. Balloon angioplasty of intracranial arteries for stroke prevention. J Neuroimaging 1997;7:232–235.

83. Takis C, Kwan ES, Pessin MS, et al. Intracranial angioplasty: experience and complications. AJNR Am J Neuroradiol 1997;18:1661–1668.

84. The EC-IC Bypass Study Group. Failure of extracranial-intracranial arterial bypass to reduce the risk of ischemic stroke. N Engl J Med 1985;313:1191–1200.

85. Gumerlock M, Ono H, Neuwelt E. Can a patent extracranial-intracranial bypass provoke the conversion of an intracranial arterial stenosis to a symptomatic occlusion? Neurosurgery 1983;12:391–400.

86. Furlan A, Little J, Dohn D. Arterial occlusion following anastomosis of the superficial temporal artery to middle cerebral artery. Stroke 1980;11:91–95.

87. Day A, Rhoton A, Quisling R. Resolving siphon stenosis following endarterectomy. Stroke 1980;11:278–281.

88. Bladin PF, Berkovic SF. Striatocapsular infarction. Neurology 1984;34:1423–1430.

89. Jansen O, von Kummer R, Forsting M, Hacke W, Sartor K. Thrombolytic therapy in acute occlusion of the intracranial internal carotid artery bifurcation. AJNR Am J Neuroradiol 1995;16:1977–1986.

90. Zeumer H, Freitag HJ, Zanella F, et al. Local intra-arterial thrombolytic therapy in patients with stroke:urokinase versus recombinant tissue plasminogen activator (rt-PA). Neuroradiology 1993;35:159–162.

91. Gonner F, Remonda L, Mattle H, et al. Local intra-arterial thrombolysis in acute ischemic stroke. Stroke 1998;29:1894–1900.

92. Russo L. Carotid system transient ischemic attacks: clinical, racial, and angiographic correlations. Stroke 1981;12:470–473.

93. Bauer R, Sheehan S, Wechsler N, et al. Arteriographic study of sites, incidence, and treatment of arteriosclerotic cerebrovascular lesions. Neurology 1962;12:698–711.

94. Kieffer S, Takeya Y, Resch J, et al. Racial differences in cerebrovascular disease: angiographic evaluation of Japanese and American populations. AJR Am J Roentgenol 1967;101:94–99.

95. Brust R. Patterns of cerebrovascular disease in Japanese and other population groups in Hawaii: an angiographic study. Stroke 1975;6:539–542.

96. Kubo H. Transient cerebral ischemic attacks: an arteriographic study. Naika 1968;22:969–978.

97. Feldmann E, Daneault N, Kwan E, et al. Chinese-white differences in the distribution of occlusive cerebrovascular disease. Neurology 1990;40:1541–1545.

98. Bogousslavsky J, Barnett JHM, Fox AJ, et al. Atherosclerotic disease of the middle cerebral artery. EC-IC Bypass Study Group. Stroke 1986;17:1112–1120.

99. Yoo K-M, Shin H-K, Chang H-M, Caplan LR. Middle cerebral artery occlusive disease: the New England Medical Center Stroke registry. J Stroke Cerebrovasc Dis 1998;7:344–351.

100. Hinton R, Mohr JP, Ackerman R, et al. Symptomatic middle cerebral artery stenosis. Ann Neurol 1979;5:152–157.

101. Corston RN, Kendall BE, Marshall J. Prognosis in middle cerebral artery stenosis. Stroke 1984;15:237–241.

102. Moulin DE, Lo R, Chiang J, et al. Prognosis in middle cerebral artery occlusion. Stroke 1985;16:282–284.

103. Feldmeyer JJ, Merendaz C, Regli F. Stenosis symptomatiques de l'artere cerebrale moyenne. Rev Neurol (Paris) 1983;139:725–736.

104. Naritomi H, Sawada T, Kuriyama Y, et al. Effect of chronic middle cerebral artery stenosis on the local cerebral hemodynamics. Stroke 1985;16:214–219.

105. Jain K. Some observations on the anatomy of the middle cerebral artery. Can J Surg 1964;7:134–139.

106. Kaplan H. Anatomy and Embryology of the Arterial System of the Forebrain. In P Vinken, G Bruyn (eds), Handbook of Clinical Neurology, Vol 11. Amsterdam: North Holland, 1972;1–23.

107. Hier DB, Gorelick PB, Shindler AG. Topics in behavioral neurology and neuropsychology. Boston: Butterworth, 1987.

108. Fisher CM. Left hemiplegia and motor impersistence. J Nerv Ment Dis 1956;123:201–218.

109. Hier DB, Mohr JP. Incongruous oral and written naming: evidence for a subdivision of the syndromes of Wernicke's aphasia. Brain Lang 1977;4:115–126.

110. Sevush S, Roeltgen D, Campanella D, et al. Preserved oral reading in Wernicke's aphasia. Neurology 1983;33:916–920.

111. Awada A, Poncet M, Signoret J. Confrontation de la Salpetriere 4 Mai 1983: troubles des compartement soudains avec agitation chez un homme de 68 ans. Rev Neurol (Paris) 1984;140:446–451.

112. Schmidley J, Messing R. Agitated confusional states in patients with right hemisphere infarctions. Stroke 1984;15;883–885.

113. Caplan LR, Kelly M, Kase CS, et al. Infarcts of the inferior division of the right middle cerebral artery. Neurology 1986;36:1015–1020.

114. Adams H, Damasio H, Putnam S, et al. Middle cerebral artery occlusion as a cause of isolated subcortical infarction. Stroke 1983;14:948–952.

115. Weiller C, Ringelstein EB, Reiche W, et al. The large striatocapsular infarct: a clinical and pathological entity. Arch Neurol 1990;47:1085–1091.

116. Caplan LR. The large striato-capsular infarct: a clinical and pathophysiologic entity: critique. Neurology Chronicle 1991;1:12–13.

117. Damasio A, Damasio H, Rizzo M, et al. Aphasia with nonhemorrhagic lesions in the basal ganglia and internal capsule. Arch Neurol 1982;89:15–20.

118. Naesser M, Alexander M, Estabrooks N, et al. Aphasia with predominantly subcortical lesion sites. Arch Neurol 1982;39:2–14.

119. Heinsius T, Bogousslavsky J, van Melle G. Large infarcts in the middle cerebral artery territory. Etiology and outcome patterns. Neurology 1998;50:341–350.

120. Hier DB, Mondlock J, Caplan LR. Recovery of behavioral abnormalities after right hemisphere stroke. Neurology 1983;33:345–350.

121. Schwab S, Rieke K, Aschoff A, et al. Hemicraniotomy in space-occupying hemisopheric infarction: useful early intervention or desperate activism. Cerebrovasc Dis 1996; 6:325–329.

122. Schwab S, Steiner T, Aschoff A, et al. Early hemicraniectomy in patients with complete middle cerebral artery infarction. Stroke 1998;29:1888–1893.

123. Tomsick T, Brott T, Barsan W, et al. Prognostic value of the hyperdense middle cerebral artery sign and stroke scale score before ultraearly thrombolytic therapy. AJNR Am J Neuroradiol 1996;17:79–85.

124. Caplan LR, Brass CM, DeWitt LD, et al. Transcranial Doppler ultrasound: present status. Neurology 1990;40:696–700.

125. Alexandros AV, Bladin CF, Norris JW. Intracranial blood flow velocities in acute ischemic stroke. Stroke 1994;25:1378–1383.

126. Segura T, Serena J, Molins A, Davalos A. Clusters of microembolic signals: a new form of cerebral microembolism presentation in a patient with middle cerebral artery stenosis. Stroke 1998;29:722–724.

127. Masuda J, Yutani C, Miyashita T, Yamaguchi T. Artery-to-artery embolism from a thrombus formed in a stenotic middle cerebral artery: report of an autopsy case. Stroke 1987;18:680–684.

128. Wong KS, Lam WWM, Liang E, et al. Variability of magnetic resonance angiography and computed tomography angiography in grading middle cerebral artery stenosis. Stroke 1996;27:1084–1087.

129. Mori E, Yoneda Y, Tabuchi M, et al. Intravenous recombinant tissue plasminogen activator in acute carotid artery territory stroke. Neurology 1992;42:976–982.

130. Trouillas P, Nighogossian N, Getenet J, et al. Open trial of intravenous tissue plasminogen activator in acute carotid territory stroke. Stroke 1996;27:882–890.

131. Wolpert SM, Bruckman H, Greenlee R, et al. Neuroradiologic evaluation of patients with acute stroke treated with recombinant tissue plasminogen activator. AJNR Am J Neuroradiol 1993;14:3–13.

132. del Zoppo GJ, Higashida R, Furlan AJ, et al. PROACT: a phase ll randomized trial of recombinant pro-urokinase by direct arterial delivery in acute middle cerebral artery stroke. Stroke 1998;29:4–11.

133. Mori T, Fukuoka M, Kazita K, Mori K. Follow-up study after intracranial percutaneous transluminal cerebral balloon angioplasty. AJNR Am J Neuroradiol 1998;19:1525–1533.

134. Chimowitz MI, Kokkinos J, Strong J, et al. The Warfarin-Aspirin Symptomatic Intracranial Disease Study. Neurology 1995;45:1488–1493.

135. Critchley M. The anterior cerebral artery, and its syndromes. Brain 1930;53:120–165.

136. Uihlein A, Thomas R, Cleary J. Aneurysms of the anterior communicating artery complex. Mayo Clin Proc 1967;42:73–87.

137. Gacs G, Fox A, Barnett HJM, et al. Occurrence and mechanisms of occlusion of the anterior cerebral artery. Stroke 1983;14:952–959.
138. Bogousslavsky J, Regli F. Anterior cerebral artery territory infarction in the Lausanne Stroke Registry. Clinical and etiologic patterns. Arch Neurol 1990;47:144–150.
139. Brust JC. Anterior Cerebral Artery. In HJM Barnett, JP Mohr, B Stein, F Yatsu (eds), Stroke: Pathophysiology, Diagnosis and Management (3rd ed). New York: Churchill Livingstone, 1998;401–425.
140. Nagaratnam N, Davies D, Chen E. Clinical effects of anterior cerebral artery infarction. J Stroke Cerebrovasc Dis 1998;7:391–397.
141. Rhoton AL, Sacki N, Pearlmutter D, Zeal A. Microsurgical anatomy of common aneurysm sites. Clin Neurosurg 1978;26:248–306.
142. Gorczyca W, Mohr G. Microvascular anatomy of Heubner's recurrent artery. J Neurosurg 1976;44:359–367.
143. Caplan LR, Schmahmann JD, Kase CS, et al. Caudate infarcts. Arch Neurol 1990;47:133–143.
144. Dunker R, Harris A. Surgical anatomy of the proximal anterior cerebral artery. J Neurosurg 1976;44:359–367.
145. Chamarro A, Marshall RS, Valls-Sole J, et al. Motor behavior in stroke patients with isolated medial frontal ischemic infarction. Stroke 1997;28:1755–1760.
146. Geschwind N, Kaplan E. A human cerebral deconnection syndrome. Neurology 1962;12:675–695.
147. Geschwind N. Disconnection syndromes in animals and man. Brain 1965;88:237–294, 585–644.
148. Rubens A. Aphasia with infarction in the territory of the anterior cerebral artery. Cortex 1975;11:239–250.
149. Alexander M, Schmitt M. The aphasia syndrome of stroke in the left anterior cerebral artery territory. Arch Neurol 1980;37:97–100.
150. Ross E. Left medial parietal lobe and receptive language functions: mixed transcortical aphasia after left anterior cerebral artery infarction. Neurology 1980;30:144–151.
151. Fisher CM. Abulia minor versus agitated behavior. Clin Neurosurg 1983;31:9–31.
152. Fesenmeier JT, Kuzniecky R, Garcia J. Akinetic mutism caused by bilateral anterior cerebral tuberculous arteritis. Neurology 1990;40:1005–1006.
153. Fisher CM. Intermittent interruption of behavior. Trans Am Neurol Assoc 1968;93:209–210.
154. Brion S, Jedynak C-P. Trouble du tranfer inter-hemispherique a propos de trois observations de tumeurs du corps calleux. Le signe de al main etrangere. Rev Neurol (Paris) 1972;126:257–266.
155. Goldberg G, Mayer NH, Toglia JU. Medial frontal cortex infarction and the alien hand sign. Arch Neurol 1981;38:683–686.
156. Geschwind DH, Iacoboni M, Mega MS, et al. Alien hand syndrome: interhemispheric motor disconnection due to a lesion in the midbody of the corpus callosum. Neurology 1995;45:802–808.
157. Freeman FR. Akinetic mutism and bilateral anterior cerebral artery occlusion. J Neurol Neurosurg Psychiatry 1971;34:693–694.
158. Borggreve F, De Deyn PP, Marien P, et al. Bilateral infarction in the anterior cerebral artery vascular territory due to an unusual anomaly of the circle of Willis. Stroke 1994;25:1279–1281.
159. Ferbert A, Thorn A. Bilateral anterior cerebral territory infarction in the differential diagnosis of basilar artery occlusion. J Neurology 1992;239:162–164.
160. Caplan LR, Helgason CM. Caudate Infarcts. In G Donnan, B Norrving, J Bamford, J Bogousslavsky (eds), Lacunar and Other Subcortical Infarctions. Oxford: Oxford University Press, 1995;117–130.
161. Saris S. Chorea caused by caudate infarction. Arch Neurol 1983;40:590–591.
162. Alexander GE, DeLong MR, Strick PL. Parallel organization of functionally segregated circuits linking basal ganglia and cortex. Ann Rev Neurosci 1986;9:357–381.
163. Alexander GE, Delong MR. Microstimulation of the primate neostriatum: I. Physiological properties of striatal microexcitable zones. J Neurophysiol 1985;53:1417–1432.
164. Caplan LR. Intracranial branch atheromatous disease. Neurology 1989;39:1246–1250.
165. Rhoton A, Fuji K, Fradd B. Microsurgical anatomy of the anterior choroidal artery. Surg Neurol 1979;12:171–187.
166. Mohr JP, Steinke W, Timsit SG, et al. The anterior choroidal artery does not supply the corona radiata and lateral ventricular wall. Stroke 1991;22:1502–1507.
167. Takahashi S, Suga T, Kawata Y, Sakamoto K. Anterior choroidal artery:angiographic analysis of variations and anomalies. AJNR Am J Neuroradiol 1990;11:719–729.
168. Cooper I. Surgical occlusions of the anterior choroidal artery in Parkinsonism. Surg Gynecol Obstet 1954;99:207–219.
169. Helgason C, Caplan LR, Goodwin V, et al. Anterior choroidal territory infarction: case reports and review. Arch Neurol 1986;43:681–686.
170. Ward T, Bernat J, Goldstein A. Occlusion of the anterior choroidal artery. J Neurol Neurosurg Psychiatry 1984;47:1046–1049.
171. Masson M, DeCroix JP, Henin D, et al. Syndrome de l'artere choroidienne anterieure: etude clinique et tomodensitometrique de 4 cas. Rev Neurol (Paris) 1983;139:553–559.
172. Decroix JP, Graveleau PH, Masson M, Cambier J. Infarction in the territory of the anterior choroidal artery: a clinical and computerized tomographic study of 16 cases. Brain 1986;109:1071–1085.
173. Helgason CM. Anterior Choroidal Artery Territory Infarction. In G Donnan, B Norrving, J Bamford, J Bogousslavsky (eds), Lacunar and Other Subcortical Infarctions. Oxford: Oxford University Press, 1995;131–138.
174. Frisen L. Quadruple sector anopia and sectorial optic atrophy: a syndrome of the distal anterior choroidal artery. J Neurol Neurosurg Psychiatry 1979;42:590–594.
175. Helgason C, Wilbur A, Weiss A, et al. Acute pseudobulbar mutism due to discrete bilateral capsular infarction in the territory of the anterior choroidal artery. Brain 1988;111:507–524.
176. Damasio H. A computed tomographic guide to the identification of cerebral vascular territories. Arch Neurol 1983;40:138–142.
177. Bruno A, Graff-Radford NR, Biller J, Adams HP. Anterior choroidal artery territory infarction: a small vessel disease. Stroke 1989;20:616–619.
178. Mayer JM, Lanoe Y, Pedetti L, Fabry B. Anterior choroidal-artery territory infarction and carotid occlusion. Cerebrovasc Dis 1992;2:315–316.
179. Leys D, Mounier-Vehier F, Lavenu I, et al. Anterior choroidal artery territory infarcts. Study of presumed mechanisms. Stroke 1994;25:837–842.

Chapter 7

Large Vessel Occlusive Disease of the Posterior Circulation

Following the suggestion of American[1–4] and British[1,5] authors in the late 1950s and early 1960s, physicians lumped posterior circulation ischemia under the catchall terms *vertebrobasilar insufficiency* (VBI) or *vertebrobasilar territory infarction*. Various treatments were tried in groups of patients with VBI.[1,6] As in the case of large, heterogeneous groups of patients with anterior and posterior circulation disease lumped under the categories of transient ischemic attack (TIA), progressing, or so-called completed stroke, no single treatment strategy proved helpful for the group as a whole. With the advent of more angiography, better surgery, and safe, noninvasive diagnostic techniques, physicians and surgeons began to consider treatment of individual patients with anterior circulation disease, depending on the (1) nature, severity, and location of their vascular lesions; (2) degree of infarction; (3) hematologic findings; and (4) general health of the patient.

The same strategy should be applied to patients with vertebrobasilar disease because this category is even more heterogeneous than anterior-circulation ischemic disease.[1,7,8] This chapter follows this idea and categorizes posterior circulation occlusive disease, depending on the causative vascular lesions. Remember that in the posterior circulation, considerably more tissue is fed by small, penetrating arteries, so the proportion of small-artery to large-artery disease is higher than in the anterior circulation. Lacunes and penetrating branch territory infarcts within the vertebrobasilar system are considered in Chapter 8. A monograph devoted entirely to posterior circulation disease discusses this topic in much more detail than is possible in this chapter.[1]

Occlusion or Severe Stenosis of the Subclavian and Innominate Arteries

The extracranial vertebral arteries (ECVAs) arise from the proximal subclavian arteries. Thus, disease of the subclavian or innominate arteries before the ECVA origins can lead to changes in vertebral artery (VA) flow. Reivich et al.[9] and others[10–12] brought this practical fact to the attention of physicians when they recognized the subclavian steal syndrome. In this syndrome, obstruction to the proximal subclavian artery led to a low-pressure system within the ipsilateral VA and in blood vessels of the ipsilateral upper extremity. Blood from a higher-pressure system, the contralateral VA and basilar artery, was diverted and flowed retrograde down the ipsilateral VA into the arm (Figure 7-1). Figure 7-2 shows an arteriogram from a patient with subclavian steal. In the nearly 3 decades since the description of this syndrome, knowledge of its natural history, diagnosis, and treatment has greatly expanded.

Most often, subclavian artery disease is detected when patients with coronary or peripheral vascular occlusive disease in the legs are referred to ultrasound laboratories for noninvasive testing. Most patients with subclavian artery disease are asymptomatic. In those with symptoms, most complaints relate to arm ischemia. Fatigue, aching after exercise, and coolness are described. In a large series of patients with subclavian steal, studied in 1988 by Hennerici and colleagues, one-third of patients reported pain, numbness, or fatigue in the arm. Only 15 of 324 patients (4.8%), however, had objective physical signs of brachial ischemia or embolism.[13]

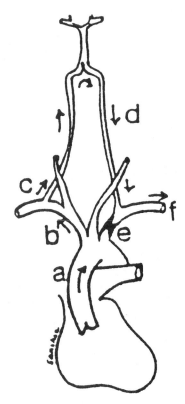

Figure 7-1. Subclavian steal: (a) aortic arch, (b) innominate artery, (c) right vertebral artery, (d) left vertebral artery, (e) occlusion of subclavian artery proximal to the left vertebral artery, (f) subclavian artery. Arrows represent direction of flow.

Neurologic symptoms are not common unless there is accompanying carotid artery disease. Among 155 patients, 116 patients (74%) with a unilateral subclavian steal shown by ultrasonography had no neurologic symptoms.[13]

JK, a 53-year-old laborer, noted occasional dizziness, sometimes with diplopia and fuzzy vision, when he worked. The attacks were brief, and always went away within seconds when he stopped working. For 6 months, his left hand felt cool and occasionally ached after he exercised.

The most frequent symptoms of subclavian artery disease relate to the ipsilateral arm and hand. Coolness, weakness, and pain on use of the arm are common, but may not be severe enough for the patient to consult a doctor. When there is impair-

ment of VA flow (decreased antegrade flow or retrograde flow), patients may report spells of dizziness. Dizziness is by far the most common neurologic symptom of subclavian steal syndrome, and usually has a spinning or vertiginous character. Diplopia, decreased vision, oscillopsia, and staggering occur but less frequently, often accompanying the dizziness. The attacks are brief and may occasionally be brought on by exercising the ischemic arm, a diagnostic point that is sometimes useful during examination. In most patients, however, exercise of the ischemic limb does not provoke neurologic symptoms or signs.

On examination of JK, the left radial pulse was smaller in volume and delayed relative to the carotid and right radial pulses. Blood pressure was 160/90 mm Hg in the right arm, and 120/50 mm Hg in the left. The left hand felt cool. There was a loud bruit in the left supraclavicular region that decreased slightly as the blood pressure cuff on the left arm was inflated to a pressure exceeding 120 mm Hg. There also was a loud, high-pitched focal bruit at the right carotid bifurcation. Neurologic examination was normal.

The diagnosis of subclavian artery occlusive disease can usually be made by physical examination. Invariably, there is a difference in the wrist and the antecubital pulses in the two arms. The pulse in the affected limb is of smaller volume and is delayed relative to the contralateral arm. Blood pressure is also reduced asymmetrically. In my experience, however, the pulse asymmetry has usually been more obvious than the blood pressure difference. I do not know of a single case of subclavian steal syndrome in which the pulse was symmetric and a blood pressure difference was prominent. I believe that it is more important to carefully feel both wrist pulses simultaneously than it is to routinely measure blood pressure in both arms. A supraclavicular bruit may be present. When the bruit originates from an ECVA stenosis without subclavian narrowing, inflating a blood pressure cuff above systolic pressure may augment the bruit by directing more blood into the ECVA. When the bruit is caused by subclavian or innominate artery stenosis, inflating the cuff reduces flow into the arm, so the bruit becomes softer.

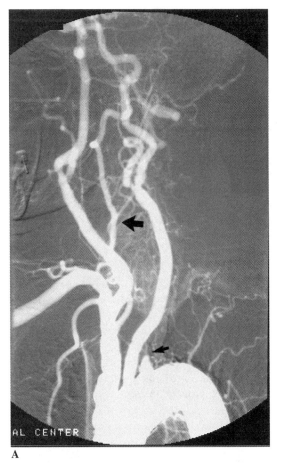

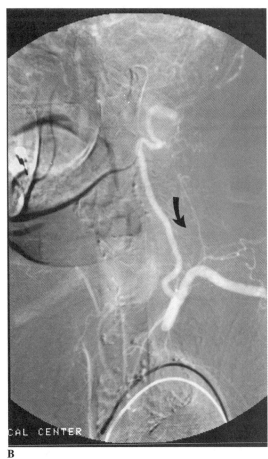

A   B

Figure 7-2. (A) Subtraction arch angiogram from a patient with subclavian steal syndrome. Arch angiogram, early phase. The right subclavian artery and right vertebral artery (*large arrow*) fill normally. The left subclavian artery is occluded just above its origin (*small arrow*). **(B)** Arch angiogram, later films. The left vertebral artery is opacified after filling from the right intracranial vertebral artery, and blood is flowing retrograde down the left vertebral artery into the left subclavian artery beyond the occlusion (*arrow*). (Reprinted with permission from LR Caplan. Posterior Circulation Disease: Clinical Findings, Diagnosis, and Management. Boston: Blackwell, 1996.)

Atherosclerosis of the proximal subclavian artery is usually associated with occlusive disease in other large arteries, typically the coronary, lower extremity, and other extracranial arteries. In JK, the loud, focal, right carotid bruit indicated important concomitant right internal carotid artery (ICA) disease. Other diseases, especially Takayasu's disease and temporal arteritis,[14] can lead to subclavian stenosis. Baseball pitchers and cricket bowlers are also at risk for developing innominate and subclavian artery disease because of their arm mechanics during throwing. A cervical rib or chronic use of an arm crutch can also lead to stenosis or aneurysmal dilation of the subclavian artery. Clots can form in

the diseased vessel and periodically embolize to individual finger arteries, causing a syndrome that can be confused with unilateral Raynaud's syndrome. When the lesion affects the innominate artery, signs and symptoms of decreased carotid artery flow can also occur. Innominate artery disease is much less common than subclavian artery disease.[15,16] Figure 7-3 is a magnetic resonance angiography (MRA) of a patient with severe innominate artery stenosis.

A high proportion of patients with innominate artery disease are cigarette smokers. In series of patients with innominate disease, women are more often affected than men, in contrast to

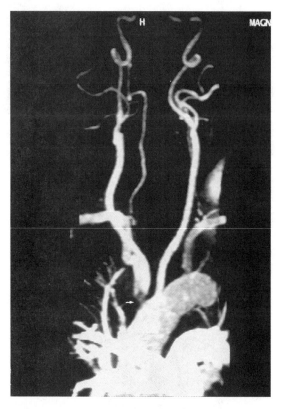

Figure 7-3. Gadolinium-enhanced magnetic resonance angiography of the aortic arch region shows a severe stenosis of the proximal innominate artery (*arrow*).

patients with carotid, subclavian, and peripheral vascular occlusive disease, in which there is a male preponderance.[15] Although right subclavian steal is much less frequent than left, it is more serious and more important to treat. Two early cases, reported by Symonds, describe right subclavianartery occlusion with spread of clot into the innominate and carotid arterial systems.[17] Since then, occasional patients who had recurrent arm and brain ischemia, caused by embolization of floating thrombi within the innominate artery, have been reported.[1,18,19]

An illustrative case report described the events in a well-known professional baseball pitcher.[20] Symptoms began when the pitcher noted his throwing arm suddenly went "dead" and his first three digits felt numb. Angiography showed complete occlusion of the right subclavian artery just proximal to the medial edge of the first rib. Five days later while exercising, he suddenly developed

a left hemiplegia and confusion.[20] Subsequent angiography showed that the clot had propagated proximally to block the innominate artery, and had embolized into ICA branches intracranially.[20]

I saw a patient who presented with a confusing constellation of symptoms and signs that included (1) transient right monocular vision loss, (2) coldness of the right arm, (3) left upper-extremity weakness, (4) double vision, (5) dizziness, (6) ataxia, and (7) a left homonymous hemianopia. Evaluation, including magnetic resonance imaging (MRI) and angiography, showed a stenosis of the innominate artery with a superimposed thrombus. Infarcts were present within the right MCA territory, right posterior cerebral artery (PCA) territory, and cerebellar territory supplied by the superior cerebellar artery (SCA). The patient had embolized through the right carotid artery branch of the innominate artery, to the ipsilateral eye and the MCA, and through the ipsilateral subclavian-ECVA to the distal basilar artery and its PCA and SCA branches. The array of ipsilateral arm and eye ischemia, accompanied by anterior and posterior circulation ischemia (or both), is diagnostic of innominate artery disease.

Although frequent attacks of posterior circulation ischemia may occur in patients with subclavian steal, development of a posterior circulation stroke is rare.[1,13,21] There is usually much smoke but little fire. I could find only two documented, reported examples of serious brain stem or cerebellar infarction in patients with subclavian steal, and each followed severe hypotension. Among more than 400 patients with posterior circulation TIAs and ischemic strokes in the New England Medical Center Posterior Circulation Registry, only two had symptoms (TIAs) attributable to significant subclavian or innominate artery disease.[1]

> Noninvasive testing of JK's arms showed reduced left forearm blood flow measured by oscillography. Duplex ultrasonography showed severe stenosis 2 cm above the origin of the left subclavian artery. Continuous wave (CW) Doppler examination at C2 revealed a reversal of flow in the left ECVA. Transcranial Doppler (TCD) blood-flow velocities were normal. MRI was normal. Angiography confirmed a high-grade stenosis of the left subclavian artery, with retrograde flow down the left VA on

delayed films. A moderately severe stenosis (2.5 mm residual lumen) of the right ICA and slight stenosis of the left ICA at their origins were also evident. The intracranial arteries were normal. He was treated with aspirin (300 mg daily) and was urged to limit vigorous exercising of the left arm. The episodes of dizziness persisted for 3 months and then stopped. He has been followed for symptoms of anterior circulation ischemia.

Noninvasive testing of flow in the arm should allow the diagnosis of subclavian artery stenosis. Helpful are oscillographic measurements of forearm blood flow, venous occlusive plethysmography of the arm,[22] and analysis of the relative velocities of pulse-wave propagation in the two arms.[23]

Doppler sonography gives an accurate indication of flow in the proximal ECVA system. Hennerici et al. studied the accuracy of CW Doppler in detecting innominate and subclavian artery lesions.[16] All 21 patients with Doppler-detected innominate artery stenosis and all 66 patients with subclavian steal had angiography that confirmed the ultrasound findings.[16] In patients with slight or moderate subclavian-artery stenosis, reduction of flow is found in the ECVA during systole. The flow, however, is usually antegrade. With increasingly severe subclavian stenosis, blood flow reverses during systole, but remains cephalad in diastole, or blood flow is persistently decreased.[13,24–27] The subclavian arteries are often well shown by duplex sonography and CW Doppler.[28] The left subclavian artery B-mode images are usually obtained 1–4 cm above the subclavian artery origin. Duplex scanning of the right subclavian artery is more problematic because the proximal right subclavian artery makes a posterolateral curve.[28] TCD recordings give information about the intracranial effects of the proximal arterial disease.[13,26,27] Hennerici et al. reported the TCD findings in 50 patients with subclavian steal: 47 unilateral and three bilateral.[13] Most patients had normal brachial artery flow velocities and retrograde flow, irrespective of the flow pattern in the proximal ECVA. MRA can also show the innominate and subclavian arteries as well as the ECVAs, especially when arch films are taken after gadolinium infusions. Figure 4-16 is a gadolinium-

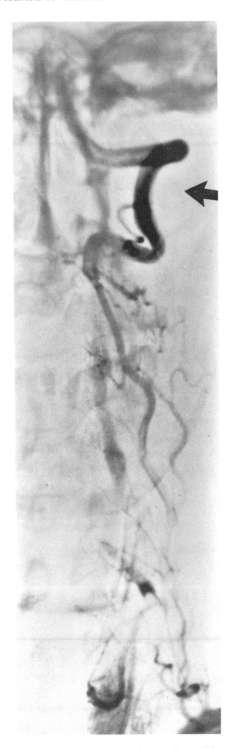

Figure 7-4. Subclavian artery angiogram shows filling of the distal extracranial vertebral artery from collaterals (*arrow*). (Reprinted with permission from LR Caplan. Posterior Circulation Disease: Clinical Findings, Diagnosis, and Management. Boston: Blackwell, 1996.)

enhanced MRA that shows normal subclavian, innominate, and vertebral arteries.

When angiography is performed, it is especially important to obtain delayed films of ECVA flow; otherwise, the retrograde phase of flow might be missed. It is also important to assess the carotid arteries carefully because often there is associated occlusive disease in other arteries.

Subclavian artery disease is usually relatively benign. The spells of posterior circulation ischemia and the arm symptoms often improve with time, as collateral circulation to the arm develops. Operations on the proximal subclavian or innominate artery, when performed by thoracotomy, are more serious operative procedures than vascular surgery involving only a neck incision. Sometimes, the intriguing radiologic demonstration of reversal of VA flow seduces surgeons into repairing the subclavian disease (by repair of the subclavian artery or ligation of the proximal ECVA) but neglecting the more serious concomitant ICA disease. When the patient is incapacitated by arm ischemia (e.g., if the syndrome occurs in a golfer or a pitcher) repair is indicated. When the disease affects the right innominate or subclavian artery, serious carotid-territory infarction can ensue, so repair is in order. In most other patients, I suggest watchful waiting. I try to reduce risk factors, such as smoking, hypertension, and hyperlipidemia, and observe the patient for attacks related to the anterior circulation.

Occlusion or Severe Stenosis of the Vertebral Artery

Proximal Vertebral Artery Disease in the Neck

The most frequent location for atherosclerotic disease of the ECVAs is at their origin from the subclavian arteries. Atherosclerosis at this site shares epidemiologic features with its close cousin, atherosclerosis of the ICA origin. In fact, the two sites are frequently affected in the same individuals.[29,30] My colleagues and I have found that stenosis at the ECVA origins is found less often in African-Americans and Asians than in whites.[1,31] ECVA was the most common site of atherosclerotic narrowing in the New England Medical Center Posterior Circulation Registry series of more than 400 patients with vertebrobasilar TIAs and strokes.[1]

> LM, a 63-year-old white man, had repeated attacks of spinning dizziness during the past 2 weeks. In some spells, the only symptom was dizziness. In others, diplopia and staggering occurred. In one attack, his right limbs felt transiently weak. The attacks were brief, lasting 30 seconds to 4 minutes. They tended to occur while he was quietly resting, and never occurred during exertion. He also had occasional left occipital headaches.

The most frequently reported symptom during TIAs caused by ECVA-origin disease is dizziness. The attacks are indistinguishable from those described by patients with subclavian steal, except that ECVA-origin TIAs are not precipitated by effort or by arm exertion. Although dizziness is the most common symptom, it is seldom the only neurologic symptom. Usually, in at least some attacks, dizziness is accompanied by other definite signs of hindbrain ischemia. Diplopia, oscillopsia, weakness of both legs, hemiparesis, or numbness are often mentioned if the patient is closely questioned. Fisher stated that he had not seen a patient with spells of unaccompanied dizziness lasting 6 weeks or more that were caused by documented VA disease.[32] In the years since this report, I have also not seen such a patient. Because dizziness is a common neurologic symptom and is in most cases not caused by cerebrovascular disease, I seldom diagnose VA disease in patients with repeated, unaccompanied dizziness. True vertigo, present only on rising and retiring, and true positional vertigo are never caused by ECVA-origin disease. In patients with risk factors for stroke and unaccompanied spells of dizziness, I usually order ultrasound or MRA to detect lesions of the VA in the neck or intracranially.

VA atheromas often originate in the subclavian artery and spread to the proximal few centimeters of the ECVA. They may also arise at the origin of the ECVA. Little has been written about the morphology of VA-origin lesions. Although ulceration and plaque hemorrhage are commonly recognized when carotid endarterectomy specimens are examined, ECVA lesions are said to be fibrous and smooth and seldom ulcerate.[33,34] Scant pathologic data about ECVA-origin lesions exist because ECVA surgery is usually performed by using a bypass, so the vessel is not available for pathologic examination. Careful necropsy examinations of the ECVAs have not been reported subsequent to recognition of the importance of plaque ulceration and hemorrhage. ICA and ECVA-origin lesions cannot be assumed to be morphologically identical. The geometry of the two origins is quite different. The ECVA arises at nearly 90 degrees from the subclavian artery, whereas the ICA is almost a direct 180 degree extension of the common carotid artery (CCA). Caliber and flow disparities between the ICA and ECVA origins also exist. Only a small fraction of subclavian flow goes into each ECVA, a much smaller vessel, whereas a high proportion of CCA blood goes into the ICA, a vessel of nearly the same size.

In 1989, Pelouze reported a man with multiple attacks of vertigo and brain stem ischemia, which continued despite prescription of aspirin.[35] Angiography showed irregular stenosis near the ECVA origin and a B-mode scan suggested an ulcerated plaque. An ECVA endarterectomy was performed, and the surgical specimen showed an ulcerated, irregular plaque that represented the source of multiple intracranial posterior circulation emboli.[35] The question of the presence of ECVA-origin plaque ulceration is of great importance, but remains unsolved until more necropsy or surgical specimens are carefully examined. Do small platelet-fibrin and erythrocyte-fibrin emboli arise frequently from the proximal ECVA and embolize to distal arteries in the posterior circulation? Would agents that reduce platelet aggregability or anticoagulants (or both) be effective for patients with ECVA-origin TIAs?

Two important anatomic facts explain why ECVA-origin lesions seldom cause chronic, hemodynamically significant low flow to the vertebrobasilar system:

1. The VAs are paired vessels that unite to form a single basilar artery; only rarely is there complete atresia of one VA, although asymmetries are frequent.
2. The ECVA gives off numerous muscular and other branches as it ascends in the neck. In contrast, there are no nuchal branches of the ICA.

In the VA system, there is much more potential for development of adequate collateral circulation. Figure 7-4 shows collaterals filling the distal ECVA in a patient with ECVA-origin occlusion. Even when there is bilateral occlusion of the VAs at their origins, patients do not usually develop posterior circulation infarcts.[1,36,37] ECVA-origin disease is more benign than ICA-origin disease from a hemodynamic aspect.

Embolization of white platelet-fibrin and red erythrocyte-fibrin thrombi from atherostenotic occlusive lesions is the most important presentation of ECVA-origin disease.[1,37–40] During a period of 2 weeks, I cared for three patients with intra-arterial posterior circulation embolism arising from an occlusive lesion at the ECVA origin.[40] A similar situation is well known in the anterior circulation. A patient is admitted with a small MCA-territory infarct, and ultrasound or angiography shows an occlusion at the ICA origin. The recently formed occlusive thrombus has fragmented and embolized distally. Among 407 patients in the New England Medical Center Posterior Circulation Registry, 80 patients had severe stenosis or occlusion of the proximal ECVA. In 45 (56%) of these 80 patients, embolization from the VA lesion was the most likely cause of brain ischemia.[37] Only 13 out of 80 patients (16%) were considered to have hemodynamic-related TIAs. Twelve of these 13 patients had severe bilateral VA occlusive disease. The only patient with unilateral VA disease had bilateral ICA occlusions.[37] Intra-arterial embolism to the intracranial posterior circulation arteries occurs much more often than is presently recognized.

Neurologic examination of LM was normal. A high-pitched focal bruit was audible in the left supraclavicular fossa, and a soft bruit was heard over the right posterior mastoid region. MRI was normal. Noninvasive testing confirmed a reduction in flow in the left ECVA. Angiography showed a severe stenosis of the left ECVA origin (Figure 7-5). Intracranial films showed good basilar artery filling. The right VA was normal. He was treated with warfarin and had no further attacks. Six months later, B-mode, CW Doppler, and color Doppler flow imaging (CDFI) suggested complete occlusion of the proximal

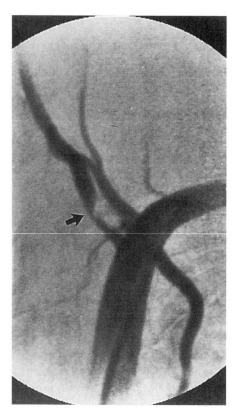

Figure 7-5. Subclavian angiogram shows severe stenosis of the left vertebral artery origin (*arrow*). The artery is dilated distal to the stenosis (poststenotic dilatation).

ECVA with no antegrade flow. Warfarin was stopped a month later without subsequent ischemic spells.

In patients with proximal ECVA disease, a bruit can often be heard over the supraclavicular region. Physicians should auscultate by moving the stethoscope bell to listen over the posterior cervical muscles and mastoid. Sometimes, as in the patient LM, a bruit is heard over the contralateral side because of increased collateral blood flow. B-mode scans can image the proximal VA in the segment between the origin of the artery until its entrance into the foramen transversaria of the cervical vertebrae.[1,27,28] CDFI is also helpful in showing ECVA flow patterns. CW Doppler insonation in the low neck and at the C2 region is the most effective means of monitoring ECVA blood flow. In the presence of a severe occlusive lesion at the ECVA origin, blood flow is

usually retrograde or to-and-fro above the occlusive lesion. Perhaps MRA, especially with gadolinium enhancement, may prove effective in imaging disease of the ECVA origin, obviating the need for invasive catheter angiography.

Data about the natural history of disease of the ECVA origin and the response of patients with this lesion to various treatments are insufficient to warrant firm conclusions as to the best therapy. Moufarrij and colleagues reviewed their experience with VA lesions. Long-term follow-up of their series of more than 80 patients with greater than 75% stenosis of the ECVA origin showed that only two patients had brain stem strokes. These two patients also had basilar artery stenosis.[41]

Vascular surgeons have shown that they can bypass ECVA-origin lesions with low morbidity and mortality.[1,34,42–45] No data exist about the effectiveness or lack thereof of antiplatelet aggregating agents or warfarin in patients with proximal ECVA disease. In the preceding case of LM, I chose warfarin to prevent thrombosis and subsequent embolization in a vessel with low-antegrade blood flow. If the lesion had been less stenotic, I would have chosen aspirin to prevent fibrin-platelet emboli. In some patients, I have chosen surgical reconstruction. Angioplasty is another therapeutic technique that has been used in some patients with ECVA-origin stenosis. Clearly, more data are needed regarding the natural history of ECVA-origin disease and its response to medical and surgical treatments. The advent of MRA and wider application of noninvasive techniques to the posterior circulation may provide groups of patients with ECVA-origin disease who can be followed prospectively and studied to determine the relative use of various therapies.

Intracranial Vertebral Artery Disease

Severe atherosclerotic narrowing is rare in the cervical portions of the VAs, except at their origins. Plaques are relatively routinely observed opposite osteophytes but rarely narrow the vessel.[1,33] The distal ECVA is vulnerable to trauma,[1] dissections,[1,46–48] and fibromuscular dysplasia. VA dissections are discussed in Chapter 11. The distal cervical ECVA is occasionally severely narrowed in patients with temporal arteritis[49] and in women taking high estrogen-content contraceptive pills.[50]

Atherosclerosis of the intracranial vertebral arteries (ICVAs) is most severe in the distal segment of the arteries, often at the vertebrobasilar junction.[1,51,52] Narrowing often extends into the proximal portion of the basilar artery. Less often, stenosis involves the ICVA just after it penetrates the dura to enter the cranium. In contrast to patients with proximal ECVA disease, there is no single typical patient with ICVA occlusive disease. Therefore, four different patient examples are presented and discussed herein.

Patient 1

A 57-year-old white man, WA, had a transient attack of dizziness and diplopia when he arose from a nap. Awakening the next day, he felt dizzy, as if the room were rocking or wavering like a ship. He felt a series of sharp, painful jabs in his left eye. His left face felt strangely numb. He veered to the left when he tried to sit or stand. His left arm was clumsy. His voice was hoarse, and he gagged as he tried to swallow water. Vomiting and hiccups developed as the morning progressed, so he went to the hospital. Examination showed diminished pain and temperature sensation on the left face and right body, including the limbs; nystagmus, worse on looking leftward; diminished left corneal reflex; left ptosis and a smaller left pupil; clumsiness of the left hand and foot; and decreased palatal motion on the left.

The most frequent findings in patients with ICVA occlusion are related to ischemia of the lateral medulla, the lesion illustrated by this patient.[1] In patients with lateral medullary infarction, the most common vascular lesion is occlusion of the proximal or middle portion of the ICVA.[1,53] Penetrating branches to the lateral medulla arise from the middle and distal two-thirds of the ICVAs and penetrate through the lateral medullary fossa to reach and supply the lateral medullary tegmentum.[1,54,55] The medial branches of the posterior inferior cerebellar arteries (PICAs) supply only a small portion of the dorsal medullary tegmentum.[55] The ICVA occlusive lesions decrease flow in these penetrators. Less often, lateral medullary infarction

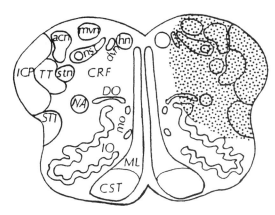

Figure 7-6. Dorsal lateral medullary infarct (Wallenberg's syndrome). (acn = accessory cuneate nucleus; CRF = central reticular formation; CST = corticospinal tract; DO = dorsal accessory olivary nucleus; dvn = dorsal vagal nucleus; hn = hypoglossal nucleus; ICP = inferior cerebellar peduncle; IO = inferior olivary nucleus; ML = medial lemniscus; mo = medial accessory olivary nucleus; mvn = medial vestibular nucleus; nst = nucleus of the solitary tract; STT = spinothalamic tract; stn = spinal trigeminal nucleus; TT = trigeminal tract; NA = nucleus ambiguus.)

is caused by occlusion of the small medullary branches or the medial PICA branch. Important symptoms and signs of lateral medullary infarction can be understood best by recalling the anatomic nuclei and tracts in the lateral medulla (Figure 7-6).

1. Nucleus and descending spinal tract of V: Symptoms include sharp jabs or stabs of pain in the ipsilateral eye and face and a feeling of numbness of the face; examination usually confirms decreased pinprick and temperature sensations on the ipsilateral face, and a reduced corneal reflex.

2. Vestibular nuclei and their connections: Feelings of dizziness or instability of the environment result from dysfunction of the vestibular system and may invoke vomiting; careful examination usually documents nystagmus with coarse rotatory eye movements when looking to the ipsilateral side and small-amplitude faster nystagmus when looking contralaterally[1]; sometimes, the eyes forcibly deviate to the side of the lesion, so-called ocular lateral pulsion.[1,56-57]

3. Spinothalamic tract: Lesions of this structure usually produce diminished pinprick and temperature sensation in the contralateral limbs and body; this loss of function is seldom spontaneously rec-

ognized or reported by patients and is usually noticed only after detection on examination. At times, the pinprick and temperature loss extends to the contralateral face because of involvement of the crossed quintothalamic tract, which appends itself medially to the spinothalamic tract.[1,58] Rarely, the loss of pain and temperature sensation is totally contralateral and involves the face, arm, trunk, and leg.[1,58]

4. Restiform body (inferior cerebellar peduncle): Symptoms include veering or leaning toward the side of the lesion and clumsiness of the ipsilateral limbs; on examination, there frequently is hypotonia and exaggerated rebound of the ipsilateral arm, but frank intention tremor is not common; on standing or sitting, patients often lean or tilt to the side of the lesion.

5. Autonomic nervous system nuclei and tracts: The descending sympathetic system traverses the lateral medulla in the lateral reticular formation; dysfunction causes an ipsilateral Horner's syndrome; the dorsal motor nucleus of the vagus is sometimes affected, leading to tachycardia and a labile increased blood pressure.

6. Nucleus ambiguus: When the infarct extends medially, it often affects this nucleus, causing hoarseness and dysphagia. The pharynx and palate are weak on the side of the lesion, sometimes causing patients to retain food within the piriform recess of the pharynx. A crow-like cough represents an attempt to extricate food from this area. At times, there is also ipsilateral facial weakness, perhaps related to ischemia of the caudal part of the VII-nerve nucleus, just rostral to the nucleus ambiguus, or involvement of corticobulbar fibers going toward the VII-nerve nucleus.[1]

7. Abnormal respiratory control: Initiation and control of respiration are known to involve the lateral pontine and medullary tegmentum. Poliomyelitis and bilateral medullary infarcts are well known to cause decreased respiratory drive.[59] Levin and Margolis described a single patient with failure of automatic respirations ("Ondine's curse"—sleep-related apnea) caused by a one-sided lateral medullary infarct.[60] Bogousslavsky et al. described in detail the clinical and autopsy findings in two patients with one-sided lateral medullopontine infarction who had respiratory failure.[61] Hypoventilation is probably related to involvement of the nucleus of the solitary tract, nucleus ambiguus,

nucleus retroambiguus, and nuclei parvocellularis and gigantocellularis.[1,61]

When infarction is limited to the lateral medulla, prognosis for recovery is good.[1,62] Three exceptions exist[1,63]:

1. Some patients also have infarction in the ipsilateral inferior cerebellum, a region fed by the PICA; when the infarct is large, headache, head tilt, and stupor can result. A posterior fossa pressure cone can develop and cause death from medullary compression.[1]

2. Some patients with lateral medullary infarcts die suddenly; although the etiology of sudden death is uncertain, it is most likely caused by sudden increase in vagal tone (secondary to involvement of the dorsal motor nucleus of the vagus), or to involvement of automatic respiratory centers.

3. Some patients with one-sided lateral medullary infarcts have occlusive lesions in both ICVAs. Development of symptomatic ischemia, in the lateral medulla contralateral to the infarct, has a serious prognosis because of the frequency of autonomic dysfunction and loss of automatic control of respiration. Some patients with bilateral ICVA disease have a poor prognosis once symptoms develop.[1,51,52,64] Because of these important problems, it has been my practice to evaluate patients with lateral medullary infarcts for cerebellar infarction and cerebellar mass effect using MRI, to study the ICVAs noninvasively using MRA and TCD, and to monitor respiration early in the course of the illness.

In some patients with ICVA occlusion, ischemia of the medial medulla accompanies the lateral medullary infarct. This phenomenon is explained by an ICVA occlusion, which blocks the anterior spinal artery orifices.[65] In addition to the signs already mentioned, a hemiparesis affects the contralateral arm and leg because of ischemia to the medullary pyramid. Ipsilateral weakness of the tongue and contralateral loss of position sense are less frequent findings and are explained by involvement of the hypoglossal nerve and the medial lemniscus.[66–68] Occlusion of the distal portion of the ICVA that blocks the orifice of the anterior spinal artery can cause infarction, limited to the medial medulla, without associated lateral medullary infarction.[68]

In WA, B-mode and CW Doppler of the neck VA were normal. TCD showed an increase in blood-flow velocities in the left ICVA. Right ICVA pressures were normal. MRA showed severe stenosis of the left ICVA, just after the artery entered the cranium.

TCD can give accurate indications of occlusive lesions, involving the ICVAs, using insonation through a suboccipital foramen magnum window.[26,27] After the TCD and MRA results, the patient was treated with warfarin. The arterial stenosis is being followed by serial TCD examinations.

Patient 2

A 48-year-old woman, AD, suddenly felt dizzy and unsteady on her feet. She vomited and was unable to walk. When examined, the only positive findings were gait ataxia and slight conjugate gaze paresis to the left. CT was normal. The next morning, she was sleepy and reported severe headache. Her neck was stiff and she preferred to stay stationary in bed. A complete left conjugate gaze paresis to oculocephalic maneuvers was evident, and the left corneal reflex was reduced. Both plantar responses were extensor. CT showed a large area of hypodensity in the left cerebellum. The fourth ventricle was not visible, and the lateral ventricles were enlarged. MRI confirmed a large PICA-territory cerebellar infarct (Figure 7-7). She became stuporous and difficult to arouse. She was treated with intravenous steroids and mannitol, but did not awaken. Soft, necrotic, cerebellar tissue was removed through a left posterior fossa craniotomy, after which she made an excellent recovery.

The most common vascular lesion found in patients with cerebellar infarction is occlusion or severe stenosis of the ICVA.[1,69–72] Often, the occlusion is caused by embolism, the thrombus arising from a source in the heart, or proximal vascular system.[72] The syndrome of cerebellar infarction is often difficult to diagnose. Symptoms can resemble labyrinthitis and can appear deceptively slight. Gait ataxia and vomiting are often accompanied by dizziness, closely mimicking the findings in patients with cerebellar hemorrhage.[1,73] Frequently, no signs of lateral medullary ischemia are evident. Initial CT scan, as in this case, may be normal. It is important to make certain that the fourth ventricle is of normal size and is in normal position. In retrospect, this was not done in this patient. Review of the initial films revealed slight rightward deviation and tilting of the fourth ventricle. MRI is more accurate in detecting early cerebellar ischemia. Especially important for localization are T2-weighted sagittal sections. On sagittal films, localization of the vascular territory involved is relatively easy. Lesions above the horizontal fissure are in the SCA territory. Lesions below the fissure are localized to anterior inferior cerebellar artery (AICA) or PICA territories, depending on anterior or posterior localization on the inferior surface of the cerebellum. Figure 7-8 shows a PICA-territory infarct on a T2-weighted sagittal section.

Swollen cerebellar lesions may compress the cerebellopontine angle, leading to involvement of the ipsilateral fifth, sixth, seventh, and eighth cranial nerves. Compression of the medulla and pons

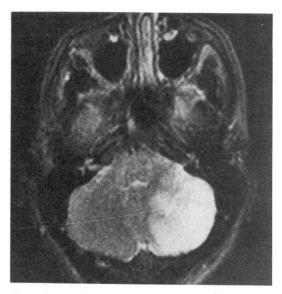

Figure 7-7. Magnetic resonance imaging T2-weighted axial image shows large posterior inferior cerebellar artery territory infarct.

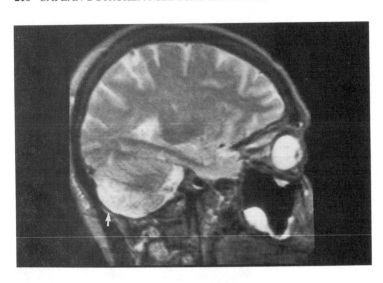

Figure 7-8. Magnetic resonance imaging T2-weighted sagittal view: arrow points to posterior inferior cerebellar territory infarct.

is the probable cause of conjugate-gaze paresis to the ipsilateral side. This finding is especially important because the presence of a conjugate-gaze palsy, without contralateral hemiplegia, is virtually diagnostic of a cerebellar space-taking lesion. With more severe compression, the plantar responses become extensor, systolic pressure rises, diastolic pressure falls, the pulse may slow, and respiration may cease.

As the cerebellum swells, hypodensity usually appears on repeat CT. Posterior fossa cisterns are compressed, and the ventricles become enlarged because of compression of the fourth ventricle. On MRI, compression of the contralateral vermis and brain stem are usually evident. Without treatment, death often ensues.[1,74–76] Preferred therapy is decompression of the swollen cerebellum. In some patients, medical decompression using steroids and osmotic agents has been helpful. Success has also been achieved in some patients by placing a ventricular drain in the lateral ventricles.[77,78] It is often difficult to separate brain stem pressure caused by cerebellar infarction, from brain stem ischemia caused by the propagation of clot into the basilar artery. MRI scans are helpful in making this distinction, but MRA or catheter angiography (or both) are often necessary to visualize the vascular lesions.

Patient 2, AD, is an example of a large cerebellar infarct. In other patients, cerebellar infarcts are quite small and cause little or no abnormal neurologic signs. Embolism from the heart or ECVA can cause cerebellar infarction by blocking the ICVA, PICA, or SCA. Cardiac evaluation and MRA or standard angiography can usually delineate the nature of the causative vascular disease.

Patient 3

A 65-year-old man, BE, had transient headache and dizziness on two occasions, 7 and 10 days before admission. On the day of admission, he suddenly became blind and agitated. When examined 5 hours later, he could not recall events of the past 3 weeks. He could form no new memories and had a complete right hemianopia. No other abnormalities of brain stem or central nervous system function were evident. CT revealed infarcts in the left occipital and temporal lobes in the distribution of the left PCA. MRI also showed a small infarct in the left cerebellum, in PICA territory. Angiography revealed occlusion of the left ICVA and embolic amputation of the left PCA. All other vessels were normal or showed only minor atheroma. Cardiac evaluation was normal.

This patient had an ICVA occlusion, followed by an embolus to the distal basilar artery system. In retrospect, the two episodes of dizziness probably represented transient cerebellar or medullary ischemia. When the vertebrobasilar system has been studied at necropsy, embolic occlusions are common in the PCAs.[1,79] These emboli may arise from recent occlusion within the ECVAs or the ICVAs.[1,39,40,80] Koroshetz and Ropper studied 12 patients with PCA infarcts and brain stem symptoms.[80] They found that three patients had donor sites for intra-arterial embolism in the ICVA. The three other patients had lesions of the ICVAs and the ECVAs. All of the patients had intra-arterial embolism as the cause of PCA infarction.[80] Documentation of artery-to-artery emboli, from freshly occluded VAs, has made me prescribe heparin or warfarin for such patients during the time it takes for the clot to solidify and attach to the artery (2–4 weeks). Insufficient data exist to determine the risk to benefit ratio of anticoagulants for preventing embolization and progressing infarction in patients with recent ICVA occlusions. Thrombolysis is another potential therapeutic strategy to treat recent ICVA occlusion, although there are no published data.

Patient 4

A 60-year-old hypertensive, diabetic African-American man, EO, noted diplopia and dizziness after arising from a nap. The symptoms were transient. Two days later, however, he staggered and had double vision. On examination, he had gait ataxia, nystagmus, and slight left facial weakness. When he stood, he became dizzy, felt weak, and his vision dimmed. He was treated with heparin and bed rest. Six days later, he gradually became stuporous and quadriplegic. He died soon after of pneumonia. Necropsy revealed bilateral occlusion of the ICVAs and extensive necrosis of the cerebellar hemispheres, medulla, and pons.

Bilateral ICVA disease is relatively common. Among 430 patients in the New England Medical Center Posterior Circulation Registry, 21% had severe ICVA occlusive disease[51] and 42 patients (10%) had bilateral severe ICVA occlusive disease.[52] The diagnosis of bilateral ICVA occlusion is often difficult.[1,64] Early symptoms may be deceptively mild and are usually referable to the cerebel-

lum and lateral medulla, like those seen in Patients 1 (WA) and 2 (AD). Because of a low-flow system, the symptoms are often positionally sensitive, worsening when the patient sits or stands or when blood pressure falls spontaneously or after treatment. Usually, TIAs continue and are multiple and stereotyped.[52] Symptoms and signs may also gradually progress.[64] Heparin is most often ineffective because the progressive ischemia is caused by reduced brain stem perfusion. Cerebellar and pyramidal signs and symptoms predominate. At times, ischemia of the PCA territories also leads to abnormalities of vision, memory, and behavior. Bilateral ICVA occlusive lesions are most common in hypertensive and diabetic patients.[52] Death caused by extensive hindbrain ischemia can result.[64] Sundt,[81] Ausman,[82] Roski and colleagues,[83] and others reported the success of posterior circulation bypass treatment for patients with bilateral ICVA lesions. A variety of different shunts have been used, depending on the location of the blockage. The most common procedures involve anastomosis of the occipital artery to the PICA, or the superficial temporal artery to the AICA, SCA, or PCA. Before such a shunt is performed, angiography with full visualization of the ECVAs and ICVAs is critical. ICA injections should also be made to detect retrograde flow from the posterior communicating arteries into the basilar system. Alternative strategies to augment brain stem perfusion are ICVA endarterectomy[84] and angioplasty.[85]

Patients 1 through 4 illustrate serious posterior circulation infarction caused by ICVA disease. In some patients, this vascular lesion is tolerated without symptoms or with only minor TIAs. As a general rule, however, the more distally located a vascular lesion is along the path from the proximal subclavian-vertebral junction to the distal basilar artery, the more likely it is to cause infarction. The more proximal the lesion, the more likely it is to be benign.

Little is known about optimal treatment of lesions of the ICVA. Allen and others have performed direct endarterectomies on the ICVA, usually in its proximal portion.[84] Interventional radiologists have the capability to perform angioplasties on the ICVA. I have been involved in the treatment of three patients with bilateral ICVA occlusive disease in whom unilateral ICVA angioplasty effectively stopped TIAs.[85] Thrombolytic treatment could also lyse ICVA thrombi if given early enough after occlusion. In the patient examples and discussion, I have emphasized the need for vigilance to detect large cerebellar infarcts and decompress these lesions. I often use short-term heparin or warfarin therapy for patients with ICVA occlusions in an attempt to prevent clot propagation and embolization. In some patients with severe ICVA stenosis I have used longer-term warfarin (6 months to 1 year), keeping the international normalized ratio (INR) between 2 and 3. I follow patients with ICVA stenosis with serial TCD, and MRA examinations for progression of the vascular lesion to complete occlusion or for recanalization with disappearance of critical stenosis. I stop anticoagulants approximately a month after documented occlusion or reestablishment of wide patency. I have no data that support these choices of treatment, but they make good sense to me at the present time. I anxiously await careful prospective studies of treatment of patients with ICVA disease.

Occlusion or Severe Stenosis of the Basilar Artery

In a landmark report, Kubik and Adams called attention to the clinical and pathologic features of occlusion of the basilar artery.[86] Characterized by quadriparesis and cranial nerve abnormalities, which allowed for accurate diagnosis during life, the disorder was then considered invariably fatal. We now know that the outcome of patients with basilar-artery occlusive disease is quite variable. Some patients die or are left severely disabled, whereas others survive with little or no deficit.[1,87] Prognosis depends on the rapidity of the occlusion, location and extent of the thrombosis, presence of occlusive disease in other posterior circulation arteries, and development of adequate collateral circulation.

> A 63-year-old man, OL, was unable to rise from bed because of weakness in both his legs. He had a myocardial infarction 5 years earlier. During the past 2 weeks, he had two transient episodes of diplopia, one accompanied by momentary buckling of the legs. During the past month, he had occasional, severe, occipital headaches. For the past 3 days, he had noted weakness of his left leg and diplopia but refused to seek medical care.

Atherosclerosis commonly affects the first few centimeters of the basilar artery. Stenosis can also occur in the middle and distal segments.[1,88,89] Patients with basilar-artery atherosclerosis have a high frequency of atherosclerosis elsewhere, especially in the coronary, carotid, and iliofemoral arteries. In Kubik and Adams' original report,[86] most patients developed signs abruptly without previous warnings. Their paper preceded recognition of the frequency and importance of TIAs, however, and emanated from the pathology laboratory. Careful questioning of most patients with basilar-artery occlusive disease elicits descriptions of attacks of temporary brain stem dysfunction before their strokes, as in patient OL. The most common symptoms during these TIAs are (1) diplopia; (2) dizziness, most often without true spinning; (3) weakness of both legs; or (4) weakness alternating between different limbs in different attacks. As in occlusive disease of other large extracranial and intracranial arteries, some patients develop prominent headache during the weeks before and during development of a critical decrease in blood flow. With basilar-artery occlusive disease, the headache is usually occipital, often spreading to the vertex of the head.

> On examination, OL's limbs were weak, more so on his left side. He could not move his right arm and leg, but could lift the left heel off the bed to a height of 15 cm for 5 seconds before it would fall. He could adduct the left shoulder toward him by sliding it along the bed, but could not lift the arm or move his fingers. Both plantar responses were extensor. Pinprick and touch perception were normal. He could not look to the right. On gaze to the left, only the left eye moved but it showed abducting nystagmus. No adduction of the right eye on attempted left gaze occurred. The voice was dysarthric, and secretions pooled in the back of his throat.

The basilar artery forms from the merging of the two ICVAs at the medullopontine junction. The basilar artery ends at the junction of the pons and midbrain. The major territory of supply of the basilar artery is the pons, especially the basis pontis. The tegmentum of the pons has a rich, collateral supply of vessels but depends primarily on the SCAs, vessels that originate from the rostral basilar artery just before it bifurcates. Occlusion of the basilar artery often causes ischemia in the pontine base bilaterally, sometimes extending into the medial tegmentum on one or both sides. Figure 7-9 shows an example of the distribution of ischemia in basilar-artery occlusion, patterned after Kubik and Adams.[86] Note that the medulla and cerebellar hemispheres are usually spared, in contrast to the situation when one or both ICVAs are blocked. Blockage of the midbasilar artery at the orifice of the AICAs often is accompanied by infarction in the anterior inferior cerebellum on one or both sides.[1,90,91] Figure 7-10 is a necropsy specimen of the pons in a patient with basilar artery occlusion, which shows a pattern similar to Figure 7-9.

Visualizing the anatomic regions of damage helps in predicting and understanding the usual neurologic signs and symptoms that accompany basilar-artery occlusion:

1. Paralysis of the limbs: Weakness is usually bilateral but may be asymmetric, as in patient OL's presentation; stiffness, hyperreflexia, and extensor plantar reflexes are found on examination of the weak limbs. Some patients present with a hemiparesis, but also usually have weakness and reflex changes in the limbs contralateral to the hemipare-

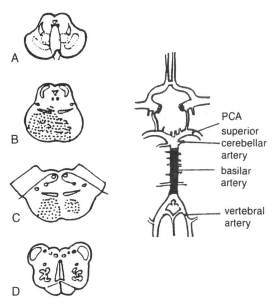

Figure 7-9. Pons with infarct caused by occlusion of the basilar artery: (**A**) midbrain, (**B**) upper pons, (**C**) lower pons, and (**D**) medulla. (PCA = posterior cerebral artery.) (Adapted from C Kubik, R Adams. Occlusion of the basilar artery: a clinical and pathological study. Brain 1946;69:73–121.)

Figure 7-10. Myelin-stained section of the pons shows a large infarct limited to the paramedian portion of the base in a patient with basilar artery occlusion. (Reprinted with permission from LR Caplan. Posterior Circulation Disease: Clinical Findings, Diagnosis, and Management. Boston: Blackwell, 1996.)

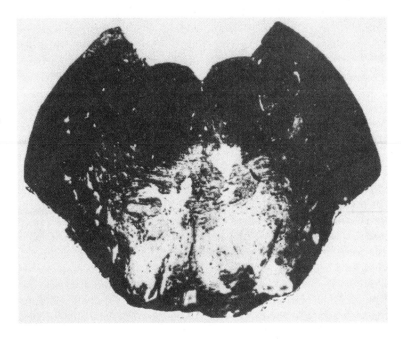

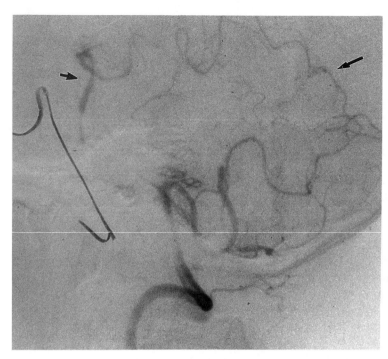

Figure 7-11. Vertebral angiogram, lateral view: Basilar artery is occluded; rostral basilar artery is filled (*short arrow*) from collaterals going around the cerebellum (*long arrow*) from the posterior inferior cerebellar artery to the superior cerebellar artery branches.

sis on examination.[1] Hemiparesis was more common than quadriparesis in patients with basilar artery occlusion studied in the New England Medical Center Posterior Circulation Registry.[1]

2. Bulbar or pseudobulbar paralysis of the cranial musculature: The infarct can directly involve cranial motor nuclei, causing paralysis of the face, palate, pharynx, neck, or tongue on one or both sides. The IX–XII nerve nuclei are located within the medullary tegmentum, which is usually below the level of the infarct. Weakness of the cranial musculature innervated by these nuclei causes dysarthria, dysphonia, hoarseness, dysphagia, and tongue weakness. These are common findings in patients with basilar artery occlusion and pontine infarction. The pontine lesion interrupts corticofugal descending fibers destined for these cranial-nerve nuclei. The resulting weakness is referred to as *pseudobulbar* because it involves the descending pathways controlling the bulbar nuclei rather than the nuclei themselves. Exaggerated jaw and facial reflexes, increased gag reflex, and easily induced emotional incontinence with excessive laughing or crying accompany the weakness. In some cases, the limb and bulbar paralysis is so severe that the patient cannot communicate verbally or by gesture. Such patients have been referred to as *locked-in*

because of their loss of motor function.[1] Eye movement or eye-blinking signals can sometimes be arranged, which clearly prove the patient is alert and intellectually preserved despite the paralysis.

3. Absence of sensory or cerebellar abnormalities: The infarct usually affects the midline and paramedian structures in the basis pontis. Collateral circulation is generally through the circumferential vessels, which course around the lateral portions of the brain stem, and supply the lateral base, tegmentum, and cerebellum. Figure 7-11 shows collaterals filling the cerebellar arteries in a patient with basilar artery occlusion. The cerebellar hemispheres are mostly nourished by the PICA, which originates before the basilar artery, and the SCA, which is preserved when the basilar-artery clot does not extend to the distal basilar artery. The spinothalamic tracts and the cerebellum are often spared from the ischemia.

4. Abnormalities of eye movement: The sixth-nerve nuclei, medial longitudinal fasciculi (MLF), and pontine lateral gaze centers are located in the paramedian pontine tegmentum, and therefore are vulnerable to ischemia in this region. Lesions of the sixth nerve or nucleus cause paralysis of abduction of the eye. An MLF lesion produces a defect in adduction of the ipsilateral eye on gaze directed to

the opposite side and nystagmus of the contralateral abducting eye. This syndrome, called an *internuclear ophthalmoplegia*, can be bilateral. Lesions of the paramedian pontine tegmentum may also affect the paramedian pontine reticular formation (PPRF), the so-called pontine lateral gaze center, which mediates gaze to the same side. A lesion of this region causes an ipsilateral conjugate-gaze paresis. A unilateral lesion can affect both the PPRF and the MLF on the same side. The resulting syndrome was present in patient OL, and has been called the *one and one-half syndrome* by Fisher [1,92] because only one-half of gaze (scoring 1 for gaze to each side) is preserved. OL had paralysis of right gaze caused by a lesion of the right PPRF and paralysis of the adducting right eye on gaze to the left caused by involvement of the right MLF.

5. Nystagmus: The vestibular nuclei and their connections are also commonly affected, causing vertical and horizontal nystagmus.

6. Other eye signs: Ptosis, small pupils, and ocular skewing are also often found in patients with basilar-artery occlusion.

7. Coma: If the lesion interrupts function of the medial pontine tegmentum bilaterally, coma may develop.[1,93] Reduced consciousness is a poor prognostic sign, but care must be taken in differentiating reduced alertness from the locked-in state.

CT of OL was normal. MRI on the first day showed ischemia in the mid and lower pons bilaterally in the basis pontis. The basilar-artery flow void was absent in the lower pons. Heparin was given intravenously in a continuous-drip infusion. During the first 24 hours, the patient developed increased weakness of the right leg. He remained stable thereafter, and by day 10 he could lift both arms and speak more clearly. MRA on day 2 was technically poor but suggested a basilar artery occlusion. Catheter angiography on day 10 showed slight irregularity without stenosis of the ECVAs at their origins. The basilar artery was completely occluded just after its origin. An ICA injection opacified the rostral basilar artery through the posterior communicating artery. By day 14, he could sit with help and had no blood pressure drop or increased weakness when he did

so. Heparin was stopped after coumadin had achieved an INR of 2.5. He recovered partially during rehabilitation and had no further worsening of signs or symptoms.

CT is not sensitive in imaging brain stem infarcts, although this capability has improved with newer-generation scanners. CT is, however, reliable in excluding primary brain stem hemorrhage, one of the differential diagnostic considerations. MRI provides better imaging of brain stem and cerebellar infarcts.[94–96] In the patient just described, OL, and in others with bilateral abnormalities of brain stem function, the principal differential diagnosis is between basilar-artery obstruction and obliteration of basilar branch arteries bilaterally, despite a patent basilar artery.[97] This distinction can usually be made by vascular imaging tests, CTA, MRA, and catheter angiography.

When OL presented, the lack of a history of prior stroke and the extensive nature of the bilateral signs made it highly probable that the lesion involved the main basilar artery. He had persistent neurologic signs for more than 72 hours, so he was not a candidate for thrombolysis. If he had presented within 24 hours, I would have considered catheter angiography followed by intra-arterial thrombolysis if his basilar artery were occluded. I would have performed MRA as a screening test as soon as he presented before performing angiography.

I gave heparin intravenously after the CT scan excluded hemorrhage. I prefer not to do invasive studies early in the course of fluctuating brain stem ischemia, performing angiography only when the diagnosis remains uncertain, or when intra-arterial treatment (thrombolysis, angioplasty, or both) is considered. Reduced perfusion of the brain stem is a major problem. Attention must be given to maximizing blood flow. I keep patients at bed rest with their heads flat. Blood pressure should not be lowered unless it is in the malignant range, and cardiac failure should be treated. Dehydration and hypovolemia should be avoided. During the initial course of the ischemia (up to 2 weeks), patients may develop additional symptoms when they sit, stand, or are merely propped up in bed.[98] I observe patients carefully when they sit or stand, checking their pulse and blood pressure and noting any change in neurologic function. Ambulation should be gradual and carefully supervised. TCD is some-

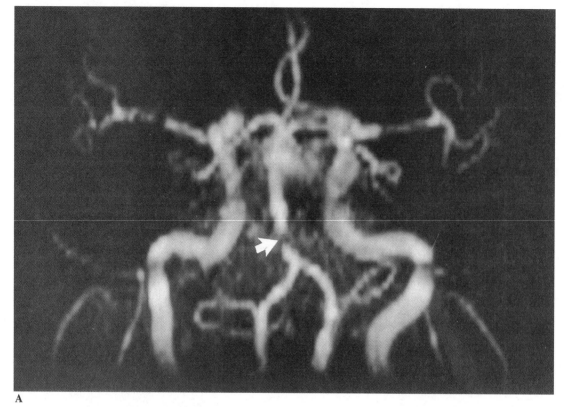

A

Figure 7-12. Basilar artery disease shown by magnetic resonance angiography. **(A)** The proximal basilar artery shows a short flow void (*arrow*), indicating severe focal stenosis at this region. (Reprinted with permission from LR Caplan. Posterior Circulation Disease: Clinical Findings, Diagnosis, and Management. Boston: Blackwell, 1996.) **(B)** Basilar artery occlusion. The basilar artery ends abruptly (*arrow*) after the anterior inferior cerebellar artery branches and the remainder of the artery is not well seen.

times not accurate in showing basilar-artery disease because the lesion is often beyond the range of the suboccipital probe. MRI can suggest basilar-artery occlusion by the absence of the usual basilar-artery flow void. MRA is often able to define basilar-artery disease.[99-101] Figure 7-12 shows MRAs of patients with basilar artery stenosis and occlusion.

When there is strong clinical suspicion that the vascular lesion affects the main basilar artery, or when the clinical picture is confusing and preliminary vascular imaging studies do not clarify the nature of the vascular lesion, I use angiography to help decide the next therapeutic step. Catheter angiography is usually deferred 4–10 days while the patient continues to receive heparin until the clinical course appears stable. If the patient with ischemia has not stabilized and continues to deteriorate despite heparin, I then suggest angiography earlier. If MRA or angiography shows a

complete basilar-artery occlusion, I continue heparin, followed by warfarin, for a total of 6–8 weeks, and use aspirin or other antiplatelet aggregants thereafter. If there is a severe stenosis of the basilar artery without occlusion, I usually use long-term warfarin treatment in an attempt to prevent occlusion. If there is only minor plaque disease in the major basilar artery, I select agents, such as aspirin or clopidogrel or aspirin with dipyridamole, which decrease platelet aggregation and agglutination.

In patients with no obvious intrinsic lesions by angiography, it is important to think of the possibility of embolism and be certain that studies are adequate to exclude a cardiogenic embolus or embolism from the aorta or the proximal innominate, subclavian or VAs. Angioplasty has occasionally been performed to open basilar-artery stenotic lesions, but this procedure can result in obliteration

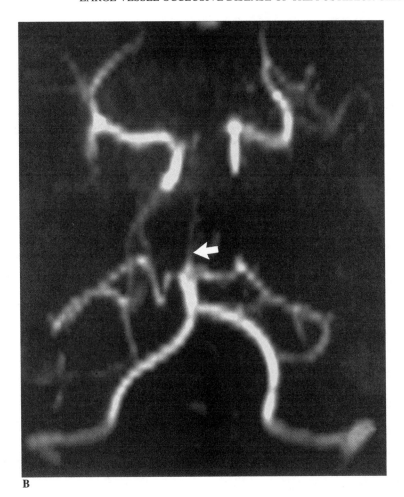

B

of paramedian and other arteries that penetrate from the basilar artery.

> A 38-year-old man, PG, was discovered comatose by his son. That morning he had been normal, according to his wife, who recalled no recent signs of ill health in her husband. He had no history of heart or vascular disease. On examination, his pupils were dilated and fixed at 8 mm each. His eyes were deviated down and outward. Lateral motion in each eye was obtained by oculocephalic maneuvers. No abnormal motor signs were evident.

The bilateral III nerve dysfunction and coma suggested a midbrain lesion. This could be caused by a large supratentorial space-taking lesion with midbrain compression or by an intrinsic lesion within the midbrain. Because of the lack of history, absence of stroke risk factors, and limitation of the neurologic examination by coma, I believed it mandatory to order urgent neuroimaging tests.

> The CT in patient PG was normal with and without contrast. MRI could not be performed urgently. The next day, diffusion-weighted and T2-weighted images showed infarction in the paramedian thalamus and midbrain tegmentum. MRA was normal. An echocardiogram showed a left atrial myxoma.

In most patients with basilar artery occlusion, the thrombus is limited to the proximal basilar artery. In some patients, the occlusion extends to the distal basilar-artery segment; in other patients, more often in African-Americans, occlusion or severe stenosis can affect predominantly the distal basilar artery.[1,31,88] Occlusion of the distal basilar artery is most often caused by embolism from the heart or the proximal VA system. Emboli small enough to pass through

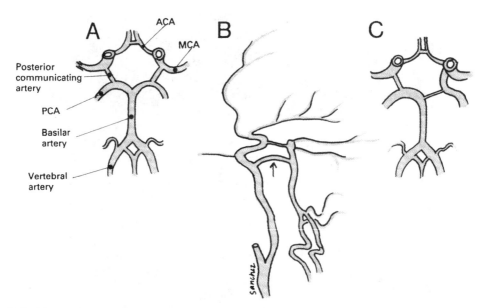

Figure 7-13. (**A**) Normal circle of Willis, basal view; (**B**) primitive trigeminal artery (*arrow*), lateral view; (**C**) origin of posterior communicating artery from the internal carotid artery. (ACA = anterior cerebral artery; MCA = middle cerebral artery; PCA = posterior cerebral artery.)

the VAs do not usually lodge in the proximal basilar artery, a vessel larger than each ICVA, but travel to the distal basilar artery or PCA branches. The distal basilar artery supplies the midbrain and diencephalon through small vessels that pierce the posterior perforated substance. Signs of dysfunction in this territory include[1,102–104]:

1. Pupillary abnormalities: The lesion may interrupt the afferent reflex arc by interfering with fibers going toward the Edinger-Westphal nucleus. The III-nerve nucleus can also be involved, as well as the rostral descending sympathetic system. The pupils are usually abnormal and can be small, mid-position, or dilated, depending on the level and extent of the lesion. Decreased pupillary reactivity and eccentricity of the pupil are also found.

2. Eye movement abnormalities: Vertical gaze abnormalities are common in patients with rostral brain stem lesions. Paralysis of upward or downward gaze is common. The eyes may also be skewed and may be deviated at rest, most often downward and inward. Hyperconvergence, retractory nystagmus, and pseudo VI-nerve paresis are other oculomotor abnormalities.

3. Altered level of alertness: Hypersomnolence or frank coma can result from bilateral paramedian rostral brain stem dysfunction. After the

acute phase, the patient may remain relatively inert and apathetic.

4. Amnesia: Memory loss can accompany thalamic infarction. Patients are unable to form new memories and may not be able to recall events just preceding their stroke. There may be an array of other behavioral abnormalities, including agitation, hallucinations, and abnormalities that mimic lesions of the frontal lobe.

In PG, the bilateral III-nerve palsies identified a midbrain lesion that was confirmed by MRI. Because the most frequent cause is embolic, the cardiac and vascular investigations are important. Identification of the left atrial myxoma led to successful removal of the cardiac tumor. The patient awakened on day 4 after his stroke and was left with a bilateral III-nerve palsy as his only important, persistent, neurologic sign.

Occlusion or Severe Stenosis of the Posterior Cerebral Arteries

The PCAs are the major terminal branches of the basilar artery. In approximately 30% of patients, one basilar communicating segment is hypoplastic, and the PCA is derived primarily from the ipsilat-

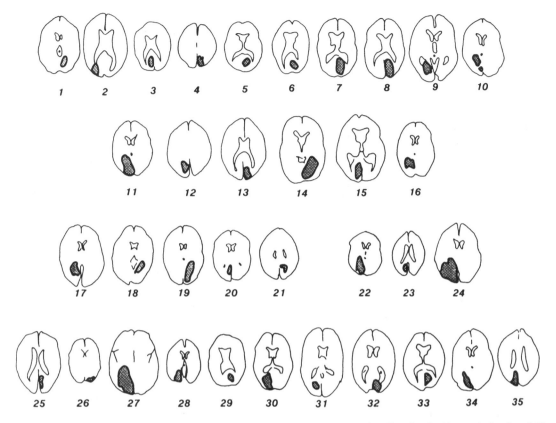

Figure 7-14. Montage of posterior cerebral artery infarcts on computed tomography. (Reprinted with permission from MS Pessin, E Lathi, M Cohen, et al. Clinical features and mechanism of occipital infarction. Ann Neurol 1987;21:290–299.)

eral ICA through its posterior communicating artery branch. Figure 7-13 illustrates the fetal-type PCA and a retained, primitive ICA-basilar artery communication, a trigeminal artery. Intrinsic atheromatous disease of the PCA most often affects the origin of the vessel. Its epidemiology is similar to disease of the proximal MCA. Most often, infarcts in the PCA territory are caused by emboli to the posterior circulation.[1,39,79,80,105,106] Castaigne and colleagues in a necropsy study identified 30 infarcts within PCA territory.[79] The most common mechanism of infarction was embolism from a proximal occlusive lesion within the vertebrobasilar system (15 out of 30, 50%). In eight patients, clot propagated from the basilar artery into the PCA. Only three patients had thrombosis of the PCA engrafted on previous atherosclerotic narrowing.[79]

Pessin, myself, and colleagues studied the mechanism of infarction in 35 patients with hemianopia and a unilateral infarct on CT limited to the PCA territory on one side.[105] Figure 7-14 is a montage of the

CT lesions from this study. The most frequent mechanism of infarction was embolism. A cardiac source of embolism was present in 10 patients (28.5%), and intra-arterial embolism arising from proximal posterior circulation lesions was found in six patients (17%). In 11 other patients, the clinical and angiographic findings suggested embolism, but no definite donor site was established. Among the 35 patients, 27 (77%) had embolic occlusion of PCA branches.[105] Among 79 patients with PCA-territory infarction in the New England Medical Center Posterior Circulation Registry, embolism was the most likely stroke mechanism in 65 patients (82%).[106] Series of patients with PCA-territory infarcts reported by other centers have shown that embolism is the predominant cause of these infarcts.[1,106]

An analogy can be drawn between the two brain circulations. In the anterior circulation, emboli usually lodge in MCA branches, leading to cortical infarcts; in the posterior circulation, emboli traverse the vertebral and basilar arteries and ultimately lodge in PCA branches, producing cortical infarcts. Intrinsic disease of the MCA and PCA does occur, but is far less common than cardiogenic or artery-to-artery embolization. When intrinsic atherosclerosis of the PCA is present, the clinical presentation usually consists of transient hemianopic visual symptoms, sometimes accompanied by transient hemisensory symptoms on the same side.[107]

A 64-year-old African-American woman, MA, awakened and realized she could not see to her left. She was able to read and could clearly identify objects in the room, but found it necessary to turn to the left to "see better." She also noted a dull pain behind her right eye. She was not aware of any difficulty with her limbs, walking, or thinking. During the past few weeks, she had several attacks of diminished vision to her left, each lasting a few minutes. On examination, there was a left homonymous hemianopia with slight sparing of the most central portion of the left visual field. The patient could read, note the color and nature of objects and pictures, draw common objects, copy drawings, and accurately bisect lines scattered on a page. Motor, sensory, reflex functions, and gait were normal.

After giving off penetrating branches to the midbrain and thalamus, the PCA supplies branches to the occipital lobes and supplies the medial and inferior portions of the temporal lobes. Headache in patients with PCA disease is often retro-orbital or above the eye, probably reflecting the fact that the upper surface of the tentorium is innervated by the first division of the fifth nerve. Infarction in the cerebral territories of the PCA most often affects vision and somatic sensation, but seldom causes paralysis.[1,105,106–111]

Visual Field Abnormalities

The single most common finding in patients with PCA-territory infarction is a hemianopia.[1,109,110] Hemianopia is caused by infarction of the striate visual cortex on the banks of the calcarine fissure, a region supplied by the calcarine branch of the PCA,

or it is caused by interruption of the geniculocalcarine tract as it nears the visual cortex. If just the lower bank of the calcarine fissure is involved, the lingual gyrus, a superior quadrant-field defect, results. An inferior quadrantanopia results if the lesion affects the cuneus on the upper bank of the calcarine fissure.

When infarction is restricted to the striate cortex and does not extend into the adjacent parietal cortex, the patient is fully aware of the visual defect. Usually described as a void, blackness, or limitation of vision to one side, patients usually recognize that they must focus extra attention to the hemianopic field. When given written material or pictures, patients with hemianopia caused by occipital lobe infarction are able to see and interpret the stimuli normally, although it may take them a bit longer to explore the hemianopic visual field. Hemianopia and visual neglect are not synonymous, nor is visual neglect merely a more-or-less severe form of hemianopia. In patients with occipital lobe infarcts, physicians can reliably map out the visual fields by confrontation. At times, the central or medial part of the field is spared, so-called macular sparing. Optokinetic nystagmus is normal. Some patients, although they accurately report motion or the presence of objects in their hemianopic field, cannot identify the nature, location, or color of that object.

In contrast, patients with infarction in the parietal lobe, most often in MCA territory, who have preservation of geniculocalcarine fibers and the striate cortex, have visual neglect. Their findings are quite different from those in patients with medial occipital infarction. Patients with visual neglect are usually unaware of their visual-field defect. They often (1) ignore objects in the abnormal visual field; (2) do not notice words in their impaired field, often reading only half of a headline or paragraph; (3) miss objects in pictures in the neglected field; and (4) have reduced optokinetic nystagmus to the side of the visual defect. Poor drawing and copying are also commonly associated with visual neglect. When the parieto-occipital and temporal branches of the PCA are involved, leading to large infarcts in the entire PCA territory, a hemianopia and visual neglect are present. More often, in isolated infarcts of the striate cortex, patients have a hemianopia without neglect. In my experience, visual neglect without a hemianopia is always caused by infarction within the MCA territory.

Somatosensory Abnormalities

The lateral thalamus is the site of the major somatosensory relay nuclei, the ventroposteromedial and lateral nuclei. Ischemia to these nuclei or white matter tracts carrying fibers from the thalamus to somatosensory cortex (postcentral gyrus and the sensory 2 region in the parietal operculum) produce changes in sensation, usually without paralysis. Patients describe paresthesias or numbness in the face, limbs, and trunk. On examination, their touch, pinprick, and position senses are reduced. The combination of hemisensory loss, with hemianopia and without paralysis, is virtually diagnostic of infarction in the PCA territory. The occlusive lesion is within the PCA, before the thalamogeniculate branches to the lateral thalamus.[111] Rarely, occlusion of the proximal portion of the PCA can cause a hemiplegia.[1,112–115] Penetrating branches from the most proximal portion of the PCA penetrate into the midbrain to supply the cerebral peduncle. PCA-origin occlusions cause hemiplegia caused by midbrain peduncular infarction accompanied by a hemisensory loss caused by lateral thalamic infarction and hemianopia caused by occipital lobe infarction. The resultant neurologic deficit is not easily distinguished clinically from MCA or anterior choroidal artery territory infarcts, but separation is made readily by CT and MRI results. Figure 7-15 from Hommel et al.[115] shows the proximal branches of the PCA.

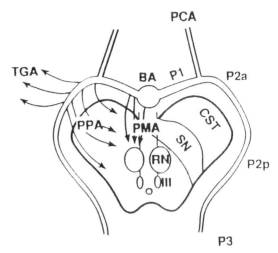

Figure 7-15. Axial diagram of the midbrain arteries. (BA = basilar artery; CST = corticospinal tract in the cerebral peduncle; PCA = posterior cerebral artery; PMA = paramedian arteries; PPA = peduncular perforating arteries; P1 = proximal segment of the PCA; P2a = anterior segment of the P2 part of the PCA; P2p = posterior segment of the P2 part of the PCA; P3 = P3 part of the PCA; RN = red nucleus; SN = substantia nigra; TGA = thalamogeniculate arteries; III = oculomotor nucleus.) (Reprinted with permission from M Hommel, G Besson, P Pollak, et al. Hemiplegia in posterior cerebral artery occlusion. Neurology 1990;40:1496–1499.)

Cognitive and Behavioral Abnormalities

When the left PCA territory is infarcted, several additional findings may occur:

1. Alexia without agraphia: Infarction of the left occipital lobe and splenium of the corpus callosum is associated with a remarkable clinical syndrome, first described by Dejerine,[116] and later amplified by Geschwind and Fusillo.[117] Because the left visual cortex is infarcted, patients see with their right occipital lobe and their left visual field. To name what they see, the information must be communicated from the right occipital cortex to the language region in the left temporal and parietal lobes. Infarction of the corpus callosum or adjacent white matter paths interrupts communication between the right occipital cortex and the left hemisphere. Patients have difficulty naming what they see. The most conspicuous abnormality is in reading. Although usually able to name individual letters or numbers, the patient cannot read words or phrases. Because the speech cortex is normal, they retain the ability to speak, repeat speech, write, and spell aloud. Although they are able to write a paragraph, they often cannot read it back moments later. Usually accompanying the dyslexia is a defect in color naming.[1,117] Patients can match colors and shades, proving that their perception of colors is normal. They can also describe the usual color of familiar objects and can even color correctly when given an array of crayons. Nonetheless, they are unable to give a color its correct name.

2. Anomic or transcortical sensory aphasia[118]: Some patients with left PCA-territory infarction have difficulty naming objects. Others can repeat, but not understand, spoken language.

3. Gerstmann's syndrome: PCA-territory infarction can undercut the angular gyrus, leading to a host of findings, usually lumped together as Gerstmann's syndrome.[1] These findings include (1) diffi-

culty telling right from left, (2) difficulty in naming digits on their own or on others' hands, (3) constructional dyspraxia, (4) agraphia, and (5) difficulty in calculating. In any single patient, all features may appear together or one or more may occur in isolation. Gerstmann's syndrome also occurs when the angular gyrus region is infarcted during left MCA-territory infarction.

4. Altered memory: A defect in acquisition of new memories is common when both medial temporal lobes are damaged,[1,119] but also occurs in lesions limited to the left temporal lobe.[1,117,120–123] The memory deficit in unilateral lesions is usually not permanent, but has lasted up to 6 months. Patients cannot recall recent events and when given new information, they cannot recall it moments later. They often repeat statements and questions spoken only minutes before.

5. Associative visual agnosia[1,124,125]: Some patients with left PCA territory infarction have difficulty understanding the nature and use of objects presented visually. They can trace with their fingers and copy objects, demonstrating that visual perception is preserved. They can often name objects if the objects are presented in their hand and explored by touch or when verbally described. One patient, when shown a pair of scissors, had no idea what it was. When the instrument was placed in her hand, she was able to name it. When asked to list five objects that might be used for cutting, she included scissors, indicating that the name of the object was available to the patient.[120]

Infarcts of the right PCA territory are often accompanied by prosopagnosia, difficulty in recognizing familiar faces.[1,125–127] At times, patients cannot recognize their spouses, children, or even their own images in a mirror. Despite the seeming inability to recognize, match, or identify faces, physiologic tests of autonomic function are consistent with familiarity on a subconscious level.[127] Disorientation to place and an inability to recall routes, read, or revisualize the location of places on maps are also common findings in patients with right PCA-territory infarcts.[128] Patients with right occipito-temporal infarcts also may have difficulty revisualizing what a given object or person should look like. Dreams may also be devoid of visual imagery. Visual neglect is much more common after lesions of the right PCA territory.

When the PCA territory is infarcted bilaterally, the most common findings are cortical blindness, amnesia, and agitated delirium.[1,102] Most often, bilateral PCA-territory infarction is caused by embolism with blockage of the distal basilar artery bifurcation. Cortically blind patients cannot see or identify objects in either visual field, but have preserved pupillary light reflexes.[129] Some patients with cortical blindness do not volunteer or admit they cannot see and seem to avoid barriers in their way. Amnesia caused by bilateral medial temporal-lobe infarction may be permanent and closely resembles Korsakoff's syndrome.[119] Also, infarcting the hippocampus, fusiform, and lingual gyri, usually bilaterally, leads to an agitated hyperactive state that could be confused with delirium tremens.[1,102,130,131] When infarction is limited to the lower banks of the calcarine fissures bilaterally, the major findings are prosopagnosia and defective color vision.[1,110,125,132,133]

> CT showed an infarct in patient MA in the medial occipital lobe on the right. Angiography was not performed. Extracranial Doppler examination at C2 did not show reversed VA flow on either side. TCD showed a focal region of increased blood-flow velocity in the right PCA. MRI showed that the occipital infarct involved striate cortex above and below the calcarine fissure. MRA showed a focal narrowing of the right PCA. Cardiac echo and rhythm monitoring were normal. She was discharged on aspirin therapy. The findings did not change during the ensuing years of follow-up.

CT can accurately reflect the vascular territory involved. In this patient, it confirmed that the lesion was in the territory of the calcarine branch of the right PCA.[1,134,135] CT also verified that the lesion was ischemic and not caused by intracerebral hemorrhage. MRI is probably better able to image small associated lesions in the thalamus, midbrain, and more proximal brain stem and cerebellum, thus helping to localize the offending vascular lesion. Sagittal T2-weighted MRI sections through the medial occipital lobes can also identify the location of the lesions in relation to the calcarine fissure and the optic radiations, and thereby help prognosticate recovery of visual field defects. The occipital lobe is a site of predilection for amyloid angiopathy. Hemorrhage from amyloid angiopathy often occurs in the absence of hypertension and can mimic an ischemic stroke. Little is known at present about optimum therapy for patients with intrinsic disease of the PCA. When infarction is limited to branches of the PCA, cardiogenic embolism should be considered and appropriate investigations performed to exclude it.

In patient MA, there was no clinical or laboratory evidence to suggest cardiac-origin embolism. Noninvasive studies gave no evidence for an ECVA occlusion in the neck, a potential source of intra-arterial embolism to the PCA. If ECVA occlusion had been suggested by noninvasive tests, or if epidemiologic and ecologic factors had favored a ECVA-origin lesion, a gadolinium-enhanced MRA examination of the subclavian ECVA-origin region or catheter angiography would have been ordered. She was African-American and had no history of coronary or peripheral vascular disease, and did not have hypercholesterolemia. These factors weighed against the likelihood of a proximal ECVA lesion.[31] The absence of brain stem symptoms and normal ICVA blood-flow velocities on TCD examination argued against an ICVA occlusion. The TCD findings of a focal increase in blood-flow velocity in the right PCA strongly favored a focal lesion involving the PCA. Intracranial MRA excluded an ICVA lesion and identified the intrinsic lesion within the right PCA. The preceding spells of left visual field loss favored an intrinsic right PCA occlusive lesion. Even if more extensive infarction were to occur in the right PCA territory, the likelihood of serious disability was small. The risk to the patient of further, serious, neurologic disability did not, in my opinion, warrant invasive diagnostic procedures or hazardous therapy. I elected to prescribe aspirin.

Differential Diagnosis of Posterior Circulation Ischemia

Advances in technology, especially the introduction of MRI, echocardiography, ultrasound, TCD, and MRA, have now made it possible to investigate patients with posterior circulation ischemia safely and quickly and identify the causative vascular mechanism. Diffusion and perfusion-weighted MRI can also be helpful within the posterior circulation by showing regions that are hypoperfused

and identifying infarcts earlier than T2-weighted standard MRI scans.

I have found it useful to divide the posterior circulation into smaller territories that refect the vascular distribution of the main arteries. The ICVAs join at the medullo-pontine junction to form the basilar arteries. The territory usually perfused by the ICVAs includes the medulla and the cerebellum supplied by the PICA branch of the ICVAs. This region is designated as *proximal intracranial posterior circulation territory*. The basilar artery bifurcates at the ponto-mesencephalic junction. The territory supplied by the basilar artery, including the pons and the portion of the cerebellum supplied by the AICA branch, is designated as *middle intracranial posterior circulation territory*. The portion of the posterior circulation supplied by the distal basilar artery and its SCA, PCA, and penetrating artery branches is referred to as *distal intracranial posterior circulation territory*. The distal territory includes the midbrain, thalamus, SCA-supplied cerebellum, and the occipital and temporal lobe regions supplied by the PCAs. Figure 7-16, modeled after a figure in the Duvernoy atlas,[55] shows these posterior circulation territories.

Designation of brain territory is made by using clinical and imaging data. For example, suppose a patient has clinical findings of a left lateral medullary syndrome and a right hemianopia. MRI shows only a left occipital-lobe infarct. This patient must have proximal and distal intracranial posterior circulation territory ischemia. Moreover, the left proximal-territory lesion means that the left ICVA must have been involved at some point. The combination of proximal and distal-territory infarction is most often explained by an embolus that first landed at the ICVA and then traveled to the basilar bifurcation region, or an occlusive lesion of the ICVA with distal embolism. Designation of territory tells the clinician the rostrocaudal localization of the vascular lesion. Vascular diagnostic technology, including extracranial and transcranial ultrasound, CTA, MRA, standard angiography, and echocardiography can then be used to define the causative vascular lesions.

Treatment has lagged far behind advances in diagnostic technology. I hope that in the near future, trials of various therapies in patients with documented vascular lesions will shed more light on treatment.

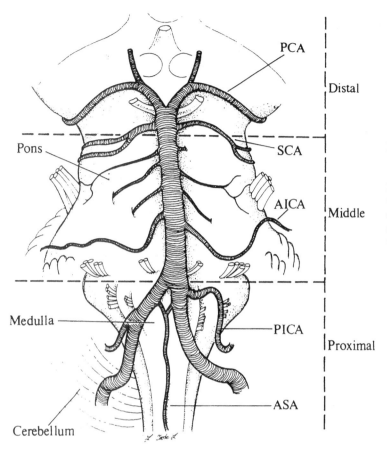

Figure 7-16. Sketch of the base of the brain shows the intracranial vertebral and basilar arteries and their branches. The brain regions are divided into proximal, middle, and distal intracranial territories. (AICA = anterior inferior cerebellar artery; ASA = anterior spinal artery; PCA = posterior cerebral artery; PICA = posterior inferior cerebellar artery; SCA = superior cerebellar artery.) (Drawing by Laurel Cook-Lowe. Reprinted with permission from LR Caplan. Posterior Circulation Disease: Clinical Findings, Diagnosis, and Management. Boston: Blackwell, 1996.)

References

1. Caplan LR. Posterior Circulation Disease. Clinical Findings, Diagnosis, and Management. Boston: Blackwell, 1996.
2. Millikan C, Siekert R. Studies in cerebrovascular disease. The syndrome of intermittent insufficiency of the basilar arterial system. Mayo Clin Proc 1955;30:61–68.
3. Denny-Brown D. Basilar artery syndromes. Bull N Engl Med Center 1953;15:53–60.
4. Fang H, Palmer J. Vascular phenomena involving brainstem structures. Neurology 1956;6:402–419.
5. Williams D, Wilson T. The diagnosis of the major and minor syndromes of basilar insufficiency. Brain 1962;85:741–774.
6. Millikan C, Siekert R, Shick R. Studies in cerebrovascular disease: the use of anticoagulant drugs in the treatment of insufficiency or thrombosis within the basilar arterial system. Mayo Clin Proc 1955;30:116–126.
7. Caplan LR. Vertebrobasilar disease: time for a new strategy. Stroke 1981;12:111–114.
8. Caplan LR. Vertebrobasilar disease: should we continue the double standard of managing patients with brain ischemia? Heart Stroke 1993;2:377–381.
9. Reivich M, Holling E, Roberts B, et al. Reversal of blood flow through the vertebral artery and its effects on cerebral circulation. N Engl J Med 1961;265:878–885.
10. Heyman A, Young W, Dillon M, et al. Cerebral ischemia caused by occlusive disease of the subclavian or innominate arteries. Arch Neurol 1964;10:581–589.
11. North R, Fisher W, DeBakey M, et al. Brachial-basilar insufficiency syndrome. Neurology 1962;12:810–820.
12. Patel A, Toole J. Subclavian steal syndrome: reversal of cephalic blood flow. Medicine (Baltimore) 1965;44:289–303.
13. Hennerici M, Klemm C, Rautenberg W. The subclavian steal phenomenon: a common vascular disorder with rare neurologic deficits. Neurology 1988;38:669–673.
14. Pollock M, Blennerhassett J, Clark A. Giant cell arteritis and the subclavian steal syndrome. Neurology 1973;23:653–657.
15. Brewster DC, Moncure AC, Darling C, et al. Innominate artery lesions: problems encountered and lessons learned. J Vasc Surg 1985;2:99–112.
16. Hennerici M, Aulich A, Sandemann W, Freund H-J. Incidence of asymptomatic extracranial occlusive disease. Stroke 1981;12:750–758.
17. Symonds C. Two cases of thrombosis of subclavian artery with contralateral hemiplegia of sudden onset, probably embolic. Brain 1927;50:259–260.

18. Martin R, Bogousslavsky J, Miklossy J, et al. Floating thrombus in the innominate artery as a cause of cerebral infarction in young adults. Cerebrovasc Dis 1992;2:177–181.

19. Ferriere M, Negre G, Bellecoste JF, et al. Thrombus flottant sous-clavier responsible d'un syndrome encephalo-digital, deux observations. La Presse Med 1984;13:27–29.

20. Fields WS, LeMak NA, Ben-Menachem Y. Thoracic outlet syndrome: review and reference to a stroke in a major league pitcher. AJNR Am J Neuroradiol 1986;7:73–78.

21. Baker R, Rosenbaum A, Caplan L. Subclavian steal syndrome. Contemp Surg 1974;4:96–104.

22. Ekestrom S, Eklund B, Liljequist L, et al. Noninvasive methods in the evaluation of obliterative disease of the subclavian or innominate artery. Acta Med Scand 1979; 206:467–471.

23. Berguer R, Higgins R, Nelson R. Noninvasive diagnosis of reversal of vertebral artery blood flow. N Engl J Med 1980;302:1349–1351.

24. Von Reutern GM, Pourcelot L. Cardiac cycle-dependent alternating flow in vertebral arteries with subclavian artery stenosis. Stroke 1978;9:229–236.

25. Liljequist L, Ekestrom S, Nordhus O. Monitoring direction of vertebral artery blood flow by Doppler shift ultrasound in patients with suspected subclavian steal. Acta Chir Scand 1981;147:421–424.

26. von Reutern G-M, von Budingen H-J. Ultrasound diagnosis of cerebrovascular disease. Doppler sonography of the extracranial and intracranial arteries, duplex scanning. Stuttgart: Georg Thieme, 1993;129–175.

27. von Budingen H-J, Staudacher T. Evaluation of Vertebrobasilar Disease. In DW Newell, R Aaslid (eds), Transcranial Doppler. New York: Raven Press, 1992;167–195.

28. Ackerstaff RGA. Duplex Scanning of the Aortic Arch and Vertebral Arteries. In EF Bernstein (ed), Vascular Diagnosis (4th ed). St Louis: Mosby, 1993;315–321.

29. Fisher CM, Gore I, Okabe N, et al. Atherosclerosis of the carotid and vertebral arteries: extracranial and intracranial. J Neuropathol Exp Neurol 1965;24:455–476.

30. Hutchinson E, Yates P. Carotico-vertebral stenosis. Lancet 1957;1:2–8.

31. Gorelick PB, Caplan LR, Hier DB, et al. Racial differences in the distribution of posterior circulation occlusive disease. Stroke 1985;16:785–790.

32. Fisher CM. Vertigo in cerebrovascular disease. Arch Otolaryngol 1967;85:529–534.

33. Moosy J. Morphology, sites, and epidemiology of cerebral atherosclerosis. Res Publ Assoc Res Nerv Ment Dis 1966; 51:1–22.

34. Imparato A, Riles T, Kim G. Cervical vertebral angioplasty for brainstem ischemia. Surgery 1981;90:842–852.

35. Pelouze GA. Plaque ulcerie de l'ostium de l'artere vertebrale. Rev Neurol 1989;145:478–481.

36. Fisher CM. Occlusion of the vertebral arteries. Arch Neurol 1970;22:13–19.

37. Wityk RJ, Chang H-M, Rosengart A, et al. Proximal extracranial vertebral artery disease in the New England Medical Center Posterior Circulation Registry. Arch Neurol 1998;55:470–478.

38. George B, Laurian C. Vertebrobasilar ischemia with thrombosis of the vertebral artery: report of two cases with embolism. J Neurol Neurosurg Psychiatry 1982;45:91–93.

39. Caplan LR, Tettenborn B. Embolism in the Posterior Circulation. In R Bergner, LR Caplan (eds), Vertebrobasilar Arterial Disease. St. Louis: Quality Medical Publishers, 1991;50–63.

40. Caplan LR, Amarenco P, Rosengart A, et al. Embolism from vertebral artery origin occlusive disease. Neurology 1992;42:1505–1512.

41. Moufarrij N, Little JR, Furlan AJ, et al. Vertebral artery stenosis: long term follow-up. Stroke 1984;15:260–263.

42. Callow A. Surgical management of varying patterns of vertebral artery and subclavian artery insufficiency. N Engl J Med 1964;270:546–552.

43. Roon A, Ehrenfeld W, Cooke P, et al. Vertebral artery reconstruction. Am J Surg 1979;138:29–36.

44. Berguer R. Surgical Indications for Reconstruction of the Vertebral Artery. In R Berguer, LR Caplan (eds), Vertebrobasilar Arterial Disease. St. Louis: Quality Medical Publishers, 1991;201–210.

45. Kieffer E, Koskas F, Bahnini A, et al. Long-term Results After Reconstruction of the Cervical Vertebral Artery. In LR Caplan, EG Shifrin, AN Nicolaides, WS Moore (eds), Cerebrovascular Ischaemia, Investigations and Management. London: Med-Orion, 1996;617–625.

46. Caplan LR, Zarins C, Hemmatti M. Spontaneous dissection of the extracranial vertebral arteries. Stroke 1985;16: 1030–1038.

47. Caplan LR, Tettenborn B. Vertebrobasilar occlusive disease, review of selected aspects: 1. Spontaneous dissection of extracranial and intracranial posterior circulation arteries. Cerebrovasc Dis 1992;2:256–265.

48. Mokri B, Houser OW, Sandok BA, Piepgras DG. Spontaneous dissections of the vertebral arteries. Neurology 1988;38:880–885.

49. Wilkinson I, Russel R. Arteries of the head and neck in giant cell arteritis. Arch Neurol 1972;27:378–391.

50. Bickerstaff E. Neurological Complications of Oral Contraceptives. Oxford: Clarendon Press, 1975.

51. Muller-Kuppers M, Graf KJ, Pessin MS, et al. Intracranial vertebral artery disease in the New England Medical Center Posterior Circulation Registry. Eur Neurol 1997;37:146–156.

52. Shin H-K, Yoo K-M, Chang HM, Caplan LR. Bilateral intracranial vertebral artery disease in the New England Medical Center Posterior Circulation Registry. Arch Neurol 1999;56:1353–1358.

53. Fisher CM, Karnes W, Kubik C. Lateral medullary infarction: the pattern of vascular occlusion. J Neuropathol Exp Neurol 1961;20:323–379.

54. Stephens RB, Stilwell DL. Arteries and Veins of the Human Brain. Springfield, IL: Charles C Thomas, 1969.

55. Duvernoy HM. Human Brainstem Vessels. Berlin: Springer, 1978.

56. Kommerall G, Hoyt W. Lateropulsion of saccadic eye movements. Arch Neurol 1973;28:313–318.

57. Meyer K, Baloh R, Krohel G, et al. Ocular lateropulsion: a sign of lateral medullary disease. Arch Opthalmol 1980;98:1614–1616.

58. Matsumoto S, Okuda B, Imai T, Kameyama M. A sensory level on the trunk in lower lateral brainstem lesions. Neurology 1988;38:1515–1519.

59. Devereaux M, Keane J, Davis R. Automatic respiratory failure associated with infarction of the medulla: report of

two cases with pathologic study of one. Arch Neurol 1973;29:46–52.

60. Levin B, Margolis G. Acute failure of automatic respirations secondary to a unilateral brainstem infarct. Ann Neurol 1977;1:583–586.
61. Bogousslavsaky J, Khurma R, Deruaz JP, et al. Respiratory failure and unilateral brainstem infarction. Ann Neurol 1990;28:668–673.
62. Currier R, Giles C, Westerberg M. The prognosis of some brainstem vascular syndromes. Neurology 1958;8:664–668.
63. Caplan LR, Pessin M, Scott RM, et al. Poor outcome after lateral medullary infarcts. Neurology 1986;36:1510–1513.
64. Caplan LR. Bilateral distal vertebral artery occlusion. Neurology 1983;33:552–558.
65. Hauw J, Der Agopian P, Trelles L, et al. Les infarctes bulbaires. J Neurol Sci 1976;28:83–102.
66. Sawada H, Seriu N, Udaka F, Kameyama M. Magnetic resonance imaging of medial medullary infarction. Stroke 1990;21:963–966.
67. Tyler KL, Sandberg E, Baum KF. Medial medullary syndrome and meningovascular syphilis: a case report in an HIV-infected man and a review of the literature. Neurology 1994;44:2231–2235.
68. Kim JS, Kim HG, Chung CS. Medial medullary syndrome: report of 18 new patients and a review of the literature. Stroke 1995;26:1548–1552.
69. Sypert G, Alvord E. Cerebellar infarction: a clinicopathological study. Arch Neurol 1975;32:351–363.
70. Amarenco P, Hauw JJ, Henin D, et al. Les infarctus du territoire de l'artere cerebelleuse postero-inferieure: etude clinico-pathologique de 28 cas. Rev Neurol 1989;145:277–286.
71. Amarenco P, Hauw JJ, Gautier JC. Arterial pathology in cerebellar infarction. Stroke 1990;21:1299–1305.
72. Amarenco P, Caplan LR. Vertebrobasilar occlusive disease, review of selected aspects: 3. mechanisms of cerebellar infarctions. Cerebrovasc Dis 1993;3:66–73.
73. Fisher CM, Picard E, Polak A, et al. Acute hypertensive cerebellar hemorrhage: diagnosis and surgical treatment. J Nerv Ment Dis 1965;140:38–57.
74. Lehrich J, Winkler G, Ojemann R. Cerebellar infarction with brainstem compression: diagnosis and surgical treatment. Arch Neurol 1970;22:490–498.
75. Fairburn B, Oliver L. Cerebellar softening: a surgical emergency. BMJ 1956;1:1335–1336.
76. Hornig CR, Rust DS, Busse O, et al. Space-occupying cerebellar infarction. Clinical course and prognosis. Stroke 1994;25:372–374.
77. Seelig J, Selhorst J, Young H, et al. Ventriculostomy for hydrocephalus in cerebellar hemorrhage. Neurology 1981;31:1537–1540.
78. Rieke K, Krieger D, Adams H-P, et al. Therapeutic strategies in space-occupying cerebellar infarction based on clinical, neuroradiological and neurophysiological data. Cerebrovasc Dis 1993;3:45–55.
79. Castaigne P, Lhermitte F, Gautier J, et al. Arterial occlusions in the vertebral-basilar system. Brain 1973;96:133–154.

80. Koroshetz WJ, Ropper AH. Artery-to-artery embolism causing stroke in the posterior circulation. Neurology 1987;37:292–296.
81. Sundt T, Whisnant J, Piepgras D, et al. Intracranial bypass grafts for vertebral-basilar ischemia. Mayo Clin Proc 1978;53:12–18.
82. Ausman J, Diaz F, de los Reyes R, et al. Anastomosis of occipital artery to AICA for vertebrobasilar junction stenosis. Surg Neurol 1981;16:99–102.
83. Roski R, Spetzler R, Hopkins L. Occipital artery to posterior-inferior cerebellar artery bypass for vertebrobasilar ischemia. Neurosurgery 1982;10:44–49.
84. Allen G, Cohen R, Preziosi T. Microsurgical endarterectomy of the intracranial vertebral artery for vertebrobasilar transient ischemic attacks. Neurosurgery 1981;81:56–59.
85. Takis C, Kwan ES, Pessin MS, Jacobs DH, Caplan LR. Intracranial angioplasty: experience and complications. AJNR Am J Neuroradiol 1997;18:1661–1668.
86. Kubik C, Adams R. Occlusion of the basilar artery: a clinical and pathologic study. Brain 1946;69:73–121.
87. Caplan LR. Occlusion of the vertebral or basilar artery. Stroke 1979;10:272–282.
88. Pessin MS, Gorelick PB, Kwan ES, et al. Basilar artery stenosis: middle and distal segments. Neurology 1987;37:1742–1746.
89. LaBauge R, Pages C, Marty-Double JM, et al. Occlusion du tronc basilaire. Rev Neurol 1981;137:545–571.
90. Amarenco P, Hauw JJ. Cerebellar infarction in the territory of the anterior inferior cerebellar artery: a clinicopathological study of 20 cases. Brain 1990;118:139–155.
91. Amarenco P, Rosengart A, DeWitt LD, et al. Anterior inferior cerebellar artery territory infarcts. Mechanisms and clinical features. Arch Neurol 1993;50:154–161.
92. Fisher CM. Some neuro-ophthalmological observations. J Neurol Neurosurg Psychiatry 1967;30:383–392.
93. Chase T, Moretti L, Prensky A. Clinical and electroencephalographic manifestations of a vascular lesion of the pons. Neurology 1968;18:357–368.
94. Kistler J, Buonanno F, DeWitt D, et al. Vertebral-basilar posterior cerebral territory stroke: delineation by proton nuclear magnetic resonance imaging. Stroke 1984;15:417–426.
95. Simmons Z, Biller J, Adams HP, et al. Cerebellar infarction: comparison of computed tomography and magnetic resonance imaging. Ann Neurol 1986;19:291–293.
96. Biller J, Yuh W, Mitchell GW. Early diagnosis of basilar artery occlusion using magnetic resonance imaging. Stroke 1988;19:297–306.
97. Fisher CM. Bilateral occlusion of basilar artery branches. J Neurol Neurosurg Psychiatry 1977;40:1182–1189.
98. Caplan LR, Sergay S. Positional cerebral ischemia. J Neurol Neurosurg Psychiatry 1976;39:385–391.
99. Bogousslavsky J, Regli F, Maeder P, et al. The etiology of posterior circulation infarcts: a prospective study using magnetic resonance imaging and magnetic resonance angiography. Neurology 1993;43:1528–1533.
100. Roether J, Wentz K-U, Rautenberg W, et al. Magnetic resonance angiography in vertebrobasilar ischemia. Stroke 1993;24:1310–1315.

101. Wentz K-U, Rother J, Schwartz A, et al. Intracranial vertebrobasilar system: MR angiography. Radiology 1994;190: 105–110.

102. Caplan LR. Top of the basilar syndrome: selected clinical aspects. Neurology 1980;30:72–79.

103. Mehler MF. The rostral basilar artery syndrome: diagnosis, etiology, prognosis. Neurology 1989;39:9–16.

104. Mehler MF. The neuro-ophthalmologic spectrum of the rostral basilar artery syndrome. Arch Neurol 1988;45: 966–971.

105. Pessin MS, Lathi E, Cohen M, et al. Clinical features and mechanism of occipital infarction. Ann Neurol 1987;21: 290–299.

106. Yamamoto Y, Georgiadis AL, Chang HM, Caplan LR. Posterior cerebral artery territory infarcts in the New England Medical Center (NEMC) Posterior Circulation Registry. Arch Neurol 1999;56:824–832.

107. Pessin MS, Kwan E, DeWitt LD, et al. Posterior cerebral artery stenosis. Ann Neurol 1987;21:85–89.

108. Caplan LR. Posterior Cerebral Artery. In J Bogousslavsky, LR Caplan (eds), Stroke Syndromes. Cambridge: Cambridge University Press, 1995;290–299.

109. Mohr JP, Pessin MS. Posterior Cerebral Artery Disease. In HJM Barnett, JP Mohr, BM Stein, F Yatsu (eds), Stroke Pathophysiology, Diagnosis, and Management (3rd ed). New York: Churchill Livingstone, 1998;481–502.

110. Caplan LR. Visual Perceptual Abnormalities (Cerebral). In J Bogousslavsky, LR Caplan (eds), Stroke Syndromes. Cambridge: Cambridge University Press, 1995;57–67.

111. Georgiadis AL, Yamamoto Y, Kwan ES, et al. Anatomy of sensory findings in patients with posterior cerebral artery (PCA) territory infarction. Arch Neurol 1999;56: 835–838.

112. Benson DF, Tomlinson EB. Hemiplegic syndrome of the posterior cerebral artery. Stroke 1971;2:559–564.

113. Caplan LR, DeWitt LD, Pessin MS, et al. Lateral thalamic infarcts. Arch Neurol 1988;45:959–964.

114. Hommel M, Besson G, Pollak P, et al. Hemiplegia in posterior cerebral artery occlusion. Neurology 1990;40: 1496–1499.

115. Hommel M, Moreaud O, Besson G, Perret J. Site of arterial occlusions in the hemiplegic posterior cerebral artery syndrome. Neurology 1991;41:604–605.

116. Dejerine J. Contribution a l'etude anatomo-pathologique et clinique des differnetes varietes de cecite verbale. Memoires de la Societe Biologique 1892;4:61–90.

117. Geschwind N, Fusillo M. Color naming defect in association with alexia. Arch Neurol 1966;15:137–146.

118. Kertesz A, Sleppard A, MacKenzie R. Localization in transcortical sensory aphasia. Arch Neurol 1982;39:475–479.

119. Victor M, Angevine J, Mancall E, et al. Memory loss with lesion of hippocampal formation. Arch Neurol 1961;5: 244–263.

120. Caplan LR, Hedley-White T. Cueing and memory dysfunction in alexia without agraphia. Brain 1974;97:251–262.

121. Benson F, Marsden C, Meadows J. The amnestic syndrome of posterior cerebral artery occlusion. Acta Neurol Scand 1974;50:133–145.

122. Mohr JP, Leicester J, Stoddard L, et al. Right hemianopia with memory and color deficits in circumscribed left posterior cerebral artery territory infarction. Neurology 1971; 21:1104–1113.

123. Ott B, Saver JL. Unilateral amnestic stroke. Six new cases and a review of the literature. Stroke 1993;24:1033–1042.

124. Rubens A, Benson F. Associative visual agnosia. Arch Neurol 1971;24:305–316.

125. Grusser OJ, Landis T. Visual Agnosias and Other Disturbances of Visual Perception and Cognition. Boston: CRC Press, 1991.

126. Damasio A, Damasio H, Van Hoesen G. Prosopagnosia: anatomic basis and behavioral mechanisms. Neurology 1982;32:331–341.

127. Tranel D, Damasio AR. Autonomic recognition of familiar faces by prosopagnosics: evidence of a knowledge without awareness. Neurology 1985;35(Suppl 1):119–120.

128. Fisher CM. Disorientation to place. Arch Neurol 1982;39: 33–36.

129. Symonds C, McKenzie I. Bilateral loss of vision from cerebral infarction. Brain 1957;80:415–455.

130. Medina J, Rubino F, Ross E. Agitated delirium caused by infarctions of the hippocampal formation and fusiform and lingual gyri: a case report. Neurology 1974;24:1181–1183.

131. Horenstein S, Chamberlain W, Conomy J. Infarction of the fusiform and calcarine regions: agitated delirium and hemianopia. Trans Am Neurol Assoc 1962;92:357–367.

132. Meadows J. Disturbed perception of colors associated with localized cerebral lesions. Brain 1974;97:615–632.

133. Damasio A, Yamada T, Damasio H, et al. Central achromatopsia: behavioral, anatomic,and physiologic aspects. Neurology 1980;30:1064–1071.

134. Kinkle W, Newman R, Jacobs L. Posterior Cerebral Artery Branch Occlusions: CT and Anatomical Considerations. In R Berguer, R Bauer (eds), Vertebrobasilar Arterial Occlusive Disease. New York: Raven Press, 1984;117–133.

135. Goto K, Tagawa K, Uemma K, et al. Posterior cerebral artery occlusion. Radiology 1979;132:357–368.

Chapter 8
Penetrating and Branch Artery Disease

Occlusions or stenoses of large extracranial and intracranial arteries are traditional lesions generally recognized by physicians and surgeons caring for stroke patients. Abnormalities in larger arteries are easily confirmed by angiography and noninvasive tests and are readily verified by gross inspection of arteries removed at surgery or necropsy. In contrast, lesions in microscopic intracranial arteries, although acknowledged as genuine pathologic findings, are a more controversial cause of stroke. Fisher (Figure 1-2) reviewed the history of lacunar infarctions,[1] defined the nature and etiology of the vascular pathology causing lacunes,[2] and described many clinical syndromes that can be readily and reliably diagnosed as lacunar. Fisher almost single-handedly brought this disorder to the attention of the neurologic community. Yet, many still fail or refuse to integrate the concept of lacunar infarction into their differential diagnosis of stroke, and others are skeptical that lacunes can be diagnosed clinically. Even in the year 2000, lacunes remain controversial.[3]

Besson and Hommel[3] and Hauw[4] reviewed the history of the development of the lacunar infarction concept. Durand-Fardel first introduced the term *lacunes* in 1843 to describe small holes, usually found in the striatum, which contain fine meshwork of tissues and vessels.[5] The clinical findings in patients with lacunar infarction were first described by Ferrand,[6] working in the laboratory of Pierre Marie, and by Marie himself.[7] These French authors noted that lacunes were most often located in the lentiform nuclei, thalamus, pons, internal capsule, and cerebral white matter. Hemiplegia was the major finding in acute lacunar infarction. The clinical condition of multiple lacunes was termed *état lacunaire* by Marie and was characterized by pseudobulbar

palsy and an abnormal small-stepped gait. Foix and colleagues added clinical details about the findings in capsular and pontine lacunar infarcts.[8–10] Little was added after Foix until Fisher's work on the pathology and clinical findings in lacunar infarction.[3,4]

Pathology

Lacunes are small, discrete, often irregular lesions, ranging from 1 to 20 mm in size. Only 17% of lacunes are smaller than 1 cm.[1] Inspection of the tiny cavities usually reveals fine strands of connective tissue resembling cobwebs. Marie recognized that true lacunes had to be differentiated from dilatated perivascular spaces, so-called *état criblé*, and from postmortem holes produced by gas bacilli (*état vermoulu*).[7] Gas cavities are usually numerous, perfectly round, with no cobwebs, and often retain a characteristic bad smell. These distinctions are important today because studies show that magnetic resonance imaging (MRI) often reveals the dilatated perivascular *état criblé* lesions as discrete loci of increased signal.[11] The most common locations of lacunar infarcts are the putamen and the pallidum, followed by the pons, thalamus, caudate nucleus, internal capsule, and corona radiata. More rare are lacunes in the cerebral peduncles, pyramids, and white matter. These lesions are not found in the cerebral or cerebellar cortices.

Serial sections of the penetrating arteries that supply the territory of lacunar infarcts reveal a characteristic vascular pathology.[2] These tiny vessels often have focal enlargements and small hemorrhagic extravasations through the walls of the arteries. Subintimal foam cells sometimes obliter-

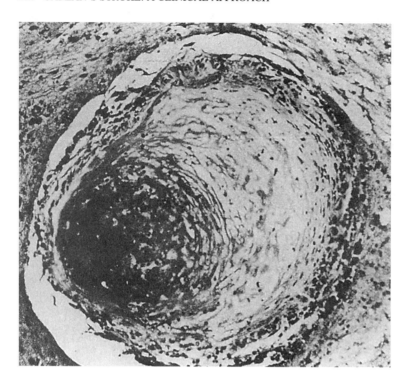

Figure 8-1. Small penetrating artery showing lipohyalinosis and fibrinoid necrosis; lumen is considerably compromised. (Courtesy of C. Miller Fisher, M.D.)

ate the lumens, and pink-staining fibrinoid material lies within the vessel walls (Figure 8-1). The arteries in spots are often replaced by whorls, tangles, and wisps of connective tissue that obliterate the usual vascular layers. Fisher called these processes *segmental arterial disorganization, fibrinoid degeneration*, and *lipohyalinosis*. Fisher also recognized that sometimes larger deep infarcts, which he dubbed *giant lacunes*, could be caused by occlusion of parent vessels, such as the middle cerebral artery (MCA) stem, causing obstruction of the orifices of lateral lenticulostriate arteries.[12]

Fisher,[13,14] Cole and Yates,[15] and Rosenblum[16] recognized that small aneurysmal dilatations of these lipohyalinotic penetrating arteries could potentially rupture, causing intracerebral hemorrhage (ICH). These lesions were probably similar to those recognized by Charcot and Bouchard[17] as the cause of parenchymatous bleeding. The distribution of deep hypertensive hemorrhages was the same as the locations of lacunes (putamen, capsule, thalamus, and pons). Lipohyalinotic arteries could occlude, leading to lacunar infarction, or rupture, causing ICH.[13] Fisher reviewed the charts of 114 patients who had lacunes at necropsy. All but three patients had hypertension defined by a prior history of this disease, ele-

vated blood pressure recorded on examination, or heart weight exceeding 400 g without other explanation.[1] Fisher attributed segmental arterial disorganization and lipohyalinosis to hypertension.

Foix and Hillemand,[9,10,18–20] Stopford,[21,22] and Düret[23,24] defined the territories of arteries that branched from the parent cerebral and basilar arteries. More recently, Pullicino reviewed in detail the anatomy of these arteries[25] and their usual territories of supply.[26] Foix recognized that infarcts were often limited to the territories of one of these branches. The orifices of these branches were often obstructed by a pathology different from lipohyalinosis. Fisher and Caplan,[27] Fisher,[28] and Caplan[29] described the vascular pathology in these branches. Fisher and Caplan[27] reported vascular lesions causing ischemia limited to the territory of basilar artery branches, separating this vasculopathy from lipohyalinosis. This pathology is referred to as *intracerebral branch atheromatous disease* (Figures 8-2 through 8-4).[29] The orifices of the penetrating branches could be blocked by atheroma in the parent artery, atheroma could originate in the parent artery and extend into the branch (so-called junctional plaques), or *microatheroma* could arise at the origin of the branch itself. Thrombus was often superimposed on

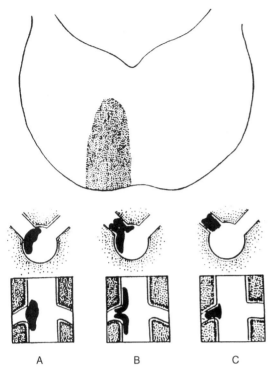

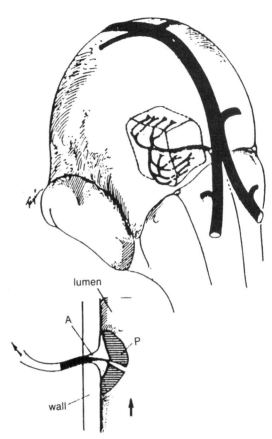

Figure 8-2. Top drawing shows an infarct (*stippled area*) in the left basis pontis. Bottom drawings show (**A**) plaque within parent artery, blocking the orifice of the branch; (**B**) plaque within the parent artery, extending into the branch (junctional plaque); (**C**) microatheroma, formed within the branch and blocking it.

Figure 8-3. Basilar branch occlusion: The diagram at the bottom shows a close-up of the artery shown within the cube above. A plaque (*arrow*) is seen extending into the branch. (A = atheroma; P = plaque.) (Reprinted with permission from CM Fisher, LR Caplan. Basilar artery branch occlusion: a cause of pontine infarction. Neurology 1971;21:900–905.)

the atheromas. This vasculopathy can be called microatheroma and is clearly distinct on pathologic grounds from the arteriopathy underlying lacunes.[30] Pontine infarcts are the most frequent pathologic lesion found in necropsies of diabetics and must, in most cases, be caused by atheromatous branch disease.[31] Infarcts limited to the territories of the anterior choroidal arteries (AChA) and the thalamogeniculate arteries are also most often explained by atheromatous branch disease. Microatheromas, parent-artery plaques, and occlusion of parent arteries by in situ thrombosis or embolism probably explain deep infarcts in normotensive patients. Although lipohyalinosis and microatheroma are readily separated by meticulous pathologic examination, the distinction is nearly impossible clinically. Boiten categorized 100 patients with lacunes into two separate groups.[32] One group had atherosclerotic risk factors and single symptomatic lacunes;

the other group had hypertension, multiple lacunes (some of which were asymptomatic) and white matter lucency on neuroimaging scans. He posited that the former group had atheromatous branch disease and the latter group had lipohyalinosis.[32] Because the prognosis for branch occlusions and lacunes is probably identical and treatment is similar, there is little practical reason to clinically separate lacunes from branch infarcts.

General Clinical Findings

A 56-year-old African-American man, RB, awakened with weakness of his right arm.

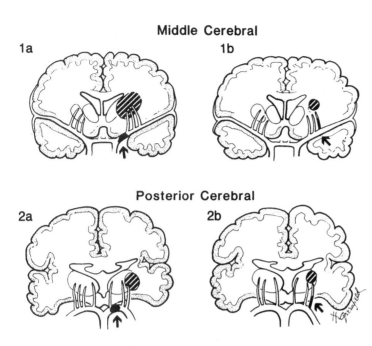

Figure 8-4. Mechanisms of deep infarction: (**1a**) basal ganglionic capsular infarct resulting from middle cerebral arteryt occlusion (*arrow*), (**1b**) smaller deep capsular infarct owing to lenticulostriate artery occlusion (*arrow*), (**2a**) lateral thalamic infarct owing to posterior cerebral artery occlusion (*arrow*), (**2b**) lateral thalamic infarct resulting from thalamogeniculate artery occlusion (*arrow*). (Reprinted with permission from LR Caplan, LD DeWitt, MS Pessin, et al. Lateral thalamic infarcts. Arch Neurol 1988;45:959–964. Copyright © American Medical Association.)

As he stood to go to the bathroom, he became aware that his right leg was also weak. He called his wife, who noted that his voice was slightly thick. He did not have a headache, nor did he feel dizzy or otherwise unwell. As the day progressed, the weakness in his arm and leg seemed to fluctuate. By nightfall, however, he could not move his right arm or right leg. He had no prior history of stroke, heart disease, or claudication and did not recognize any warnings days before the episode. Two months earlier, a physician told him that his blood pressure was high and "bore watching," but prescribed no medication.

Fisher repeatedly emphasized in his writings that hypertension was the major cause of fibrinoid degeneration and lipohyalinosis, the arteriopathy that leads to lacunar infarcts. Others have noted a lower frequency of hypertension in patients, in which computed tomography (CT) verified the diagnosis of lacunar infarcts (52.5%,[33] 57%,[34] 65%,[35] 72%[36]). Seventy-five percent of patients clinically diagnosed as having lacunar infarcts in the Harvard Stroke Registry had hypertension.[37] In a necropsy study, 64% of patients with lacunes at postmortem had a history of hypertension.[38] For a more thorough evaluation, Fisher used pathologic criteria to diagnose lacunes and hypertension (heart weight >400 g with no other cause), and carefully searched hospital and doctors' notes for past blood-pressure recordings. Although clearly not all patients with deep infarcts are hypertensive, a diagnosing physician should be wary of attributing a lesion to small vessel occlusive disease if there is no past or current evidence of hypertension or diabetes. I have also seen normotensive patients with elevated hematocrits who have a clinical picture of lacunar infarction, possibly caused by clotting within small arteries. Fisher found severe large vessel atherosclerosis in 64% of the 114 patients with lacunes, a frequency far exceeding the usual 9% found in a population without lacunes.[1] Thus, hypertension definitely predisposes patients to premature atherosclerosis of large extracranial and intracranial arteries. Large and small vessel diseases frequently coexist, so the mere presence of clinical, noninvasive, or angiographic evidence of atherosclerotic stenosis does not exclude a lacunar etiology of stroke.

Lacunes are small and deep. Because there is no accompanying over-distension of superficial arteries and deep arteries have no pain fibers, headache caused by vascular distension does not occur in patients with lacunes. These small lesions produce no mass effect that might cause headache or decreased alertness. Lacunes are far from the cortex and do not produce seizures[37] or affect the surface-recorded electroencephalogram (EEG).[39] The presence of decreased alertness, unaccustomed headache, or seizures argue against a lacunar etiology of a stroke.

The course of illness in patients with lacunar infarction is also different from patients with large artery occlusive disease and cerebral embolism.[37,40] Prior transient ischemic attacks (TIAs) occur in approximately 20% of patients with lacunes,[40–42] a frequency far below that for large vessel disease but more than in cerebral embolism. When TIAs do occur in patients with lacunar infarcts, they span a shorter time interval and are more stereotyped than in other ischemic etiologies. Brief, stereotyped TIAs may occur many times during a day. The deficit often evolves gradually in patients with lacunar infarcts, with frequent fluctuations and progression during the initial 72 hours of the stroke. Sudden deficits, maximal at onset, are less frequent than in patients with other etiologies of ischemic stroke. Gradual worsening of paralysis over a few days is a characteristic course in some patients with pure motor hemiparesis caused by lacunar infarction.

> On examination of patient RB, the blood pressure was 165/95 mm Hg. He was alert and understood, repeated, and used language normally. The patient read, wrote, and spelled words correctly. His voice was slightly slurred. His right face, shoulder, arm, hand, thigh, and foot were moderately weak. Deep tendon reflexes were exaggerated on the right, and the right plantar response was extensor. He felt touch normally in his right limbs and could identify accurately the nature of objects in his right hand. He could also localize spots touched on his right limbs. Visual fields were normal.

Lacunes have a predilection for particular anatomic sites—those nourished by penetrating arteries. Some of these deep lesions produce characteristic clinical syndromes, whereas others are clinically silent or produce findings difficult to distinguish from superficial infarction. In a necropsy series of 167 patients with lacunes, 93 patients (56%) had no

reported related symptoms.[38] Anatomic localization is probably most helpful in the diagnosis of lacunes. RB had paralysis of face, arm, and leg with exaggerated reflexes and an extensor toe sign. A lesion of the motor cortex causing these findings would have to extend from the face area near the sylvian fissure, a region fed by the MCA, to the paramedian frontal lobe foot area, which is fed by the anterior cerebral artery. Such a lesion would invariably affect language, sensation, or vision. A sizable superficial or deep frontal-lobe lesion would not only produce motor dysfunction, but would also likely cause conjugate eye deviation to the side of the lesion and abulia. Marie emphasized hemiplegia as the sign of lacunar infarction.[7] Fisher termed the syndrome of isolated weakness of face, arm, and leg *pure motor hemiplegia*,[12] and taught that these findings are diagnostic of lacunar infarction in the pons or internal capsule. Some authors,[35,43,44] using radioisotope studies or CT, found lesions other than lacunes in patients with pure motor hemiplegia. MRI is even more sensitive and shows cortical lesions in some patients clinically thought to have a lacunar syndrome. Remember that Fisher examined the patients intensively. When he called the patient's syndrome *pure motor*, he had compulsively tested sensation, visual fields, and cortical function and found them normal. Fisher also demanded that weakness include face, arm, and leg and that hypertension be present to make the diagnosis of a pure motor stroke. Patient RB fulfills Fisher's criteria for pure motor hemiplegia. Were patients with CT lesions, other than lacunes, examined in the same compulsive and thorough manner as an important requisite for the clinical diagnosis of lacunes in these other radiographic studies? I advise a strategy similar to that taught in high school geometry: Try to prove your original diagnostic impression wrong. Seek out features (i.e., sensory, visual, or intellectual abnormalities) that would disprove your diagnosis. Mental status testing is key because most pure-motor hemiplegia patients with lesions other than lacunes have some aberration in alertness, behavior, or intellect that suggests frontal lobe disease.

Even when the lacunar syndromes are apparently pure, some patients have a small hematoma as the cause of the syndrome. Small putaminal, capsular, and pontine hematomas are known to cause pure motor hemiparesis and other syndromes most often caused by lacunar infarction.[40,42,45,46] Before clinicians can be secure in their diagnosis of lacunar infarction, I believe neuroimaging tests (CT or MRI), which show a lacune or exclude parenchymatous hemorrhage and surface infarction, are mandatory. Diffusion-weighted MRI has the capacity for separating recent lacunar infarcts from old lesions.

Location of Lesions and Clinical Syndromes

Hemispheral Lesions within the Anterior Circulation

Probably the most commonly recognized clinical syndrome in patients with lacunes in the cerebral hemispheres is pure-motor hemiparesis. Patient RB had this syndrome. The causative lesion is usually found in the internal capsule. The three types of capsular lesions causing pure-motor hemiparesis distinguished by Rascol and colleagues are (1) large lesions spanning the anterior and posterior limbs of the capsule, caused by occlusion of large lateral lenticulostriate arteries; (2) capsulopallidal infarcts located predominantly in the posterior limb of the capsule in the territory of medial lenticulostriate arteries; and (3) lesions in the anterior limb and caudate nucleus in the supply region of the recurrent artery of Heubner.[40,42] MRI studies show that patients with pure-motor hemiparesis can also have lesions in the midbrain, pons, and medulla, affecting descending corticospinal fibers in the cerebral peduncle, basis pontis, or medullary pyramid.[47,48]

Motor weakness does not always equally affect the face, arm, and leg. Often, the face is at least partially spared.[40] At times, almost a pure monoparesis of the arm or leg is present with only minimal weakness or hyperreflexia of the other limb. In the Stroke Data Bank, the clinical findings related to the degree of involvement of face, arm, and leg did not correlate with the location of the lesion in the internal capsule.[40,49] Mohr summarized,

> There no longer seems much reason to adhere to the older dogma[50] that the motor fibers occupy the anterior half of the posterior limb of the internal capsule. . . . Further, the available case material does not document a series of cases with an homunculus whose face is anterior and whose leg is posterior in the plane of the internal capsule.[40]

In some patients with lacunar infarction, the clinical picture includes a combination of weakness, pyramidal signs, cerebellar-type ataxia, and incoordination of the limbs on one side of the body. This syndrome was first called *homolateral ataxia and crural paresis* in patients in whom the predominant involvement was in the lower limbs.[51] Later, Fisher dubbed the syndrome *ataxic hemiparesis*, indicating that the arm and leg could be variously involved, but the major signature of the syndrome was the combination of cerebellar and motor signs in the limbs on the same side of the body.[52] In some patients, there are also sensory symptoms ipsilateral to the motor abnormalities.[53] The relative severity of ataxia compared to weakness varies considerably, as does the relative involvement of arm compared to leg. Localization of lesions causing ataxic hemiparesis varies widely. Many lesions are in the posterior limb of the internal capsule. Lacunes in the midbrain and pons, however, can also cause this clinical syndrome.

At times, the clinical findings show abnormalities of motor function on one side of the body, but there is no true paralysis, reflexes are not exaggerated, and the plantar response is flexor. I refer to these findings as a *nonpyramidal hemimotor syndrome*. Some lesions that cause these clinical findings involve the striatum and the globus pallidus. Decreased spontaneous and associated movements, clumsiness, slight increased resistance to passive movement, and slowness of the affected limbs are often found. Some patients have a minor degree of hemi-parkinsonism. Others have a movement disorder with choreic features. Some patients with hemichorea have had striatal infarcts.[54,55]

Sometimes, the predominant dysfunction in patients with hemispheral lacunes is bulbar. Dysarthria, dysphagia, and even mutism may occur, caused by interruption of corticobulbar fibers in the white matter underlying the motor cortex, capsule, striatum, or pons. Limb symptoms may be minor or absent. Tapping the corner of the mouth may show heightened contraction of the orbicularis oris, orbicularis oculi on the side of the bulbar dysfunction, or on both sides of the face. Often, the tongue and face are weak on one side. In patients with predominantly bulbar signs, the lesions are often bilateral and the syndrome is pseudobulbar.[56] The initial lesion sometimes produces no symptoms or only minor hemimotor signs. When the contralateral side of the brain becomes involved, the bilateral disturbance in corticobulbar fibers causes predominantly bulbar abnormalities, especially dysarthria and dysphagia, sometimes with exaggerated laughing and crying.

In Chapter 6, I discuss caudate[57] and AChA-territory infarcts.[58–60] Infarcts in these regions can be quite small, readily qualifying as lacunes, or they can be more extensive, deep infarcts. Caudate lesions can be limited to the caudate nucleus or extend into the anterior limb of the internal capsule and anterior putamen.[57] AChA-territory infarcts can involve the globus pallidus or the posterior limb of the internal capsule.[56,58–60] Infarcts in these areas are probably caused by intracranial-branch atheromatous disease, affecting one or more of Heubner's arteries and the AChA.[29]

Involvement of small penetrating branches of these arteries is probably most often caused by microatheromas or lipohyalinosis. Neuropathologic studies of patients with lesions in the distribution of Heubner's artery and the AChA are too scanty to document or refute this hypothesis.[29] Some patients with caudate infarcts have prominent dysarthria and cognitive and behavioral abnormalities, especially abulia and restlessness.[57] Some patients with left caudate infarcts have aphasia, usually slight and transient. In a necropsy series of patients with lacunes found at postmortem, aphasia with right hemiparesis was one of the most frequent clinical syndromes correlating with lacunar infarction.[38] The responsible lesions were in the striatum and anterior limb of the internal capsule or the thalamus.

Posterior Circulation, Brain Stem, Thalamic Lacunes, and Branch Occlusions

Pons and Medulla

Lacunes and branch-territory infarcts are often found in the pons.[47,48,61,62] In a prospective study of MRI scans in 100 patients hospitalized with lacunar infarcts in Grenoble, France, 38 of the lesions (25%) were in the pons.[47] Among 12 patients in another series studied acutely with MRI, 6 of 11 lesions were located in the pons and had symptoms appropriate to that localization.[63] The most common site of the pontine lesions is in the basis pontis on one side, most often medially in the distribution of one of the paramedian branches of the basilar artery.[61,62] Few necropsy specimens of patients with infarcts in this location have been studied.

The pathology in some has been lipohyalinosis and segmental arterial disorganization of penetrating arteries within the basis pontis.[2,12]

In three patients, arterial lesions involving basilar-artery branches were studied in more detail by serially sectioning the pons, with the basilar artery and its branches still attached to the pons.[27,28] In one patient, an atheromatous plaque within the basilar artery obstructed the intramural part of the 0.5-mm–diameter basilar-artery branch.[27] Distally, in the blocked branch, there was a mass of agglutinated platelets, which arose as a tiny intra-arterial embolus from the lesion in the parent artery or formed in situ because of reduced flow. In another patient, a plaque arising in the lumen of the basilar artery extended into the mouth of a 0.5-mm–diameter branch, forming a junctional plaque.[27] In a third patient, basilar-artery branches were blocked bilaterally.[28] At the orifice of a basilar branch in this patient, a microdissection made a crevice in a plaque, and a superimposed thrombus obstructed the branch. The mechanisms of blockage of branches are depicted in Figures 8-2 through 8-4. Flat or elevated plaques in the parent basilar artery can block the orifices of branches or provide a nidus for small embolic fragments that extend into the branches. A dilated dolichoectatic basilar artery can also distort branch orifices.

Infarction of the medullary pyramid can give rise to a pure-motor hemiparesis, often sparing the face.[12,61,64–66] Lesions are basomedial in the territory of anterior spinal artery branches. The three major syndromes in the pons related to infarcts in the basis pontis are pure-motor hemiparesis, ataxic hemiparesis, and dysarthria-clumsy hand syndromes.[67,68] Pure-motor hemiplegia is probably the most common of the syndromes and occurs most often when the pontine infarcts are in the paramedian basis pontis. In some patients, additional findings help identify the pontine locus. An ipsilateral VI-nerve palsy or intranuclear ophthalmoplegia are occasionally associated with the contralateral hemiparesis.[27,61,67] Involvement of the tegmentum and base can include the paramedian pontine reticular formation, causing a conjugate-gaze palsy toward the side of the lesion, accompanied by contralateral limb weakness and pyramidal signs. At times, although there is no gaze palsy, conjugate-gaze movements are asymmetric with slight abnormalities of ipsilateral conjugate gaze. Involvement of the medial lemniscus, as well as pyramidal tract fibers, leads to some sensory symptoms and signs on the side of the hemiparesis.[67,68] Usually, these are minor paresthesias and a slight loss of vibration sense, with preserved pinprick and temperature sensation.

The basis pontis carries fibers crossing into the brachium pontis, traveling toward the cerebellum. Interruption of pontocerebellar fibers can cause cerebellar-type incoordination and ataxia. Ataxic hemiparesis is often caused by a pontine lesion.[51,52,61,62,67,68] The infarcts that cause ataxic hemiparesis are usually smaller and more rostral, dorsal, and lateral than the lesions associated with pure-motor hemiparesis.[61,62,68] Subtle, minor incoordination of the ipsilateral limbs can provide a clue to this localization because pontocerebellar-crossing fibers are involved bilaterally, to some extent. The dysarthria clumsy-hand syndrome is usually caused by a small lacune in the more dorsal portion of the basis pontis, affecting corticobulbar fibers near the medial lemniscus.[61,62,68,69] Often, associated facial and tongue weakness is severe, but examination of the hand and arm is nearly normal, despite the patient's report of awkwardness.

Occasionally, lacunes are located in the medial or lateral pontine tegmentum in the distribution of branches that penetrate horizontally from long, circumferential arteries or penetrate from the base of the pons.[61,62,70] These lacunes are the ischemic counterpart of lateral tegmental brain stem hematomas.[71] These lesions usually involve the sensory lemniscus that has formed from the joining of the medial lemniscus and lateral spinothalamic tracts in the rostral pons. Or these lesions may involve the medial lemniscus or the spinothalamic tract before formation of the sensory lemniscus. A pure, sensory, strokelike syndrome occurs with subjective paresthesias or numbness (or both) in the contralateral face, arm, and leg. Dizziness, gait ataxia, dysarthria, and nystagmus are variable accompaniments.[70,72,73]

Midbrain

In the midbrain, penetrating-artery lesions involve primarily the cerebral peduncle and the paramedian zones. Few examples have been reported in detail.[61,74–76] Some infarcts in this distribution are caused by occlusion of the parent posterior cerebral artery (PCA).[77] The distribution of the penetrating branches of the PCA is diagrammed in Figure 7-12.

One clinical syndrome includes a third nerve palsy ipsilaterally, caused by involvement of the fascicles of the third nerve within the midbrain, accompanied by a contralateral hemiparesis (Weber's syndrome). In some patients, involvement of the red nucleus, as well as the cerebral peduncle on the same side, gives rise to a combination of motor weakness and tremor. The tremor usually develops as the hemiparesis improves and is present at rest and on intention. The affected arm is usually also quite incoordinated and ataxic. Few cases of midbrain branch lesions with neuropathologic confirmation have been reported.[77,78]

Thalamus

Thalamic lacunes are quite common. In the MRI study of Hommel and colleagues, thalamic lesions accounted for 14% of the lacunes.[47] Penetrating-artery territory infarcts are located paramedially in the distribution of the various thalamoperforating arteries and laterally in the distribution of the thalamogeniculate artery or the lateral posterior choroidal artery. The two most important and consistent paramedian thalamoperforating arteries are the polar (tuberothalamic) artery and the thalamic-subthalamic arteries.[61,78–86] The polar artery arises on each side from the middle third of the posterior communicating artery and supplies the anteromedial and anterolateral thalamic nuclei. At times, this vessel is absent, in which case its territory is supplied by the thalamic-subthalamic arteries. The predominant findings in infarcts fed by the thalamoperforating arteries are cognitive and behavioral, but the syndromes do differ, depending on the artery involved.[61,81,83,85,86] Unilateral anterolateral thalamic infarction in the distribution of the polar artery on the left or right side usually causes abulia, facial asymmetry, transient minor contralateral motor abnormalities and, at times, aphasia (left lesions) or visual neglect (right lesions). Abulia, with slowness, decreased amount of activity and speech, and long delays in responding to queries or conversation, is the predominant abnormality. Some patients are disorganized and dress in a slovenly manner. Usually, in patients with unilateral lesions, abulia, cognitive, and behavioral changes improve after 3–6 months. Occasionally, bilateral infarcts are found in the territory of the polar artery of each side.[87] This means that bilateral arteries probably occasionally arise from a single or loop artery, or a common rete. When the polar artery is affected bilaterally, the behavioral abnormality is more severe and persistent. Memory may also be affected.[87] The behavioral effects are probably explained by the synaptic corticothalamic relationship with the frontal lobe and other cortical regions.

The thalamic-subthalamic arteries originate from the proximal PCAs and supply the most posteromedial portion of the thalamus near the posterior commissure. The right- and left-sided arteries may arise separately, but can originate from a single unilateral artery or a common pedicle.[61,78,79] Unilateral lesions are usually characterized by paresis of vertical gaze (upward or both upward and downward) and by amnesia. Motor and sensory signs and symptoms are absent. The pathway for vertical gaze includes the rostral interstitial nucleus of the medial longitudinal fasciculus and connections between the two eyes for vertical eye movements, which travel through the commissures at the diencephalic-mesencephalic junction. A unilateral lesion interrupts these commissural fibers, thus causing conjugate vertical-gaze palsy.[88] Memory loss may be severe, with profound difficulty in forming new memories and encoding recent events. The amnesia often improves within 6 months in unilateral infarct patients. Bilateral butterfly-shaped paramedian posterior thalamic infarction can result from a branch occlusion of a single supplying artery or pedicle, although scant necropsy data are available from well-studied cases.[61,78,80,89] Hypersomnolence and bilateral third-nerve palsies can occur in patients with bilateral infarcts.[89] The same syndrome can result from occlusion of the rostral basilar artery, as discussed in Chapter 7.

Lacunes and branch-territory infarcts are especially common in the lateral thalamus. This region, including the somatosensory nuclei (ventral posterior lateral and ventral posterior medial) and the ventral lateral and ventral anterior nuclei, is supplied by the thalamogeniculate group of arteries. These vessels arise from the PCA and are the posterior circulation counterpart of the lenticulostriate branches of the MCA. Occlusion of these arteries or their branches leads to a variety of different clinical syndromes.[61,90]

Larger lateral thalamic infarcts were first described by Dejerine and Roussy, and the clinical findings have long been referred to as *le syndrome thalamique*.[91] The essential features of this syndrome, almost always caused by atheromatous-branch disease in my experience, are contralateral hemisensory symptoms accompanied by contralateral limb ataxia. At times, there are jumpy adventitious hemichoreic movements of the contralateral arm, and the hand may tend to assume a fisted posture. Some patients have a transient hemiparesis at onset that improves quickly.

Usually, the sensory phenomena are mostly paresthesias, which involve the face, neck, trunk, and limbs. Sensory loss is usually slight. The sensory signs relate to ischemia of the somatosensory nuclei. The ataxia is caused by interruption of cerebellofugal fibers going to the ventral anterior and ventral lateral nuclei. Also interrupted are fibers from the striatum (the ansa lenticularis), which are projected toward these motor nuclei. Dystonia, chorea, and hemiparkinsonian-like features are probably caused by interruption of these extrapyramidal-system projections. Pain in the affected limbs and trunk may develop months after the original stroke and was one of the cardinal features mentioned by Dejerine and Roussy.[91] Many patients never have pain. Pain is almost never noted at or shortly after onset.

Occlusion of branches of the thalamogeniculate arteries supplying the somatosensory nuclei is responsible for the vast majority of patients with so-called pure sensory stroke.[92–95] In this condition, the patient has somatosensory complaints without other signs or symptoms. Most often, the patient describes numbness, tingling, or pins-and-needles sensations in the face, limbs, and trunk. All hemicorporeal sensations are represented in the thalamic somatosensory relay nuclei. In the somatosensory cortex, the hand and face have large representations, whereas little space is accorded to the trunk, scalp, and other regions not capable of fine sensory distinctions. Thus, numbness of the inner mouth, eye, ear, scalp, chest, back, abdomen, and genitalia is much more common in thalamic lacunes than in superficial lesions of the parietal cortex.[93,94]

After a few days, the somatic sensations may take on an unpleasant quality and may be characterized as burning, tightness, or soreness.[93,94] Sensory symptoms may be transient or permanent, even when lacunar infarction is present on MRI. Usually, subjective sensory complaints are more prominent than objective loss of sensation. Many patients with pure sensory stroke have no detectable loss of threshold to any sensory modality, whereas others show only a minimal qualitative or quantitative difference between the two sides of the body. Motor, visual, and intellectual functions are normal. Occasionally, pure sensory stroke can be caused by a lateral or medial tegmental pontine or midbrain infarct.[61,70,72,73,96]

Occlusion of thalamogeniculate branches, on occasion, can cause a syndrome referred to as *sensory motor stroke*.[97] This condition is characterized by the sensory symptoms and signs described in relation to pure sensory stroke. These symptoms are accompanied by paresis and pyramidal signs in the same limbs as the sensory symptoms. Few such cases have been studied at necropsy. In one well-studied case, the responsible infarct involved the somatosensory nuclei. Pallor of the adjacent posterior limb of the internal capsule was evident.[97] Review of the drawings from the original Dejerine-Roussy article clearly shows that lateral thalamic infarcts often affect the adjacent internal capsule.[61,90,91] The thalamogeniculate arteries must sometimes supply this zone, contrary to the teachings in some neuroanatomy texts. Ischemia of the internal capsule is probably responsible for the transient paresis found in some patients with lateral thalamic infarcts and for the motor abnormalities in patients with sensory motor stroke.

Infarcts in the territory of the medial and lateral posterior choroidal arteries are the least well known and most rarely reported of all thalamic infarcts. The lateral posterior choroidal arteries supply mostly the pulvinar, a portion of the lateral geniculate body, and the anterior nucleus. The medial arteries supply the habenula, anterior pulvinar part of the center median nucleus, and the paramedial nuclei.[61] There have been few clinical pathologic and clinical neuroimaging reports of patients with posterior choroidal territory infarcts.[61,86,98,99]

Hemianopia, hemisensory symptoms, and behavioral abnormalities may occur in patients with posterior choroidal artery territory infarcts. The most specific and well-defined abnormality relates to the visual fields. The posterior choroidal arteries and their lateral choroidal artery branches supply a portion of the lateral geniculate body reciprocal to that supplied by the AChAs. The characteristic visual field defect in patients with posterior choroidal artery territory infarcts is a sectoranopia, involving a wedge-shaped defect on each side of the horizontal meridian.[99,100] In contrast, the visual field defect in patients with AChA-territory infarcts can include loss of the upper and lower quadrants, with sparing of vision in a line along the median horizontal meridian. Patients with posterior choroidal

territory infarcts can also have an upper or lower quadrantanopia.[86]

Laboratory Investigations in Patients Suspected of Having Lacunar Strokes

Having described the known lacunar syndromes and their usual responsible lesions, I return to patient RB, who had hypertension and the clinical findings of pure motor hemiparesis.

> In RB, the complete blood cell count was normal. EEG showed minor symmetric slowing. CT showed a small infarct in the posterior limb of the internal capsule on the left and a tiny lesion in the right putamen. MRI also showed these lesions and another tiny lacune in the right thalamus. Magnetic resonance diffusion-weighted scans showed a bright lesion in the posterior limb of the left internal capsule. Magnetic resonance angiography and ultrasound of the carotid and vertebral arteries were normal.

Because lacunes are small and deep in the hemisphere or are located in the brain stem, they usually do not have a major influence on the EEG recorded from the convexity.[39] CT findings depend on the location and size of the lesion. Pontine lacunes are seldom imaged by CT, but can nearly always be seen on MRI scans.[61] Pure motor hemiplegia probably has the highest frequency of CT positivity among the lacunar syndromes. Rascol et al. found hypodense lesions on CT in 29 of 30 patients with pure motor stroke.[42] They divided the lesions into large capsulo-putamino-caudate infarcts, and smaller capsulo-pallido or capsulo-caudate infarcts.[42] Some patients with larger infarcts had angiographic abnormalities in the lenticulostriate arteries. Others have reported MCA occlusive disease in patients with large basal ganglionic and capsular infarctions.[29,101–104] In contrast, patients with pure sensory stroke seldom have lesions visible on CT.[93]

MRI is undoubtedly superior to CT in imaging small brain stem and thalamic infarcts.[47,48,61,63,105] Rothrock and colleagues evaluated 31 patients with the clinical diagnosis of lacunar infarction. Twenty-three patients (74%) had appropriate lesions on MRI.[63] When CT and MRI were performed, MRI was superior in imaging lesions appropriate to the symptoms. In another study among 110 patients, MRI was effective in imaging one or more possibly responsible lacunar infarcts in 89 patients.[47] When gadolinium-diethylene-triamine penta-acetic acid enhancement is given, acute lacunar infarcts are generally enhanced.[105] Use of enhancement may be helpful when the clinicians find more than one lesion and are uncertain of the age of the lesions. Generally, only acute lesions are enhanced. Diffusion-weighted MRI is especially useful in showing lacunar infarcts soon after symptoms begin, and in separating recent infarcts from old infarcts. Only recent lesions are shown well on diffusion-weighted MRI. CT or MRI is essential for excluding small hemorrhages from the differential diagnosis; such hemorrhages can cause findings identical to lacunar syndromes. By imaging hemosiderin, MRI is more effective than CT in determining whether old lesions were small hematomas or lacunar infarcts.

Angiographic abnormalities have been shown in some patients with lacunar infarcts, and include carotid artery and MCA disease.[104] Some large artery lesions are probably incidental and unrelated to the cause of the stroke. Necropsy studies have shown that most patients with hypertension and lacunes have a high incidence of coexisting atherosclerosis. Angiography in apparently healthy prisoners[106] also shows a high frequency of atherosclerosis. Thus, the finding of atherosclerotic occlusive disease in larger extracranial and intracranial arteries does not prove an etiologic relationship to the lacunar infarct. In some cases, blockage of parent arteries can produce infarction in territories of lenticulostriate, thalamogeniculate, and pontine penetrating arteries. Figure 8-4 diagrammatically depicts the vascular lesions in occlusion of penetrating and parent arteries. The lesion in the parent artery can be a plaque, in situ thrombosis, or an embolus.[29] Parentartery lesions are especially important to consider in patients with lacunes exceeding 20 mm, which involve the basal ganglia and capsule. In my experience, the clinical syndrome usually includes more features than the usual lacunar syndrome.[29,103] Echocardiography and cardiac rhythm monitoring are also important to exclude cardiac-origin embolism to parent arteries in some patients. The larger deep infarcts are less often caused by lipohyalinosis.

Neuroimaging, preferably with MRI, is important in every patient. The need for thorough laboratory testing depends on the (1) presence of appropriate risk factors, such as hypertension, polycythemia, or diabetes; (2) typicality of the neurologic findings; (3) thoroughness of the neurologic examination and the experience of the examining physician[107]; and (4) the neuroimaging results. If the patient has no evidence of past or present hypertension, physicians should be skeptical of lipohyalinosis as the cause of infarction. Atypical neurologic findings or the presence of unaccustomed headache, reduced alertness, or seizures argue for more complete laboratory investigations. At times, unexpected superficial infarcts, small hemorrhages, and even nonvascular conditions, such as tumors, are discovered by CT or MRI.

When the clinical diagnosis is uncertain, extracranial and transcranial ultrasound, computed tomography angiography, magnetic resonance angiography, or standard angiography may be indicated. Generally, after preliminary evaluation, which should include a detailed history and examination, blood studies, EEG, and either CT or MRI, physicians are able to place the patient with brain ischemia into one of three categories: (1) high certainty of lacune; (2) lesion consistent with a lacune but not diagnostic (atypical lacune); or (3) findings not compatible with a lacunar etiology. Examples of possible findings in these three groups are listed in Table 8-1. Patients in categories two and three require more evaluation than those in category one.

> RB was kept on bed rest. Weakness began to improve during the second week, when he was transferred to a rehabilitation hospital. While he was at the rehabilitation hospital, he was referred to an internist who carefully followed him and instituted antihypertensive treatment.

Treatment

No treatment has been shown to modify the course of lacunar infarction. The morphologic nature of lipohyalinosis and fibrinoid degeneration, both of which involve lesions of the vessel wall and not the arterial intima, make it theoretically unlikely that thrombolytic agents, anticoagulants, or agents that decrease platelet aggregation would be effective treatments. Anecdotal reports indicate that anticoagulants are not effective.[108] My own experience confirms that patients continue to progress while

Table 8-1. Findings in Patients with Suspected Lacunar Infarction

	Diagnosis Highly Probable	Diagnosis Likely but Uncertain	Lacune Unlikely or Excluded
Ecology	Hypertension	Diabetic Mild hypertension	No hypertension
Neurologic signs	Paralysis of right face, arm, leg	Paralysis (right) arm > leg	Paralysis of right hand
	No other findings	No other signs	Aphasia
Other symptoms	None	Slight unaccustomed headache	Severe headache
			Seizure at onset
Laboratory	Compatible small deep infarct on MRI or CT	Normal CT	Hypodensity (left) frontal region or other cortical zone on CT; hemorrhage on CT or MRI

CT = computed tomography; MRI = magnetic resonance imaging.

receiving heparin. The disease is far beyond the reach of the surgeon's knife.

Infarction is most likely related to impaired blood flow beyond the region of penetrating artery obstruction. Logical treatment is optimization of blood pressure, blood volume, and blood flow. Because the lesion is caused by hypertension, the most logical therapy to prevent new lipohyalinotic disease is to carefully control the blood pressure. Overzealous reduction of blood pressure during the acute ischemia, however, can decrease flow in collateral arteries and expand the region of infarction.[27,28] I prefer to wait until after the first 2–3 weeks of the stroke to institute major reductions in blood pressure. I try to maximize blood flow during the first days and keep the patient at rest with the head flat to augment cranial flow. If the vascular etiology of the lesion is parent-vessel disease and not lipohyalinosis, then treatment of that condition is appropriate.

Some authors and physicians do not include lacunar infarction in their differential diagnosis of brain ischemia because they believe clinical recognition of the disorder is unreliable. I believe that its inclusion is important for two reasons. First, the disorder is common; to omit a lesion found in 10% of all brains is foolhardy. Second, recognition of this etiology has a direct behavioral result—that is, no aggressive diagnostic testing, and no anticoagulant or surgical treatment is prescribed. Randomized trials of various treatments are needed in patients with well-defined lacunar infarction to test these hypotheses. The investigation and treatment of other causes of cerebral ischemia—large artery occlusive disease, brain

embolism, and systemic hypotension—are quite different. In addition, technologic advances, especially MRI, have greatly improved the clinical diagnosis of lacunar infarction.

Chronic Small Vessel Disease

The disorder that leads to single lacunar infarcts often involves multiple penetrating arteries. As a result, multiple lacunar infarcts are often found in the brain at necropsy or are visible on MRI scans. In the necropsy study of Tuszynski and colleagues, 169 patients had 327 lacunes, an average of 1.9 lacunes per patient.[38] Less than one-half of the patients (46%) had only one lacune, 16% had two, and 38% had three or more lacunes. Investigators in the past[1–7] found an even higher frequency of multiple lesions, but more widespread control of hypertension has likely altered this tendency. Most often, lacunes involve the striatum, capsule, thalamus, cerebral white matter, and pons. When extensive, they give the deeper portions of the brain a Swiss cheese–like appearance. This condition was often referred to as *état lacunaire* after Pierre Marie.[7] Traditionally, the clinical findings have been described as including (1) pseudobulbar abnormalities of speech, swallowing, and emotional control; (2) small stepped gait; (3) parkinsonian-like rigidity; (4) hyperreflexia; (5) extensor plantar reflexes; (6) dementia with slow thinking and responses; and (7) variable weakness and sensory signs and symptoms. More recent experience, especially from CT and MRI, raises questions about this traditional view. First, many patients with multiple lacunes seem quite well preserved and function normally. Second, patients with the syndrome described almost always have associated, rather severe changes in the cerebral white matter and ventricular enlargement. Most clinicians and investigators are inclined to ascribe the dementia and clinical signs more to the white matter disease (dubbed *leuko-araiosis* by Hachinski)[109] than to the lacunes. The combination of lacunes, white matter gliosis, and atrophy almost invariably occur together and are associated with widespread abnormalities of penetrating small arteries.[110] The combination should be considered a chronic brain microvasculopathy.

The chronic white matter changes were initially described by Otto Binswanger.[111,112] Olszewski, in a review of the history and pathology of the condition, used the term *subcortical arteriosclerotic encephalopathy*.[113,114] Babikian and Ropper reviewed the pathologic features in more than 40 cases described in the literature,[115] and other reviews discuss the usual pathologic findings.[116,117] Grossly visible in the cerebral white matter are confluent areas of soft, puckered, and granular tissue. These areas are patchy and emphasize the occipital lobes and periventricular white matter, especially anteriorly and close to the surface of the ventricles.[115–117] The cerebellar white matter is also often involved. The ventricles are enlarged, and, at times, the corpus callosum is small. The volume of white matter is reduced, but the cortex is generally spared. There are nearly always some lacunes. These were present in one series in 39 of 42 necropsy cases of Binswanger's disease.[115] Microscopic study shows myelin pallor. Usually, the myelin pallor is not homogeneous, but islands of decreased myelination are surrounded by normal tissue. At times, the white matter abnormalities are so severe that necrosis and cavitation occur. Gliosis is prominent in zones of myelin pallor. The walls of penetrating arteries are thickened and hyalinized. Occlusion of the small arteries is rare.[116] Occasional patients with Binswanger white matter changes have had amyloid angiopathy as the underlying vascular pathology.[117–120] In these patients, arteries within the cerebral cortex and leptomeninges are thickened and contain a congophilic substance that stains for amyloid. Arteries within the white matter and basal ganglia are also concentrically thickened.

Similar microangiopathic abnormalities in the cerebral white matter and lacunar infarcts can also be found as a familial condition. This disorder, dubbed CADASIL (*c*erebral *a*utosomal *d*ominant *a*rteriopathy with *s*ubcortical *i*nfarcts and *l*eukoencephalopathy), was first described in France as an autosomal dominant inherited condition.[121–124] The penetrating arteries in patients with CADASIL show concentric thickening of vascular walls associated with fibrous proliferation and hyaline degeneration of the intima, and sometimes reduplication of the internal elastic lamella.[123,124] The vessels contain a substance that is *p*-aminosalicylic acid–positive but is not amyloid.

The clinical picture in patients with microangiopathies is quite variable. Most patients have some abnormalities of cognitive function and behavior.[114–117] Most often, patients become slow and abulic. Memory loss, aphasic abnormalities, and visuospatial dysfunction are also found. Pseudobulbar palsy, pyramidal signs, extensor plantar reflexes, and gait abnormalities are also common. The clinical findings often progress gradually or stepwise, with worsening during periods of days to weeks. Often, there are long plateau periods of stability of the findings.[114,117] Many patients also have acute lacunar strokes.

Patients with amyloid angiopathy most often present with recurrent brain hemorrhages, predominantly in the cerebral white matter. They also become demented. CADASIL has a rather early age of onset. The average is approximately 40 years of age.[124] Acute strokes and progressive cognitive, behavioral, and motor signs predominate. Depression and headache, often meeting criteria for migraine, are also frequently present in patients with CADASIL and their relatives.[124,125] Tournier-Lasserve and colleagues have shown linkage of the CADASIL disease gene to the D19S226 locus on chromosome 19q12.[126]

CT often shows periventricular hypodensity. On MRI, the findings are more obvious and dramatic, with zones of periventricular increased density on T2-weighted images and patchy white matter changes.[115,117,127] Figure 8-5 is an MRI of a patient with Binswanger white matter abnormalities. I prefer not to use the term *leuko-araiosis* for these white matter changes. *Leuko-araiosis* is a general term and many patients with white matter abnormalities do not have vascular disease. Several different patterns of white matter abnormalities include (1) caps that occur around the ventricular system, especially in the

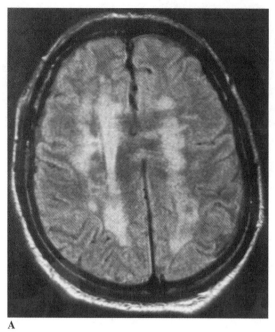 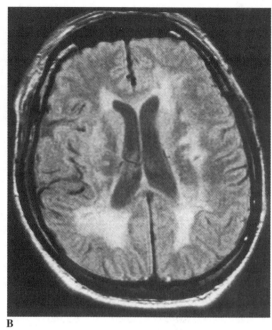

A B

Figure 8-5. Magnetic resonance imaging T2-weighted images. Axial sections **(A)** and **(B)** show increased signal around the ventricles and large areas of abnormal signal in the white matter of the centrum semiovale in a patient with Binswanger's disease.

region of the anterior horns and occipitally; (2) a rim of abnormal white matter signal often surrounds the ventricle diffusely or more focally; and (3) discrete, small foci or patchy or confluent regions of abnormal signal are also noted and vary from single to many lesions. Awad and colleagues attempted to correlate these various lesions with the neuropathology.[11] In general, diffuse periventricular rims represent gliosis that is probably caused by transependymal flow of cerebrospinal fluid.[11] Tiny foci often are caused by état criblé. Lesions in the centrum semiovale and corona radiata are generally regions of chronic partial ischemia.[11] Some studies indicate that hemorheologic changes in the blood, with increased fibrinogen levels and increased whole blood viscosity, may be prevalent in patients with chronic microangiopathies.[117,128] Increased blood viscosity and slow flow through the microvasculature could compound the vascular lesions, leading to hypoperfusion in the territories of deep penetrating arteries.[117] Blood pressure monitoring in patients with microangiopathic white matter disease and lacunar infarcts in Japan showed that these patients had high-average ambulatory blood pressures and reduced nighttime dips in

blood pressure.[129] Suboptimal treatment of hypertension can clearly contribute to worsening of the white matter abnormalities.

Treatment of the chronic microangiopathies is unknown. Impressed by the preliminary data about hyperviscosity, I have begun to treat these patients by attempting to reduce their hematocrits (by blood donation and stopping smoking) and by reducing their fibrinogen levels by prescribing eicosapentaenoic-rich fish oil preparations and other strategies. I also encourage liberal fluid intake.

This microvasculopathy must be differentiated from multiple infarcts caused by large artery occlusive disease and from multiple cerebral emboli as causes of vascular dementia. In these two other conditions, most of the infarcts are cortical or cortical and subcortical, and the history usually includes acute strokes. In these latter causes of vascular dementia, extracranial and transcranial ultrasound, echocardiography, cardiac rhythm monitoring, hematologic screening for coagulopathies, and vascular imaging studies usually show a cardiac-origin embolic source or multiple large artery occlusive disease.

References

1. Fisher CM. Lacunes, small deep cerebral infarcts. Neurology 1965;15:774–784.
2. Fisher CM. The arterial lesions underlying lacunes. Acta Neuropathol 1969;12:1–15.
3. Besson G, Hommel M. Historical Aspects of Lacunes and the "Lacunar Controversy." In PM Pullicino, LR Caplan, M Hommel (eds), Cerebral Small Artery Disease. New York: Raven Press, 1993;1–10.
4. Hauw J-J. The History of Lacunes. In G Donnan, B Norrving, J Bamford, J Bogousslavsky (eds), Lacunar and Other Subcortical Infarcts. Oxford: Oxford University Press, 1995;3–15.
5. Durand-Fardel M. Traite des ramollisements du cerveau. Paris: Bailliere, 1843.
6. Ferrand J. Essai sur l'hemiplegie des vieillards: les lacunes de desintegration cerebrale. Paris: Thesis, 1902.
7. Marie P. Des foyers lacunaires de desintegration et des differents autres etats cavitaires du cerveau. Rev Med (Paris) 1901;21:281.
8. Foix C, Levy M. Les ramollisements sylviens. Rev Neurol 1927;43:1–51.
9. Foix C, Hilleman P. Contribution a l'etude des ramollisements protuberantiels. Rev Med 1926;43:287–305.
10. Caplan LR. Charles Foix—the first modern stroke neurologist. Stroke 1990;21:348–356.
11. Awad I, Johnson PC, Spetzler RF, Hodak JA. Incidental subcortical lesions identified on magnetic resonance imaging in the elderly: II. Postmortem pathological correlations. Stroke 1986;17:1090–1097.
12. Fisher CM. Pure motor hemiplegia of vascular origin. Arch Neurol 1965;13:30–44.
13. Fisher CM. Pathological observations in hypertensive cerebral hemorrhage. J Neuropathol Exp Neurol 1971;30:536–550.
14. Fisher CM. Cerebral miliary aneurysms in hypertension. Am J Pathol 1972;66:313–324.
15. Cole F. Yates P. Intracerebral microaneurysms and small cerebrovascular lesions. Brain 1966;90:759–767.
16. Rosenblum WJ. Miliary aneurysms and "fibrinoid" degeneration of cerebral blood vessels. Hum Pathol 1977;8:133–139.
17. Charcot J, Bouchard C. Nouvelles recherches sur la pathogenie de l'hemorrhagie cerebrale. Arch Phys Norm Pathol 1868;1:110–127, 643–665.
18. Foix C, Hilleman P. Irrigation de la protuberance. Compt Rendu Soc Biol (Paris) 1925;42:35–37.
19. Foix C, Hilleman P. Les arteres de l'axe encephalique jusqu'a diencephale inclusivement. Rev Neurol 1925;41:705–739.
20. Foix C, Hilleman P. Irrigation du bulbe. Compt Rendu Soc Biol (Paris) 1924;42:33–35.
21. Stopford J. The arteries of the pons and medulla oblongata: I. J Anat Physiol 1915;50:131–164.
22. Stopford J. The arteries of the pons and medulla oblongata: II. J Anat Physiol 1916;50:255–280.
23. Düret H. Conclusion d'un memorie sur la circulation bulbaire. Arch Phys Norm Pathol 1873;50:88–89.
24. Düret H. Recherches anatomiques sur la circulation de l'encephale. Arch Phys Norm Pathol 1874;1:60–91, 316–353.
25. Pullicino PM. The Course and Territories of Cerebral Small Arteries. In PM Pullicino, LR Caplan, M Hommel (eds), Cerebral Small Artery Disease. New York: Raven Press, 1993;11–39.
26. Pullicino PM. Diagrams of Perforating Artery Territories in Axial, Coronal, and Sagittal Planes. In PM Pullicino, LR Caplan, M Hommel (eds), Cerebral Small Artery Disease. New York: Raven Press, 1993;41–72.
27. Fisher CM, Caplan LR. Basilar artery branch occlusion: a cause of pontine infarction. Neurology 1971;21:900–905.
28. Fisher CM. Bilateral occlusion of basilar artery branches. J Neurol Neurosurg Psychiatry 1977;40:1182–1189.
29. Caplan LR. Intracranial branch atheromatous disease: a neglected, understudied and underused concept. Neurology 1989;39:1246–1250.
30. Ostrow PT, Miller LL. Pathology of Small Artery Disease. In PM Pullicino, LR Caplan, M Hommel (eds), Cerebral Small Artery Disease. New York: Raven Press, 1993;93–123.
31. Peress N, Kane W, Aronson S. Central nervous system findings in a tenth-decade autopsy population. Prog Brain Res 1973;40:473–484.
32. Boiten J. Lacunar stroke: a prospective clinical and radiologic study. Maastricht: Thesis, 1991.
33. Norrving B, Cronqvist S. Clinical and radiologic features of lacunar versus nonlacunar minor stroke. Stroke 1989;20:59–64.
34. Pullicino P, Nelson R, Kendall B, et al. Small deep infarcts diagnosed on computed tomography. Neurology 1980;30:1090–1096.
35. Weisberg L. Computed tomography and pure motor hemiparesis. Neurology 1979;29:490–495.
36. Donnan G, Tress B, Bladin P. A prospective study of lacunar infarction using computed tomography. Neurology 1982;32:47–56.
37. Mohr JP, Caplan LR, Melski J. The Harvard Cooperative Stroke Registry: a prospective registry. Neurology 1978;28:754–762.
38. Tuszynski MH, Petito CK, Levy DB. Risk factors and clinical manifestations of pathologically verified lacunar infarctions. Stroke 1989;20:990–999.
39. Caplan LR, Young R. EEG findings in certain lacunar stroke syndromes. Neurology 1972;22:403.
40. Mohr JP. Lacunes. Stroke 1982;13:3–11.
41. Miller V. Lacunar stroke, a reassessment. Arch Neurol 1983;40:129–134.
42. Rascol A, Clanet M, Manelfe C, et al. Pure motor hemiplegia: CT study of 30 cases. Stroke 1982;13:11–17.
43. Nelson R, Pullicino P, Kendall B, et al. Computed tomography in patients presenting with lacunar syndromes. Stroke 1980;11:256–261.
44. Richter R, Bruse J, Bruun B, et al. Frequency and course of pure motor hemiparesis: a clinical study. Stroke 1977;8:58–60.
45. Gobernado JM, de Molina AR, Gimeno A. Pure motor hemiplegia due to hemorrhage in the lower pons. Arch Neurol 1980;37:393.
46. Mori E, Tabuchi M, Yamadori A. Lacunar syndrome due to intracerebral hemorrhage. Stroke 1985;16:454–459.
47. Hommel M, Besson G, LeBas JF, et al. Prospective study of lacunar infarction using magnetic resonance imaging. Stroke 1990;21:546–554.

48. Besson G. Les infarctus lacunaires: evaluation clinique et par l'imagerie par resonance magnetique. Grenoble, France: Theses, 1989.

49. Kase CS, Wolf PA, Hier DB, et al. Lacunar infarcts: clinical and CT aspects: the Stroke Data Bank experience. Neurology 1986;36:178–179.

50. Dejerine J, Dejerine-Klumpke H. Anatomie des Centres Nerveux, Vol 2. Paris: Rueff, 1901;128–157.

51. Fisher CM, Cole M. Homolateral ataxia and crural paresis, a vascular syndrome. J Neurol Neurosurg Psychiatry 1965;28:48–55.

52. Fisher CM. Ataxic hemiparesis. Arch Neurol 1978;35:126–128.

53. Helgason CM, Wilbur AC. Capsular hypesthetic ataxic hemiparesis. Stroke 1990;21:24–33.

54. Goldblatt D, Markesbury W, Reeves AG. Recurrent hemichorea following striatal lesions. Arch Neurol 1974;32:51–54.

55. Kase C, Maulsby G, DeJaun E. Hemichorea-hemiballism and lacunar infarction in the basal ganglia. Neurology 1981;31:452–455.

56. Helgason C, Wilbur A, Weiss A, et al. Acute pseudobulbar mutism due to discrete bilateral capsular infarction in the territory of the anterior choroidal artery. Brain 1988;111:507–524.

57. Caplan LR, Schmahmann JD, Kase CS, et al. Caudate infarcts. Arch Neurol 1990;47:133–143.

58. Fisher FM. Capsular infarcts. Arch Neurol 1979;36:65–73.

59. Helgason C, Caplan LR, Goodwin J, Hedges T. Anterior choroidal artery territory infarction: case reports and review. Arch Neurol 1986;43:681–686.

60. Mohr JP, Steinke W, Timsit SG, et al. The anterior choroidal artery does not supply the corona radiata and lateral ventricular wall. Stroke 1991;22:1502–1507.

61. Caplan LR. Posterior circulation disease. Clinical findings, diagnosis, and management. Boston: Blackwell, 1996.

62. Bassetti C, Bogousslavsky J, Barth A, Regli F. Isolated infarcts of the pons. Neurology 1996;46:165–175.

63. Rothrock JF, Lyden PD, Hesselink JF, et al. Brain magnetic resonance imaging in the evaluation of lacunar stroke. Stroke 1987;18:781–786.

64. Leestra JE, Noronha A. Pure motor hemiplegia, medullary pyramid lesion, and olivary hypertrophy. 1976;39:877–884.

65. Ropper AH, Fisher CM, Kleinman GM. Pyramidal infarction in the medulla: a cause of pure motor hemiplegia sparing the face. Neurology 1979;29:91–95.

66. Milandre L, Arnaud O, Khalil R. Infarction of the medullary pyramid identified on MRI. Cerebrovasc Dis 1992;2:183–184.

67. Kataoka S, Hori A, Shirakawa T, Hirose G. Paramedian pontine infarction, neurological/topographical correlation. Stroke 1997;28:809–815.

68. Kim JS, Lee JH, Im JH, Lee MC. Syndromes of pontine base infarction, a clinical-radiological correlation study. Stroke 1995;26:950–955.

69. Fisher CM. A lacunar stroke, the dysarthria-clumsy hand syndrome. Neurology 1967;17:614–617.

70. Helgason CM, Wilbur AC. Basilar branch pontine infarctions with prominent sensory signs. Stroke 1991;22:1129–1136.

71. Caplan LR, Goodwin J. Lateral segmental brainstem hemorrhages. Neurology 1982;32:252–260.

72. Shintani S, Tsuroka S, Shiigai T. Pure sensory stroke caused by a pontine infarct. Clinical, radiological, and physiological features in four patients. Stroke 1994;25:1512–1515.

73. Kim JS, Bae YH. Pure or predominant sensory stroke due to brainstem lesion. Stroke 1997;28:1761–1764.

74. Ho K-L. Pure motor hemiplegia due to infarction of the cerebral peduncle. Arch Neurol 1982;39:524–526.

75. Bogousslavsky J, Maeder P, Regli F, et al. Pure midbrain infarction: clinical syndromes, MRI, and etiologic patterns. Neurology 1994;44:2032–2040.

76. Martin PJ, Chang H-M, Wityk R, Caplan LR. Midbrain infarction: associations and aetiologies in the New England medical Center Posterior Circulation Registry. J Neurol Neurosurg Psychiatry 1998;64:392–395.

77. Hommel B, Besson G, Pollak P, et al. Hemiplegia in posterior cerebral artery occlusion. Neurology 1990;40:1496–1499.

78. Castaigne P, Lhermitte F, Buge A, et al. Paramedian thalamic and midbrain infarcts: clinical and neuropathological study. Ann Neurol 1981;10:127–148.

79. Percheron G. Les arteres du thalamus humain. II: Arteres et territoires thalamique paramedians de l'arterie basilarie communicante. Rev Neurol (Paris) 1976;132:309–324.

80. Bogousslavsky J, Miklossy J, Deruaz J, et al. Unilateral left paramedian infarction of thalamus and midbrain: a clinicopathological study. J Neurol Neurosurg Psychiatry 1986;49:686–694.

81. Graff-Radford NR, Damasio H, Yamada T, et al. Non haemorrhagic thalamic infarction. Brain 1985;108:495–516.

82. Bogousslavsky J, Regli F, Assal G. The syndrome of tuberothalamic artery territory infarction. Stroke 1986;17:434–441.

83. Bogousslavsky J, Regli F, Uske A. Thalamic infarcts: clinical syndromes, etiology, and prognosis. Neurology 1988;38:837–848.

84. Tatemichi T, Steinke W, Duncan C, et al. Paramedian thalamo-peduncular infarction: clinical syndromes and magnetic resonance imaging. Ann Neurol 1992;32:162–171.

85. Bogousslavsky J, Caplan LR. Vertebrobasilar occlusive disease, review of selected aspects. III: thalamic infarcts. Cerebrovasc Dis 1993;3:193–205.

86. Bogousslavsky J. Thalamic infarcts in Lacunar and Other Subcortical Infarcts. In G Donnan, B Norrving, J Bamford, J Bogousslavsky (eds), Oxford: Oxford University Press, 1995;149–170.

87. Kaplan RF, Estol CJ, Damasio H, et al. Bilateral polar artery thalamic infarcts. Neurology 1991;41(Suppl 1):329.

88. Wall M, Slamovits TL, Weisberg LA, Trufant SA. Vertical gaze ophthalmoplegia from infarction in the area of the posterior thalamo-subthalamic paramedian artery. Stroke 1986;17:546–555.

89. Meissner I, Sapir S, Kokmen E, Stein SD. The paramedian diencephalic syndrome: a dynamic phenomenon. Stroke 1987;18:380–385.

90. Caplan LR, DeWitt LD, Pessin MS, et al. Lateral thalamic infarcts. Arch Neurol 1988;45:959–964.

91. Dejerine J, Roussy G. Le syndrome thalamique. Rev Neurol 1906;14:521–532.

92. Fisher CM. Pure sensory stroke involving face, arm, and leg. Neurology 1965;15:76–80.
93. Fisher CM. Thalamic pure sensory stroke: a pathologic study. Neurology 1978;28:1141–1144.
94. Fisher CM. Pure sensory stroke and allied conditions. Stroke 1982;13:434–447.
95. Fisher CM. Lacunar strokes and infarcts: a review. Neurology 1982;32:871–876.
96. Hommel M, Besson G, Pollak P, et al. Pure sensory stroke due to a pontine lacune. Stroke 1989;20:406–408.
97. Mohr JP, Kase C, Meckler R, et al. Sensorimotor stroke. Arch Neurol 1977;34:734–741.
98. Mohr JP, Timsit S. Choroidal Artery Disease. In HJM Barnett, JP Mohr, BM Stein, F Yatsu (eds), Stroke, Pathophysiology, Diagnosis, and Management (3rd ed). New York: Churchill Livingstone, 1998;503–512.
99. Besson G, Bogousslavsky J, Regli F. Posterior choroidal-artery infarct with homonymous horizontal sectoranopia. Cerebrovasc Dis 1991;1:117–120.
100. Frisen I, Holmegaard L, Rosencrantz M. Sectorial optic atrophy and homonymous, horizontal sectoranopia; a lateral posterior choroidal artery syndrome. J Neurol Neurosurg Psychiatry 1978;41:374–380.
101. Adams H, Damasio H, Putnam S, et al. Middle cerebral artery occlusion as a cause of isolated subcortical infarction. Stroke 1983;14:948–952.
102. Maki G, Mihara H, Shizuka M, et al. CT and arteriographic comparison of patients with transient ischemic attacks: correlation with small infarcts of basal ganglia. Stroke 1983;14:276–280.
103. Caplan LR, Babikian V, Helgason C, et al. Occlusive disease of the middle cerebral artery. Neurology 1985; 35:975–982.
104. Bogousslavsky J, Regli F, Maeder P. Intracranial large-artery disease and "lacunar" infarction. Cerebrovasc Dis 1991;1:154–159.
105. Miyashita K, Naritomi H, Sawada T, et al. Identification of recent lacunar lesions in cases of multiple small infarction by magnetic resonance imaging. Stroke 1988;29: 834–839.
106. Faris A, Poser C, Wilmore D, et al. Radiologic visualization of neck vessels in healthy men. Neurology 1963;13:386–396.
107. Lodder J, Bamford J, Kappelle J, Boiten J. What causes false clinical prediction of small deep infarcts. Stroke 1994;5:86–91.
108. Dobkin B. Heparin for lacunar stroke in progression. Stroke 1983;14:421–423.
109. Hachinski V, Potter P, Merskey H. Leuko-araiosis. Arch Neurol 1987;44:21–23.
110. Okeda R. Morphometrische Vergleichsuntersuchungen an Hirnarterien bei Binswangerscher Encephalopathie und Hochdruckencephalopathie. Acta Neuropathol (Berlin) 1973;26:23–43.
111. Binswanger O. Die abgrenzung der allgemeinen progressiven paralyse. Klin Wochenschr 1894;49:1103–1105; 1895;50:1137–1139; and 1895;52:1180–1186.
112. Blass JP, Hoyer S, Nitsch R. A translation of Otto Binswanger's article: the delineation of the generalized progressive paralysis. Arch Neurol 1991;48:961–972.
113. Olszewski J. Subcortical arteriosclerotic encephalopathy. World Neurol 1965;3:359–374.
114. Caplan LR, Schoene WC. Clinical features of subcortical arteriosclerotic encephalopathy (Binswanger's disease). Neurology 1978;28:1206–1215.
115. Babikian V, Ropper AH. Binswanger disease: a review. Stroke 1987;18:1–12.
116. Fisher CM. Binswanger's encephalopathy: a review. J Neurol 1989;236:65–79.
117. Caplan LR. Binswanger's disease—revisited. Neurology 1995;45:626–633.
118. Gray F, Dubas F, Roullet E, Escourolle R. Leukoencephalopathy in diffuse hemorrhagic cerebral amyloid angiopathy. Ann Neurol 1985;18:54–59.
119. Dubas F, Gray F, Roullet E, Escourolle R. Leukoencephalopathies arteriopathiques. Rev Neurol 1985;141:93–108.
120. Loes D, Biller J, Yuh WT, et al. Leukoencephalopathy in cerebral amyloid angiopathy: MR imaging in four cases. AJNR Am J Neuroradiol 1990;11:485–488.
121. Tournier-Lasserve E, Iba-Zizen I-T, Romero N, Bousser M-G. Autosomal dominant syndrome with stroke-like episodes and leukoencephalopathy. Stroke 1991;22:1297–1302.
122. Mas JL, Dilouya A, de Recondo J. A familial disorder with subcortical ischemic strokes, dementia, and leukoencephalopathy. Neurology 1992;42:1015–1019.
123. Baudrimont M, Dubas F, Joutel A, et al. Autosomal dominant leukoencephalopathy and subcortical ischemic stroke: a clinicopathological study. Stroke 1993;24:122–125.
124. Davous P. CADASIL: a review with proposed diagnostic criteria. Eur J Neurology 1998;5:219–233.
125. Dichgans M, Mayer M, Uttner I, et al. The phenotypic spectrum of CADASIL: clinical findings in 102 cases. Ann Neurol 1998;44:731–739.
126. Tournier-Lasserve E, Joutel A, Melki J, et al. Cerebral autosomal dominant arteriopathy with subcortical infarcts and leukoencephalopathy maps on chromosome 19q12. Nat Genet 1993;3:256–259.
127. Chabriat H, Levy C, Taillia H, et al. Patterns of MRI lesions in CADASIL. Neurology 1998;51:452–457.
128. Schneider R, Ringelstein EB, Zeumer H, et al. The role of plasma hyperviscosity in subcortical arteriosclerotic encephalopathy (Binswanger's disease). J Neurol 1987;234:67–73.
129. Yamamoto Y, Akiguchi I, Oiwa K, et al. Adverse effect of nighttime blood pressure on the outcome of lacunar infarct patients. Stroke 1998;29:570–576.

Chapter 9
Brain Embolism

Embolism is the most common cause of brain ischemia. A variety of embolic particles arise from the heart, aorta, and cervicocranial arteries to reach the intracranial arteries. Doctors in the past thought that release of embolic materials into the circulation was unusual and had a high hit rate—that is, that emboli reaching intracranial arteries had a strong likelihood of causing stroke and brain infarction. Newer diagnostic testing, including emboli monitoring using transcranial Doppler ultrasound (TCD), has shown high rates of brain embolism.[1–6] Embolic particles are often found in the circulation, but the hit rate is low.

Clinical Findings

Embolism requires a donor source and a recipient artery. The clinical presentation of a patient with brain embolism relates to the recipient site; symptoms and signs depend on the size of the embolus, location of the recipient artery, and how long the embolus continues to block blood flow at the recipient site. The recipient artery, of course, cannot distinguish the source of the embolic material, nor do the clinical neurologic findings differ among emboli of cardiac, intra-arterial, or venous origin.

A 31-year-old carpenter, TL, was evaluated after the sudden onset of confusion and right-hand weakness. The symptoms began suddenly at work. Three years earlier, he had what he called a minor stroke, characterized by numbness and weakness of the left arm and leg. Cerebral angiography was normal, but he was given war-farin during the 2 years after this event. Approximately 3 months after stopping coumadin, he had a brief attack of dizziness and veered to the left when he walked for approximately 1 week. He gave no history of cardiac or vascular disease, and examination of the heart and neck arteries was normal, except for a slight tachycardia. Blood pressure was 130/60 mm Hg. On neurologic examination, his speech was fluent but contained many paraphasic errors. He had difficulty repeating spoken language and read, wrote, and spelled poorly. His right arm was weak, and he could not recognize objects placed in his right hand. His left plantar response was extensor.

TL's recent event most likely involved the left cerebral hemisphere convexal surface, including the precentral and postcentral gyri and the inferior parietal lobe. The event that occurred 3 years before was also of sudden onset and involved the right cerebral hemisphere. The dizziness and veering to one side probably represented ischemia in the left cerebellum. The three events in three different locations and vascular territories makes embolism the most likely diagnosis, but the source is not obvious from the clinical data.

Embolic strokes most often begin suddenly. The clinical signs evolve during seconds or a few minutes. The deficit may begin during physical activity but more often occurs during rest or activities of daily life.[2,7,8] Traditionally, the neurologic deficit in patients with embolic stroke is described as *maximal at onset*. As soon as an embolus blocks a recipient brain artery, collateral circulation begins to develop and some improvement may occur. Unlike thrombi formed locally at sites of prior atherosclerotic narrowing, emboli are only loosely adherent to vessel walls. They readily fragment, dislodge, and move to more distal arteries. The breakup and distal movement of emboli strongly affect the subsequent clinical course. Movement of emboli most often occurs during the first 48 hours after symptom onset.

Fragmentation and distal movement of emboli (recanalization) before the development of irreversible brain damage allow reperfusion of ischemic brain tissue and is usually accompanied by clinical improvement. In some patients, however, the embolus or its fragments block an important distal branch, leading to further ischemia and worsening of symptoms. For example, a patient with an embolus to the left mainstem middle cerebral artery (MCA) might have the sudden onset of aphasia and right hemiplegia and hemisensory loss. When the embolus passes and the lenticulostriate arteries supplying the internal capsule and basal ganglia regions are reperfused, the hemiparesis might improve. Increased cortical blood flow could improve speech. If the embolus passed into the inferior division of the MCA supplying the temporal lobe and occluded a temporal artery branch, the patient might then develop a fluent Wernicke-type aphasia. When there is further worsening after initial improvement in patients with embolism, the worsening usually occurs in a single step and nearly always occurs during the first 48 hours. Multiple, stepwise worsening; gradual, smooth worsening; and delayed worsening are unusual. Late worsening after 48 hours is explained by the development of brain edema or hemorrhage into the area of infarction because hemorrhagic transformation often occurs between days 2 and 7 after stroke onset.

Another pattern quite characteristic of brain embolism has been called *spectacular shrinking deficit* by Mohr.[9,10] This term describes sudden, complete or nearly complete clearing of sudden-onset severe neurologic signs. Most often, the patient has had rapid recanalization of a mainstem MCA or basilar artery embolus.[10]

Approximately four out of every five emboli that arise from the heart go into the anterior circulation equally divided between the two sides. The remaining one-fifth of emboli go into the posterior circulation,[2,7,8,11] a rate approximately equal to the proportion of the blood supply that goes into the vertebrobasilar arteries. The recipient artery destination depends on the size and nature of the particles. Calcific particles from heart valves and mitral annular calcifications are less mobile and adapt less well to the shape of their recipient artery than red (erythrocyte-fibrin) and white (platelet-fibrin) thrombi. The circulating bloodstream seems able to somehow bypass, obstructing cholesterol crystal emboli, especially in the retinal arteries.

Within the anterior and posterior circulations, there are predilection sites for the destination of embolic particles.[12,13] Large emboli entering a common carotid artery (CCA) could become lodged in the CCA or internal carotid artery (ICA), especially if atheromatous plaques had already narrowed the lumens of these arteries. If the emboli successfully traversed the ICAs in the neck, the next common lodging place is the intracranial bifurcation of the ICAs into the anterior cerebral arteries (ACAs) and MCAs. Arterial bifurcations are common resting places for emboli. Emboli that pass through the carotid intracranial bifurcations most often go into the MCAs and their branches.[12] Gacs et al. showed that balloon emboli placed in the circulation nearly always followed the same pathway and ended up in the MCAs and their branches. Embolism in experimental animals caused by the introduction of silicone cylinders or spheres, elastic cylinders, and autologous blood clots also showed a high incidence of MCA-territory localization.[13] Emboli often pass into the superior and inferior divisions of the MCA and their cortical branches. The superior division supplies the cortex and white matter above the sylvian fissure, including the frontal and superior parietal lobes. The inferior division supplies the area below the sylvian fissure, including the temporal and inferior parietal lobes. TL's recent event most likely involved the inferior division of the left MCA. His first attack probably involved the right MCA. Emboli seldom go into the MCA penetrating artery (lenticulostriate arteries) branches because these arteries originate at a nearly 90-degree angle from the parent arteries. Embolism into the MCAs can cause a variety of patterns of infarction. Cortical and cortical-subcortical infarcts are most common.[2] In young patients with blocked mainstem MCA, the rapid development of collateral circulation over the convexity of the brain often leads to sparing of the superficial territory of the MCA.

The lenticulostriate branches are blocked by the embolus in the mainstem MCA, and collateral circulation to the deep MCA territory is poor. The resultant infarct is limited to the basal ganglia and surrounding white matter and is usually called a *striatocapsular infarct*. Occasionally, emboli block an ACA or its distal branches, causing an infarct in the paramedian area of one frontal lobe.

Emboli that enter the posterior circulation can block the vertebral arteries in the neck or intracranially. Emboli that are able to pass through the intracranial vertebral arteries (ICVAs) usually pass through the proximal and middle portions of the basilar artery, which are wider than the ICVAs. The basilar artery becomes more narrow as it courses craniad. Emboli often block the distal basilar artery bifurcation (top-of-the-basilar) or one of its branches—the penetrating arteries to the medial portions of the thalami and midbrain, the superior cerebellar artery (SCA), which supplies the upper surface of the cerebellum, and the posterior cerebral arteries (PCAs), which supply the lateral portions of the thalami and the temporal and occipital lobe territories of the PCAs. The most frequent brain areas infarcted are the (1) posterior inferior portion of the cerebellum in the territory of the posterior inferior cerebellar artery branch of the ICVA, (2) the superior surface of the cerebellum in the territory of the SCA, and (3) the thalamic and hemispheral territories of the PCAs.[14] TL's second attack probably represented cerebellar ischemia.

The nature of the clinical neurologic signs depends on the location of the occluded artery and is similar to the signs described in Chapters 6 and 7. An occluded ACA causes leg weakness, abulia, and left-arm apraxia. When the occluded vessel is the upper trunk of the left MCA, Broca's aphasia and weakness of the right side of the face and the right hand and arm result. An occluded left MCA inferior trunk causes Wernicke's aphasia and a right homonymous hemianopia. An occluded PCA causes a homonymous hemianopia, whereas an embolus at the top of the basilar artery can cause cortical blindness, lethargy or agitation, and abnormal eye movements. At times, emboli may be large enough to occlude a normal or an already stenotic ICA, MCA stem, ICVA, or basilar artery, causing more severe neurologic deficits.

Emboli of cardiac origin are often larger than those arising in the cervicocranial arteries, so the infarcts are, on average, larger than artery-to-artery embolic infarcts.[15–18] In the Stroke Data Bank, the average volume of infarction on computed tomography (CT) in patients with cardiac origin embolism was 2.4 times greater than in patients with intra-arterial embolism, a highly significant difference ($p < .01$).[19] In a study of more than 2,000 stroke patients, the average size of brain infarcts caused by cardiac-source embolism was 73.7 cm^3 versus 48.9 cm^3 for nonembolic infarcts.[18] Decreased level of consciousness early during the course of the stroke, a finding probably related to the size of infarction among other factors, was also significantly more common in Stroke Data Bank patients with cardiogenic embolism, as compared with those with intra-arterial embolism (29.8% vs 6.1%, $p < .01$).[19]

TL had no history of systemic embolism. Embolism to systemic arteries has always been considered an important criterion for the clinical diagnosis of brain embolism. Necropsy studies of patients with brain embolism of cardiac origin nearly always show embolic infarcts in other organs, especially the spleen and kidneys. In contrast, the frequency of clinical recognition of systemic embolism is quite low. The frequency of diagnosis of systemic embolism in various stroke registries was 2% in the Harvard Stroke Registry, 2.3% in the Michael Reese Stroke Registry, 3.6% in the Stroke Data Bank, and 3% in the Lausanne Stroke Registry.[11] Eight percent, the highest frequency of systemic embolism, was found in a study of 60 patients with cardiogenic brain embolism in whom two patients had kidney embolism and three patients had peripheral limb embolism.[20]

Embolism to the brain that causes ischemia usually produces transient or persistent neurologic symptoms. The brain is like litmus paper and is sensitive to perturbations. Systemic embolism also causes ischemia, but the symptoms are much less specific. Embolism to a limb might cause arm pain, leg cramps, or other transient discomfort. These symptoms are common and usually result from activity, positioning of the limb, or some other banal, everyday occurrence. Similarly, embolism to the intestinal tract might cause stomach cramps, bowel irregularity, or a stomachache. These are rather common and nonspecific symptoms. Embolism to the kidneys or spleen causes flank or abdominal discomfort and is rarely diagnosed as related to systemic embolism. Hematuria and sudden-onset severe limb ischemia are probably the only two situations that usually lead to recognition of systemic embolism, especially in patients with known heart disease.

Imaging and Laboratory Findings Related to the Recipient Artery and Its Supply

Brain imaging using CT, magnetic resonance imaging (MRI), or both, and vascular imaging using CT angiography (CTA), magnetic resonance angiography (MRA), standard catheter angiography, and TCD can yield information in relation to the recipient artery and the presence, location, and size of embolic brain infarcts.

> CT scan in TL showed a region of lucency involving the left angular and postcentral gyri. Within the lucent areas were small regions of stippling caused by hemorrhagic transformation. There were also small, old infarcts in the right frontal lobe and left cerebellum. Hematologic, serologic, and coagulation studies were normal. MRI confirmed the same regions of infarction. The hemorrhagic changes in the recent inferior parietal lobe infarct were more evident on MRI than CT. Angiography on the third hospital day revealed a sharp cutoff of the left angular artery. The proximal arteries were normal.

Neuroimaging with CT and MRI can suggest brain embolism. Because emboli most often lodge in distal arteries that supply cortical zones, embolic infarcts are often V-shaped and abut on the superficial cortical surface. Multiple cortical infarcts in various vascular supply regions suggest cardiac-origin embolism. Ringelstein and colleagues analyzed the CT pattern of infarction among 60 patients with cardiogenic embolism.[21] Most infarcts were large and cortically based (41 lesions). Some patients had small cortical, subcortical, and insular infarcts. A few patients had deep infarcts in the striatocapsular region.[21] Multiple cortical and cortical-subcortical infarcts in different vascular territories are especially suggestive of brain embolism from a cardiac or aortic source. At times, acute emboli are imaged as hyperdense arteries on noncontrast CT.[22,23] Newer diagnostic testing, including emboli monitoring using TCD, has shown high rates of brain embolism.[1–6] Most often, the hyperdensity takes the course and shape of the MCA.[22,23] Occasionally, calcific fragments can also be seen within arteries on noncontrast CT scans.

Embolic infarcts may be pale, spotted with small petechial hemorrhages, or frankly hemorrhagic. Fisher and Adams extensively studied their necropsy material to define the mechanism of hemorrhagic infarction in the brain.[24,25] Obstruction of a nutrient artery causes brain ischemia to neurons and ischemic damage to the blood vessels within the area of ischemia. When the obstructing embolus moves distally, the previously ischemic region is reperfused with blood. The damaged capillaries and arterioles within that region are no longer competent, and blood leaks into the surrounding infarcted tissue. An example of this is shown in Figure 9-1 from the Fisher and Adams study. This patient had an embolus that initially blocked the mainstem MCA before its lenticulostriate branches, causing ischemia to the basal ganglia, internal capsule, and the superficial cortical territories supplied by the MCA. The embolus then moved and had passed beyond the lenticulostriate branches at necropsy but continued to obstruct the MCA more distally. The reperfused deep basal ganglionic region was hemorrhagic at necropsy, whereas the superficial territory of the MCA, which was never reperfused, showed a bland infarct.

The essential cause of hemorrhagic infarction is reperfusion of previously ischemic tissue. The other stroke mechanism that causes hemorrhagic infarction is systemic hypoperfusion. After cardiac arrest or shock, the reinstitution of effective circulation after a prolonged period of brain hypoperfusion can cause hemorrhage within border-zone infarcts. Hemorrhagic changes are extremely common in patients with brain embolism. In two series, investigators prospectively studied the frequency of hemorrhagic infarction on sequential brain-imaging scans.[26,27] Yamaguchi et al. compared the findings on CT scans performed 3–10 days after stroke in 120 patients who had embolic brain infarcts with 109 patients whose infarcts were believed to be caused by local thrombotic occlusive disease.[26] Hemorrhagic infarcts were found in 45 patients (40%) with embolic infarcts, as compared with two patients (1.8%) with local thrombosis-related infarcts. Okada and colleagues performed CT scans every 10 days in 160 patients who had presumed embolic brain infarcts.[27] Hemorrhagic infarction

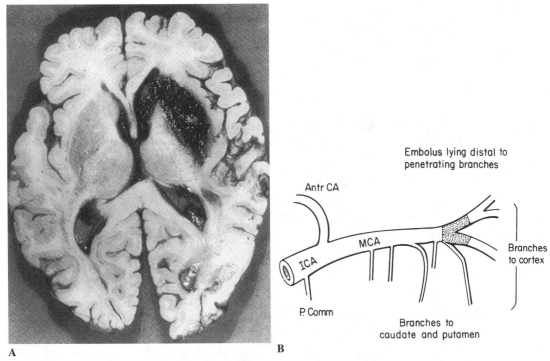

Figure 9-1. (A) Coronal section of the brain at necropsy shows a hemorrhagic infarction on the right involving the caudate nucleus and putamen, regions supplied by the lenticulostriate branches of the right middle cerebral artery. **(B)** Intracranial internal carotid artery (ICA) and its branches at necropsy. An embolus (*hatched region*) was found in the distal portion of the mainstem middle cerebral artery (MCA) beyond the lenticulostriate branches that supply the caudate nucleus and putamen. At one time, this embolus must have blocked these penetrating branches and then moved more distally in the artery. (Antr CA = anterior cerebral artery; P. Comm = posterior communicating artery.) (Reprinted with permission from CM Fisher, RD Adams. Observations on Brain Embolism with Special Reference to Hemorrhagic Infarction. In AJ Furlan [ed], The Heart and Stroke. London: Springer, 1987;17–36.)

was found on CT at some time during the course in 65 patients (40.6%). Hemorrhagic changes were found on the initial CT scan performed during the first 4 days in only 10 patients (6%), whereas the remainder of the hemorrhagic infarcts were found on follow-up CT scans.[27] Studies at the New England Medical Center in Boston showed that all patients with cerebral and cerebellar hemorrhagic infarcts reported had embolic causes.[28,29] MRI is more sensitive than CT in showing hemorrhagic changes, therefore sequential MRI probably would show a frequency greater than 50% for hemorrhagic changes in patients with embolic brain infarcts.

In most patients, hemorrhagic infarction consists of diapedesis of red blood cells into infarcted tissue. The appearance is that of scattered petechial hemorrhages or a confluent purpuric pattern scattered throughout the infarct.[30] In some brain infarcts,

especially large ones involving more than one lobe, localized homogeneous collections of blood (hematomas) can develop within the region of hemorrhagic infarction.[30] In the majority of patients with hemorrhagic infarcts, the hemorrhagic transformation does not cause worsening of the clinical symptoms and signs. The hemorrhagic changes are usually found on routine follow-up scans. Bleeding into dead tissue does not alter clinical findings unless a large space-occupying hematoma develops.

Experience with acute angiography since the late 1980s has shown a high rate of demonstration of intracranial emboli in patients with cardiac-origin sources and extracranial occlusive disease.[31–33] CTA, MRA, and standard catheter angiography, especially if performed within 48 hours of stroke onset, often allow visualization of emboli. A sudden sharp, abrupt termination of a distal or medium-sized ves-

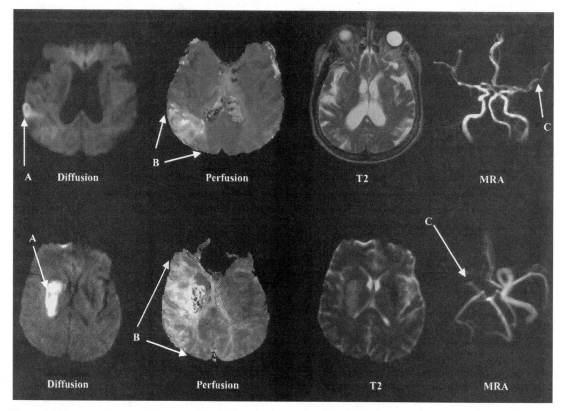

Figure 9-2. Comprehensive magnetic resonance studies of two patients with brain embolism. In the top row, the magnetic resonance angiography (MRA) (*far right*) shows reduced flow in the right middle cerebral artery (*arrow*); although the T2-weighted magnetic resonance imaging is normal, the diffusion-weighted image (**A**) at the far left shows an infarct (*arrow*), and the perfusion image (**B**) shows a region of decreased perfusion that is more extensive than the infarct on the diffusion-weighted image (*two arrows*). In the bottom row, the right middle cerebral artery is occluded on MRA (*far right arrow at* [**C**]). A striato-capsular infarct is faintly visible on the T2-weighted image but is more obvious on the diffusion image. A very large area of perfusion abnormality exists (**B**). (Submitted by Drs. Rafael Llinas and Italo Linfante, Beth Israel Deaconess Hospital)

sel without visible atherosclerosis or a filling defect in the lumen of a symptomatic recipient artery are diagnostic of embolization. Figure 9-2 shows acute MR studies in two patients studied with standard T2-weighted MRI, diffusion-weighted MRI (DWI), perfusion MRI, and MRA examinations. In each patient, the vascular occlusive embolus was shown on MRA, and the perfusion abnormality exceeded the diffusion abnormality, indicating the presence of brain tissue that was ischemic but not yet infarcted. Disappearance of the obstruction in subsequent films or on later angiograms substantiates the diagnosis. Dalal et al. reported nine patients that had emboli seen on initial angiography but later disappeared.[34] Others have documented disappearance or movement of emboli.[35] The finding of a normal artery that

supplies a region of cortical and subcortical infarction is also highly suggestive of embolism.

TCD ultrasound insonation of patients with sudden-onset hemispheric strokes has shown frequent MCA occlusion. Sequential TCD examinations that show clearing of an obstruction suggest embolism.[36] A new capability has entered the diagnostic arsenal of clinicians—emboli monitoring using TCD. Ultrasound probes are positioned over brain arteries, most often the MCA and PCA on each side. When particles pass through the arteries being monitored, they produce an audible chirping noise and high-intensity transient signals (HITS) are visible on an oscilloscope. The signal character depends on the nature of the particles (gas, thrombus, calcium, cholesterol crystal, and so forth), par-

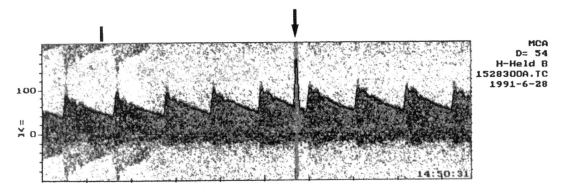

Figure 9-3. Transcranial Doppler recording over the middle cerebral artery (MCA). A single high-intensity transient signal is recorded (*arrow*).

ticle size, and particle transit time. Figure 9-3 shows a microembolic signal captured by TCD monitoring. Monitoring probes can be placed on the neck and brain arteries. Emboli that arise from the heart or aorta should go equally to each side, proportionately to the anterior and posterior circulation arteries, and the signals should appear in the neck before appearing intracranially. In contrast, emboli that originate in a neck artery should go only to the intracranial arterial branches on the side of the donor artery. Embolic signals do not appear in the neck. For example, emboli from the left ICA generate embolic signals detectable in the left MCA and not in the neck, PCAs, or right-sided arteries. This technique allows better identification of the nature of embolic materials and their sources. This technique also allows some quantification of the emboli load and a means of monitoring the effect of various therapies on lessening that load.

In one study, Daffertshofer and colleagues monitored 280 patients with acute MCA-territory ischemic events, as well as 118 asymptomatic controls, for periods of 30–60 minutes.[5] Only two controls (1.7%) had microembolic signals. No microembolic signals were detected among 78 patients who had no identified sources of embolism, whereas 12.9% of patients with sources of emboli had microembolic signals.[5] Microemboli were found more often in patients with vascular sources of embolism, such as ICA stenosis (17.1%), as compared with 6.2% in patients with cardiac sources of embolism. One-fifth of patients with ICA stenosis greater than 70% had microem-

bolic signals, as compared with 13% in patients with less than 70% ICA stenosis.[5]

Sliwka et al., during a 6-month period, monitored 109 consecutive patients with atrial fibrillation or other potential cardiac sources of embolism.[6] Nine of the patients had insufficient temporal windows and could not be monitored with TCD. Microembolic signals were detected in 36 of the 100 patients successfully monitored. The average number of microembolic signals was 2.69 ± 2.70 per 30 minutes (range, 1–12). Patients with atrial fibrillation who had coronary atherosclerotic heart disease with ejection fractions of less than 30%, dilatated cardiomyopathy, or mitral stenosis had the highest percentage of microemboli detection.

Georgiadis and colleagues monitored 300 patients with potential cardiac sources of emboli and 100 patients with severe ICA disease using TCD.[37] They found the following frequencies of microembolic signals among their monitored patients: 43%, infective endocarditis; 34%, left ventricular aneurysm; 26%, intracardiac thrombus; 26%, dilatated cardiomyopathy; 21%, nonvalvular atrial fibrillation; 15%, native valvular disease; 55% prosthetic valves; 28%, ICA disease (52% symptomatic ICA disease, 7% asymptomatic disease); and 5% among controls.

Echocardiography showed an enlarged heart with a reduced ejection fraction suggestive of a cardiomyopathy. Myocardial biopsy later revealed cardiac sarcoidosis. During the next year, TL had no further brain emboli while taking warfarin.

Table 9-1. Types of Embolic Materials

Cardiac	Arterial
Red erythrocyte-fibrin thrombi	Red erythrocyte-fibrin thrombi
White platelet-fibrin thrombi	White platelet-fibrin thrombi
Bacteria-endocarditis	Cholesterol crystals
Fibrin strands and bland vegetations	Atheromatous plaque debris
Calcium (valves and mitral annulus calcification)	Calcium
Myxoma and other tumor particles	Tumor particles
	Air
	Fat
	Talc and microcrystalline cellulose (drug injection)

Source: Modified with permission from LR Caplan. Of birds and nests and brain emboli. Rev Neurol 1991;147:265–273.

In this case, the negative hematologic studies, absence of risk factors for atherosclerosis, and normal proximal extracranial and intracranial arteries suggested brain embolism despite the absence of known cardiac disease. Cardiac evaluation finally clarified the diagnosis.

Sources of Emboli

The majority of emboli to the brain arise from the heart, aorta, and cervicocranial arteries. Figure 2-2 illustrates these major sources. A variety of particles with different physical properties can arise from the heart, arteries, or circulation.[1,2,38] Table 9-1 lists the various particles that arise from cardiac and intra-arterial sources. Occasionally, foreign materials, such as air, fat, and cancer cells, enter the circulation and embolize to various systemic organs.[2]

Cardiac Sources

In the 1950s, the only two cardiac disorders accepted as having an important risk of causing embolism were rheumatic mitral stenosis with atrial fibrillation and recent myocardial infarction. Many cardiac lesions and disorders carry a risk of cardiac thrombosis and embolism. More modern cardiac diagnostic testing has made it possible to diagnose cardiac disorders more definitively and to attempt to quantify the risk of embolism. Cardiac disorders that carry a risk of brain embolism can be divided into six groups. These six groups are (1) arrhythmias, especially atrial fibrillation and sick sinus syndrome; (2) valvular heart diseases, especially mitral stenosis, prosthetic heart valves, infective endocarditis, and marantic endocarditis; (3) ventricular myocardial abnormalities, especially related to coronary artery disease, myocarditis, and other dilated cardiomyopathies; (4) lesions within the cavity of the ventricles, especially tumors, such as myxomas and thrombi; (5) shunts, especially intra-atrial septal defects and patent foramen ovale (PFO) that allow passage of emboli forming in the peripheral veins to enter the systemic circulation, causing so-called paradoxical embolism; and (6) atrial lesions, such as dilatated atria, atrial infarcts and thrombi, and atrial septal aneurysms. Table 9-2 lists the major cardiac donor sources of embolism.

Virchow, in 1856, described three antecedent conditions for the development of thrombi within the chambers of the heart.[39] These three conditions are (1) a region of circulatory stasis, (2) injury to the endothelial surfaces of the heart, and (3) increased blood coagulability. In areas of stasis, a low shear rate and other factors activate the classical coagulation cascade, leading to the formation of erythrocyte-fibrin thrombi. Stasis occurs most often in the atria and atrial appendages in patients with atrial fibrillation. Stasis also occurs in the ventricular chambers in patients with global and focal regions of decreased myocardial contractility. Altered myocardial endothelium occurs in patients with myocardial infarcts, ventricular aneurysms, inflammatory and other myocardiopathies, and endocardial disorders. Valvular endothelium can be damaged by many different conditions. Loss of a protective endothelial surface exposes circulating blood to the underlying tissues and causes platelet activation, adhesion, and secretion, as well as activating the coagulation cascade. Studies have begun to show increased platelet activation and blood coagulability in patients with cardiac-source embolism.[40–43]

Arrhythmias

Atrial Fibrillation. Atrial fibrillation is one of the most common cardiac disorders. Approximately

0.4% of the population has atrial fibrillation, and the disorder becomes much more common as patients age. Perhaps as many as 5% of individuals older than 60 years have atrial fibrillation. Epidemiologic studies performed since the 1970s have firmly established that atrial fibrillation is an important risk factor for stroke, that stroke is most often caused by cardiogenic embolism, and that standard antithrombotic treatment substantially reduces the frequency of brain embolism in patients with atrial fibrillation.[44] The etiology of atrial fibrillation and associated cardiac and other medical factors affect the risk of stroke in patients with atrial fibrillation.[44,45] In the Framingham Study, the presence of rheumatic heart disease and atrial fibrillation conveyed 17.6 times the risk of stroke compared with the lone atrial fibrillation rate of 5.6 times.[46] Advanced age, congestive heart failure, history of hypertension, previous myocardial infarction, and prior thromboembolism increase the risk of stroke in patients with atrial fibrillation. These features should be known from the medical history. A collaborative analysis of five atrial fibrillation stroke prevention studies analyzed the contribution of various historical risk factors on the development of stroke during follow-up.[47] The relative risks (RR) determined by multivariate analysis of all the data were history of previous stroke or transient ischemic attack (TIA) (RR, 2.5), diabetes mellitus (RR, 1.7), history of hypertension (RR, 1.6), and increasing age (RR, 1.4 for each decade).[47–49] These calculated relative risks were for the occurrence of any stroke and were not limited to those attributable to cardiogenic embolism.

Echocardiography findings are also helpful in assessing the risk of brain embolism in individual patients with atrial fibrillation.[50–52] Transesophageal echocardiography (TEE) can detect left atrial and left atrial appendage thrombi. In patients with atrial fibrillation who do not have valvular disease, thrombi often form in, and dislodge from, the left atrial appendage, whereas patients with atrial fibrillation and valvular disease have more left atrial thrombi. In patients with valvular disease and atrial fibrillation, thrombi have been detected in 9–29% of patients, compared with 10% prevalence in patients without valvular disease.[2] Small thrombi less (than 2 mm) and those that have already dislodged are not readily detected. Left atrial enlargement and abnormal left

Table 9-2. Some Cardiac Sources of Emboli

Coronary artery disease
    Mural thrombi
    Ventricular aneurysms
    Hypokinetic zones
Arrhythmias
    Atrial fibrillation
    Sick sinus syndrome
Valvular disease
    Mitral stenosis, rheumatic
    Aortic stenosis, rheumatic
    Bicuspid aortic valve
    Mitral annulus calcification
    Calcific aortic stenosis
    Mitral valve prolapse
    Bacterial endocarditis
    Nonbacterial thrombotic endocarditis
Cardiomyopathies or endocardiopathies
    Endocardial fibroelastosis
    Alcoholic cardiomyopathy
    Cocaine cardiomyopathy
    Myocarditis
    Sarcoidosis
    Fabry's disease
    Amyloidosis
Intracardiac lesions
    Myxomas
    Fibroelastomas
    Malignant cardiac tumors
    Metastatic tumors
    Ball-valve thrombi
Septal abnormalities (paradoxical embolism)
    Atrial septal defects
    Patent foramen ovale
    Atrial septal aneurysms

atrial appendage function, as determined by Doppler TEE, also convey an increased risk for cardioembolic stroke.[53,54] The presence of mitral annulus calcification (MAC) and left ventricular dysfunction also increases the risk of stroke in patients with atrial fibrillation.[2]

Spontaneous echo contrast (also called *smoke*) is probably one of the most important factors that predict the likelihood of cardiogenic embolism in patients with atrial fibrillation.[55–58] First described in patients with mitral valve disease, *spontaneous echo contrast* refers to swirling hazes of echogenicity within the cardiac chambers. The echogenic swirls can move repeatedly within the cavity and may disappear when blood flow increases or when local stasis resolves. The intensity can vary from a faint cloud-like appearance to bright echo contrast. Spontaneous echo contrast is probably caused by the interaction between plasma proteins and erythrocytes at low shear rates. The major determinants of spontaneous echogenicity are the hematocrit, fibrinogen levels, and slow intracardiac flow. Chimowitz and colleagues showed that the presence of spontaneous echo contrast was highly associated with prior strokes in patients who had either atrial fibrillation or mitral valve stenosis.[58]

Table 5-7 reviews the results of the major trials of anticoagulation and antiplatelet aggregants in patients with atrial fibrillation who do not have valvular disease. Warfarin is approximately 50% more effective than aspirin in reducing the rate of stroke in patients with atrial fibrillation without valvular disease.[59] Aspirin is also an effective treatment; aspirin probably conveys a stroke risk reduction of 20–25% with no clear relationship to aspirin dose. Treatment should be decided on an individual basis. Clinicians should weigh the risk of stroke without warfarin versus the risk of important hemorrhage during warfarin treatment.

Sick Sinus Syndrome. Although sinus node dysfunction has been recognized clinically since the beginning of the twentieth century, identification of the malfunctioning atrium as a source of embolism was first recognized during the 1970s.[60,61] A variety of names are used for this condition, including *sick sinus syndrome*, *sinoatrial disorder*, and *bradycardia-tachycardia syndrome*. Essential for the diagnosis is demonstration of sinus node dysfunctioning. Patients often present with slow or fast cardiac rhythms, or both. Lown characterized the disorder as consisting of chaotic atrial activity, changing p-wave contour, and bradycardia, admixed with multiple and recurrent ectopic beats and runs of atrial and nodal tachycardia.[62] Many patients also have atrial fibrillation or flutter with a relatively slow ventricular response (<70 beats/minute).[63] An analysis of cardiovascular disease in Rochester, Minnesota showed that 2.9% of men and 1.5% of women aged 75 years or older had the sick sinus syndrome.[64] Systemic emboli mostly to the brain occurred in approximately 14–18% of patients with the sick

sinus syndrome.[65,66] Patients with tachyarrhythmias are more likely to embolize than those with just bradyarrhythmias. As in patients with atrial fibrillation, increasing age is associated with an increased frequency of embolism. The use of pacemakers (atrial single-chamber pacing or ventricular single-chamber pacing) does not seem to reduce the frequency of stroke or stroke death.[67]

As in patients with atrial fibrillation, dysfunction of the left atrium probably promotes thrombus formation. Tachycardia may precipitate dislodging of thrombi from the heart into the systemic circulation. Activation of platelets and increased blood coagulability probably contribute to the likelihood of thromboembolism. Although no formal, prospective, randomized trials of anticoagulation or aspirin therapy have been performed in patients with sinus node dysfunction, the therapeutic responses and treatment considerations are probably the same as those for patients with atrial fibrillation.

Cardiac Valve Disease. One-fifth to one-tenth of all patients with cardiac valve disease have cardioembolic strokes.[68] Abnormalities of valve surfaces and changes in valve function and cardiac physiology, which result from valve disease, promote the formation of white platelet-fibrin thrombi and red clots on valve surfaces and in the adjacent heart chambers. Stenotic valves have decreased pliability and irregular surfaces; progressive commisural adhesions and valve leaflet dystrophic calcification develop, leading to progressive narrowing of the cross-sectional area of valve orifices. Valvular outlet obstruction causes increased turbulence of blood flow. The intensity of turbulence is markedly increased in the jet stream of blood distal to the stenotic valve.[69] Platelets are activated in regions of increased turbulence; the amount of thrombus formed is directly related to valve orifice turbulence.

Distal to stenotic valves, blood flow consists of a central jet stream surrounded by annular eddies that course between the outflow tract walls and the mainstream. These eddies permit blood to remain closer to the irregular valve surfaces than occurs in regions of normal laminar flow. Platelets activated by the turbulent jet stream have prolonged contact with dystrophic irregular valve surfaces, causing adhesion of platelet-fibrin thrombi to valve surfaces, further platelet activation, and formation of thrombi. Valve incompetence also prolongs the time that blood is in contact with abnormal valve surfaces and also promotes thrombus formation. Valve disease often leads to atrial and ventricular enlargement. Left atrial enlargement is especially common in patients with mitral stenosis and mitral insufficiency and can be severe. Enlargement of the left atrium is accompanied by stasis and thrombus formation, especially in the left atrial appendage and in patients who develop atrial fibrillation.

Rheumatic Mitral Valve Disease. Although the incidence of rheumatic fever and rheumatic heart disease has dramatically declined, rheumatic heart disease is still an important cause of brain embolism. The mitral valve is most often involved. Second in frequency is involvement of the mitral and aortic valves. Isolated rheumatic aortic valve disease is unusual, and the pulmonic and tricuspid valves are seldom the site of important clinical rheumatic valvulitis.

Embolization, especially to the brain, may be the earliest clinical indication of rheumatic mitral stenosis. The frequency of embolism in patients with mitral stenosis ranges in series from 10% to 20%.[70–72] Approximately 50–75% of emboli detected clinically involve the brain. Embolism is most common in patients with mitral stenosis. Although embolism does occur in patients with mitral stenosis who have normal sinus rhythm, the development of atrial fibrillation greatly increases the risk of embolism. In 194 patients with rheumatic heart disease and systemic embolism, Daley et al. found a mitral valve lesion in 97%, atrial fibrillation in 90%, and either a mitral valve lesion or atrial fibrillation in 100%.[73] In a study of 754 patients with chronic rheumatic heart disease followed for more than 5,000 patient-years, the incidence of embolism was 1.5% per patient-year.[70] Embolism was seven times more frequent in patients with atrial fibrillation than in those with sinus rhythm. A third of recurrences of embolism occurred during the first month, and two-thirds of recurrences were during the first year after the onset of atrial fibrillation.[70]

Anticoagulants clearly reduce the frequency of recurrent embolism.[74] Mitral valvuloplasty, the predominant treatment of mitral stenosis during the 1960s and 1970s, did not greatly influence the frequency of embolism. The atrial appendage was sometimes removed to prevent lodging of thrombi in this region. Modern diagnostic technology, espe-

cially echocardiography, has revolutionized the diagnosis of patients with mitral stenosis and other rheumatic valve lesions. Quantification of the valve orifice, as well as the effects of the mitral valve disease on the left atrium and left ventricle, is readily possible. These measurements can be performed sequentially to study disease progression and response to treatment. Left atrial and left atrial appendage thrombi are also reliably detected. Superimposed bacterial endocarditis can precipitate brain embolism, although the occurrence of endocarditis in patients with isolated mitral stenosis is unusual.

Rheumatic mitral regurgitation is a less frequent cause of brain embolism than mitral stenosis. Among 500 individuals with mitral valve disease, 66% were predominantly stenotic.[40] Twenty-one percent had predominant regurgitation and 13% were mixed. Among individuals with embolism in one series, 93% had predominant mitral stenosis and only 7% had mitral insufficiency.[74] Mitral insufficiency is often accompanied by progressive left ventricular hypertrophy. Mitral valve repair and mitral valve replacement are probably important considerations in the prevention of embolism in patients with rheumatic mitral insufficiency.

Aortic Valve Disease. In most patients, the cause of acquired aortic valve disease is not determined. Progressive calcific aortic stenosis often develops in patients with congenital bicuspid aortic valves and can also follow rheumatic valvulitis. Calcific degenerative changes are usually well developed during the fourth and fifth decades of life in patients with bicuspid valves, whereas idiopathic calcific aortic stenosis is more prevalent during the sixth to eighth decades.[75] Idiopathic calcific aortic valve disease of the elderly may be caused by an atherosclerotic degenerative process, although definite proof of this hypothesis is not yet available. Microthrombi with evidence of organization have been found at necropsy in 53% of stenotic aortic valves.[69] Changes in the aortic valve are progressive. Thickening of previously diseased valves is thought to result from the deposition of fibrin. Fibrin deposits become organized and calcified with resultant distortion of the normal valve architecture. Bicuspid and calcific aortic valves are not able to open freely. Narrowing and irregularity of the valve orifice contributes to turbulent blood flow. Abnormal flow and valve surfaces activate platelets and induce fibrin deposition, accounting for the prevalence of microthrombi along valve surfaces.

Embolism is a much less common occurrence in patients with aortic valve disease when compared with mitral valve disease. Some clinical and necropsy studies show that embolism from calcific aortic valves is probably not rare. Soulie et al. found emboli in 33% of 81 patients with calcific aortic stenosis.[76] In another autopsy study, calcific emboli were found in 37 of 165 patients (22%) with calcific aortic stenosis.[77] Thirty-two emboli were found in the coronary arteries, 11 in the renal vessels, one in the central retinal artery, and one in the MCA. Although the MCA was occluded by a calcific embolus in one patient, no neurologic signs were recorded, and no infarct was found.[77] During life, calcific emboli have often been identified in the eye because of their typical morphology on funduscopic examination of the retina. Calcific retinal emboli appear as white, irregular, immovable densities and are usually distinguishable from bright cholesterol crystals and fibrin-platelet plugs.

In all clinical studies, symptoms that reflect embolization occur more often after cardiac procedures (catheterization and surgery) than occur spontaneously. Aortic valve surgery is especially associated with a high frequency of embolism. Embolism is also more common in patients with bacterial endocarditis superimposed on bicuspid or calcific aortic valves than it is in noninfected valves. The discrepancy between the relatively high frequency of calcific emboli found at necropsy and in the eye and the low frequency of clinically symptomatic brain and visceral organ ischemic events is probably explained by the small size of the embolic particles and the fact that visceral emboli are much harder to diagnose than brain emboli.

Hypertrophic cardiomyopathy, also called *idiopathic hypertrophic subaortic stenosis*, has become more frequently recognized since the advent of echocardiography. This disorder is characterized by disproportionate and asymmetric hypertrophy of the left ventricular myocardium in the region of the ventricular septum, as compared with the left ventricular free wall. Septal hypertrophy is associated with systolic anterior motion of the mitral valve and variable left ventricular outflow obstruction, depending on myocardial contractility. Structural abnormalities of the mitral valve often accompany the hypertrophic cardiomyopathy.[78] The rate of stroke in patients with hypertrophic cardiomyopathy is low. Stroke rarely occurs early in the course of the disease. When stroke occurs, it is usually a result of embolism in relation to atrial fibrillation, bacterial endocarditis, mitral valve dysfunction, or mitral annular calcification. Atrial fibrillation tends to develop late in patients with hypertrophic cardiomyopathy and is often accompanied by left atrial enlargement.[79,80] MAC is also associated with idiopathic hypertrophic subaortic stenosis.[81]

Little has been written about embolism in patients with aortic insufficiency. Aortic regurgitation is caused by dysfunction of the aortic valve leaflets or aortic root. Rheumatic valvulitis and infective endocarditis are probably the most common causes of aortic leaflet disease causing aortic insufficiency, whereas Marfan syndrome, aortic dissection, and annuloaortic ectasia caused by aging and hypertension are the usual causes of aortic root disease. Syphilis was formerly a common cause of aortic valve insufficiency but is rare. Rheumatic aortic valvulitis and vegetations on the aortic valve are potential sources of brain and systemic embolism in patients with aortic regurgitation.

Mitral Valve Prolapse. Barlow and Bosman, in an early report of the midsystolic click–mitral valve prolapse (MVP) syndrome, reported a 23-year-old woman who had transient left arm weakness. Evaluation showed MVP.[82,83] No details of the neurologic symptoms or signs were included, and the relationship of the neurologic event to her heart condition was not considered.[82,83] Since then, a number of case control and necropsy studies have shown that patients with MVP may have cardiogenic embolism, but this is not common. Cerebrovascular events in patients with MVP have a relatively low recurrence rate, even without treatment. MVP is the single most frequently diagnosed cardiac valvular abnormality. Estimates of prevalence range from 5% to 21%, with the rate being slightly higher in girls and women.[84] The basic pathologic process is disruption of collagen and infiltration of the valve by a myxomatous substance rich in mucopolysaccharide. The mitral valve is often thickened and the chordae tendineae and mitral annulus may also contain myxomatous deposits, which can cause elongation of the chordae, sometimes with rupture and dilatation of the mitral valve annulus. Abnormal mitral valve leaflet motion can cause fibrosis and thickening of the endocardial surface of the valve leaflets.[85] The tricuspid and aortic valves sometimes also show myxomatous degeneration. When there is enough slippage, so that a portion of the mitral valve fails to coapt against the rest of the leaflet, then mitral regurgitation develops. Patients with MVP sometimes have abnormal left ventricular contractions. At necropsy, thrombi have been found, especially in the angle between the posterior leaflet of the mitral valve and the left atrial wall.[83,86,87] Transformation of the normally rigid valve into loose myxomatous tissue results in stretching of the valve leaflets, loss of endothelial continuity, and rupture of subendothelial connective tissue fibers. These changes could promote the formation of platelet-fibrin thrombi on the valve surface.

MVP is diagnosed by echocardiography when there is abnormal posterior movement of the coapted anterior or posterior leaflets (or both) of 2 mm or more, and one or both of the mitral valve leaflets are displaced during systole into the left atrium above the plane of the mitral annulus.[83] Midsystolic "buckling" or pansystolic "hammocking" of the valve leaflets is also sometimes found.[83] Mitral valve thickening and redundancy and the presence of mitral regurgitation are important additional criteria for the presence of important myxomatous mitral valve changes.[88,89] Approximately 8% of patients with MVP develop severe mitral regurgitation, which leads to congestive heart failure and necessitates mitral valve replacement. Atrial fibrillation can occur at any time but is more common in older patients, especially those with mitral regurgitation and large left atria. Myxomatous valves can become infected during bacteremia but the frequency of infective endocarditis is low. MVP occurs in patients with inherited connective tissue disorders, such as Marfan syndrome, Ehlers-Danlos syndrome, and osteogenesis imperfecta.[83]

The first report of a possible relation between MVP and brain ischemia was by Barnett in 1974.[90] The initial report outlined four patients, but Barnett and his colleagues later expanded the number of cases to 14 patients.[87,91] All patients were relatively young (10–48 years old), and none had cardiovascular risk factors or occlusive vascular lesions. Barnett and colleagues later published a case-control series that provided further evidence of a relationship between MVP and brain ischemia in young patients.[92]

Among six series of patients with MVP and brain ischemic events reviewed by Lauzier and Barnett,[83] there were 114 patients, including 46 men and 68 women. Two-thirds of the events were strokes. The remainder were TIAs. Single attacks were more common than multiple ischemic events. Sixteen of the patients had an arrhythmia detected by rhythm monitoring, including eight with atrial fibrillation.

Abnormalities of platelet function have been shown in patients with MVP and thromboembolism. Shortened platelet survival time, an increase in circulating platelet aggregates, and increased levels of beta-thromboglobulin and platelet factor IV were found in patients with MVP.[83] Interaction of circulating platelets with abnormal endocardial and valve structures in patients with myxomatous valve degeneration causes increased platelet aggregation, adhesion, and secretion. Platelet fibrin aggregates adhere to abnormal valve surfaces and later embolize or promote formation of erythrocyte-fibrin clots.

The recurrence rate of stroke in patients with MVP is low. In patients with mitral regurgitation and large left atria, and in those with atrial fibrillation and atrial or valvular thrombi shown by echocardiography, warfarin anticoagulation is probably indicated. In patients who do not have atrial fibrillation, endocarditis, or severe mitral insufficiency, the treatment of choice is probably an antiplatelet aggregant, such as aspirin or clopidogrel.

Mitral Annulus Calcification. MAC is a degenerative disorder of the fibrous support structure of the mitral valve that occurs rather commonly in the elderly, especially in women. In the original description of MAC, four of the 14 patients described by Korn and colleagues had brain infarcts, and three of those four had multiple infarcts.[93] The first important description of MAC as a potential cause of stroke was by DeBono and Warlow.[94] These authors studied 151 patients with retinal or brain ischemia and found MAC in eight patients, as compared with no instances of MAC in age and sex-matched controls who did not have brain or eye ischemia.[94]

During the years 1979–1981, 426 men and 733 women in the Framingham Study Cohort (average age, 70 years) who did not have strokes had M-mode echocardiograms.[95] Among these 1,159 patients, 44 men (10.3%) and 116 women (15.8%) had MAC. During 8 years of follow-up, 51 patients without

MAC (5.1%) had strokes, as compared with 22 patients with MAC (13.8%); MAC was associated with a 2.10 RR of stroke (95% confidence interval, 1.24–3.57, $p = .006$).[95] A continuous relation was found in this study between frequency of stroke and severity of MAC; each millimeter of thickening on the echocardiogram represented an RR of stroke of 1.24. Even when patients with atherosclerotic heart disease and congestive heart failure were excluded, patients with MAC still had stroke risk that was two times as high as those without MAC.[95]

Calcification has a predilection for the posterior portion of the mitral annulus ring. Calcific masses often extend as far as 3.5 cm into the adjacent myocardium and often project superiorly toward the atrium and centrally into the cavity of the left ventricle.[93] Ulceration and extrusion of the calcium through the overlying cusp into the ventricular cavity is found in some patients with MAC studied at necropsy, and thrombi are sometimes attached to the ulcerated regions.[96] Thrombi attached to calcified mitral annuli have also been shown by echocardiography. Embolic material in patients with MAC can be calcium (as shown in calcific aortic stenosis) or thrombus.

MAC is common, especially in older women, and is often accompanied by mitral regurgitation and atrial fibrillation. Bacterial endocarditis can be superimposed. Hypertension, coronary atherosclerotic heart disease, and occlusive cerebrovascular disease are also often present in the population of patients with MAC. There are no data on the use of any prophylactic treatment on the prevention of brain or arterial embolism in patients with MAC.

Prosthetic Cardiac Valves. Advances in cardiac diagnosis and surgery have led to increasingly frequent replacement of heart valves. There are more than 80 different models of prosthetic valves, and more than 60,000 valve replacements are performed annually in the United States alone.[97] Mechanical valves are made primarily with metal and carbon alloys and are quite thrombogenic. Bioprosthetic valves are most often heterografts derived from pig or cow pericardial or valve tissues mounted on metal supports. Homografts, in the form of preserved human valves, are occasionally used for valve replacements. Bioprosthetic valves have low thrombogenic tendencies (but still higher than native valves), so long-term anticoagulation is ordinarily not prescribed. Bioprosthetic valves are less durable than mechanical valves.[97]

Valve thrombosis is an important complication in patients with both mechanical and bioprosthetic valves. Important valve thrombosis causes pulmonary congestion, reduced cardiac output, and brain and systemic embolism. The frequency of prosthetic-valve thrombosis is estimated to be between 0.1% and 5.7% per year.[98,99] Alteration of blood flow related to mechanical valves, as well as the inherent thrombogenicity of the materials used, promotes thrombosis and thromboembolism. Hematologic studies in patients with mechanical valves show elevation of platelet-specific proteins, which indicate platelet activation and decreased platelet survival.[100]

The pathophysiologic events that promote thromboembolism begin during heart surgery. Prosthetic materials and injured perivalvular tissues cause platelet activation as soon as circulation is restored. Dacron sewing rings, common to all prosthetic valves, form a fertile nidus for platelet activation and adhesion. Prosthetic material also activates the intrinsic pathway of the coagulation cascade. These events promote the formation of red erythrocyte-fibrin thrombi. Degenerative changes in bioprosthetic valves can also stimulate deposition of white platelet-fibrin thrombi. Late thrombosis is also found in the cusp sinuses of bioprosthetic mitral valves that have undergone fibrosis and calcification.[101]

Embolism is an important complication in patients with mechanical and bioprosthetic valves. The frequency of major embolism in patients with mechanical valves is estimated to be 4% per year if no antithrombotic therapy is used.[102] This frequency is reduced to approximately 2% per year by medications that decrease platelet aggregation, and to 1% per year with warfarin anticoagulation.[102] Most symptomatic emboli go to the brain. Patients with mitral mechanical valves have a slightly higher frequency of embolization than those with aortic valves, probably related to the higher frequency of associated atrial fibrillation and large left atria in patients with mitral valve prostheses. Patients with bioprosthetic valves also have a risk of embolism. In one series of 128 patients with porcine bioprosthetic valves inserted during 5–8 years of follow-up, two of 43 patients with aortic valve replacement, nine of 62 with porcine mitral valves, and four of 18 with both mitral and aortic prosthetic valves had clinical thromboemboli.[103] Most patients with thromboemboli in this series had atrial fibrillation or heart block.[103] Large left atria, atrial fibrillation, left ventricular dysfunction, and infective endocarditis are important associated conditions in patients with prosthetic valves that cause thromboembolism.

Anticoagulation is recommended for all patients with prosthetic heart valves. Patients with bioprosthetic valves are usually treated for the first 3 months after surgery using a target international normalized ratio (INR) of 2.0–3.0. Oral anticoagulant therapy reduces the incidence of embolism in patients with mechanical valve prostheses and the intensity of anticoagulation has been recommended to be higher than that used with bioprosthetic valves (INR of 2.5–4.9). Patients with caged-ball prostheses may require a higher intensity of anticoagulation than those with bileaflet disk valves and those with single-tilting disk valves. Adding antiplatelet medications, such as dipyridamole, aspirin, or clopidogrel, can further reduce the frequency of embolism. Aspirin and lower-intensity anticoagulation (INR of 2.0–3.0) are probably as effective as high-intensity anticoagulation and have less risk of serious bleeding. Because prosthetic valves induce formation of white platelet-fibrin and red erythrocyte-fibrin clots, the use of combined antiplatelet aggregant and anticoagulant therapy makes sense. Pregnant women with prosthetic valves should be treated with heparin or low-molecular-weight heparin because the incidence of thromboemboli is increased while pregnant and also in the puerperium.

Infective Endocarditis. The clinical spectrum of endocarditis has changed dramatically. Compared with series of endocarditis patients performed in the 1960s, series of patients with infective endocarditis performed in the 1990s contain older patients, more drug addicts, more examples of tricuspid valve involvement (usually in intravenous drug addicts), and more patients with infection of prosthetic valves. Diagnostic capabilities have also changed. Echocardiography and newer brain and cerebrovascular imaging techniques allow better clarification of the cardiac and brain pathology and pathophysiology. Brain ischemia, intracerebral hemorrhage, subarachnoid hemorrhage, encephalopathy, and meningitis were the major neurologic complications found in series of patients with native valve and prosthetic valve endocarditis.[104–109]

Brain ischemia is invariably caused by embolism. Approximately one-fifth of patients with endocarditis develop brain infarcts. At necropsy, small, usually multiple, cortical or subcortical bland infarcts are found. The larger infarcts are usually found in patients with *Staphylococcus aureus* endocarditis. Ischemia can take the form of TIAs that involve the brain or retina. Brain ischemia may be the presenting sign of endocarditis and is most common early in the course of the disease. Ischemic strokes can also occur days after antibiotic treatment has begun. Monitoring of patients with endocarditis using TCD shows that microemboli continue to occur even after antibiotic treatment, although more emboli are detected before and shortly after antibiotics are given. Brain ischemia was described in 17%,[105] 19%,[106] and 15%[109] of patients in various infective endocarditis series.

Brain hemorrhage is much less frequent than ischemia, but the effects of hemorrhage can be devastating and fatal. Intracerebral hemorrhage was found in 6%,[105] 7%,[106] 2.8%,[108] and 5.6%[109] of patients in various endocarditis series. Series that included modern brain imaging and necropsy studies clarified the mechanisms of intracerebral hemorrhage in endocarditis.[107,110,111] Some patients bleed into bland infarcts. This usually takes the form of hemorrhagic infarction—petechial and larger regions of hemorrhagic mottling within infarcts, without formation of frank, discrete hematomas. In some patients, large hematomas develop. Hematomas are often found in patients treated with anticoagulants. In other patients, intracerebral hemorrhage results from rupture of a septic arteritis caused by embolization of infected material to the artery with necrosis of the arterial wall.[110,111] In a minority of patients, intracerebral hemorrhage is caused by rupture of a mycotic aneurysm into the brain substance. Brain hemorrhage, similar to the situation in patients with brain ischemia, is most common at or near presentation and is less common after effective antibiotic treatment. Many patients who develop brain hemorrhage have had an attack of transient or persistent brain ischemia in the hours or days before the hemorrhage. This prodromal ischemia is explained by an arterial embolus causing brain infarction. Hemorrhage into an infarct or rupture of the artery that received the infected embolus causes the hemorrhage, which often proves fatal.[110,111]

The need for angiography to detect mycotic aneurysms and the indications for surgical treatment of aneurysms found by angiography are controversial topics. In a review by Hart et al., among 2,119 patients with endocarditis, only 5% of patients with brain hemorrhages had identified mycotic aneurysms.[110] Mycotic aneurysms are caused by embolization of infected material into the wall and adventitia of brain arteries. The aneurysms usually occur distally along arteries and tend to be multiple. The location of aneurysms in patients with infective endocarditis is similar to those found in patients with atrial myxomas, probably because of similar embolic etiologies. In contrast, ordinary saccular "berry" aneurysms occur proximally along the basal arteries of the circle of Willis. Angiography of patients without brain hemorrhage seldom shows mycotic aneurysms. Mycotic aneurysms have been shown to disappear in some patients on sequential angiography performed after bacteriologic cure.[112–114] Mycotic aneurysms can rupture, however, sometimes after bacteriologic cure, and re-rupture can prove fatal. The decision as to whether to perform angiography and surgical treatment if an aneurysm is found must rest on the clinical findings in individual patients.

Diffuse brain-related symptoms, usually referred to as *encephalopathy*, are common in patients with endocarditis. Symptoms include lethargy and decreased level of consciousness, confusion, agitation, poor concentration, and memory loss. Encephalopathy has different explanations. Often, the encephalopathy is toximetabolic and explained by systemic factors, such as azotemia, pulmonary dysfunction, hyponatremia, and so forth. In many patients, encephalopathy is a toxic effect related to fever and the acute infection. Patients with *S. aureus* acute endocarditis are more often toxic than in endocarditis caused by other organisms. Necropsy, CT, and MRI studies of patients with encephalopathy often show multiple, small, scattered brain infarcts, microabscesses, or both.[107,115] Encephalopathy usually develops during uncontrolled infection with virulent organisms, supporting the role of microscopic septic emboli as the cause.[107]

Meningitis also occurs in patients with endocarditis. Meningeal infection is caused by embolization of infected vegetations to meningeal arteries. The presentation is often headache with fever. Because the usual infecting organism is not virulent, the patient is not as ill as in other acute forms of bacterial meningitis. Meningitis occurred in 6.4%[104] and 1.1%[105] in two series of patients with endocarditis.

Valvular vegetations in patients with infective endocarditis are composed of platelets, fibrin, erythrocytes, and inflammatory cells attached to damaged endothelium of native and prosthetic valves. Organisms are enmeshed within the fibrinous material, often deep within the vegetations, explaining why antibiotics have difficulty sterilizing the lesions. Vegetations range in size from several millimeters to several centimeters, and their potential for embolization relate to their size and friability. The mitral valve is most often involved. Mitral valve disease, however, is also more frequent than other valve disease. In the past, the predominant underlying valve disease was rheumatic; calcified valves, MVP, and prosthetic valves now make up a higher proportion of cases than in the past. The neurologic complications of native valve and prosthetic valve endocarditis are the same.[105,107,108]

Laboratory studies are helpful in diagnosis, but the clinical findings remain protean, and most important for recognition of infective endocarditis is a strong clinical suspicion. The disease should be suspected in any patient with unexplained fever and a heart murmur. Multiple blood cultures are important in all patients suspected of having infective endocarditis. The spinal fluid may be normal or contain slightly increased protein levels and increased numbers of erythrocytes and leukocytes. Usually, the pleocytosis is moderate (<300 cells/ cc) and may be predominantly lymphocytic or polymorphonuclear unless a clinical picture of meningitis is present, in which case there may be more white blood cells. The frequency of detection of vegetations on echocardiography depends on the technique used and the frequency of examinations. Infective vegetations appear as bright, usually mobile echo-dense lesions attached to valve leaflets. Lesions smaller than 2 mm are not reliably identified by echocardiography. In the series of Hart et al. (using M-mode and two-dimensional transthoracic echocardiography), vegetations were found on 41% of initial echocardiograms in patients with *S. aureus* endocarditis, compared with 57% of initial studies in patients with streptococcal species endocarditis.[106] Transesophageal echocardiography is likely to show vegetations more often than transthoracic echocardiography.

An echocardiogram that fails to show a vegetation does not exclude the diagnosis of endocarditis.

The most important treatment is the rapid introduction of specific antimicrobial drugs. Most neurologic complications occur before or near the time of diagnosis and initial antibiotic treatment. Recurrent strokes do occur after bacteriologic cure, but rarely. In one series among 147 patients discharged from the hospital after treatment of infective endocarditis, 15 developed strokes after discharge; all except one of the stroke patients had prosthetic valve endocarditis.[105] Strokes in this series occurred long after discharge (median, 22 months) and were better explained by recurrence of endocarditis, complications of anticoagulants, and noninfective disease of the prosthetic valves than by cerebrovascular complications of the original endocarditic episode.[105] Native valve endocarditis is not an indication for anticoagulation, even when brain or systemic embolism has occurred. Controversy surrounds the issue of maintenance of anticoagulation in patients who have mechanical valve endocarditis, but most clinicians favor cautious continuation of anticoagulants unless a brain hemorrhage develops. When a hemorrhagic infarct or brain hemorrhage develops, anticoagulation with warfarin is usually stopped for 1–2 weeks. In patients with a major risk of recurrent embolization, it may be safe to use heparin beginning soon after the hemorrhage is discovered and later switch back to warfarin. Cardiac surgery to debride or replace infected valves is performed for cardiac indications. These include mostly heart failure related to valve dysfunction, lack of control of infection, valve infection with fungal or other virulent organism not controllable by antimicrobial drugs, and valve or chordae tendineae rupture.

Noninfective Fibrous and Fibrinous Endocardial Lesions (Including Valve Strands). In a variety of other circumstances, fibrous valve thickening, often with grossly visible vegetations that contain mixtures of platelets and fibrin, are found on the heart valves and adjacent endocardium in patients who have no evidence of rheumatic fever or bacterial endocarditis. The first detailed description of such lesions was by Libman and Sacks, who reported four patients studied clinically and pathologically with an "atypical verrucous endocarditis."[116] Necropsy showed fibrous thickening of

valves with vegetations, especially along the closure lines of the valves and on valve leaflets. The vegetations spread to the papillary muscles and ventricular endocardium. Only one patient had prominent clinical neurologic abnormalities, a unilateral paralysis and seizures, which developed shortly before death. The authors speculated that these findings might be caused by emboli from the valvular vegetations. Libman and Sacks were uncertain of the diagnosis but noted that the clinical picture resembled some of the erythematous diseases. The next year, Klemperer, Pollack, and Baehr published the pathologic findings in disseminated lupus erythematosus.[117] In 1935, Baehr and colleagues published a series of 23 patients who had acute disseminated lupus erythematosus, among whom 13 patients had a nonrheumatic verrucous endocarditis similar to that described by Libman and Sacks.[118] These clinical and pathologic reports brought the disease systemic lupus erythematosus (SLE), known previously as predominantly a skin disorder, to the attention of the medical community as an acute disseminated systemic disease. Gross, a younger colleague of Libman and Sacks at Mount Sinai Hospital in New York in 1940, reported a detailed study of 27 hearts, 23 of which were fatal cases of SLE.[119] Gross pointed out that the patients in the original report from the Mount Sinai Hospital had the typical clinical findings of lupus erythematosus and suggested that the verrucous endocardial lesions were diagnostic of that disease.[119] Libman and Sacks[116] and Gross[119] were aware that similar endocarditic lesions also occurred in terminal or cachectic diseases, such as carcinoma, tuberculosis, and leukemia, and were called *nonbacterial thrombotic endocarditis*. Since these early reports, similar lesions of the cardiac valves and endocardium are known to occur in patients with SLE, the antiphospholipid antibody (APLA) syndrome, and marantic nonbacterial thrombotic endocarditis (NBTE). All likely have a similar pathogenesis.

Valvular lesions are common in patients with SLE. Roldan et al. performed TEE on 69 SLE patients on two occasions, averaging 29 months between echocardiograms.[120] Valvular abnormalities were found in 61% of patients on the initial TEE and in 53% on the second echocardiographic study. Valve thickening (61%), vegetations (43%), valve regurgitation (25%), and stenosis (4%) were found on the initial echocardiograms. The mitral valve was most often involved, followed closely by involvement of the aortic valve; tricuspid valve disease occurred occasionally, but pulmonic valve involvement was rare. The combined incidence of stroke, peripheral embolism, heart failure, and superimposed infective endocarditis was 22% in those with valvular disease found on TEE.[120]

APLA syndrome has become recognized since the 1970s as a prothrombic syndrome separate from SLE. The APLA syndrome is characterized by frequent fetal loss, strokes, myocardial infarcts, phlebothrombosis, pulmonary emboli, and thrombocytopenia. Serologic testing reveals positive assays for the lupus anticoagulant, anticardiolipin antibodies, or both. Echocardiographic studies have shown that there is a relatively high frequency of cardiac valvular lesions in patients with APLA syndrome, and that the valve lesions are indistinguishable from those found in patients with SLE. Barbut et al. studied the prevalence of antiphospholipid antibodies among 87 patients in whom echocardiography showed mitral or aortic regurgitation, or both[121]; 26 patients (30%) had immunoglobulin G or M anticardiolipin antibodies. Focal cerebral ischemic events occurred in eight of these patients (seven judged embolic), including seven of the immunoglobulin G anticardiolipin-positive patients.[121] Barbut and colleagues studied 21 patients with APLA antibodies who had focal cerebral ischemic events.[122] Twelve of 14 stroke patients (86%), and three of seven non–stroke lesion patients (42%) had echocardiographic evidence of mitral or aortic valve abnormalities. Eight of the 21 patients with APLA had SLE in this study.[122] In a large cooperative study performed by the Antiphospholid Antibodies in Stroke Study Group among 128 patients who had brain or ocular ischemia and were APLA positive, 16 patients (12.5%) had mitral valve abnormalities on echocardiograms, and two patients had aortic valve lesions.[123] Phospholipids are important constituents of cardiac valve endothelium, blood platelets, vascular endothelium, and coagulation proteins. At present, assays for antiphospholipid antibodies only include testing for lupus anticoagulant and anticardiolipin antibodies. Some patients with the clinical features of the APLA syndrome have valve vegetations and cardiogenic brain embolism, but antibody assays are negative.

Hypercoagulability and NBTE have long been known to occur in patients with cancer and other debilitating chronic diseases. Most often, the cancers are mucinous adenocarcinomas.[124] In one study of 20 cancer patients who had thromboembolic disease of the brain and other organs, 16 patients (80%) had NBTE at necropsy.[125] Edoute et al. performed prospective echocardiograms on 200 cancer patients and found a 19% frequency of NBTE.[126] The valve lesions equally involved the mitral and aortic valves. Elevated plasma D-dimer levels, a marker for hypercoagulability, was also often found in cancer patients with clinical thromboembolism.[126] NBTE is characterized by friable white or tan vegetations, usually along lines of valve closure. The vegetations can be large. Microscopy usually shows degenerating platelets interwoven with strands of fibrin and some leukocytes, forming eosinophilic masses of tissue.

All three conditions—SLE, APLA syndrome, and NBTE—are associated with hypercoagulability, strokes, and thrombocytopenia. The cardiac valve and endothelial lesions in these three conditions are similar and probably indistinguishable grossly and microscopically. Platelet deposition, incorporation of fibrin, and the formation of platelet thrombi on valve and endocardial surfaces are common to all three conditions. Treatment of these conditions has not been formally studied. In theory, drugs that alter platelet aggregation, secretion, and adhesion might be effective. In patients with SLE and APLA syndrome who have hypercoagulability, heparin and warfarin compounds are usually prescribed to treat the hypercoagulablity and prevent venous and arterial occlusions.

Noninfective valve lesions are also found in patients with carcinoid tumors (probably causally related to elevated serotonin levels in the blood) and after the use of some drugs (ergotamine, methysergide, dexfenfluramine, and fenfluramine and phentermine).[127] The valve and endocardial lesions that result are similar to each other morphologically and consist of fibrotic thickening of the valves with reduced pliability.

Echocardiographic examinations often show strands of mobile tissue attached to valve surfaces. The cause and significance of these strands remain uncertain. In 1856, Lambl had originally described such filamentous outgrowths from the ventricular surfaces of the aortic valves sometimes found at necropsy,[128] so these fibrous strand-like lesions have often been called *Lambl excrescences*. Later,

Magarey found similar filiform strands on the atrial surface of mitral valves.[129] The strands, which were composed of a cellular connective tissue core covered by endothelium, were usually less than 1 mm thick and ranged in length from 1 to 10 mm.[129] Magarey related the strands to mitral valve thickening and posited that they originated from fibrinous deposits on valve surfaces.[129] Freedberg et al. reviewed retrospectively a series of 1,559 patients with TEEs during a 2-year period and found mitral valve strands in 63 patients (4%) and aortic valve strands in 26 patients (1.7%).[130] Strands were found in 10.6% of patients referred because of suspected recent embolic events, compared with 2.3% of those referred for other indications.[130]

Roberts and colleagues compared the frequency of strands among patients referred for TEE because of brain ischemia and those referred for other indications.[131] An association between brain ischemia and strands was found (odds ratio, 4 to 4; 95% confidence interval, 2.0–9.6).[131] The association was strongest for younger patients and those with mitral and aortic valve strands. Cohen et al. found strands in 22.5% of 338 brain ischemia patients versus 12.1% of 276 patients who had no history of brain ischemia (odds ratio, 2 to 1; 95% confidence interval, 1.3–3.4; $p < .005$).[132] The risk of recurrent stroke in patients with strands was low.[132] Strands are often found in patients with mitral valve thickening.[132,133] Strands probably form because of a degenerative process that causes fibrinous deposits on valve surfaces. Emboli can arise from the abnormal valves, strands, or thrombi formed on the surface of the valve or on the strands. In some patients, strands may share a pathogenesis with valve lesions found in patients with SLE, APLAs, and cancer. Treatment of patients with strands has not been formally studied but anticoagulants were unsuccessful in preventing brain emboli in two reported patients[134] and are probably also not effective in patients with NBTE. Antiplatelet aggregants, or a combination of antiplatelet aggregants and anticoagulants, might be more effective in preventing thrombus formation and embolism than either agent alone.

Myocardial and Cardiac Chamber Lesions

Myocardial Infarction and Coronary Artery Disease. Systemic embolism is apparent clinically in approximately 3% (range, 0.6–6.4%) of patients with acute myocardial infarction.[2] Most clinically detected emboli involve the brain. Most strokes that occur in patients with acute myocardial infarcts are caused by embolization of thrombi formed in the left ventricle, but some strokes are caused by left atrial thrombi, hypotension, and extracranial occlusive vascular disease. Coronary artery thrombosis can cause an increase in acute phase reactants, including serine protease coagulation proteins. Venous thromboses and occlusion of atherostenotic craniocervical arteries develop in the days and weeks after myocardial infarction because of this hypercoagulability.

Left ventricular thrombi are detected in 20–40% of patients with acute anterior myocardial infarcts, but are unusual in patients with inferior infarction.[135,136] Most thrombi form on the apical wall of the left ventricle in regions of reduced ventricular contractility. Mural thrombi are more likely to form in patients with transmural and large anterior myocardial infarcts than in those with small infarcts. Areas of decreased ventricular contractility, low ejection fraction, and development of a left ventricular aneurysm predispose to thrombus formation. Figure 9-4 shows a large thrombus in the left ventricle of a patient with a fatal recent myocardial infarct. Cardiac thrombi most often develop within the first 3 days after myocardial infarction, especially in those patients with large infarcts. Systemic embolization occurs, on average, 14 days after myocardial infarction and is unusual after 4–6 weeks.[137] Anticoagulants reduce the frequency of stroke in patients with acute myocardial infarcts. Among 999 patients with acute myocardial infarction, short-term warfarin treatment for 28 days reduced the rate of stroke (0.8% vs 3.8% in nonanticoagulated controls, $p < .001$).[138]

Regions of decreased ventricular contraction and frank ventricular aneurysms often persist after acute myocardial infarction. In the Coronary Artery Surgery Study (CASS), 7.6% of patients had angiographically defined left ventricular aneurysms.[139] Although aneurysms are relatively common and mural thrombi often form within aneurysms, the risk of stroke is relatively low, at approximately 5%.[140] The risk of stroke in patients with impaired left ventricular function after myocardial infarction is substantial. In one study of 2,231 patients with left ventricular dysfunction after acute myocardial infarction who were followed for an average of 42 months, 103 patients (4.6%) developed strokes.[141]

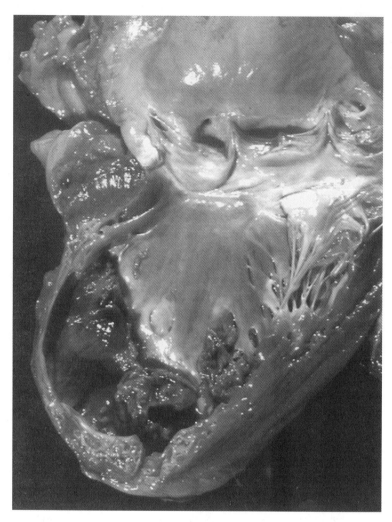

Figure 9-4. Heart at necropsy in a patient with a massive brain embolus. A large clot overlying a recent myocardial infarct exists.

Patients with ejection fractions of less than 28% were at highest risk, and for every absolute decrease of 5% in the left ventricular ejection fraction, the risk of stroke increased by 18%.

Some patients with brain embolism are unexpectedly found to have thrombi within their left ventricles. Some of these patients do not have a history of acute myocardial infarction, and the cardiac cavity lesions are often first thought to represent myxomas or other cardiac tumors. Sequential echocardiography shows that these thrombi can gradually regress or suddenly disappear,[2] often without development of neurologic or other symptoms of embolism. Thrombus formation, spontaneous endogenous fibrinolysis, and fragmentation of thrombi are dynamic processes. Thrombolytic treatment of patients with cardiac thrombi poses

the theoretical risk of fragmentation of large thrombi into portions that could embolize and cause stroke and systemic embolism. Thrombi may disappear during anticoagulation without symptoms or signs of embolism.

Myocardiopathies. Conditions that affect the endocardium and myocardium promote the formation of cardiac mural thrombi and systemic and brain embolism. The three most important factors that determine thrombus formation are (1) involvement of the endocardial surface, (2) ventricular contractility and blood flow and ejection patterns within the ventricles, and (3) activation of platelets and the coagulation system. Among the three categories of cardiomyopathies—dilatated, restrictive, and hypertrophic—mural thrombus formation and embolism are most common among the dilated cardiomyopathies. Intraventricular thrombus formation is enhanced by stasis of blood and the loss of normal subendocardial trabeculation. The network of subendocardial trabeculae functions as many small compartments that produce high levels of force within the ventricle, propelling blood away from the endocardial surface.[142]

Conditions as diverse as muscular dystrophies, cardiac amyloidosis, peripartum cardiomyopathy, Fabry's disease, cocaine-related cardiomyopathy, noncompaction of the myocardium, and cardiac sarcoidosis are sources of cardiac-origin embolism.[2] Mural thrombi form mostly within the trabeculae carneae near the cardiac apex. Atrial fibrillation develops in some patients with cardiomyopathies and further increases the frequency of embolism. Embolism is unusual in patients with hypertrophic cardiomyopathies unless they develop atrial fibrillation.

Cardiac Myxomas and Other Tumors. Although cardiac tumors are rare, they are an important cause of embolism. Myxomas are the most common heart tumor. Most myxomas originate from the interatrial septum at the edge of the fossa ovalis, but some originate from the posterior or anterior atrial walls or the auricular appendage.[143] Approximately 75% are located in the left atrium and 15–20% in the right atrium.[143] Approximately 6–8% of myxomas are found in the ventricles equally divided between the left and right ventricles.[143] Myxomas rarely arise from the heart valves. Biatrial myxomas have been described, in which case the tumor usually projects into the contralateral atrium through a PFO. Myxomas project from their endocardial attachments into cardiac chambers. Myxomas are most often found in patients between the ages of 30 and 60 years; women are affected slightly more than men, and instances of familial occurrence of myxomas have occurred.

Embolism occurs in 30–50% of patients with cardiac myxomas.[143,144] Most emboli arise from the left atrium and travel to the brain or systemic organs. Occasionally, right atrial myxomas cause systemic embolism in the presence of a PFO. Emboli consist of tumor fragments, thrombus, or both.

Occasionally, patients with brain emboli from myxomas have subarachnoid or intracerebral hemorrhage. Bleeding is related to the development of hemorrhagic infarction or rupture of aneurysms.

Embolism from myxoma tissue to the wall of brain arteries causes aneurysms that are identical to mycotic aneurysms found in patients with bacterial endocarditis. Usually, the aneurysms are relatively small, multiple, and on peripheral branches of brain arteries. Some aneurysms are quite large. The peripheral location of aneurysms in patients with myxomas and endocarditis differs from that usually found in patients with saccular ("berry") aneurysms. Delayed progressive brain ischemia and enlargement of aneurysms can develop after the initial embolic event. Although delayed growth and rupture of aneurysms and metastatic tumor growth do occur, their frequency is low. In a review of 35 patients followed at the Mayo Clinic after surgical removal of atrial myxomas, none had subsequent delayed neurologic events attributable to their myxomas.[145] Recurrent cardiac tumors after surgery can, however, give rise to recurrent embolization.

Papillary fibroelastomas are another type of cardiac tumor that often give rise to brain embolism.[146,147] The lesions consist of multiple papillary fronds that radiate from an avascular fibrocollagenous core attached by a short pedicle to the endothelium. They most often arise from the aortic valves.[147] Angina and coronary ischemia are caused by embolism to the coronary arteries. Multiple brain infarcts usually occur before the diagnosis is made by echocardiography. Rhabdomyomas are often multiple, arise from the ventricular myocardium, and project into the ventricular cavity. Tuberous sclerosis and neurofibromatosis predispose to the development of cardiac rhabdomyomas.

Emboli are often composed of tumor fragments. Theoretically, white platelet-fibrin nidi might develop on the surface and crevices of cardiac tumors, as might red erythrocyte-fibrin thrombi. For this reason, agents that affect platelet aggregation and function and standard anticoagulants might have some therapeutic effect, but no studies of their use in patients with myxomas or other cardiac neoplasms have been performed. The only definitive treatment is surgery.

Paradoxical Embolism and Cardiac Septal Lesions

Emboli entering the systemic circulation through right-to-left shunting of blood are becoming more frequently recognized because of more extensive cardiac testing of stroke patients. By far, the most common potential intracardiac shunt is a residual

PFO. The high frequency of PFOs in the normal population makes it difficult to be certain in an individual stroke patient with a PFO whether paradoxical embolism through the PFO was the cause of their stroke or whether the PFO was merely an incidental finding. Autopsy series have shown that approximately 30% of adults have a probe patent PFO at necropsy.[148] Hagen et al. studied 956 patients with clinically and pathologically normal hearts and found a PFO in 27.3%.[148] The frequency of PFOs declined with age—34.3% during the first three decades of life, 25.4% during the fourth through eighth decades, and 20.2% during the ninth and tenth decades. The average diameter of PFOs was 4.9 mm, and the size tended to increase with age.[148] Echocardiographic studies have shown that PFOs are found more often in patients with stroke than in controls, and PFOs are more common in patients with an undetermined cause of stroke ("cryptogenic stroke") than in those in whom another etiology has been defined.[149–151]

I use the following five criteria for paradoxical embolism: (1) situations that promote thrombosis of leg or pelvic veins (e.g., sitting in one position for a long period, recent surgery, and so forth); (2) increased coagulability (e.g., the use of oral contraceptives, presence of Leiden factor with resistance to activated protein C, dehydration); (3) sudden onset of stroke during sexual intercourse, straining at stool, or other activity that includes a Valsalva's maneuver or promotes right-to-left shunting of blood; (4) pulmonary embolism within a short time before or after the neurologic ischemic event; and (5) the absence of other putative causes of stroke after thorough evaluation. When at least four of these criteria are met, the diagnosis of paradoxical embolism is highly probable.

One typical patient was a 29-year-old woman who, with her husband and four children, returned home from a trip. The day was hot and she had nothing to drink during the 8-hour car ride. Much of the ride was spent disciplining the children while she kneeled on her seat facing the children, who cavorted in the back of the station wagon. When she and her husband got home, they fed the children and put them to bed. She showered and, immediately thereafter, had sex with her husband.

At the point of climax, she became unable to speak and her right arm was weak and numb. Examination showed a right hemiparesis and aphasia. CT showed a left-upper division MCA-territory infarct. Echocardiography showed a large PFO with increased flow during a Valsalva's maneuver. The heart and aorta were otherwise normal, and an MRA examination of the cervicocranial arteries was normal. She made a good recovery but had residual right hand numbness and dysnomia.

Gautier and colleagues reported on 29 patients with paradoxical embolism and reviewed 31 patients reported by others.[152] Situations that promoted venous occlusions among these 60 patients included surgery, postpartum, lower extremity injury, and jugular vein catheterization. Strokes occurred after sex, straining at stool, weight lifting, vigorous nose blowing, asthmatic attacks, gymnastics, decompressing the ears, and martial arts. Venous thrombosis was detected in few patients, and few had clinical pulmonary emboli. Pulmonary radionuclide scans, angiography, and necropsy showed pulmonary emboli in many patients.[152] The most common territory of stroke was the MCA, which was involved in 25 patients. Fifteen patients had vertebrobasilar-territory embolic infarcts.[152] Thirty-seven and one-half percent of posterior circulation infarction is more than expected, because only 20% of blood flow to the brain goes through the posterior circulation. A study of the distribution of microemboli in patients with PFOs also showed that there is an unexplained predilection for embolic material to go to posterior circulation arteries.[153]

Paradoxical embolism also occurs through ventricular septal defects, atrial septal defects, and pulmonary arteriovenous fistulas. Figure 9-5 shows various mechanisms of paradoxical embolism. Venous thrombosis can be detected if studies are performed early in the course. Some venous thrombi involve the pelvic veins and might be detected by abdominal and pelvic imaging techniques.

The advent of TEE has undoubtedly facilitated recognition and quantification of PFOs and atrial septal defects. TCD has also been used effectively to diagnose the presence of right-to-left cardiac or pulmonary shunting.[154–156] The technique involves injection of a small amount of saline, which has been agitated vigorously with a small amount of air, or mixed with a polygeline contrast agent, and injected into a cubital vein.[155] During and after the injection, the MCA is insonated using TCD. Appearance of microbubbles in the MCA within the first 3–5 cardiac cycles (<10 seconds) indicates the presence of right-to-left shunting of blood. The test is usually done with and without a Valsalva's maneuver. The technique has the advantage of being able to be used at the bedside because TCD is portable. Figure 9-6 shows a shower of HITS in an MCA after air bubble injection in a patient with a large PFO.

Predictors for the likelihood of paradoxical embolism through PFOs have been sought using TEE.[157,158] In one study, the presence of an atrial septal aneurysm accompanying the PFO was an important finding, favoring the presence of paradoxical embolism.[157] In another study, PFOs were significantly larger, and more microbubbles were present in patients with cryptogenic stroke than in those with identified causes of stroke.[158] Electrocardiographic findings can also suggest the presence of PFOs and ostium secundum atrial septal defects. An M-shaped notch on the ascending branch or on the peak of the R-wave in inferior electrocardiographic leads (II, III, aVF) is often found in patients with PFOs or atrial septal defects.[159] This notched pattern has been called *crochetage* because of its resemblance morphologically to a crochet needle.

Atrial septal aneurysms have recently received increased attention in relation to their possible role in contributing to brain embolism. Fusion of the septum primum closes the foramen ovale and leads to a depression on the right side of the interatrial septal wall. Bulging of the septum primum tissue of the atrial septum through the fossa ovalis into either the right or left atria is called an *atrial septal aneurysm*.

A strong association exists between atrial septal aneurysms and interatrial shunts. Cabanes et al. studied the frequency of atrial septal aneurysms, PFO, and MVP among 100 fully evaluated stroke patients younger than 55 years and 50 controls.[160] Atrial septal aneurysms were found in 28% of stroke patients and 8% of controls. A PFO was found in 72% of patients with atrial septal aneurysms and 25% of patients without atrial septal aneurysms. The presence of an atrial septal aneurysm (odds ratio, 4 to 3; 95% confidence interval, 1.3–14.6, p = .01) or a PFO (odds ratio, 3 to 9; 95% confidence interval, 1.5–10.0, p = .003) was strongly associated with

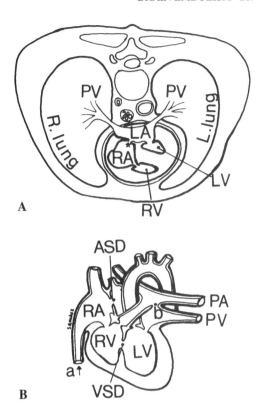

Figure 9-5. Common routes of paradoxical embolism. **(A)** Cross section through the thorax shows patent foramen ovale (*asterisk*). **(B)** Right-to-left shunts, atrial septal defect (ASD), ventricular septal defect (VSD), and fistula between the pulmonary artery and pulmonary vein (b). Clot from the leg vein ascends via the inferior vena cava (a). (LA = left atrium; LV = left ventricle; PA = pulmonary artery; PV = pulmonary vein; RA = right atrium; RV = right ventricle.)

cryptogenic stroke. The stroke odds ratio of a patient with both an atrial septal aneurysm and a PFO were 33.3 times (95% confidence interval, 4.1–270.0) the stroke odds of a patient who had neither. Atrial septal aneurysms with more than 10 mm excursion were eight times more likely to be associated with stroke than those with smaller excursions.[160] The presence of MVP in this study did not increase the odds of cryptogenic stroke. The mechanism by which atrial septal aneurysms contribute to brain embolism has not been satisfactorily clarified, but these lesions can harbor thrombi. Thrombi have occasionally been found within atrial septal aneurysms by TEE and at necropsy.[2]

Some studies have analyzed the recurrence rate of stroke in patients with PFOs and the effect of various

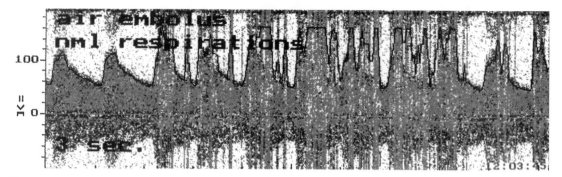

Figure 9-6. Transcranial Doppler recording over the middle cerebral artery after bubbled saline has been injected into an antecubital vein. A shower of high intensity transient signals is seen 3.5 seconds after injection.

treatments on recurrence.[2,161,162] Bogousslavsky and his Swiss colleagues studied stroke recurrence among 140 consecutive patients who had PFOs and brain ischemic events.[161] One-fourth of the patients also had atrial septal aneurysms. During a mean follow-up period of 3 years, the stroke or death rate was 2.4% per year. Only eight patients had a recurrent brain infarct (1.9% per year).[161] Ninety-two patients (66%) took aspirin (250 mg per day), whereas 37 patients (26%) were given anticoagulants, and 11 patients (8%) had surgical closure of the PFO within 12 weeks of the stroke after being treated with anticoagulants. No significant difference was found in the effect of any of the treatments on recurrence. The relatively low rate of recurrence contrasted with the severity of the initial stroke, which left disabling effects in one-half of the patients.[161] In a French multicenter study, 132 patients with PFOs, atrial septal aneurysms, or both, and cryptogenic stroke were followed for an average of 22.6 months.[162] The recurrence rate was approximately 2–3% at 2 years and was higher in patients with both PFOs and atrial septal aneurysms. Recurrences occurred in four patients who were taking antiplatelet agents, and in one patient treated with anticoagulants.[162] Lausanne investigators found no recurrence of stroke during an average follow-up of 2 years among 30 patients who had suture closure of PFOs during cardiopulmonary bypass surgery.[163] None of the patients were given antiaggregants or anticoagulants after surgery. No serious surgical complications occurred. After surgery, two patients had interatrial shunting determined by TCD and TEE, but the shunts were much smaller than before surgery.[163] PFOs have also been successfully closed using an umbrella-like device

placed through a catheter.[164] The available data regarding treatment are inconclusive, but all studies have shown a low recurrence rate (approximately 2% per year) among stroke patients with PFOs. The presence of both a PFO and an atrial septal aneurysm substantially increases the risk of stroke recurrence. Warfarin and surgical or transcatheter closure are posited to be more effective than drugs that affect platelet functions, but retrospective studies have not shown their superiority.

Most Common Cardiac Sources

Atrial arrhythmias, congestive heart failure, and akinetic regions were the most common cardiac sources of brain embolism in the Stroke Data Bank.[19] Atrial arrhythmias and left ventricular akinetic regions were the most frequent potential cardiac sources of brain emboli in the Lausanne Stroke Registry.[11] Atrial arrhythmias, myocardial abnormalities related to coronary artery disease, and congestive heart failure with low cardiac ejection fractions are probably the most important cardiac abnormalities that predispose to embolism.

Aorta

Studies of patients with stroke and TIAs have firmly established that the thoracic aorta is an important source of brain embolism. Although it was well known that the aorta was an important site of atheromatous disease, almost no mention was made of aortic atherosclerotic disease as an important cause of stroke until the 1990s. Tunick and colleagues reported four patients with unexplained brain ischemic events in whom TEE showed large, protruding, often mobile atheromas.[165,166] Tunick and colleagues then reported the TEE results among 122 patients who had stroke, TIAs, or peripheral emboli, and 122 age- and sex-matched controls.[167] Protruding atheromas were strongly related to the occurrence of embolic events (odds ratio, 3 to 2; 95% confidence interval, 1.6–6.5; p <.001), and atheromas with mobile components were only found in patients with embolic events.[167]

Observational studies and case reports alerted the medical community to the possible importance of aortic atheromas as a cause of stroke and peripheral embolism. In 1992, Pierre Amarenco and his Paris colleagues published two reports that showed definitively that aortic atheromatous disease was an important cause of stroke and could be identified clinically.[168,169] Amarenco et al. first published a necropsy study of 500 patients who had stroke or other neurologic diseases. Ulcerated aortic plaques were found in 26% of 239 patients with cerebrovascular disease, compared with only 5% of 261 patients with other neurologic diseases (p <.001).[168] The prevalence of aortic atheromas was 61% among patients with brain infarcts and no demonstrated cause and 22% among those with other defined causes (p <.001).[168] The presence of ulcerated plaques in the aortic arch did not correlate with the presence of carotid artery stenosis, suggesting that aortic and carotid artery disease were independent stroke risk factors. Amarenco and colleagues also reported a study of 12 consecutive patients with cryptogenic stroke studied by TEE.[169] Six patients (50%) had intraluminal echogenic masses in the aortic arch, most often at the junction of the ascending aorta and the arch. In one patient, the mass was pedunculated, but, in the other five patients, the attachment was broad-based with an irregular surface. The masses extended from 3 to 15 mm into the aortic lumens. Cholesterol emboli were found in quadriceps muscle biopsies in two patients with aortic masses.[169] Tobler et al. studied at necropsy the presence and distribution of atherosclerotic plaques in the ascending aorta.[170] Among 97 ascending aortas, 38% had atherosclerotic plaques larger than 8 mm in diameter; the average diameter of plaques was 19 mm. Most of the 66 plaques were distributed anteriorly or posteriorly

on the right side of the ascending aorta, and the upper and lower halves of the ascending aorta were equally involved.[170] Plaques were also often found in the aortic arch, especially at the orifice of the innominate artery (21% of 48 arch specimens).[170]

Two studies investigated the frequency of occurrence of vascular events in patients who had TEE-documented aortic arch atherosclerosis.[171,172] The French Study Group followed 331 patients who presented with brain infarcts for 2–4 years.[171] The frequency of subsequent brain infarction and other vascular events was closely correlated with the thickness of the aortic wall. After controlling for other confounding factors, the RR of brain infarction was 3.8 (95% confidence interval, 1.8–7.8; p = .0012) and of all vascular events 3.5 (95% confidence interval, 2.1–5.9; p <.001) in patients with aortic wall plaques larger than 4 mm.[171] In a prospective study conducted in two German university hospitals, physicians followed 136 patients with flat plaques less than 5 mm in thickness and 47 patients with thick plaques more than 5 mm thick, or complex plaques with mobile components for an average of 16 months.[173] Embolic events occurred in 15 patients; the incidence was 4.1 out of 100 patient-years in patients with flat plaques versus 13.7 out of 100 patient-years in those with complex, thick, or mobile plaques.[173] Figure 4-20 shows a protruding aortic atheroma shown by TEE. Aortic atherosclerosis is an especially important source of embolism during and after cardiac surgery. This subject is discussed in Chapter 16.

Treatment of aortic atheromatous disease is controversial. Although anticoagulants have been posited to aggravate cholesterol crystal embolism in several patients,[173] aortic thrombotic masses have disappeared after anticoagulant therapy.[174,175] By preventing the formation of thrombi over ulcerated areas of aortic atheromas, heparin, coumadin, or both could theoretically facilitate contact of the atheromatous material with the lumen and promote cholesterol embolism. Cholesterol embolism has also been described after thrombolytic treatment of patients with acute myocardial infarction[176]; similar to anticoagulants, thrombolytic agents could expose ulcerated areas to the circulation if thrombi were lysed. Intravenous thrombolytic treatment[177] and surgical removal of protruding atheromas[178] have also been reported to be successful in treating patients with aortic atheromas. Agents that affect platelet aggregation and function and combinations of anti-

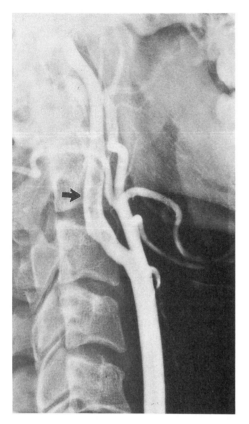

Figure 9-7. Carotid arteriogram, lateral view: Dark filling defects within the artery (*arrow*) represent luminal clots.

platelet drugs and anticoagulants might be effective in preventing embolism from aortic plaques, but they have not been systematically studied.

Arterial Sources of Embolism

Extracranial and intracranial large arteries often serve as the donor source for embolism to the brain. Arterial-source embolism is referred to as *artery-to-artery*, *intra-arterial*, or *local embolism*. The location and frequency of atherosclerotic lesions within the large arteries of the anterior and posterior circulations are discussed in Chapters 6 and 7. Ulcerated and stenotic lesions within the proximal extracranial and intracranial arteries are most often incriminated as embolic sources. Although atherosclerosis is by far the most common condition that leads to intra-arterial embolism, other vascular diseases can also serve as

donor sources. Trauma and dissections of arteries lead to local thrombus formation and embolism. Dissections are probably the second most frequent source of intra-arterial embolism. Occasionally, inflammatory diseases of the brachiocephalic branches of the aortic arch, such as temporal arteritis and Takayasu's disease, can lead to intra-arterial embolism. Thrombi sometimes form within arterial aneurysms, saccular,[179,180] and fusiform dolichocephalic aneurysms,[181] and can then break off and embolize to distal-branch arteries. Fibromuscular dysplasia is an important but relatively uncommon vascular disease that affects the pharyngeal and occasionally the intracranial portions of the carotid and vertebral arteries, which also can serve as a source of distal intra-arterial embolism. Thrombi can, on occasion, form within large arteries in the absence of important arterial disease in patients with cancer and other causes of hypercoagulability.[182] These luminal thrombi then embolize to intracranial arteries, causing strokes. Figure 9-7 shows a large thrombus within the ICA.

Imaging and Laboratory Evaluation of Potential Donor Sources

When the clinical findings, brain imaging, and vascular tests suggest brain embolism, a thorough evaluation of all potential sources—cardiac, aortic, and cerebrovascular—is usually indicated. Clinical distinction between brain embolism and in situ thrombosis is discussed in Chapter 3. Table 9-3 lists the common differential diagnostic features of these two stroke mechanisms. Some patients have more than one potential embolic donor source.

Atherosclerotic plaques and occlusive lesions often coexist in the heart, aorta, and brachiocephalic arteries. Patients with cerebrovascular occlusive lesions have a high frequency of coronary atherosclerotic heart disease, and their coronary disease is often a more serious threat for mortality and disability than cerebrovascular disease. Also, patients with coronary atherosclerotic heart disease have a high frequency of occlusive lesions within their extracranial and intracranial vascular beds. Prophylactic treatment to prevent subsequent thromboembolism should include measures to prevent embolism from all potential donor sources, not only the one that caused the present embolism.

Table 9-3. Differentiating Signs of Thrombosis and Embolism

Thrombosis	Embolism
1. Preceding brief, frequent, shotgun-like transient ischemic attacks	1. Single or infrequent but longer-lasting transient ischemic attacks or strokes
2. Transient ischemic attacks all in same vascular territory	2. Deficits maximal at onset
3. Onset of stroke after sleep	3. Onset during activity or sudden strain, cough, or sneeze
4. Postural sensitivity of the symptoms	4. Infarcts in multiple vascular territories
5. Occlusion or severe stenosis of a large artery shown by ultrasound or angiography	5. Presence of distal intra-arterial embolus by angiography or transcranial Doppler
6. Absence of distal embolus by angiography	6. Hemorrhagic cerebral infarct on computed tomography or magnetic resonance imaging
7. Infarct on computed tomography or magnetic resonance imaging near border zone of affected artery	7. Infarct on computed tomography or magnetic resonance imaging in heart of vascular territory, wedge-shaped, and abutting on cortical surface
8. Presence of risk factors for atherosclerosis: hypertension, hypercholesterolemia, angina, and so forth.	8. Presence of known cardiac, arterial, or venous source of embolus

Most patients with severe heart disease have abnormalities uncovered by history, physical examination, electrocardiograms, and chest x-ray. A TTE, including Doppler insonation and the injection of microbubbles searching for intracardiac shunts, is ordinarily indicated. Some patients, especially young adults who have a well-defined vascular donor source of embolism, such as a cervical dissection, do not need echocardiography.

When echocardiography is indicated, TTE is usually performed first. The results may be definitive, and thus a TEE would not be required. All observers agree that TEE shows many abnormalities not revealed by TTE. The use of TEE in patients with strokes and TIAs has been extensively reviewed.[183–186] TEE is more accurate than TTE in showing atrial and ventricular thrombi and in detecting and quantifying intracardiac shunts, and TEE more often shows spontaneous echo contrast than TTE.[184]

TEE sometimes fails to identify cardiac sources of emboli. Some thromboemboli are too small to be detected. An embolus that is 1–2 mm can cause a devastating neurologic deficit. A particle this size is often beyond the resolution of echocardiography. The other major reason for failure is that thrombosis and embolism are dynamic processes. When a thrombus leaves the heart to go to the brain, echocardiography may not show a thrombus within the heart if performed soon after the clinical event. Later, the thrombus may reform.

TEE also yields important information about the proximal aorta, a region not imaged by TTE. TEE is important in all patients in whom TTE suggests, but does not adequately define, the cardiac pathology and in all patients in whom other studies (cerebrovascular, hematologic, and other cardiac investigations) do not show the cause of brain embolism and brain ischemia. Radionuclide testing, including gated blood pool imaging (multigated acquisition scans), may also be helpful in selected patients, as might other cardiac imaging techniques.[187] Platelet scintigraphy is sometimes helpful in defining the presence of cardiac thrombi.[188]

TEE is the only effective, established way to image the aorta for plaques and thrombi. The ascending aorta can also be insonated using a duplex ultrasound probe placed in the right supraclavicular fossa, and the arch and proximal descending thoracic aorta can be imaged using a left supraclavicular probe.[189] The results are preliminary but promising. Most plaques are located in the curvature of the arch from the distal ascending aorta to the proximal descending aorta, regions well shown using B-mode ultrasound.[189]

The extracranial and intracranial arteries should be studied to define potential arterial donor sources of embolism, provide information about blockage of recipient arteries by emboli, or both. The four most common and effective means of studying the brachiocephalic arteries are by MRA, CTA, ultrasound, and cerebral catheter-dye angiography. Brain imaging always should accompany the vascular studies to show the location, severity, and distribution of related brain ischemia. These diagnostic tests and their use in diagnosing large artery lesions in the anterior and posterior circulations have been extensively reviewed in Chapters 4, 6, and 7.

Hematologic studies are also important in the evaluation of patients suspected of having brain embolism. Why does a patient with a chronic lesion, such as an aortic protruding atheroma, atrial fibrillation, or ICA stenosis develop a superimposed thrombus at a given time? In many patients, the explanation lies in activation of platelets, the coagulation system, or both.[190] The two processes, an intimal-endothelial lesion and heightened coagulation, interact to explain the thromboembolic event. Various conditions affect the coagulation system. Coexisting infection, cancer, dehydration, congenital or acquired hypercoagulability trauma (i.e., in patients with resistance to activated protein C) can activate the coagulation cascade that, in the presence of a suitable lesion, can lead to thrombus formation and embolism. Coagulation studies should be an integral part of the evaluation of patients with suspected brain embolism and those with potential sources of embolism who have not, as yet, had clinical events.

Treatment of Patients with Brain Embolism

Treatment of patients with brain embolism involves acute treatment of the embolic event and prophylaxis to prevent further thromboembolism. Whenever possible, clinicians should strive to prevent the first embolus. Prophylaxis of patients with atrial fibrillation using anticoagulants and prophylaxis of patients with cardiac valve disease using appropriate antibiotic treatment are important and effective measures that prevent many embolic events.

Acute Treatment of Embolic Event

Goals of treatment for the embolic event are minimization of the brain ischemia caused by the embolus and reperfusion. Brain edema is also an early occurrence in patients with embolic strokes. The edema allows recognition of ischemic tissue on diffusion-weighted MR scans. Ischemic edema can be intracellular (so-called cytotoxic edema or dry edema) or be localized, mostly in the extracellular spaces and connective tissue (vasogenic edema or wet edema). Brain edema located in the

interstices outside of cells might respond to osmotic diuretics, such as mannitol and glycerol or corticosteroids. Studies have shown that these agents are not effective, however, in series of stroke patients with large brain infarcts or hemorrhages. Most edema is probably within cells and indicates the cells are damaged. Restitution of the normal metabolic functions of these cells is likely to be more therapeutic than so-called antiedema agents. Some patients, mostly adolescents and young adults, develop sizable regions of vasogenic, extracellular brain edema, which leads to increased intracranial pressure and displacement and herniations of brain compartments. In these patients, a therapeutic trial of osmotic diuretic agents, corticosteroids, or both is warranted because the situation is often desperate. In some patients with massive brain swelling and increased intracranial pressure, removal of the skull overlying the side of the infarct (hemicraniectomy) can be life-saving, but patients may be left with severe neurologic residual deficits. Some patients make excellent recoveries after hemicraniectomies and survive with little neurologic deficit.[191,192]

The most important predictor of recovery from brain embolism is whether ischemic brain is reperfused, and how quickly. Reperfusion occurs when an occlusive embolus passes, either spontaneously or after treatment; collateral circulation to an ischemic region can also promote salvage of tissue. Many emboli pass spontaneously, usually within the first 48 hours after onset of neurologic symptoms. Vascular studies (CTA, MRA, TCD) can determine and monitor the presence of blockage of major intracranial and extracranial arteries by emboli. If the patient is seen and evaluated soon after stroke onset and embolic occlusions are identified by vascular studies, then an attempt at thrombolysis should be made unless there are contraindications or the patient already has a large brain infarct.

ML is a 46-year-old woman who suddenly developed aphasia and weakness of the right hand. She had a chronic myocardiopathy and during the preceding months reported increasing dyspnea and pedal edema. Examination 90 minutes after onset of the neurologic symptoms showed slight right-hand clumsiness and occasional word errors. She made reading, writing, and spelling errors. MR studies performed 130 minutes after onset showed an occluded left MCA on MRA, a small elliptical zone of abnormal diffusion on DWI, and a normal T2-weighted MRI scan (Figure 9-8). The studies were repeated 18 hours after intravenous recombinant tissue plasminogen activator. The MCA obstruction had improved, but there was still a residual filling defect.The infarct was seen on T2-weighted MRI and DWI but had not expanded. Perfusion imaging showed a defect larger than the infarct. On a later study, the MCA completely recanalized and the perfusion deficit cleared. The infarct remained the same but her examination returned to normal, except for minor loss of dexterity with her right hand when she played the piano.

The timing of thrombolysis is important if brain tissue is to be saved. Time = brain. Experimental studies in animals show that after 3 hours, irreversible brain ischemia (infarction) has already developed. However, salvageability of ischemic brain tissue varies considerably from patient to patient. Sometimes ischemic but salvageable brain tissue persists for many hours. This hypoperfused tissue has inadequate blood supply to function but is not irreversibly damaged. *Stunned brain* and *ischemic penumbra* are terms used for ischemic nonfunctioning brain that is not yet infarcted. The major danger of thrombolysis and of spontaneous reperfusion is that reperfusion of damaged vessels in the ischemic zone could cause major bleeding. Ideally, the decision on whether to pursue thrombolysis or other means of reperfusion, such as angioplasty, should rest on the presence of viable salvageable penumbral tissue and the extent of brain that is already infarcted, not on the time that has expired since symptom onset. The extent of infarction determines the risk of treatment; the presence and size of penumbral, stunned tissue determines the potential benefit of thrombolysis that accomplishes reperfusion. The newer magnetic resonance techniques of diffusion-weighted and perfusion MR scans performed with echo-planar equipment, when coupled with MRA, give clinicians a quantitative estimate of these factors. The case of ML illustrates the power of this imaging tool. Alternatively, clinicians esti-

mate the extent of normal, infarcted, and stunned brain supplied by the occluded artery by using brain imaging (CT and T2-weighted MRI scans), vascular studies (CTA, MRA, TCD, angiography), and neurologic examination. If the patient has a severe neurologic deficit and a large infarct is present on brain scans, then much of the brain is infarcted and there is little to gain by thrombolysis, which carries a substantial risk of hemorrhage in this circumstance. If the patient has a severe neurologic deficit and brain scans are normal, however, then there could be considerable stunned, salvageable brain, which could be restored to function if thrombolysis were successful.

Embolic occlusions respond better than thrombi formed locally in arteries that have severe atherostenosis. Recently formed thromboemboli lyse more often than older clots. Thrombi that block the extracranial or intracranial ICA rarely, if ever, respond to intravenous thrombolysis. A common situation is thrombosis of the ICA that has caused neurologic deficit by an embolus breaking off from the neck thrombus and embolizing intracranially to the MCA. Intravenous thrombolysis, in this situation, is ineffective because the drug does not reach the MCA clot because of proximal obstruction. An interventionist could pass a catheter through the clot in the neck, then manipulate the catheter to and within the MCA clot, to deliver the thrombolytic drug into the MCA clot. After lysing the intracranial clot, the catheter can be maneuvered back into the neck to lyse the neck clot and, if needed, perform an angioplasty with stenting of the atherostenotic ICA lesion. MCA branch occlusions seem to lyse best with intravenous therapy. Few patients with basilar artery thromboemboli have been studied after intravenous thrombolysis, but intra-arterial therapy of patients with basilar artery embolism is often effective. Ancrod, a substance derived from the purified protein fraction of venom from the Malayan pit viper, has defibrinolytic capabilities and has sometimes been given intravenously to acute stroke patients in an attempt to lyse thrombi.

Heparin is also used as a treatment for patients with acute thromboembolism. The posited purpose of heparinization is to prevent propagation of thrombi and breakoff of the tail of existing thrombi to prevent embolization. As far as is known, heparin does not actually lyse existing thrombi, although cardiac clots often disappear during heparin treatment. The decision to use heparin acutely to prevent

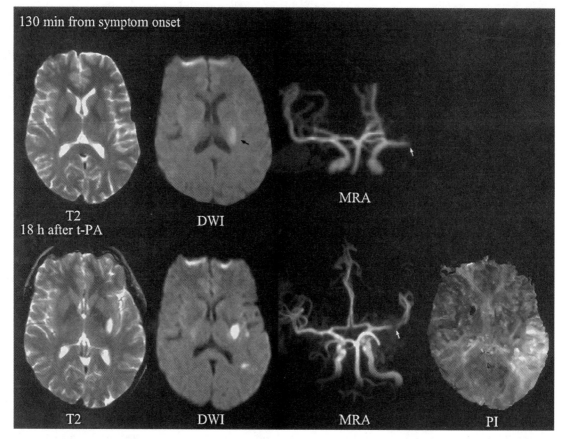

Figure 9-8. Magnetic resonance studies of a patient with a recent brain embolus. The upper row studies were performed 130 minutes after symptom onset. They show an occluded left middle cerebral artery (*small white arrow*) on magnetic resonance angiography (MRA) and a small deep infarct on diffusion-weighted image (DWI) (*small black arrow*). The T2-weighted magnetic resonance imaging is normal. The bottom row studies were performed 18 hours after intravenous recombinant tissue plasminogen activator infusion. The left middle cerebral artery has recanalized on MRA but there is a filling defect (*small white arrow*). The infarct remains small on DWI, but tiny regions of abnormality are present in the insular cortex. The infarct is also shown on the T2-weighted image. The perfusion abnormality is more extensive than the diffusion abnormality and involves considerable cerebral cortex supplied by the middle cerebral artery. (PI = perfusion imaging.) (Submitted by Drs. Rafael Llinas and Italo Linfante).

the next thromboembolic stroke involves weighing the risk of acute re-embolization versus the risk of hemorrhage related to heparin therapy. In patients with lesions with high rates of re-embolization (e.g., mitral stenosis with atrial fibrillation, atrial fibrillation with large left atria and atrial thrombi, acute myocardial infarction with mural thrombi) acute heparinization is indicated. In patients with a low risk of acute re-embolization, such as chronic atrial fibrillation or MAC, heparin can be withheld during the acute period. If the patient has a large brain infarct, then the risk of brain hemorrhage after heparin is higher than when there is little or no brain infarct. Heparin is often used after thrombolysis to maintain arterial patency.

Chronic Prophylactic Treatment to Prevent Re-embolization

Almost immediately, physicians caring for patients with brain embolism must think of preventing the next embolus. The three strategies used for prophylaxis are (1) removal of the donor source of embolism whenever possible, (2) modification of risk factors that relate to disease at the donor site, and (3) modification of coagulation functions to prevent the formation of thromboemboli. Some donor site lesions can be corrected, or at least ameliorated surgically, by using interventional radiologic techniques. Cardiac valve lesions; cardiac tumors; atrial septal defects; PFOs; and protruding, mobile, large aortic atheromas can be treated surgically. Newer interventional techniques may permit interventional percutaneous treatment of PFO and aortic atheromas. Carotid and vertebral artery lesions can be corrected surgically (endarterectomy) or by angioplasty, sometimes with stenting. Many patients with cardiac, aortic, and cerebrovascular donor site lesions have modifiable risk factors, such as smoking, hyperlipidemia, hypertension, inactive sedentary life style, and obesity. Counseling and medical treatment of these risk factors are important parts of the care of patients with brain embolism.

Manipulation of coagulation to prevent future thromboemboli is a strategy applicable to the majority of patients with brain embolism. Embolic particles are diverse. White platelet thrombi, red erythrocyte-fibrin thrombi, cholesterol crystals, calcified particles from arteries and valves, myxomatous tissue, bacteria in patients with infective endocarditis, and bland fibrous vegetations in patients with noninfective endocarditis are the most important substances. Medical prophylactic treatment against reentry of these particles into the circulation depends much on the "stuff" in the emboli rather than the source of the materials.[1,2,38] Its the bird rather than the location of the nest that is important.[38] For example, the most effective prophylaxis for prevention of embolization in patients with bacterial endocarditis is effective antibiotic sterilization of the bacterial vegetations. Cholesterol crystals, calcific particles, bacterial vegetation, and myxomatous emboli do not, as far as is known, respond to treatment with anticoagulants or drugs that modify platelet function.

The two types of medicinal agents most often used to prevent thromboemboli are standard anticoagulants (heparin, low-molecular-weight heparins, heparinoids, and warfarin compounds) and agents that alter platelet adhesion, aggregation, and secretion, such as aspirin, ticlopidine, clopidogrel, dipyridamole, and omega-3 fish oils. Chapter 5 contains a detailed discussion of the use of these compounds. White platelet-fibrin thrombi are posited to form on irregular surfaces in fast-moving bloodstreams in widely patent arteries and cavities. Red erythrocyte-fibrin thrombi, on the other hand, tend to form in regions of stasis, such as leg veins, dilatated cardiac atria, severely stenotic arteries, and so forth. At times, both white and red thrombi coexist because activated platelets are a stimulus for activation of the coagulation cascade and subsequent red-clot formation. I choose anticoagulant treatment for prophylaxis, first with heparin or low-molecular-weight heparin, and then coumadin, in patients who have lesions that promote red-clot formation and in patients whose imaging studies show thrombi. I continue coumadin as long as the situation that promotes red clots persists. These situations include persistent atrial fibrillation, myocardial aneurysm, prosthetic valves, and stenotic extracranial arteries. In patients with acute occlusive thrombi superimposed on preocclusive atherostenosis, I continue coumadin only for a short time (6–12 weeks), during which thrombi organize and no longer propagate or form fresh tails that embolize. During this time, collateral circulation has usually become maximal. Sometimes, lesions that caused the original thrombosis later improve (e.g., arterial dissections, regressing atheromas, or corrected cardiac right-to-left shunts), so anticoagulation can be stopped and replaced with antiplatelet drugs.

I use agents that alter platelet functions for patients with lesions posited to predispose to formation of white platelet-fibrin thrombi. Irregular nonstenosing atherosclerotic plaques and irregular, but nonstenotic valve surfaces are the most common situations. In patients who can tolerate aspirin, I usually prescribe 325–650 mg of coated aspirin daily. High fibrinogen levels increase whole blood viscosity and platelet aggregability and predispose to red clot formation. Drugs that lower fibrinogen levels are prescribed. In some situations, in which both red and white clots are likely to form, a combination of platelet antiaggregants and coumadin might be more effective than either agent alone.

References

1. Caplan LR. Brain embolism, revisited. Neurology 1993; 43:1281–1287.
2. Caplan LR. Brain Embolism. In LR Caplan, JW Hurst, M Chimowitz (eds), Clinical Neurocardiology. New York: Marcel Dekker, 1999.
3. Markus HS. Transcranial Doppler detection of circulating cerebral emboli, a review. Stroke 1993;24:1246–1250.
4. Sliwka U, Job F-P, Wissuwa D, et al. Occurrence of transcranial Doppler high-intensity transient signals in patients with potential cardiac sources of embolism, a prospective study. Stroke 1995;26:2067–2070.
5. Daffertshofer M, Ries S, Schminke U, Hennerici M. High-intensity transient signals in patients with cerebral ischemia. Stroke 1996;27:1844–1849.
6. Sliwka U, Lingnau A, Stohlmann W-D, et al. Prevalence and time course of microembolic signals in patients with acute strokes, a prospective study. Stroke 1997;28:358–363.
7. Mohr JP, Caplan LR, Melski JW, et al. The Harvard Cooperative Stroke Registry: a prospective registry. Neurology 1978;29:754–762.
8. Caplan LR, Hier DB, D'Cruz I. Cerebral embolism in the Michael Reese Stroke Registry. Stroke 1983;14:530–536.
9. Mohr JP, Gautier JC, Hier DB, Stein RW. Middle Cerebral Artery. In HJM Barnett, JP Mohr, BM Stein, FM Yatsu (eds). Stroke, Pathophysiology, Diagnosis, and Management, Vol 1. New York: Churchill Livingstone, 1986;377–450.
10. Minematsu K, Yamaguchi T, Omae T. Spectacular shrinking deficit: rapid recovery from a major hemispheric syndrome by migration of an embolus. Neurology 1992;42:157–162.
11. Bogousslavsky J, van Melle G, Regli F. The Lausanne Stroke Registry: Analysis of 1000 consecutive patients with first stroke. Stroke 1988;19:1083–1092.
12. Gacs G, Merer FT, Bodosi M. Balloon catheter as a model of cerebral emboli in humans. Stroke 1982;13:39–42.
13. Helgason C. Cardioembolic stroke topography and pathogenesis. Cerebrovasc Brain Metab Rev 1992;4:28–58.
14. Caplan LR. Posterior Circulation Disease, Clinical Findings, Diagnosis, and Management. Boston: Blackwell, 1996.
15. Lodder J, Krijne-Kubat B, Broekman J. Cerebral hemorrhagic infarction at autopsy: cardiac embolic cause and the relationship to the cause of death. Stroke 1986;17:626–629.
16. Hart RG, Easton JD. Hemorrhagic infarcts. Stroke 1986;17:586–589.
17. Timsit SG, Sacco RL, Mohr JP, et al. Brain infarction severity differs according to cardiac or arterial embolic source. Neurology 1993;43:728–733.
18. Bladin CF. Seizures after stroke. Melbourne, Australia: University of Melbourne, 1997. Thesis.
19. Kittner SJ, Sharkness CM, Price TR, et al. Infarcts with a cardiac source of embolism in the NINCDS Stroke Data Bank: historical features. Neurology 1990;40:281–284.
20. Ringelstein EB, Koschorke S, Holling A, et al. Computed tomographic patterns of proven embolic brain infarctions. Ann Neurol 1989;26:759–765.
21. Ringelstein EB, Koschorke S, Holling A, et al. Computed tomographic patterns of proven embolic brain infarctions. Ann Neurol 1989;26:759–765.
22. Gacs G, Fox AJ, Barnett HJ, Vinuela F. CT visualization of intracranial arterial thromboembolism. Stroke 1983;14:756–763.
23. Tomsick T, Brott T, Barsan W, et al. Thrombus localization with emergency cerebral computed tomography. Stroke 1990;21:180.
24. Fisher CM, Adams R. Observations on brain embolism with special reference to the mechanism of hemorrhagic infarction. J Neuropathol Exp Neurol 1951;10:92–93.
25. Fisher CM, Adams RD. Observations on Brain Embolism with Special Reference to Hemorrhagic Infarction. In AJ Furlan (ed), The Heart and Stroke. London: Springer, 1987;17–36.
26. Yamaguchi T, Minematsu K, Choki JI, Ikeda M. Clinical and neuroradiological analysis of thrombotic and embolic cerebral infarction. Jpn Circ J 1984;48:50–58.
27. Okada Y, Yamaguchi T, Minematsu K, et al. Hemorrhagic transformation in cerebral embolism. Stroke 1989;20:598–603.
28. Pessin MS, Estol C, Lafranchise F, Caplan LR. Safety of anticoagulation after hemorrhagic infarction. Neurology 1993;43:1298–1303.
29. Chaves CJ, Pessin MS, Caplan LR, et al. Cerebellar hemorrhagic infarction. Neurology 1996;46:346–349.
30. Garcia J, Ho K-L, Caccamo, DV. Intracerebral Hemorrhage: Pathology of Selected Topics. In CS Kase, LR Caplan. Intracerebral Hemorrhage. Boston: Butterworth–Heinemann, 1994;45–72.
31. Fieschi C, Argentino C, Lenzi G, et al. Clinical and instrumental evaluation of patients with ischemic stroke within the first six hours. J Neurol Sci 1989;91:311–322.
32. del Zoppo GJ, Poeck K, Pessin MS, et al. Recombinant tissue plasminogen activator in acute thrombotic and embolic stroke. Ann Neurol 1992;32:78–86.
33. Wolpert SM, Bruckmann H, Greenlee R, Wechsler L, Pessin MS, del Zoppo GJ. Neuroradiologic evaluation of patients with acute stroke treated with recombinant tissue plasminogen activator. The rt-PA Acute Stroke Study Group. AJNR Am J Neuroradiol 1993;14:3–13.
34. Dalal P, Shah P, Sheth S, et al. Cerebral embolism: angiographic observations on spontaneous clot lysis. Lancet 1965;1:61–64.
35. Liebeskind A, Chinichian A, Schechter M. The moving embolus seen during cerebral angiography. Stroke 1971;2:440–443.
36. Kushner MJ, Zanette EM, Bastianello S, et al. Transcranial Doppler in acute hemisphere brain infarction. Neurology 1991;41:109–113.
37. Georgiadis D, Lindner A, Manz M, et al. Intracranial microembolic signals in 500 patients with potential cardiac or carotid embolic source and in normal controls. Stroke 1997;28:1203–1207.
38. Caplan LR. Of birds and nests and brain emboli. Rev Neurol 1991;147:265–273.
39. Virchow R. Gesammelte Abhandlungen zur Wissenschaftlichenmedtezin. Frankfurt: Meidinger Sohn, 1856;219–732.
40. Hanna JP, Furlan AJ. Cardiac Disease and Embolic Sources. In LR Caplan (ed), Brain Ischemia. London: Springer, 1995;299–315.
41. Baumgartner HR, Haudenschild C. Adhesion of platelets to subendothelium. Ann N Y Acad Sci 1972;201:22–36.

42. Gustafsson C, Blomback M, Britton M, et al. Coagulation factors and the increased risk of stroke in nonvalvular atrial fibrillation. Stroke 1990;21:47–51.

43. Kumagai K, Fukunami M, Ohmori M, et al. Increased intracardiovascular clotting in patients with chronic atrial fibrillation. J Am Coll Cardiol 1990;16:377–380.

44. Wolf PA, Abbott RD, Kannel WB. Atrial fibrillation: a major contribution to stroke in the elderly. The Framingham Study. Arch Intern Med 1987;147:1561–1564.

45. Cairns JA, Connolly SJ. Nonrheumatic atrial fibrillation. Risk of stroke and role of antithrombotic therapy. Circulation 1991;84:469–481.

46. Wolf PA, Dawber TR, Thomas HE, Kannel WB. Epidemiologic assessment of chronic atrial fibrillation and risk of stroke: The Framingham Study. Neurology 1978;28:973–977.

47. Dunn M, Alexander J, DeSilva R, Hildner F. Antithrombotic therapy in atrial fibrillation. Chest 1989;95:S118–S127.

48. The Stroke Prevention in Atrial Fibrillation Investigators. Predictors of thromboembolism in atrial fibrillation: 1. Clinical features of patients at risk. Ann Intern Med 1992;116:1–5.

49. Atrial Fibrillation Investigators. Risk factors for stroke and efficacy of antithrombotic therapy in atrial fibrillation: analysis of pooled data from five randomized controlled trials. Arch Intern Med 1994;154:1449–1457.

50. Caplan LR, D'Cruz I, Hier DB, et al. Atrial size, atrial fibrillation, and stroke. Ann Neurol 1986;19:158–161.

51. The Stroke Prevention in Atrial Fibrillation Investigators. Predictors of thromboembolism in atrial fibrillation: II. Echocardiographic features of patients at risk. Ann Intern Med 1992;116:6–12.

52. DiPasquale G, Urbinati S, Pinelli G. New echocardiographic markers of embolic risk in atrial fibrillation. Cerebrovasc Dis 1995;5:315–322.

53. Vernhorst P, Kamp O, Visser CA, Verheught FWA. Left atrial appendage flow velocity assessment using transesophageal echocardiography in nonrheumatic atrial fibrillation and systemic embolism. Am J Cardiol 1993;71:192–196.

54. Garcia-Fernandez MA, Torrecilla EG, San Roman D, et al. Left atrial appendage Doppler flow patterns: implications of thrombus formation. Am Heart J 1992;124:955–965.

55. Beppu S, Nimura Y, Sakakibara H. Smoke-like echo in the left atrial cavity in mitral valve disease: its features and significance. J Am Coll Cardiol 1985;6:744–749.

56. Merino A, Hauptman P, Badiman L, et al. Echocardiographic "smoke" is produced by an interaction of erythrocytes and plasma proteins modulated by shear forces. J Am Coll Cardiol 1992;20:1661–1668.

57. Black IW, Stewart WJ. The role of echocardiography in the evaluation of cardiac sources of embolism. Echocardiography 1993;10:429–439.

58. Chimowitz MI, DeGeorgia MA, Poole RM, et al. Left atrial spontaneous echo contrast is highy associated with previous stroke in patients with atrial fibrillation or mitral stenosis. Stroke 1993;24:1015–1019.

59. Albers G. Atrial fibrillation and stroke. Three new studies, three remaining questions. Arch Intern Med 1994;154:1443–1448.

60. Rubenstein JJ, Schulman CL, Yurchak PM, et al. Clinical spectrum of the sick sinus syndrome. Circulation 1972;46:5–13.

61. Fairfax AJ, Lambert CD, Leatham A. Systemic embolism in chronic sinoatrial disorder. N Engl J Med 1976;295:190–192.

62. Lown B. Electrical reversion of cardiac arrythmias. Br Heart J 1967;29:469–489.

63. Orencia AJ, Hammill SC, Whisnant JP. Sinus node dysfunction and ischemic stroke. Heart Dis Stroke 1994;3:91–94.

64. Phillips SJ, Whisnant JP, O'Fallon WM, Frye RL. Prevalence of cardiovascular disease and diabetes mellitus in residents of Rochester, Minnesota. Mayo Clin Proc 1990;65:344–359.

65. Radford DJ, Julian DG. Sick sinus syndrome. Experience of a cardiac pacemaker clinic. BMJ 1974;3:504–507.

66. Rosenqvist M, Vallin H, Edhag O. Clinical and electrophysiologic course of sinus node disease: five-year follow-up study. Am Heart J 1985;109:513–522.

67. Bathen J, Sparr S, Rokseth R. Embolism in sinoatrial disease. Acta Med Scand 1978;203:7–11.

68. Cerebral embolism task force. Cardiogenic brain embolism. Arch Neurol 1986;43:71–84.

69. Stein PD, Sabbah HN, Pitha JV. Continuing disease process of calcific aortic stenosis. Am J Cardiol 1977;39: 159–163.

70. Szekely P. Systemic embolism and anticoagulant prophylaxis in rheumatic heart disease. BMJ 1964;1:1209–1212.

71. Keen G, Leveaux VM. Prognosis of cerebral embolism in rheumatic heart disease. BMJ 1958;2:91–92.

72. Coulshed N, Epstein EJ, McKendrick CS, et al. Systemic embolism in mitral valve disease. BMJ 1970;32:26–34.

73. Daley R, Mattingly TW, Holt CL, et al. Systemic arterial embolism in rheumatic heart disease. Am Heart J 1951;42:566–581.

74. Fleming HA, Bailey SM. Mitral valve disease, systemic embolism and anticoagulants. Postgrad Med J 1971;47:599–604.

75. Carabello BA, Crawford FA. Valvular heart disease. N Engl J Med 1997;337:32–41.

76. Soulie P, Caramanian M, Soulie J, Bader JL, Colcher E. Les embolies calcaires des atteintes orificielles calcifees du coeur gauche. Arch Mal Coeur Vaiss 1969;12:1657–1684.

77. Holley KE, Bahn RC, McGoon DC, Mankin HT. Spontaneous calcific embolization associated with calcific aortic stenosis. Circulation 1963;27:197–202.

78. Klues HG, Maron BJ, Dollar AL, Roberts WC. Diversity of structural mitral valve alterations in hypertrophic cardiomyopathy. Circulation 1992;85:1651–1660.

79. Hardarson T, De la Calzada CS, Curiel R, Goodwin JF. Prognosis and mortality of hypertrophic obstructive cardiomyopathy. Lancet 1973;1462–1467.

80. Glancy DL, O'Brien KP, Gold HK, Epstein SE. Atrial fibrillation in patients with idiopathic hypertrophic subaortic stenosis. Brit Heart J 1970;32:652–659.

81. Tajik AJ, Giuliani ER, Frye RL, et al. Mitral valve and/or annulus calcification associated with hypertrophic subaortic stenosis (IHSS). Circulation 1972;16(Suppl II):228.

82. Barlow JB, Bosman CK. Aneurysmal protrusion of posterior leaflets of the mitral valve. An auscultatory-

electrocardiographic syndrome. Am Heart J 1966;71: 166–178.

83. Lauzier S, Barnett HJM. Cerebral Ischemia with Mitral Valve Prolapse and Mitral Annular Calcification. In AJ Furlan (ed), The Heart and Stroke: Exploring Mutual Cerebrovascular and Cardiovascular Issues. London: Springer, 1987;63–100.

84. Markiewicz W, Stoner J, London E, et al. Mitral valve prolapse in one hundred presumably healthy young females. Circulation 1976;53:464–473.

85. Cheitlin MD, Byrd RC. Prolapsed mitral valve: the commonest valve disease? Curr Probl Cardiol 1984;8:3–53.

86. Ranganatham N, Silver MD, Robinson T, et al. Angiographic-morphological correlation in patients with severe mitral regurgitation due to prolapse of the posterior mitral valve leaflet. Circulation 1973;48:514–518.

87. Kostuk WJ, Boughner DR, Barnett HJM, Silver MD. Strokes: a complication of mitral-leaflet prolapse? Lancet 1977;2:313–316.

88. Marks AR, Choong CY, Sanfillipo AJ, et al. Identification of high-risk and low-risk subgroups of patients with mitral-valve prolapse. N Engl J Med 1989;320:1031–1036.

89. Nishimura RA, McGoon MD, Shub C, et al. Echocardiographically documented mitral-valve polapse: long term follow-up of 237 patients. N Engl J Med 1985;313: 1305–1309.

90. Barnett HJM. Transient cerebral ischemia: pathogenesis, prognosis, and management. Ann Royal Coll Phys Surg Can 1974;7:153–173.

91. Barnett HJM, Jones MW, Boughner DR, Kostuk WJ. Cerebral ischemic events associated with prolapsing mitral valve. Arch Neurol 1976;33:777–782.

92. Barnett HJM, Boughner DR, Taylor DW, et al. Further evidence relating mitral–valve prolapse to cerebral ischemic events. N Engl J Med 1980;302:139–144.

93. Korn D, DeSanctis R, Sell S. Massive calcification of the mitral valve, a clinicopathological study of fourteen cases. N Engl J Med 1962;267:900–909.

94. DeBono D, Warlow C. Mitral annulus calcification and cerebral or retinal ischemia. Lancet 1979;2:383–385.

95. Benjamin EJ, Plehn JF, D'Agostino RB, et al. Mitral annular calcification and the risk of stroke in an elderly cohort. N Engl J Med 1992;327:374–379.

96. Pomerance A. Pathological and clinical study of calcification of the mitral valve ring. J Clin Pathol 1970;23: 354–361.

97. Vongpatanasin W, Hillis D, Lange RA. Prosthetic heart valves. N Engl J Med 1996;335:407–416.

98. Edmunds LH Jr. Thromboembolic complications of current cardiac valvular prostheses. Ann Thor Surg 1982; 34:96–106.

99. Metzdorff MT, Grunkemeier GL, Pinson CW, Starr A. Thrombosis of mechanical cardiac valves: a qualitative comparison of the silastic ball valve and the tilting disc valve. J Am Coll Cardiol 1984;4:50–53.

100. Harker LA, Slichter SL. Studies of platelet and fibrinogen kinetics in patients with prosthetic heart valves. N Engl J Med 1970;283:1302–1305.

101. Salgado ED, Furlan AJ, Conomy JP. Cardioembolic Sources of Stroke. In AJ Furlan (ed), The Heart and

Stroke: Exploring Mutual Cerebrovascular and Cardiovascular Issues. London: Springer, 1987;47–61.

102. Cannegieter SC, Rosendaal FR, Briet E. Thromboembolic and bleeding complications in patients with mechanical heart valve prostheses. Circulation 1994;89:635–641.

103. Cohn LH, Mudge GH, Pratter F, Collins JJ Jr. Five to eight-year follow-up of patients undergoing porcine heart-valve replacement. N Engl J Med 1981;304:258–262.

104. Jones HR, Siekert RG, Geraci J. Neurologic manifestations of bacterial endocarditis. Ann Intern Med 1969;71: 21–28.

105. Salgado AV, Furlan AJ, Keys TF, et al. Neurologic complications of endocarditis: a 12-year experience. Neurology 1989;39:173–178.

106. Hart RG, Foster JW, Luther MF, Kanter MC. Stroke in infective endocarditis. Stroke 1990;21:695–700.

107. Kanter MC, Hart RG. Neurologic complications of infective endocarditis. Neurology 1991;41:1015–1020.

108. Keyser DL, Biller J, Coffman TT, Adams HP. Neurologic complications of late prosthetic valve endocarditis. Stroke 1990;21:472–475.

109. Matsushita K, Kuriyama Y, Sawada T, et al. Hemorrhagic and ischemic cerebrovascular complications of active infective endocarditis of native valve. Eur Neurol 1993;33:267–274.

110. Hart RG, Kagan-Hallet K, Joerns S. Mechanisms of intracranial hemorrhage in infective endocarditis. Stroke 1987;18:1048–1056.

111. Masuda J, Yutani C, Waki R, et al. Histopathological analysis of the mechanisms of intracranial hemorrhage complicating infective endocarditis. Stroke 1992;23:843–850.

112. Morawetz RB, Karp RB. Evolution and resolution of intracranial bacterial (mycotic) aneurysms. Neurosurgery 1984;15:43–49.

113. Moskowitz MA, Rosenbaum AE, Tyler HR. Angiographically monitored resolution of cerebral mycotic aneurysms. Neurology 1974;24:1103–1108.

114. Bingham WF. Treatment of mycotic intracranial aneurysms. J Neurosurg 1977;46:428–437.

115. Bertorini TE, Laster RE, Thompson BF, Gelfand M. Magnetic resonance inmaging of the brain in bacterial endocarditis. Arch Intern Med 1989;149:815–817.

116. Libman E, Sacks B. A hitherto undescribed form of valvular and mural endocarditis. Arch Intern Med 1924;33:701–737.

117. Klemperer P, Pollack AD, Baehr G. Pathology of disseminated lupus erythematosis. Arch Pathol 1941;32:569–631.

118. Baehr G, Klemperer P, Schifrin A. A diffuse disease of the peripheral circulation usually associated with lupus erythematosis and endocarditis. Trans Assoc Am Physicians 1935;50:139–155.

119. Gross L. The cardiac lesions in Libman-Sacks disease, with a consideration of its relationship to acute diffuse lupus erythematosis. Am J Pathol 1940;16:375–407.

120. Roldan CA, Shively B, Crawford MH. An echocardiographic study of valvular heart disease associated with systemic lupus erythematosus. N Engl J Med 1996;335: 1424–1430.

121. Barbut D, Borer J, Gharavi A, et al. Prevalence of anticardiolipin antibody in isolated mitral or aortic regurgitation, or both, and possible relation to cerebral ischemic events. Am J Cardiol 1992;70:901–905.

122. Barbut D, Borer J, Wallerson D, et al. Anticardiolipin antibody and stroke: possible relation of valvular heart disease and embolic events. Cardiology 1991;79:99–109.

123. The Antiphospholipid Antibodies in Stroke Study Group. Clinical and laboratory findings in patients with antiphospholipid antibodies and cerebral ischemia. Stroke 1990; 21:1268–1273.

124. Amico L, Caplan LR, Thomas C. Cerebrovascular complications of mucinous cancer. Neurology 1989;39: 522–526.

125. Reagan TJ, Okazaki H. The thrombotic syndrome associated with carcinoma. Arch Neurol 1974;31:390–395.

126. Edoute Y, Haim N, Rinkevich D, Brenner B, Reisner SA. Cardiac valvular vegetations in cancer patients: a prospective echocardiographic study of 200 patients. Am J Med 1997;102:252–258.

127. Connolly HM, Crary JL, McGoon MD, et al. Valvular heart disease associated with Fenflurmine-phentermine. N Engl J Med 1997;337:581–588.

128. Lambl VA. Papillare exkreszenzen an der semilunar-klappe der aorta. Wien Med Wochenscshr 1856;6:244–247.

129. Magarey FR. On the mode of formation of Lambl's excrescences and their relation to chronic thickening of the mitral valve. J Pathol Bacteriol 1949;61:203–208.

130. Freedberg RS, Goodkin GM, Perez JL, et al. Valve strands are strongly associated with systemic embolization: a transesophageal echocardiographic study. J Am Coll Cardiol 1995;26:1709–1712.

131. Roberts JK, Omarali I, Di Tullio MR, et al. Valvular strands and cerebral ischemia. Effect of demographics and strand characteristics. Stroke 1997;28:2185–2188.

132. Cohen A, Tzourio C, Chauvel C, et al. Mitral valve strands and the risk of ischemic stroke in elderly patients. Stroke 1997;28:1574–1578.

133. Lee RJ, Bartzokis T, Yeoh TK, et al. Enhanced detection of intracardiac sources of cerebral emboli by transesophageal echocardiography. Stroke 1991;22: 734–739.

134. Nighoghossian N, Derex L, Loire R, et al. Giant Lambl excrescences. An unusual source of cerebral embolism. Arch Neurol 1997;54:41–44.

135. Visser CA, Kan G, Meltzer RS, et al. Embolic potential of left ventricular thrombi after myocardial infarction: a two–dimensional echocardiographic study of 119 patients. J Am Coll Cardiol 1985;5:1276–1280.

136. Kouvaras G, Chronopoulas G, Soufras G, et al. The effects of long term antithrombotic treatment on left ventricular thrombi in patients after an acute myocardial infarction. Am Heart J 1990;119:73–78.

137. Lapeyre AC III, Steele PM, Kazmier FJ, et al. Systemic embolism in chronic left ventricular aneurysm: incidence and the role of anticoagulation. J Am Coll Cardiol 1985;6:534–538.

138. Anticoagulants in acute myocardial infarction: results of a cooperative clinical trial. JAMA 1973;225:724–729.

139. Faxon DP, Ryan TJ, Davis KB, et al. Prognostic significance of angiographically documented left ventricular aneurysm from the coronary artery surgery study (CASS). Am J Cardiol 1982;50:157–164.

140. Reeder GS, Lengyei M, Tajik AJ, et al. Mural thrombus in left ventricular aneurysm. Incidence, role of angiography, and relation between anticoagulation and embolism. Mayo Clin Proc 1981;56:77–81.

141. Loh E, Sutton M, Wun C-C, et al. Ventricular dysfunction and the risk of stroke after myocardial infarction. N Engl J Med 1997;336:251–257.

142. Oppenheimer SM, Lima J. Neurology and the heart. J Neurol Neurosurg Psychiatry 1998;64:289–297.

143. Reynen K. Cardiac myxomas. N Engl J Med 1995;333: 1610–1617.

144. Blondeau P. Primary cardiac tumors: French study of 533 cases. Thorac Cardiovasc Surg 1990;38(Suppl 2): 192–195.

145. Sandok BA, von Estorff I, Giuliani ER. Subsequent neurological events in patients with atrial myxoma. Ann Neurol 1980;8:305–307.

146. Giannesini C, Kubis N, N'Guyen A, et al. Cardiac papillary fibroelastoma: a rare cause of ischemic stroke in the young. Cerebrovasc Dis 1999;9:45–49.

147. Brown RD, Khandheria BK, Edwards WD. Cardiac papillary fibroelastoma: a treatable cause of transient ischemic attack and ischemic stroke detected by transesophageal echocardiography. Mayo Clin Proc 1995;70:863–868.

148. Hagen PT, Scholz DG, Edwards WD. Incidence and size of patent foramen ovale during the first 10 decades of life: an autopsy study of 965 normal hearts. Mayo Clin Proc 1984;59:17–20.

149. Lechat PH, Mas JL, Lascault G, et al. Prevalence of patent foramen ovale in patients with stroke. N Engl J Med 1988;318:1148–1152.

150. Di Tullio M, Sacco RL, Gopal A, et al. Patent foramen ovale as a risk factor for cryptogenic stroke. Ann Intern Med 1992;117:461–465.

151. Petty GW, Khanderia BK, Chu C-P, et al. Patent foramen ovale in patients with cerebral infarction. A transesophageal echocardiographic study. Arch Neurol 1997;54:819–822.

152. Gautier JC, Durr A, Koussa S, et al. Paradoxical cerebral embolism with a patent foramen ovale. A report of 29 patients. Cerebrovasc Dis 1991;1:193–202.

153. Venketasubramanian N, Sacco RL, Di Tullio M, et al. Vascular distribution of paradoxical emboli by transcranial Doppler. Neurology 1993;43:1533–1535.

154. Chimowitz MI, Nemec JJ, Marwick TH, et al. Transcranial Doppler ultrasound identifies patients with right-to-left cardiac or pulmonary shunts. Neurology 1991;41: 1902–1904.

155. Albert A, Muller HR, Hetzel A. Optimized transcranial Doppler technique for the diagnosis of cardiac right-to-left shunts. J Neuroimaging 1997;7:159–163.

156. Di Tullio M, Sacco RL, Venketasubramanian N, et al. Comparison of diagnostic techniques for the detection of a patent foramen ovale in stroke patients. Stroke 1993;24:1020–1024.

157. Hanna JP, Sun JP, Furlan AJ, et al. Patent foramen ovale and brain infarct. Echocardiographic predictors, recurrence, and prevention. Stroke 1994;25:782–786.

158. Homma S, Di Tullio MR, Sacco RL, et al. Characteristics of patent foramen ovale associated with cryptogenic stroke. A biplane transesophageal echocardiographic study. Stroke 1994;25:582–586.

159. Ay H, Buonanno FS, Abraham S, et al. An electrocardiographic criterion for diagnosis of patent foramen ovale associated with ischemic stroke. Stroke 1998;29:1393–1397.

160. Cabanes L, Mas JL, Cohen A, et al. Atrial septal aneurysm and patent foramen ovale as risk factors for cryptogenic stroke in patients less than 55 years of age. A study using transesophageal echocardiography. Stroke 1993;24: 1865–1873.

161. Bogousslavsky J, Garazi S, Jeanrenaud X, et al. Stroke recurrence in patients with patent foramen ovale: the Lausanne study. Neurology 1996;46:1301–1305.

162. The French Study Group on Patent Foramen Ovale and Atrial Septal Aneurysm. Recurrent cerebrovascular events in patients with patent foramen ovale or atrial septal aneurysms and cryptogenic stroke or TIA. Am Heart J 1995; 130:1083–1088.

163. Devuyst G, Bogousslavsky J, Ruchat P, et al. Prognosis after stroke followed by surgical closure of patent foramen ovale: a prospective follow–up study with brain MRI and simultaneous transesophageal and transcranial Doppler ultrasound. Neurology 1996;47:1162–1166.

164. Bridges ND, Hellensbrand W, Catson L, et al. Transcatheter closure of patent foramen ovale after presumed paradoxical embolism. Circulation 1992;86:1902–1908.

165. Tunick PA, Kronzon I. Protruding atherosclerotic plaque in the aortic arch of patients with systemic embolization: a new finding seen by transesophageal echocardiography. Am Heart J 1990;120:658–660.

166. Tunick PA, Culliford AT, Lamparello PJ, Kronzon I. Atheromatosis of the aortic arch as an occult source of multiple systemic emboli. Ann Intern Med 1991;114:391–392.

167. Tunick PA, Perez JL, Kronzon I. Protruding atheromas in the thoracic aorta and systemic embolization. Ann Intern Med 1991;115:423–427.

168. Amarenco P, Duyckaerts C, Tzourio C, et al. The prevalence of ulcerated plaques in the aortic arch in patients with stroke. N Engl J Med 1992;326:221–225.

169. Amarenco P, Cohen A, Baudrimont M, Bousser M-G. Transesophageal echocardiographic detection of aortic arch disease in patients with cerebral infarction. Stroke 1992;23:1005–1009.

170. Tobler HG, Edwards JE. Frequency and location of atherosclerotic plaques in the ascending aorta. J Thor Cardiovasc Surg 1988;96:304–306.

171. The French Study of Aortic Plaques in Stroke Group. Atherosclerotic disease of the aortic arch as a risk factor for recurrent ischemic stroke. N Engl J Med 1996;334: 1216–1221.

172. Mitusch R, Doherty C, Wucherpfennig H, et al. Vascular events during follow-up in patients with aortic arch atherosclerosis. Stroke 1997;28:36–39.

173. Bruns JL, Segel DP, Adler S. Control of cholesterol embolization by discontinuation of anticoagulant therapy. Am J Med Sci 1978;275:105–108.

174. Blackshear JL, Jahangir A, Oldenberg WA, Safford RE. Digital embolization from plaque-related thrombus in the thoracic aorta: identification with transesophageal echocardiography and resolution with warfarin therapy. Mayo Clin Proc 1993;68:268–272.

175. Freedberg RS, Tunick PA. Culliform AT, Tatelbaum RJ, Kronzon I. Disappearance of a large intraaortic mass in a patient with prior systemic embolization. Am Heart J 1993;25:445–1447.

176. Fine MJ, Kapoor W, Falanga V. Cholesterol crystal embolization: a review of 221 cases in the English literature. Angiology 1987;38:769–784.

177. Hausmann D, Gulba D, Bargheer, et al. Successful thrombolysis of an aortic-arch thrombus in a patient after mesenteric embolism. N Engl J Med 1992;327:500–501.

178. Belden JR, Caplan LR, Bojar RM, Payne DD, Blachman P. Treatment of multiple cerebral emboli from an ulcerated, thrombogenic ascending aorta with aortectomy and graft replacement. Neurology 1997;49:621–622.

179. Duncan A, Rumbaugh C, Caplan LR. Cerebral embolic disease, a complication of carotid aneurysms. Radiology 1979;33:379–384.

180. Fisher M, Davidson R, Marcus E. Transient focal cerebral ischemia as a presenting manifestation of unruptured cerebral aneurysms. Ann Neurol 1980;8:367–372.

181. Pessin MS, Chimowitz MI, Levine SR, et al. Stroke in patients with fusiform vertebrobasilar aneurysms. Neurology 1989;39:16–21.

182. Caplan LR, Stein R, Patel D, et al. Intraluminal clot of the carotid artery detected radiographically. Neurology 1984; 34:1175–1181.

183. DeRook FA, Comess KA, Albers GW, Popp RL. Transesophageal echocardiography in the evaluation of stroke. Ann Intern Med 1992;117:922–932.

184. Grullon C, Alam M, Rosman HS, et al. Transesophageal echocardiography in unselected patients with focal cerebral ischemia: when is it useful? Cerebrovasc Dis 1994;4: 139–145.

185. Daniel WG, Mugge A. Transesophageal echocardiography. N Engl J Med 1995;332:1268–1279.

186. Horowitz DR, Tuhrim S, Weinberger J, et al. Transesophageal echocardiography: diagnostic and clinical applications in the evaluation of the stroke patient. J Stroke Cerebrovasc Dis 1997;6:332–336.

187. Johnson LL, Pohost GM. Nuclear Cardiology. In RC Schlant, RW Alexander (eds), Hurst's The Heart (8th ed). New York: McGraw-Hill, 1994;2281–2323.

188. Ezekowiz MD, Wilson DA, Smith EO, et al. Comparison of indium-111 platelet scintigraphy and two-dimensional echocardiography in the diagnosis of left ventricular thrombi. N Engl J Med 1982;306:1509–1513.

189. Weinberger J, Azhar S, Danisi F, et al. A new noninvasive technique for imaging atherosclerotic plaque in the aortic arch of stroke patients by transcutaneous real-time B-mode ultrasonography. Stroke 1998;29:673–676.

190. Caplan LR, Feinberg WM, Fisher MJ, del Zoppo GJ. The Blood. In LR Caplan (ed), Brain Ischemia. Basic Concepts and Clinical Relevance. London: Springer, 1995;83–126.

191. Schwab S, Rieke K, Aschoff A, et al. Hemicraniotomy in space-occupying hemispheric infarction: useful early intervention or desperate activism. Cerebrovasc Dis 1996; 6:325–329.

192. Schwab S, Steiner T, Aschoff A, et al. Early hemicraniectomy in patients with complete middle cerebral artery infarction. Stroke 1998;29:1888–1893.

Chapter 10

Hypoxic-Ischemic Encephalopathy and Cardiac Arrests

The brain is particularly vulnerable to any decrease in its blood, oxygen, or fuel supply. Patients with hypotension or hypoxia often present to their physicians or the emergency room because of cerebral dysfunction. Most often, decreased brain perfusion is caused by cardiac disease, either arrhythmia or pump failure often caused by an acute myocardial infarction. Because circulatory failure usually leads to hypoventilation, and hypoxia soon causes diminished cardiac function, hypoxia and hypoperfusion are usually combined. The general term *hypoxic-ischemic encephalopathy* reflects the dual nature of the central nervous system stress. Pulmonary embolism is another acute disorder that causes hypotension and diminished blood oxygenation. In some patients, decreased cerebral perfusion is caused by acute blood loss or hypovolemia.

Clinical Findings

A global decrease in perfusion causes generalized nonfocal brain dysfunction. Dizziness, light-headedness, confusion, and difficulty in concentrating are common. Focal symptoms and signs, such as hemiplegia, hemianopia, and aphasia, are rarely caused by circulatory failure but are the rule in the other categories of ischemic stroke. At times, prior strokes or vascular occlusions do lead to asymmetries on neurologic examination. Examination of a patient with globally decreased cerebral perfusion usually shows an ill-appearing person with sweating, tachycardia, hypotension (especially postural), and physical examination or electrocardiographic signs of cardiac dysfunction. The two common cir-

cumstances in which neurologists might see patients with cerebral hypoperfusion resulting from systemic causes are (1) acute central nervous system symptoms in the absence of a known incident of circulatory failure and (2) after known cardiac arrest, hypotension, or cardiac surgery. In the first circumstance, the major problem is diagnosis. When there is a known cardiac arrest, the consulting physician usually asks the neurologist about the prognosis of the brain injury.

Patient 1

A 63-year-old man, LB, suddenly became agitated and restless and seemed confused. He entered the hospital 2 days before for abdominal pain, had no neurologic symptoms or abnormalities, and underwent routine gastrointestinal x-rays. A psychiatrist who was called to examine and calm the patient requested neurologic consultation because of concern about an organic cause for the behavioral change. Neurologic examination showed an agitated, restless man. He did not know his whereabouts, nor could he give any account of the previous few days. He recalled none of the three objects told to him 3 minutes before, and could not even remember that he had been given objects to recall. He spoke normally and could repeat and understand spoken language. He could write but not read. He also could not identify objects in his environment by sight and saw only parts of pictures shown to him. When the same objects were placed in his hands, he correctly named them. There were no abnormalities of motor, reflex, or somatosensory function. Gait was normal but he held his hands outstretched when he walked, as if feeling for objects and walls.

This patient had abnormalities in three major spheres—memory, vision, and behavior. These findings indicate bilateral dysfunction of the posterior portions of the cerebral hemispheres. Embolization to the rostral basilar artery, causing bilateral temporo-occipital lobe infarcts in the posterior cerebral artery (PCA) territory, could cause these findings. Alternatively, an unrecognized episode of prolonged hypotension might have led to hypoperfusion in the posterior border zone between the middle cerebral artery (MCA) and PCA territories. Distal-field infarction most often affects the posterior hemispheres, possibly because they are the regions farthest from the heart.[1]

Lesions in the posterior watershed (between the MCA and PCA) often disconnect the preserved calcarine visual cortex in the occipital lobe from the more anterior centers that control eye movements. A visual problem first described by an ophthalmologist, called *Balint's syndrome*, often results.[1–4] Patients act as if they cannot see but sometimes suprisingly notice small objects. The features of Balint's syndrome are as follows:

1. Asimultagnosia: Patients see things piecemeal; they do not see all the objects in their field of vision at one time and may notice only parts of objects. To test for this problem, physicians should ask patients to count the number of people or objects in a picture or on a table, ask patients to read a paragraph aloud to determine whether they omit words or phrases, and show patients multiple objects held up together for verbal identification.

2. Optical ataxia: Patients cannot coordinate hand and eye movements and point erratically at objects. Physicians should test for optical ataxia by asking patients to touch the noses of people in a picture or to touch the crossing point of several Xs on a page. Physicians should ask patients to trace, first with one hand and then the other, a complex drawing constructed by the examiner.

3. Apraxia of gaze: Patients are unable to gaze directly where desired. Physicians should ask patients to look at an object held to the side, then look at the examiner's nose, and then repeat the same task. Physicians should also notice how patients explore a picture.

Visual abnormalities can be more severe in either the left or the right visual field. Balint's original cases were probably caused by systemic hypoperfusion, the most common mechanism of the bilateral parieto-occipital damage. PCA infarction also can lead to Balint's syndrome. Occasionally, patients with Alzheimer's or Creutzfeldt-Jakob disease have features of Balint's syndrome but the findings develop gradually and insidiously rather than abruptly. Memory dysfunction and agitation can also be caused by bilateral PCA-territory infarcts or border-zone ischemia. These conditions are discussed in Chapter 7.

When hypotension is more severe, lesions can spread to the anterior border zones between the anterior cerebral artery (ACA) and MCA and may extend like a triangle toward the ventricle (Figure 10-1).[5,6] The areas of the motor homunculus most affected are those related to the shoulder, arm, and thigh. The face territory in the central portion of the MCA territory and the foot region in the center of the ACA supply are spared. The distribution of weakness has been likened by Mohr to a "man in a barrel."[1,7]

Among a prospective series of 34 patients with coma presumably caused by an episode of systemic hypotension, 11 had the man-in-the-barrel syndrome.[7] They moved neither arm but moved both legs spontaneously or in response to pain. The frontal eye fields are also affected, so that roving eye movements and hyperactive passive head movements (doll's eye reflexes) result. At times, perhaps because of previously asymmetric occlusive disease of extracranial and intracranial arteries, the signs can be quite asymmetric with unilateral or asymmetric arm paralysis and conjugate-eye deviation toward the side of the larger lesion. Stupor results from extensive bilateral border-zone ischemia.

LB was sedated and a computed tomography (CT) scan was ordered. The scan showed small but definite approximately symmetric hypodensities in the posterior parietal regions with sparing of the medial

Figure 10-1. Horizontal section of the cerebrum shows common patterns of hypoxic-ischemic brain damage. (a) Border-zone infarcts between anterior and middle cerebral arteries, and between middle and posterior cerebral arteries. (b) Zones of laminar necrosis within the cerebral cortex. (c) Hippocampal necrosis. (d) Necrosis of nerve cells within the globus pallidus and putamen. (Drawn by Gloria Wu, M.D. Reproduced with permission from LR Caplan, JW Hurst, MI Chimowitz. Clinical Neurocardiology. New York: Marcel Dekker, 1999.)

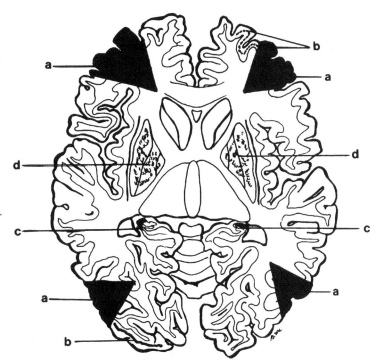

calcarine cortex and temporal lobes. An electrocardiogram showed evidence of acute myocardial infarction and multifocal, frequent, premature ventricular contractions.

CT confirmed that the lesions were between the PCA and MCA territories, supporting the diagnosis of border-zone infarction. This led to more cardiac testing, which showed an unsuspected myocardial infarction and a potentially serious arrhythmia. In retrospect, after further questioning by the patient's physician, the acute abdominal pain was probably caused by coronary disease. The diagnosis of border-zone ischemia leads to a different array of diagnostic tests than those that apply to infarction in the center of a vascular territory. I have also occasionally seen demented patients whose neurologic examination and CT scans indicated border-zone infarcts caused by repeated, unrecognized episodes of hypotension or globally decreased cerebral perfusion.

LB had a relatively slight insult and recuperated well with time. The nature of the insult and its reversibility should be emphasized. In general, it is unwise to push the patient back to work too quickly or self-confidence may be lost. Many patients are not restored mentally for months after their cardiac events but gradually regain their usual intellectual vigor over time. Time and reassurance are needed.

Patient 2

A 45-year-old previously well man, AR, collapsed at work, clutching his chest in pain. Paramedics found him pulseless minutes later and administered cardiopulmonary resuscitation (CPR) on the way to the hospital. Pulse and blood pressure were restored, but the patient lay comatose. A neurologist examined the patient the next morning, 18 hours after the arrest. The patient was sleepy but could be momentarily aroused by shouting or pinching. He would appropriately flick off painful stimuli but did not speak, obey oral commands, or answer queries. There were spontaneous restless limb movements. Blinking, swallowing, and tongue-protrusion movements were seen. Pupillary, corneal, and doll's eye reflexes were normal. Plantar responses were extensor, but there was no abnormal limb posturing.

In this patient, the consulting physician knew that the abnormal neurologic state was caused by cardiac arrest. Was the central nervous system insult likely to be lethal? What would be the quality of survival? Should orders not to resuscitate be given? This scenario is frequent in hospital practice today. Successful CPR, once rare, has become commonplace. Advances in technique, widespread teaching of medical, paramedical, and lay volunteer personnel, and the availability of special mobile equipment and facilities in some communities have saved many lives.[8–10] The heart is often able to recover from ischemia, but the brain has often been irreversibly damaged by the ischemic-anoxic insult of circulatory failure. New technology can prolong life indefinitely in a vegetative state, at great emotional, physical, and economic cost to the community and family. Physicians involved with CPR must be familiar with prognostic indicators for cerebral recovery after cardiac arrest and should consider their own ethical and moral values in applying this knowledge.

Pathology

Signs of brain dysfunction secondary to hypoxic-ischemic insults can best be remembered by visualizing the brain regions most vulnerable to circulatory failure and their pathology. The location and severity of the pathology depends on the patient's age; the completeness of the circulatory arrest; serologic factors, such as the blood sugar and pH; and the relative admixture of hypoxia and ischemia.

Severe prolonged hypoxic-ischemic insults cause necrosis of the cerebral and cerebellar cortex, cerebral edema, and injury to brain stem nuclei. The most vulnerable neurons are those in the cerebral cortex, especially in the middle laminae; pyramidal neurons in the CA1 zone of the hippocampus; neurons in portions of the amygdaloid nucleus; Purkinje cells in the cerebellar cortex; neurons in the caudate nucleus, putamen, and globus pallidus;

Table 10-1. Patterns of Hypoxic-Ischemic Injury and Their Causes

1. Diffuse cerebral cortical injury, often with laminar necrosis of the middle cortical layers, cardiac arrest, or prolonged hypotension.
2. Ischemic damage to border-zone regions, especially between the middle and posterior cerebral artery territories, and between the anterior and middle cerebral artery territories, cardiac arrest, or prolonged hypotension.
3. Necrosis of hippocampal neurons, especially in the CA1 zone, cardiac arrest, or prolonged hypotension.
4. Necrosis of basal ganglia and thalamic neurons; delayed necrosis of the basal ganglia and cerebral white matter; severe hypoxia, especially strangulation, hanging, carbon monoxide poisoning, and drowning.
5. Necrosis of Purkinje's cells in the cerebellum, prolonged ischemia.
6. Necrosis of brain stem motor and tegmental nuclei, especially cranial nerve nuclei, inferior colliculus, vestibular nuclei, and superior olive; sudden severe hypotension in infants, children, and young adults.

Source: Modified with permission LR Caplan. Cardiac Arrest and Other Hypoxic Ischemic Insults. In LR Caplan, JW Hurst, MI Chimowitz. Clinical Neurocardiology. New York: Marcel Dekker, 1999.

motor nuclei in the brain stem; and neurons in the anterior, dorsomedial, and pulvinar thalamic nuclei.[10,11] The pattern and distribution of injury also depends on the anatomy of the arterial circulation. Border zones show more injury than brain areas in the heart of the major feeding brain arteries. Selective vulnerability, arterial anatomy, and differential responses to hypoxia and ischemia explain the various patterns of brain damage seen in patients with cardiac arrest and severe hypoxia. The most common patterns are listed in Table 10-1. Acknowledgment of the anatomic patterns helps clinicians recognize the clinical syndromes and also the use of some of the investigations used in evaluating patients with hypoxic-ischemic encephalopathy.

Clinical Abnormalities and Syndromes

Brain Stem and Bihemispheral Coma

Consciousness is maintained by continuous stimulation of the cerebral hemispheres by neurons within the brain stem tegmentum. Coma develops after damage to the bilateral medial portions of the brain stem tegmentum in the pons and midbrain or when there is severe damage to the bilateral cerebral hemispheres. All patients who have had cardiac arrest have an initial period of coma. When comatose patients are first examined, there are two different patterns of findings depending on the presence or absence of brain stem reflexes. In patients with severe prolonged hypoperfusion-anoxic insults, the pupils are dilated, corneal reflexes are absent, and the eyes remain midline and do not move horizontally or vertically to doll's eye reflex or to ice water irrigation of the ear canals. Some patients have no spontaneous respirations and must be ventilated mechanically. Spontaneous limb movements, except for low-level decorticate or decerebrate movements, are absent. This state is usually referred to as *brain stem coma* because it indicates injury to brain stem tegmental nuclei. When this state is prolonged, death invariably follows.

Infants, young children, and occasionally adults have selective necrosis of their brain stem tegmental nuclei.[12,13] These patients have loss of reflex eye movements; facial, pharyngeal, and tongue weakness; and loss of the gag reflex. They usually have stiff, immobile limbs and only automatic and autonomic responses to environmental stimuli. Control of respirations is often lost, and the pulse and blood pressures may fluctuate widely. This state invariably proves fatal. Imaging may show no cerebral hemispheral abnormalities, and the brain stem may even appear normal on gross inspection at necropsy. Microscopic examination shows selective necrosis of brain stem nuclei.

Some patients with brain stem coma regain normal brain stem reflexes and spontaneous respirations and enter a state called *bihemispheral coma*. Other patients have bihemispheral coma when first examined neurologically and have not gone through a stage of brain stem coma. Patients with bihemispheral coma are unresponsive to noise, voice, or bright light. There may be some spontaneous movements of all limbs. The pupils are normal or constricted and react to light. The eyes usually remain in the midline, move from side to side, or are deviated upward. Passive movements readily elicit horizontal eye movements. Often, doll's eye movements are hyperactive, indicating lack of cerebral inhibition of the vestibulo-ocular reflex. Vertical eye movements can usually be elicited by flexing and extending the neck. In patients with forced upward eye deviation, it may be difficult to get the eyes to move fully downward on vertical doll's eyes maneuvers. The gag reflex is usually present. Some patients with bihemispheral coma have their mouths open, and some keep their jaws tightly clenched and "bulldog" down on tubes or sticks placed in their mouths, making it difficult to see the pharynx or perform the gag reflex. Watching these patients from the foot of the bed shows that they often spontaneously blink, yawn, sneeze, cough, hiccup, protrude their tongue, lick their lips, sigh, and swallow. These spontaneous mouth, face, and tongue movements are mediated through brain stem structures and indicate the brain stem is working.[14] Coma is caused by loss of the normal functions of both cerebral hemispheres.

Spontaneous limb movements and responses to pinch in the limbs vary considerably.[14] Patients who have dysfunction of the corticospinal tracts often have preserved adduction and flexion movements of the shoulders, arms, and wrists. When pinched on either the flexor or extensor surface of the arm, forearm, or hand, they flex and adduct the arm and shoulder irrespective of the site of stimulation. The flexion response brings the arm into stimuli on the flexor surface. Spontaneous or reactive extension, abducting movements of the arm or forearm, preserved movements of individual fingers, and limb withdrawal from pinch appropriate to the site of stimulation (flexion or adduction when pinched on the extensor surface, and extension or abduction when pinched on the flexor surface, movements which move the upper limb away from the stimulus) show that the corticospinal tracts are preserved and functioning. Similarly, loss of corticospinal tract function leads to extension and adduction of the lower limbs. Flexion and adduction movements, spontaneously or in response to pinch, usually indicate corticospinal tract preservation. The ability to remove or react to pinch with either the same or contralateral arm indicates that the stimulus has been perceived. Use of the arm contralateral to the pinch to ward off the noxious stimulus almost always indicates weakness of the stimulated arm. Major asymmetries of motor or sensory function usually mean asymmetric brain damage.

Patients with bihemispheral coma may remain in a vegetative state poorly responsive to environmental stimuli or they can become more alert and responsive. A number of clinical patterns of dysfunction can ensue from the bihemispheral coma stage.

As stupor lightens, agitation, restlessness, confusion, and even delirium supervene. An examination performed after the patient awakens often uncovers features of Balint's syndrome, as described in the first patient. Other patients have a selective difficulty with memory and are unable to recall recent happenings or form new lasting memories. This amnesic state clinically resembles Korsakoff's syndrome and is caused by selective vulnerability of the hippocampus and adjacent medial temporal lobe structures to hypoxic-ischemic insults.[10,11,15–18] Active memory testing is required to identify and quantify the memory loss. Physicians should give patients a 10-fact story, three objects, or three pictures, emphasizing that they will later be asked to recall the information. Patients should be asked to repeat the items to be certain that they have been registered. Later, patients should be asked to recite the items to be recalled, grading the performance (i.e., as three out of five objects after 5 minutes). Passive memory testing—asking patients what happened that morning or what they ate at their last meal—is less reliable than active memory testing.

The cerebral cortex often undergoes selective damage to the middle lamina, sparing the deeper and more superficial cortical layers.[11,19,20] This laminar necrosis frequently causes seizures. Seizures may follow severe or moderate laminar injury and may take the form of multifocal myoclonic jerks, twitches, or frank grand mal seizures. Myoclonic jerks are often exaggerated or provoked by moving or stimulating a limb. Seizures caused by diffuse hypoxic-ischemic injury are relatively resistant to treatment. Care should be taken to avoid overdosing with anticonvulsants, thus compounding the patient's stupor. If seizures create respiratory compromise, cause myoglobinuria, or release of high levels of muscle enzymes, curarization and mechanical ventilation may be necessary. Repetitive generalized myoclonus, lasting longer than 30 minutes, carries a poor prognosis in patients who survive a cardiac arrest.[21–23] In one series of 11 such patients, none regained consciousness after resuscitation and all remained comatose until death.[21] Each of these patients had extensive hypoxic-ischemic damage to the cerebral cortex, especially the hippocampus and calcarine cortices. The basal ganglia, thalamus, cerebellum, and brain stem nuclei were all severely damaged.[21]

Severe laminar necrosis can be associated with extensive loss of cortical functions, so that patients survive in a persistent vegetative state with little meaningful response to the environment but preserved brain stem function. These patients appear awake. They have sleep-wake cycles with eyes open but make no response to stimulation or to the environment.[20,24] Necropsy examinations of 10 patients with the persistent vegetative state showed extensive cortical necrosis, often laminar in distribution, and multiple microinfarcts.[20]

Prolonged partial ischemia, especially in the young, can cause damage to the basal ganglia, particularly the globus pallidus and thalamus. Strangulation and carbon monoxide poisoning produce a similar insult,[25] in which hypoxia antedates and overshadows circulatory compromise. Rigidity, decorticate posturing, and flexion of all limbs result. Although the eyes are open and fixate, patients are often mute and usually do not respond to environmental stimuli. Patients with mutism and rigidity after cardiac arrest have a poor prognosis for recovery.

Although hypoxic-ischemic cerebellar damage is commonly found at necropsy, clinical signs of cerebellar dysfunction are rare and are usually overshadowed by cerebral abnormalities. After cardiac arrest, some patients have spontaneous arrhythmic fine or coarse muscle jerking, markedly exaggerated when the limbs are used. This disorder of movements, usually called *action myoclonus* or the *Lance-Adams syndrome* after the physicians who originally described it,[26] is often accompanied by gait ataxia. The movement disorder can progress, even without further ischemic stress. Some patients, especially those with pre-existing occlusive disease of the vertebral arteries, may have prominent ataxia caused by border-zone cerebellar infarcts, mostly between the main supply of the three major circumferential cerebellar arteries.

Plum and colleagues described delayed progressive deterioration after a single hypoxic insult.[27] Three of the five patients reported deteriorated after exposure to noxious gases and had predominately hypoxic injuries. The other two patients worsened after surgery and both had hypotension and anoxia. The patients were all comatose when first examined after the insult but awakened within 24 hours and resumed relatively normal activities and functions for 4–10 days. These patients then developed cognitive and behavioral abnormalities characterized mostly by apathy, irritability, agitation, restlessness, and confusion. Walking then became clumsy and the limbs became rigid and stiff. Outcome varied from full recovery to severe disability to death. Necropsy in the two patients that died showed extensive white matter demyelination in the cerebral hemispheres. One patient also had cystic necrosis in the medial globus pallidus bilaterally.

Subsequent reports confirmed the existence of a leukoencephalopathy, often with basal ganglionic damage, which follows hypoxic-ischemic events.[28,29] The white matter damage involves rather diffuse injury to the white matter, which ranges from patchy demyelination to hemorrhagic white matter necrosis. Most reported patients have been young, and the insult has most often been predominantly hypoxic (e.g., carbon monoxide intoxication, strangulation, drowning, and gas inhalation). When initially examined after the insult, the patients were in coma, often with loss of muscle tone, quadriparesis, or involuntary movements of the limbs. Most patients who developed severe limb dysfunction with rigidity, abnormal movements, and dystonia never improved after the initial hypoxic-ischemic event, but some have had delayed deterioration, as was first reported by Plum et al. The dystonic rigid state is associated with severe damage to deep subcortical basal ganglionic and white matter tracts, usually with relative preservation of the cerebral cortex. The pathologic substrate of this syndrome presents a sharp contrast to the cerebral cortex necrosis with usual preservation of subcortical structures found in patients with the persistent vegetative state.

In two reports, two patients with delayed hypoxic leukoencephalopathy have shown a reduction of arylsulfatase-A activity to less than 50% of normal.[30,31] Although this degree of reduction does not ordinarily cause symptoms, hypoxia could cause tissue acidosis, which might potentiate myelin damage. Arylsulfatase-A is a lysosomal enzyme active in the lipid metabolism of myelin. In the presence of local tissue acidosis, this enzyme deficiency could make patients vulnerable to demyelination. Proton magnetic resonance spectroscopy

of the white matter lesions helped to identify one reported patient[31] and might be useful in evaluating other patients with hypoxic-ischemic encephalopathies. Progressive worsening is rare after cardiac arrest, although it has been described. The mechanism of progressive loss of function after single self-limited insults is uncertain.

Occasionally, patients recover from coma without obvious cerebral damage but instead have paraplegia related to hypoxic-ischemic damage to the spinal cord.[32,33] The most vulnerable spinal regions are the upper and lower thoracic and lumbar spinal cord segments. The cervical cord is usually not involved, so that the arms are normal despite severe weakness of the lower limbs. The localization of the spinal cord ischemic necrosis relates to the anatomy of the arterial supply of the spinal cord. Although arteries from each side feed into the paired posterior spinal arteries at each spinal segment, the segmental arteries that supply the single unpaired midline anterior spinal artery originate at variable levels, and one supply artery can be mostly responsible for nourishing four or five segments. The largest and most well-known artery, the artery of Adamkiewicz, originates anywhere between the ninth thoracic and second lumbar segment and supplies the lumbar spinal cord and conus medullaris. The upper and lower thoracic regions are border-zone areas between the supply of major anterior feeding arteries. The spinal damage involves mostly the anterior portion of the spinal cord, which is fed by the anterior spinal artery. The anterior horn motor neurons and the pyramidal tracts are included, but usually the posterior columns are spared. The resulting syndrome is usually a flaccid paralysis of both lower limbs. Spasticity often develops later. Control of urination and defecation is often lost and there may be a sensory level to pain and temperature on the trunk. Position and vibration sense and touch are usually preserved. Atrophy and fasciculations often develop in the thighs and legs. Spinal cord infarction is a rare but important result of cardiac arrest or prolonged systemic hypotension.

Prognosis

Often, the most important consideration in patients with potentially severe hypoxic-ischemic insults is prediction of outcome. What findings allow physi-

Table 10-2. Clinical Prognosticators in Patients Examined after Hypoxic-Ischemic Events

1. Depth and duration of coma
2. Brain stem reflexes
   a. Pupillary light reflex
   b. Corneal reflex
   c. Oculovestibular responses
3. Spontaneous respirations and requirement for a ventilator
4. Motor responses to stimuli
5. Eye positions and movements
6. Vocal responses
7. Ability to follow commands
8. Seizures, myoclonus, and other involuntary movements

Source: Reprinted with permission from LR Caplan. Cardiac Arrest and Other Hypoxic Ischemic Insults. In LR Caplan, JW Hurst, MI Chimowitz. Clinical Neurocardiology. New York: Marcel Dekker, 1999.

cians to predict the likelihood of survival and the presence, nature, and severity of residual neurologic damage? Investigators have struggled to find reliable prognosticators since the 1970s.[34–46] Table 10-2 lists the various clinical indicators that have been studied and analyzed. Persistence or absence of clinical findings has different prognostic use during the first hours, day, week, and after the first month.

Survival after cardiac arrest depends on the following three major factors: (1) the severity of the cardiac disease and hypoxic-ischemic cardiac injury, (2) the extent and reversibility of brain stem damage, and (3) cardiopulmonary and infectious complications that occur in the hospital. The heart may be even more vulnerable than the brain to hypoxia and ischemia.[44] After severe anoxia of 4 minutes' duration or longer, arrhythmias and asystole often develop, causing decreased cardiac output and decreased brain perfusion. The brain stem nuclei control automatic and autonomic functions, including control of cardiovascular functions and respirations. Survival is rare after severe damage to the bilateral brain stem tegmentum. Pulmonary embolism, congestive heart failure, recurrent cardiac arrhythmias and cardiac arrests, pneumonia, and urinary tract sepsis are frequent and often serious complications in patients after cardiac arrest, especially in those patients who remain in coma or states of reduced consciousness.

The nature and severity of persistent neurologic signs depend on the severity and location of the cerebral, cerebellar, and spinal damage. Prediction of the nature and severity of persistent neurologic deficits can only be assessed when brain stem coma has cleared and the patient is in bihemispheral coma or has awakened.

During the first minutes and hours after cardiac arrest or other hypoxic-ischemic insults, the most important signs of prognostic importance are the depth and duration of the coma, brain stem functions, and reflexes.[36–43] Sustained brain stem dysfunction causes deep, prolonged coma, an absence of brain stem reflex functions, and poor control of respirations. Patients with irreversible, severe bilateral medial tegmental brain stem damage do not survive. Testing of brain stem reflex functions is important in all comatose patients. Clinicians should note the rate, depth, and regularity of respirations and the need for mechanical ventilation. Some spontaneous movements, such as blinking, yawning, coughing, sneezing, gagging, and swallowing, use brain stem reflex functions. The presence of these movements indicates preserved brain stem function.[14]

In the series of Snyder et al., all patients who at 3 hours after cardiopulmonary arrest had no corneal reflexes or absent pupillary light reflexes died.[38,39] By 6 hours, no survivors had absence of the three brain stem reflexes studied—pupillary light response, corneal reflex, and reflex eye movements. By 24–48 hours, only 3 of 25 survivors (12%) had any brain stem reflex abnormality. In another series, 52 of 210 patients (25%) with hypoxic-ischemic coma had absent pupillary light reflex when first examined, and none of the 52 patients had a final outcome better than severe disability.[37]

Pupillary size during the initial hours after the insult is another useful prognostic indicator.[45] The pupils dilate and responses to light are lost within a few minutes of cardiac arrest. Pupillary dilatation throughout resuscitation carried a poor prognosis in one series. Drugs, especially catecholamines and atropine, can affect pupillary size, so clinicians should be cautious about using pupillary size as a prognostic sign in patients who have received drugs that affect pupillary diameter. Persistent dilation of the pupils is an ominous sign.

The depth of coma is another important indicator during the first hours after cardiac arrest. Deep coma usually means extensive brain stem dysfunction or injury to the cerebral hemispheres bilaterally. In most adults when the hypoxic-ischemic insult is severe enough to injure the brain stem and cause deep coma and loss of brain stem reflexes, the cerebral hemispheres are even more severely damaged because structures in the cerebrum are more vulnerable to hypoxia than brain stem nuclei.

During the early hours, analysis of spontaneous movements of the limbs and motor responses of the limbs to sensory stimuli is useful in prognosis. The absence of limb movement, even after pinching, is an unfavorable prognostic sign. The presence of only automatic decorticate (flexion of the upper limbs and extension of the lower limbs) or decerebrate (extension of the upper and lower limbs) responses to painful stimuli also is an unfavorable sign for survival and good recovery. Spontaneous varied limb movements and normal withdrawal of limbs to pain is a favorable sign.

Some patients have frequent myoclonic movements during the first hours after resuscitation. Sudden jerks of the limbs, face, jaw, and eyelids are common. The jerks are often bilateral and synchronous and can be accompanied by upward movement of the eyes and twitching of the eyelids. The jerks are often precipitated by touch, tracheal suctioning, insertion of catheters, and noise. The jerks can also be precipitated by a loud clap. Frequent myoclonic jerks predict death or at best a persistent vegetative state.

Roine analyzed the prognostic importance of seizures among 155 patients who survived out-of-hospital cardiac arrest in Helsinki.[34] Seizures during the first 24 hours were not prognostically useful. Fifty-three percent of patients who had seizures during the first day survived, compared with 70% of survivors who had no first-day seizures. Seizures after the first day were associated with a poor outcome, however, because only three of 15 patients (20%) with seizures after the first day recovered consciousness, and only one patient (7%) lived for one year. Status epilepticus at any time after cardiac arrest was a dire sign because all nine patients with epileptic status died.

In patients who survive the first 24 hours, prognostic indicators are somewhat different during the next few days. Absence of the normal brain stem pupillary, corneal, oculovestibular, and pharyngeal reflexes at 24 hours indicates a poor prognosis. Persistent brain stem dysfunction means brain stem

and severe hemispheral damage because the hemispheres are almost always more damaged than the brain stem. Most patients who eventually survive at 24 hours have bihemispheral coma or have become alert. The duration and depth of coma are probably the most important prognostic indicators during the first days. Prolonged bihemispheral coma is a poor prognostic indicator. In one series, day two was the most common time for patients to emerge from coma, and most patients who survived awakened by the end of day two. Only 2 of the 27 patients (7%) in deep coma through day two survived.[38] In another series, no patient in postanoxic coma after the third day survived.[41] In another series, five of 12 patients (42%) with good outcome remained in coma for 2 or more days, but all but one of the 12 patients awakened and reached their best level of function within the first week after resuscitation.[46]

Eye opening, eye movements, and motor responses are also useful prognostic indicators during the first few days. By the end of the first day, the absence of spontaneous eye opening indicates a poor prognosis. Most patients who have a good recovery begin to open their eyes and have at least intermittent visual fixation movements. The presence of eye opening, however, does not always indicate a good outcome. In one large series, spontaneous eye opening often occurred by 48 hours in patients with both good and bad outcomes. Persistent roving eye movements without visual fixation usually means severe bilateral cerebral hemispheral damage and indicates a poor outcome. Sustained upgaze also carries a poor prognosis.[47] The absence of withdrawal limb movements when painful stimuli are given is also a poor prognostic sign, as is persistence of obligatory reflex decorticate or decerebrate posturing. Most patients who have good recovery begin to obey commands during the first few days. The most reliable way of judging prognosis is to perform careful repeated neurologic examinations within the first hours and days after the insult.

Clinicians are often involved in declaring brain death after cardiac arrest. The following criteria are often used as indicators of brain death, an irreversible state in which there is no precedent for meaningful survival.[48,49] Physicians can declare death if criteria for brain death are met, despite persistence of cardiac function.

1. Coma with loss of cerebral reactivity
2. Absence of spontaneous respiration
3. Loss of brain stem reflexes (pupillary, corneal, oculovestibular, and oculocephalic)
4. Electrocerebral silence (so-called flat electroencephalogram [EEG]) for longer than 12 hours (in the absence of hypothermia or sedative drugs)

> In AR, blood sugar was 150 mg/dl on admission. The pH was 7.32 one hour after arrest. CT was normal. EEG showed diffuse delta and theta slowing but the background changed when the patient was pinched and light was shown in the face. By day three, he had awakened and spoke normally but had a severe amnestic syndrome.

The level of blood sugar at the time of arrest may be one factor that affects recovery. Myers and Yamaguchi showed that young monkeys given infusions of glucose before induced cardiac arrest had more cerebral damage than similarly studied animals infused with saline.[50] Others have corroborated these findings in adult animals and showed that more severe damage also results when glucose is given after the ischemic insult.[51] The damage may be caused by production of lactate, which can injure brain tissue. Systemic lactic acidosis can clearly compound the cerebral damage. Poor neurologic recovery after cardiac arrest was linked to higher blood sugar levels (>300 mg/dl) in one human study.[52] Theoretically, high blood calcium levels might also have a deleterious effect.

EEGs of patients in coma after cardiac arrest are usually abnormal and contain diffuse slowing in the theta and delta ranges, as well as periodic phenomena and epileptiform discharges. In the most severe injuries, the EEG may be flat-electrocerebral silence. Severe slowing or low amplitude of the background activity has a bad prognosis, especially if documented in EEGs 12 or 24 hours apart.

Some patients in deep coma from hypoxic-ischemic injury have preserved alpha activity. Alpha coma activity differs from normal rhythms as follows[53,54]:

1. It is usually faster (9–12 cycles/second), compared with the usual (8–10 cycles/second) alpha.
2. It is more frontal, central, and parietal, as compared with the usual occipital location.

3. It is usually temporary.
4. It does not respond to auditory, photic, or tactile stimuli.

Evoked-response testing may also help determine the degree of cerebral injury. Brain imaging has not been helpful during the first days after cardiac arrest, but few studies of CT or magnetic resonance imaging (MRI) have been performed during the acute period after cardiac arrest.[55–58] Many patients are too unstable to be transported to the scanners. Kjos et al. studied early CT findings in 10 patients.[55] Nine of the patients had some evidence of diffuse cerebral edema, and six patients had poor discrimination between the gray and white matter. Watershed cerebral and cerebellar infarcts and bilateral basal ganglia and thalamic hypodensities are also found in some patients. Diffuse mass effect with obliteration of basal cisterns has been described but is rare.[56] In some patients, brain edema and discrete infarcts are seen after several days.

Roine analyzed MRI findings among 155 patients resuscitated after out-of-hospital cardiac arrest and compared the findings with 88 controls.[57] Brain infarcts were more common after cardiac arrest but the difference was significant only for deep infarcts. Twenty-five percent of patients had cortical infarcts, 14% had cerebral watershed infarcts, 21% had deep cerebral infarcts, and 4% had deep watershed infarcts. The number of infarcts and multiple infarcts were more common in the resuscitated group. Two patients had diffuse hypointensity of the cerebral white matter. Severe edema on MRI or CT scans was a dire prognostic sign. Repeated MRI examinations during the course of patients with severe neurologic deficits may show high–signal-intensity cortical lesions compatible with laminar necrosis.

Single-photon emission CT can show changes in cerebral blood flow after cardiac arrest, but the changes are quite nonspecific.[59] Usually, the decreased perfusion is most severe frontally. In one study, regional blood flow was almost invariably abnormal after cardiac arrest.[34] Regional blood flow improved over time in some patients but often remained abnormal. No consistent correlation was found between blood flow and outcome.

The brains of patients considered brain dead before death is pronounced are usually soft and necrotic at autopsy. Angiography before death reveals an absence of intracranial circulation. Brain swelling is so extensive that antegrade flow of blood into the cranium is blocked. Absence of blood flow into the intracranial arteries is not c ompatible with survival. The transcranial Doppler system has been used since the early 1990s to evaluate patients for the determination of brain death.[60–62]

Treatment

Little is known about optimal treatment of patients to minimize cerebral damage after cardiac arrest, although many experimental and clinical studies deal with this problem. Certainly, it is important to maintain good cardiac output and ventilation and prevent complications of the stuporous state, such as aspiration, pneumonia, and urosepsis. Theoretical advantages can be cited for:

1. Hemodilution
2. Artificially induced hypertension to augment cerebral blood flow
3. Hypothermia
4. Barbiturate anesthesia to reduce cerebral metabolism
5. Lowering of blood sugar
6. Corticosteroids
7. GM_1 gangliosides
8. Calcium channel blockers
9. Free-radical scavengers

When many of these treatments are combined in the experimental animal, brain damage is reduced, although evidence that any single treatment is effective is scant.[63] Much more work is needed to answer the important question of how to treat patients with brain dysfunction after cardiac arrest.

References

1. Mohr JP. Neurological Complications of Cardiac Valvular Disease and Cardiac Surgery Including Systemic Hypotension. In P Vinken, G Bruyn (eds), Handbook of Clinical Neurology, Vol 38. Neurological Manifestations of Systemic Disease. Amsterdam: North Holland Publishing, 1979;143–171.
2. Balint R. Seelenlahmung des Schauens, optische Ataxie, raumliche Storung der Aufmerksamheit. Z Psychiatr Neurol 1909;25:51–81.
3. Tyler HR. Cerebral Disturbance of Vision in Neuro-ophthalmology, Vol 4. St. Louis: Mosby, 1968;266–281.
4. Hecaen H, Ajuriaguerra J. Balint's syndrome and its minor forms. Brain 1954;77:373–400.
5. Zulch K. On the Circulatory Disturbances in the Borderline Zones of the Cerebral and Spinal Vessels. In JG Greenfield, D Russell (eds), Proceedings of the Second International Congress on Neuropathology, Vol 8. Amsterdam: Excerpta Medica, 1955;894–895.
6. Romanul F, Abramowicz A. Changes in brain and pial vessels in arterial border zones. Arch Neurol 1974;11:40–65.
7. Sage JI, Van Uitest RL. Man-in-the-barrel syndrome. Neurology 1986;36:1102–1103.
8. Copley D, Mantel J, Rogers W, et al. Improved outcome for prehospital cardiopulmonary collapse with resuscitation by bystanders. Circulation 1977;56:901–905.
9. Lund I, Skulberg A. Cardiopulmonary resuscitation by lay people. Lancet 1975;2:702–704.
10. Caplan LR. Cardiac Arrest and other Hypoxic Ischemic Insults. In LR Caplan, JW Hurst, M Chimowitz (eds), Clinical Neurocardiology. New York: Marcel Dekker, 1999;1–34.
11. Adams JH, Brierley JB, Connor RCR, Treip CS. The effects of systemic hypotension upon the human brain: clinical and neuropathological observations in 11 cases. Brain 1966;89:235–268.
12. Gilles F. Hypotensive brainstem necrosis. Arch Pathol 1969;88:32–41.
13. Roland EH, Hill A, Norman MG, et al. Selective brainstem injury in an asphyxiated newborn. Ann Neurol 1988;23:89–92.
14. Fisher CM. The neurological examination of the comatose patient. Acta Neurol Scand 1969;45(Suppl 36):5–56.
15. Caronna J, Finkelstein S. Neurologic syndrome after cardiac arrest. Stroke 1978;9:517–520.
16. Volpe B, Hirst W. The characterization of an amnesic syndrome following hypoxic-ischemic injury. Arch Neurol 1983;40:436–440.
17. Cummings J, Tomiyasu U, Reed S, et al. Amnesia with hippocampal lesion after cardiopulmonary arrest. Neurology 1984;34:679–681.
18. Petito C, Feldmann E, Pulsinelli W, Plum F. Delayed hippocampal damage in humans following cardiorespiratory arrest. Neurology 1987;37:1281–1286.
19. Brierley JB, Adams JH, Graham D, et al. Neocortical death after cardiac arrest: a clinical, neurophysiological, and neuropathological report of two cases. Lancet 1971;2:560–565.
20. Dougherty J, Rawlinson D, Levy D, et al. Hypoxic-ischemic brain injury and the vegetative state: clinical and neuropathologic correlation. Neurology 1981;31:991–997.
21. Young GB, Gilbert JJ, Zochodne DW. The significance of myoclonic status epilepticus in postanoxic coma. Neurology 1990;40:1843–1848.
22. Wijdicks EFM, Parisi JE, Sharbrough FW. Prognostic value of myoclonic status in comatose survivors of cardiac arrest. Ann Neurol 1994;35:239–243.
23. Krumholz A, Stern BJ, Weiss HD. Outcome from coma after cardiopulmonary resuscitation. Relation to seizures and myoclonus. Neurology 1988;38:401–405.
24. Jennett B, Plum F. Persistent vegetative state after brain damage: a syndrome in search of a name. Lancet 1972;1:734–737.

25. Dooling E, Richardson E. Delayed encephalopathy after strangling. Arch Neurol 1976;33:196–199.

26. Lance J, Adams R. The syndrome of intention and action myoclonus as a sequel to hypoxic encephalopathy. Brain 1963;86:111–133.

27. Plum F, Posner JB, Hain R. Delayed neurologic deterioration after anoxia. Arch Intern Med 1962;110:56–67.

28. Ginsberg MD, Hedley-White T, Richardson EP. Hypoxic-ischemic leukoencephalopathy in man. Arch Neurol 1976; 33:5–14.

29. Hori A, Hirose G, Kataoka K, et al. Delayed postanoxic encephalopathy after strangulation. Arch Neurol 1991;48: 871–874.

30. Weinberger LM, Schmidley JW, Schafer IA, Raghaven S. Delayed postanoxic demyelination and arylsulfatase-A pseudodeficiency. Neurology 1994;44:152–154.

31. Gottfried JA, Mayer SA, Shungu DC, Chang Y, Duyn JH. Delayed posthypoxic demyelination: association with arylsulfatase-A deficiency and lactic acidosis on Proton MR spectroscopy. Neurology 1997;49:1400–1404.

32. Caronna J, Finkelstein S. Neurologic syndromes after cardiac arrest. Stroke 1978;9:517–520.

33. Silver JR, Buxton PH. Spinal stroke. Brain 1974;97: 539–550.

34. Roine RO. Neurological outcome of out-of-hospital cardiac arrest [doctoral thesis]. University of Helsinki, 1993.

35. Earnest MP, Breckinridge JC, Yarnell PR, Oliva PB. Quality of survival after out-of-hospital cardiac arrest: predictive value of early neurologic evaluation. Neurology 1979; 29:56–60.

36. Wijdicks E. Neurological Complications of Cardiac Arrest. In EFM Wijdicks (ed), Neurology of Critical Illness. Philadelphia: FA Davis, 1995;86–103.

37. Levy DE, Caronna JJ, Singer BH, et al. Predicting outcome from hypoxic-ischemic coma. JAMA 1985;253: 1420–1426.

38. Snyder BD, Loewenson RB, Gumnit RJ, et al. Neurologic prognosis after cardiopulmonary arrest: II. Level of consciousness. Neurology 1980;30:52–58.

39. Snyder BD, Gumnit RJ, Leppik IE, et al. Neurologic prognosis after cardiopulmonary arrest: IV. Brainstem reflexes. Neurology 1981;31:1092–1097.

40. Bates D, Caronna J, Cartlidge NEF, et al. A prospective study of nontraumatic coma: methods and results in 310 patients. Ann Neurol 1977;2:211–220.

41. Bell JA, Hodgson HJF. Coma after cardiac arrest. Brain 1974;97:361–372.

42. Longstreth WT, Diehr P, Inui TS. Prediction of awakening after out-of-hospital cardiac arrest. N Engl J Med 1983; 308:1378–1382.

43. Shewmon DA, DeGiorgio CM. Early prognosis in anoxic coma: reliability and rationale. Neurol Clin 1989;7:823–843.

44. Steen-Hansen JE, Hansen NN, Vaagenes P, Schreiner B. Pupil size and light reactivity during cardiopulmonary resuscitation. A clinical study. Crit Care Med 1988;16:69–70.

45. Bassetti C, Bomio F, Mathis J, Hess CW. Early prognosis in coma after cardiac arrest: a prospective clinical, electrophysiological, and biochemical study of 60 patients. J Neurol Neurosurg Psychiatry 1996;61:610–615.

46. Plum F. Vulnerability of the brain and heart after cardiac arrest. N Engl J Med 1991;324:1278–1280.

47. Keane JR. Sustained upgaze in coma. Ann Neurol 1981;9: 409–412.

48. Ad Hoc Committee of the Harvard Medical School. A definition of irreversible coma. Report of the Ad Hoc Committee of the Harvard Medical School to examine the definition of brain death. JAMA 1968;205:337–340.

49. Walker A. An appraisal of the criteria of cerebral death. JAMA 1977;237:982–986.

50. Myers C, Yamaguchi S. Nervous system effects of cardiac arrest in monkeys. Arch Neurol 1977;34:65–74.

51. Plum F. What causes infarction in ischemic brain? Neurology 1983;33:222–233.

52. Longstreth W, Inui T. High blood glucose level on hospital admission and poor neurological recovery after cardiac arrest. Ann Neurol 1984;15:59–63.

53. Westmoreland B, Klass D, Sharbrough F, et al. Alpha coma. Arch Neurol 1975;32:713–718.

54. Chokroverty S. "Alpha-like" rhythms in electroencephalograms in coma after cardiac arrest. Neurology 1975;25: 655–663.

55. Kjos BO, Brandt-Zawadzki M, Young RG. Early CT findings of global central nervous system hypoperfusion. AJNR Am J Neuroradiol 1983;4:1043–1048.

56. Morimoto Y, Kemmotsu O, Kitami K, et al. Acute brain swelling after out-of-hospital cardiac arrest: pathogenesis and outcome. Crit Care Med 1993;21:104–110.

57. Roine RO, Raininko R, Erkinjuntti T, et al. Magnetic resonance imaging findings associated with cardiac arrest. Stroke 1993;24:1005–1014.

58. Sawada H, Udaka F, Seriu N, et al. MRI demonstration of cortical laminar necrosis and delayed white matter injury in anoxic encephalopathy. Neuroradiology 1990; 32:319–321.

59. Roine RO, Launes J, Nikkinen P, et al. Regional cerebral blood flow after human cardiac arrest. Arch Neurol 1991; 48:625–629.

60. Caplan LR, Brass LM, DeWitt LD, et al. Transcranial Doppler ultrasound: present status. Neurology 1990;40: 696–700.

61. Kirkham F, Levin S, Padayachee T, et al. Transcranial pulsed Doppler ultrasound findings in brainstem death. J Neurol Neurosurg Psychiatry 1987;50:1504–1513.

62. Ropper A, Kehne S, Wechsler L. Transcranial Doppler in brain death. Neurology 1987;37:1733–1735.

63. Giswold S, Safar P, Rao G, et al. Multifaceted therapy after global brain ischemia in monkeys. Stroke 1984;15: 803–812.

Chapter 11
Nonatherosclerotic Vasculopathies

Many different nonatherosclerotic vascular diseases cause brain ischemia. Some of these conditions also cause ocular ischemia and intracranial hemorrhage. Some have been well characterized, whereas in others, information about pathogenesis and clinical features is mteager. Herein, I discuss the most frequent and important conditions.

Arterial Dissection

Dissection of extracranial arteries was once considered rare. Reports of Fisher, Ojemann, and colleagues in the 1970s clarified the clinical and radiologic features in patients with dissection of the internal carotid artery (ICA).[1,2] Since then, arterial dissections have been recognized more often. The extracranial ICA is the most commonly affected artery and is usually involved in its pharyngeal and distal extracranial segments well above the ICA origin. This location is unusual for atherosclerosis, which almost invariably affects the internal carotid origin or the carotid siphon. Dissections of the extracranial vertebral artery (ECVA) affect the vessel in its distal segment between its emergence from the vertebral column and its dural penetration, or in the first segment of the artery above the vertebral artery (VA) origin but before entrance into the transverse foramina.[3,4] The pharyngeal ICA and the first and third segments of the ECVA are more mobile and less firmly anchored than the origins and intracranial penetration sites of these arteries. Dissections often involve loops and redundant portions of the extracranial arteries.[5]

Most dissections involve some trauma, stretch, or mechanical stress. Trauma may be severe but can be trivial (e.g., twisting the neck to avoid a falling tree branch, lunging for a Ping-Pong ball, or turning the neck abruptly while backing up a car or skiing). Many examples of so-called spontaneous dissection are triggered by minor trauma that is forgotten or deemed inconsequential by the patient. Congenital or acquired abnormalities of the connective tissue elements in the media or elastica of the arteries and edema of the arterial wall can promote dissection; Marfan's syndrome, cystic medial necrosis, fibromuscular dysplasia, and migraine are disorders found more often than expected in patients with arterial dissections.[3] Ultrastructural connective tissue abnormalities of collagen and extracellular matrix are sometimes found in the skin of patients with extracranial arterial dissections.[6]

A tear within the arterial wall leads to bleeding. Usually, blood dissects within the media along the longitudinal course of the artery. Dissection in the plane between the media and adventitia sometimes causes aneurysmal out-pouching of the artery. Dissections also produce an intimal tear, allowing the intramural hematoma to reenter the lumen (Figure 11-1). The expanded arterial wall may encroach on the lumen. Thrombus is often present within the lumen as a result of reentry of the intramural hematoma or because of stasis of blood flow caused by luminal compromise. The intramural expansion probably also stimulates the endothelium to release factors promoting thrombosis. The luminal clot is usually loosely adherent to the intima and can readily embolize distally. In the weeks and months after dissection, the intramural blood is absorbed, and the lumen usually returns to its normal size. Aneurysmal pouches may remain as a mark of the healed lesion.

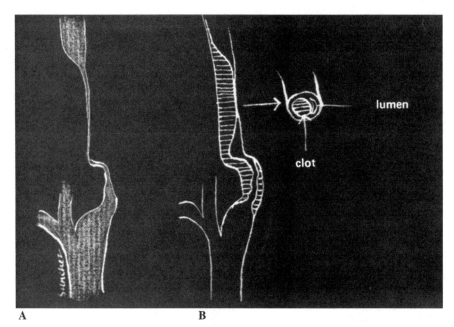

Figure 11-1. Dissection of the internal carotid artery: (**A**) angiogram shows string sign; (**B**) lumen compromised by intramural clot.

A   B

Often in carotid artery dissection, the most impressive feature is pain. Ipsilateral throbbing headache and sharp pain locally in the neck, jaw, pharynx, or face are often noted, separating dissection from ordinary atherosclerotic occlusion.[1–4,7–12] The sympathetic fibers traveling along the wall of the ICA are usually disturbed, leading to an ipsilateral partial Horner's syndrome characterized by ptosis and meiosis. Facial sweat function is preserved because the sympathetic innervation of the sweat glands travels along the external carotid artery (ECA).

Transient ischemic attacks (TIAs) are common and may involve the ipsilateral eye and brain. The spells often come more frequently than in atherosclerotic ischemia, which led Fisher to coin the term *carotid allegro.*[1] Some patients with ICA dissection have visual scintillations and bright sparkles resembling migraine, even though many have had no personal or family history of migraine. Some patients hear a pulsatile noise in the head or ear. TIAs are probably caused by luminal compromise with distal hypoperfusion, but most patients with severe strokes have evidence of embolization of clot to the middle cerebral artery (MCA) from thrombus at the site of the dissection. When the ICA dissection extends to the carotid siphon, ischemic optic neuropathy can develop as a result of decreased perfusion of arteries supplying the optic nerve.[13] When it occurs, stroke is usually noted shortly after the ICA dissection but may occur during the days and weeks after the event. Late stroke is rare but has been reported after traumatic ICA dissection.[14] At times, dissection may occur in steps. Pain in the neck may be present for days. The pain may recur days or even weeks later and be accompanied by ischemic attacks or strokes. Undoubtedly, the initial tear extended and more intramural bleeding developed when the symptoms worsened.[7] At times, both carotid arteries and even the VAs are dissected at the same time.

Ultrasound testing can suggest the presence of dissection. B-mode ultrasound can show tapering of the ICA lumen beginning well above the ICA origin, an irregular membrane crossing the lumen, and even demonstration of true and false lumens.[15] Continuous wave (CW) Doppler can show a typical pattern characterized by a high-amplitude signal with markedly reduced systolic Doppler frequencies and alternating flow directions over the region of luminal narrowing.[16] This Doppler signal probably results from abnormal vessel wall pulsations and some bidirectional movement of the blood column. Duplex scans of the VAs in the neck can also suggest dissection.[17] Typical findings are increased arterial diameter, decreased pulsatility, intravascular abnormal echoes, and hemodynamic evidence of decreased flow. Color Doppler flow imaging can also show the regions of dissection

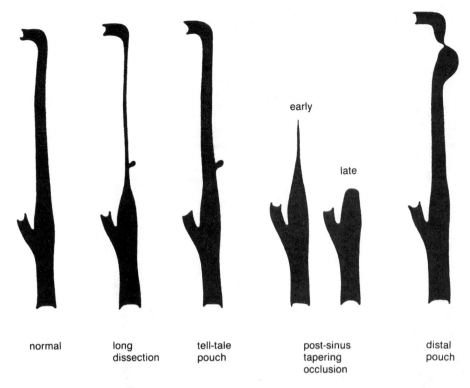

normal   long dissection   tell-tale pouch   early   late   post-sinus tapering occlusion   distal pouch

Figure 11-2. Various abnormal carotid arteriograms in patients with carotid artery dissection. (Reprinted with permission from CM Fisher, RG Ojemann, GH Robertson. Spontaneous dissection of cervicocerebral arteries. Can J Neurol Sci 1978;5:9–19.)

within the neck. Diminished flow in the high neck at the level of the atlas detected by CW Doppler and decreased flow in the intracranial VA shown by transcranial Doppler (TCD) suggest the presence of distal ECVA dissections. In patients with extracranial ICA dissections, TCD may show diminished intracranial velocities in the ICA siphon and MCA. When this occurs in young patients without risk factors for atherosclerosis or embolism with normal ICA bifurcations in the neck, the diagnosis of dissection is likely.

Diagnosis of arterial dissection has traditionally been made by standard catheter angiography. Figure 11-2 is a cartoon that illustrates various arteriographic features of carotid dissections. Figure 11-3 is a montage of angiograms in patients with extracranial ICA dissections. The most common angiographic finding is a string sign (see Figures 11-1A and 11-3A), consisting of a long, narrow column of contrast material that begins distal to the carotid bifurcation and can extend to the base of the skull.[1,2] There may also be total occlusion of the ICA. This occlusion differs from the typical atherosclerotic occlusion; ICA occlusions caused by dissection usually begin more than 2 cm distal to the origin of the ICA, spare the siphon, and have a gradually tapering segment that ends in the occlusion. There may also be localized aneurysmal sacs or outpouchings both proximal and distal along a narrowed, normal, or unusually dilatated portion of the artery. Computed tomography (CT) and magnetic resonance imaging (MRI) taken as axial cross sections through the area of dissection can show the intramural bleeding and mural expansion and can confirm the diagnosis of dissection. Figure 11-4 is an MRI cross section that shows a bilateral traumatic ICA dissection. Magnetic resonance angiography (MRA) and computed tomography angiography (CTA) can also show typical abnormalities in patients with dissections.

ICA dissection, especially with pharyngeal aneurysm formation, can also lead to dysfunction of the

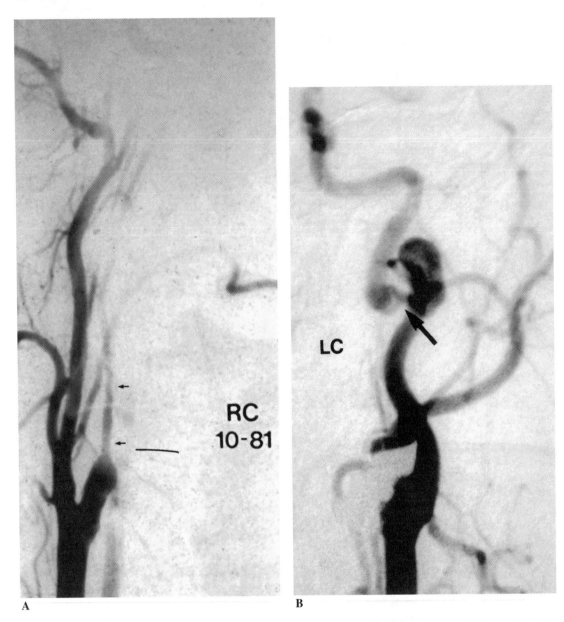

Figure 11-3. Carotid artery angiograms in patients with extracranial internal carotid artery dissections. **(A)** Abrupt change in diameter of the internal carotid artery with a long, string-like narrowing (arrows). **(B)** Aneurysmal dilatation of a tortuous carotid artery with an acute dissection. The arrow points to a region of narrowing. **(C)** Long carotid artery dissection with regions of narrowing and aneurysmal pouches. The arrowhead points to an aneurysmal dilatation at the proximal end of the dissection. The thick black arrow points to a region of narrowing of the artery and the double black arrows point to an irregular aneurysmal dilatation more distally in the pharyngeal portion of the artery. (LC = left carotid artery; RC = right carotid artery.)

lower cranial nerves at the skull base. Dysgeusia, Horner's syndrome, and weakness and atrophy of the tongue are the most common cranial-nerve signs. Tongue weakness and atrophy are caused by compression and ischemia of the hypoglossal nerve as it lies adjacent to the carotid sheath. At times, the IX, X, XI, and XII cranial nerves are involved.

ECVA dissections were first recognized in patients who had neck trauma or chiropractic manipulation.[8,18–20] VA injuries have also been

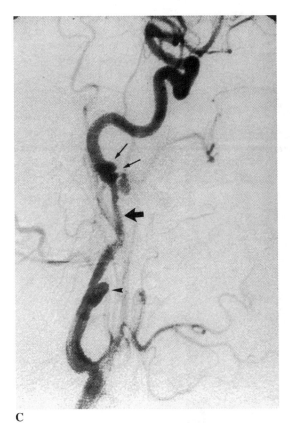

C

reported in patients who manipulate their own necks [21,22] or have maintained their necks in a fixed position for some time.[20,23–26] ECVA dissections also occur after surgery and resuscitation presumably because of sustained neck postures in patients who are anesthetized or unresponsive.[27] These lesions most often involve the distal extracranial (third segment) of the VA. Figure 11-5 is a montage of angiograms in patients with ECVA dissections. Spontaneous ECVA dissections clinically and radiologically mimic those related to trauma.[3,4,20] Pain in the posterior neck or occiput and generalized headache are common.

Pain often precedes neurologic symptoms by hours, days, and, rarely, weeks. Some patients with ECVA dissections have only neck pain and do not develop neurologic symptoms or signs. TIAs most often include dizziness, diplopia, veering, staggering, and dysarthria. TIAs are less common in ECVA dissections than ICA dissections. Infarcts usually cause signs that begin suddenly. The most common patterns of ischemic brain

damage are cerebellar infarction in posterior inferior cerebellar artery (PICA) distribution and lateral medullary infarction. As in extracranial ICA dissections, infarcts are invariably explained by embolization of fresh thrombus to the ICVA. Occasionally, dissections extend or begin intracranially. Sometimes, emboli reach the superior cerebellar arteries (SCAs), main basilar artery, or posterior cerebral arteries (PCAs). ECVA dissections can also cause cervical root pain.[28,29] Aneurysmal dilatation of the ECVA adjacent to nerve roots causes the radicular pain and can lead to radicular distribution motor, sensory, and reflex abnormalities.[28,29] Occasionally, spinal cord infarction results because of hypoperfusion in the supply zones of arteries from the ECVA that nourish the cervical spinal cord.[29,30]

Many patients with extracranial ICA and VA dissections have headache, pain, and TIAs without lasting neurologic deficits. Intracranial dissection is less common but is more serious and is almost invariably associated with severe deficits or death unless the dissection has a limited extent. Intracranial dissections can cause infarction, subarachnoid bleeding, or mass effects.[4,20,31–34] When the dissections are between the media and the intima, luminal narrowing and local hypoperfusion usually occur and lead to infarction in the regions of supply. In the anterior circulation, the supraclinoid ICA and mainstem MCA are most often involved.[31,33] Figure 11-6 is an arteriogram of an intracranial ICA dissection that extends into the MCA and anterior cerebral artery (ACA). In the posterior circulation, the intracranial vertebral arteries (ICVAs) and basilar artery are most often affected.[4,20,32] Intracranial dissections were considered in the past to always be devastating or fatal, but modern technology has led to increased recognition of patients with intracranial dissections who have only minor signs. When dissections extend between the media and the adventitia, aneurysms and tears through the adventitia may lead to subarachnoid hemorrhage (SAH), which can be repeated. At times, dissections lead to prominent aneurysmal masses, which can present as space-taking lesions that compress adjacent cranial nerves or brain parenchyma.

Occasionally, patients have chronic dissections with aneurysms and multifocal regions of dissection of various ages.[4,20,32] These patients usually

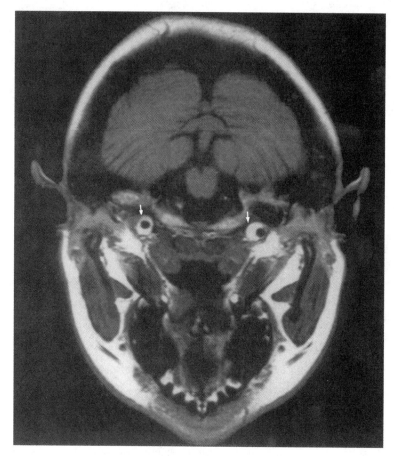

Figure 11-4. Axial cross section magnetic resonance imaging scan of a patient with bilateral extracranial internal carotid artery dissections. The arrows point to the carotid arteries. Dark flow voids represent the lumen of the arteries, and the high-intensity bright areas represent intramural hematomas. (Reprinted with permission from JS Matsumara, WH Pearce. Traumatic carotid artery dissection. N Engl J Med 1996;335:13–68. Copyright © American Medical Association.)

have abnormal arterial media and elastic membranes and the arteries show healing intramural hematomas and tears of different ages. I have cared for two such patients, one with recurrent SAH and the other with recurrent posterior-circulation TIAs and strokes.[32] In the latter patient, thrombus was visible within each bilateral ICVA-dissecting aneurysm, and symptoms stopped after treatment with warfarin and aspirin combined. Some patients with chronic or recurrent dissections have fibromuscular dysplasia. When intracranial arteries are involved, hemorrhage and local mass effect can be prominent.

Most extracranial dissections heal spontaneously with time. Their location high in the neck usually makes surgical repair difficult or impossible. When complete occlusion has occurred, the arteries often do not recanalize and remain occluded. Arteries that retain some residual lumen invariably heal and normalize. Intracranial dissec-

tions have been repaired surgically in patients with SAH, although the incidence of spontaneous healing and recurrent bleeding is unknown. Although there have been no controlled trials of medical therapy, I am impressed by many anecdotal reports and my own positive experience with anticoagulants. Prevention of embolization of thrombus at or shortly after the dissection should prevent stroke. Anticoagulants have not seemed to increase the extent of the dissections, which is a major theoretical concern. Because the risk of embolization is only during the acute period, I use heparin followed by warfarin. I try to maximize cerebral blood flow (CBF) during the acute period to augment collateral circulation. Healing of dissections can be monitored using MRI, MRA,[35] CTA,[36] and ultrasound. I stop anticoagulants after 6 weeks in patients with dissected arteries that remain occluded. I continue anticoagulants in patients with patent arteries until luminal stenosis improves

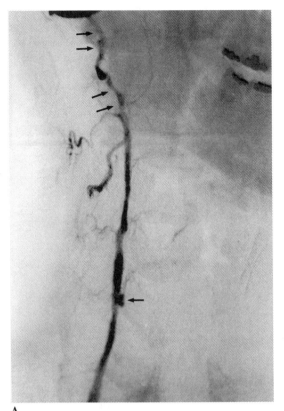

A

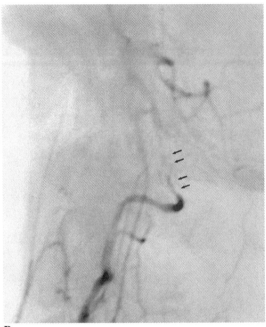

B

Figure 11-5. Extracranial vertebral artery dissections. **(A)** Vertebral angiogram, lateral view. A long vertebral artery dissection shows regions of irregular narrowing (*top arrows*) and an aneurysmal pouch (*lower arrow*). **(B)** Vertebral angiogram, lateral view. Dissection in the distal extracranial vertebral artery with narrowing and near occlusion of the artery (*arrows*). Flow above the dissection is severely compromised. **(C)** Vertebral angiogram, anteroposterior view. The distal extracranial vertebral artery is narrowed and flow is compromised (*short arrows*). Dye refluxes into the contralateral intracranial vertebral artery (*long arrow*).

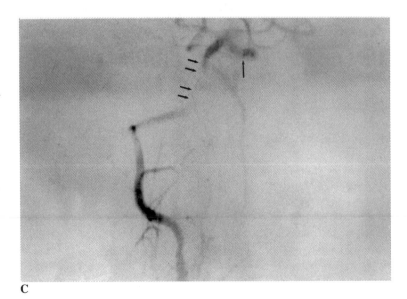

C

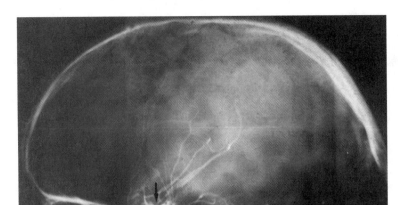

Figure 11-6. Intracranial internal carotid artery dissection in a child. (**A**) Carotid angiogram, lateral view. The arrow points to the dissection within the intracranial internal carotid artery. (**B**) A magnified close-up view shows the dissection. The white arrow shows that the middle cerebral artery is occluded. The open arrowhead points to an occluded anterior cerebral artery.

A

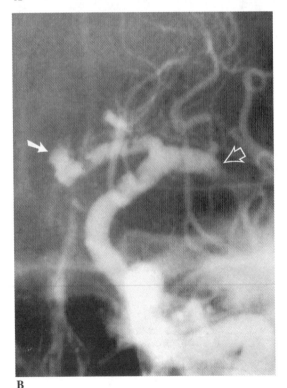

B

to the point that flow is not significantly obstructed. I monitor the patient using ultrasound or MRA. When arterial blood flow is improved, I switch to drugs that modify platelet function, such as aspirin, clopidogrel, or dipyridamole.

Fibromuscular Dysplasia

First recognized in the renal circulation, fibromuscular dysplasia is known to affect many other systemic arteries, including extracranial and cerebral arteries. It is a nonatheromatous multifocal condition that can involve any or all of the three layers of the arterial wall. In the cerebral circulation, it is reported in only 0.6% of nonselected consecutive cerebral arteriograms.[37,38] No data exist on its true incidence in patients evaluated for stroke. This blood vessel abnormality is most commonly described in middle-aged women.[38] Bilateral ICA involvement is common (86%); abnormalities usually involve the pharyngeal portion of the artery and extend from the level of C1 proximally 7–8 cm, with sparing of the carotid bifurcation and the intracranial carotid artery. Twenty percent of patients have coexistent ECVA fibromuscular disease.[38]

The most common form of fibromuscular dysplasia affects the media. Constricting bands composed of fibrous dysplastic tissue and proliferating smooth-muscle cells in the media alternate with areas of luminal dilatation related to medial thinning and disruption of the elastic membrane.[39,40] These abnormalities produce the characteristic string-of-beads appearance on arteriography (Figure 11-7). Hypertrophy of fibrous tissues in the adventitia or intima can cause segmental areas of stenosis. Occasionally, patients have had band-like shelves or diaphragms within greatly enlarged carotid bulbs in the neck; superimposed thrombi were present in these "megabulbs."[41] Some patients with fibrous septa have had typical string-of-beads abnormalities in the pharyngeal carotid arteries on angiography but some have not had other obvious changes characteristic of fibromuscular dysplasia.[41] *Fibromuscular dysplasia* is probably not a single disease but may be a general term for a variety of different conditions that affect the arterial walls.

Although most fibromuscular dysplasia vascular lesions are asymptomatic, this vascular abnormality can cause brain ischemia. Fibromuscular dysplasia is frequently associated with aneurysms of the intracranial arteries. In one series of 37 patients with fibromuscular dysplasia, 19 patients had a total of 25 aneurysms.[42] The diagnosis of fibromuscular dysplasia is occasionally made at the time of evaluation of SAH. Fibromuscular dysplasia also predisposes patients to arterial dissections with related stroke syndromes. In other patients, fibromuscular dysplasia affecting an artery appropriate to explain the CT and clinical findings is the only abnormality uncovered. The lumen is not often severely compromised. The mechanism of the distal ischemia in this circumstance is unknown. Functional changes in vessel contraction (vasoconstriction) could lead to distal hypoperfusion. Altered blood flow with stasis could lead to thrombus formation and distal intra-arterial embolism. Any medium-sized muscular intracranial artery can be affected. The most prominent clinical features are TIAs and strokes of minor or moderate severity. Fatal or severe strokes are unusual. Headache, syncope, and Horner's syndrome are also frequent accompanying symptoms.

Most research and clinical interest have been directed at atherosclerotic disease of the intima and subintima of arteries. Little is known about the other portions of the arterial wall. Clearly, disease of the artery walls can lead to altered contractility, dilatation with aneurysm formation, and tears with intramural hematomas. The disorder called *fibromuscular dysplasia* is pathologically heterogenous and may occur as a result of a variety of different etiologies that share abnormalities of connective tissue. The collagen, elastic tissue, and extracellular matrix can be involved. Knowledge of these disorders of vascular connective tissue is rudimentary.

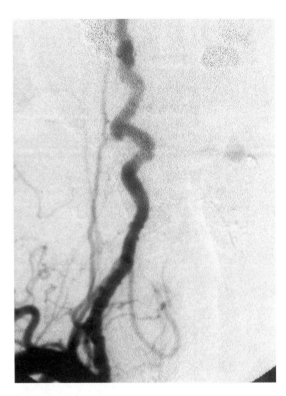

Figure 11-7. Carotid arteriogram, lateral view, shows typical sausage-like string-of-beads effect in a patient with fibromuscular dysplasia.

Angioplasty, often with stenting, has been used to dilate arteries harboring fibromuscular dysplasia lesions. In a series of patients with stroke presumably caused by fibromuscular dysplasia, the recurrence rate is quite low even without therapy.[39] Insufficient data are available to warrant rational therapeutic suggestions. I usually prescribe antiplatelet aggregating agents but rarely use anticoagulants or recommend surgical repair or mechanical dilation of the arteries. I often prescribe calcium channel blockers to prevent vasoconstriction. If the patient is hypertensive, the renal arteries should be studied. When fibromuscular dysplasia is found on angiography, CTA, MRA, or standard arteriography is warranted to exclude associated intracranial aneurysms.

Heritable Disorders of Connective Tissue

Heritable disorders of connective tissue are a group of hereditary disorders that are usually rec-

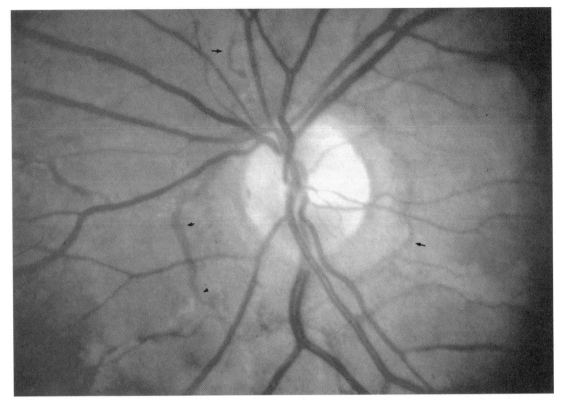

Figure 11-8. Angioid streaks (*arrows*) in the retina in a patient with pseudoxanthoma elasticum. (Courtesy of Thomas Hedges III, M.D., New England Medical Center.)

ognizable in childhood and involve the skin, vascular system, and skeletal tissues. The full spectrum of these disorders is still unraveling and little in-depth analysis has been made of the neurologic and cerebrovascular features.

Pseudoxanthoma elasticum (PXE) has an estimated prevalence of approximately 1 in 160,000 and has both autosomal dominant and recessive hereditary patterns.[43,44] The most easily recognized abnormalities are skin changes.[43–46] The skin of the face, neck, axilla, antecubital, inguinal, and periumbilical regions first becomes thickened and grooved. Yellowish papules and plaques are seen in these areas and also on the mucosa of the lips, palate, buccal area, vagina, and rectum. Later, the skin becomes lax and redundant. Angioid streaks, which are reddish-brown or gray, radiate from the optic disk and are usually wider than veins. Figure 11-8 is a fundus photograph that shows angioid streaks in a patient with PXE. The abnormality of

connective and elastic tissue causes tortuosity of vessels, premature vascular calcification, intimal thickening, microaneurysms, and fusiform aneurysms. Gastrointestinal bleeding is common and is a result of the vascular changes.[45] Premature occlusive vascular disease affects the coronary, peripheral limb, retinal, and cerebral arteries. The degenerative vascular changes begin with fragmentation and calcification of the internal elastic lamina and are followed by extensive intimal and medial calcification.[45] The arteries of the aortic arch and intracranial arteries are involved. One patient had occlusion of both ICAs at the skull base and a carotid-cavernous fistula.[47] Hypertension and mitral valve prolapse (MVP) are common,[44] and SAH and intracerebral hemorrhage (ICH) occur. The cerebrovascular lesions most often consist of lacunar infarcts and white matter ischemia of the microangiopathic Binswanger type. Cortical infarcts are less common.

Ehlers-Danlos syndrome describes a group of clinically and genetically heterogenous conditions that share defects in collagen.[48] The skin is hyperextensible and easily bruised, and the joints show hypermobility. Cardiac and cerebrovascular lesions are common and include MVP and tricuspid valve prolapse, septal defects, and dilatation of the aortic root and pulmonary arteries.[49] Intracranial aneurysms, carotid-cavernous fistulae, and arterial dissections have been reported.[48,50,51] Rupture of various systemic and cerebral vessels leads to frequent bleeding and SAH.

Marfan's syndrome is an autosomal-dominant hereditary disorder that is probably more common than other hereditary disorders and occurs in approximately 4–6 per 100,000 individuals.[52] The underlying nature of the condition is not known, but the vascular abnormalities relate to abnormal collagen and elastin. The phenotype of long limbs, pectus chest deformity, arachnodactyly, and joint laxity is easily recognizable. Subluxation of the lens occurs in more than one-half of the patients, and ophthalmologic examination is helpful in diagnosis. The diameter of the aortic root is invariably enlarged, and aortic regurgitation and MVP are common. Aortic aneurysms and dissections are also frequent clinical problems in patients with Marfan's syndrome.

Dilatative Arteriopathy

Some patients with dilatative arteriopathy are prone to elongated, ectatic, tortuous intracranial arteries. This abnormality can be found in children and often involves multiple arteries.[53–56] Hereditary factors probably play an important role, especially in the young. In one reported family, three brothers had large fusiform basilar artery aneurysms and alpha-glucosidase deficiency.[55] In an 11-year-old girl who died from a ruptured dolichoectatic basilar artery aneurysm, necropsy showed that the artery had large gaps in the internal elastic lamina with only short segments of elastica remaining in some regions.[54] Pathologic examination in other young patients with dolichoectasia has shown deficiencies in the muscularis and internal elastic lamina with irregular thickness of the media, multiple gaps in the internal elastica, and regions of fibrosis. At times, the intima is thickened, and there is severe

elastic tissue degeneration and an increase in the vasa vasorum. When the abnormality is severe, the elongated dilatated arteries are called *dolichoectatic* or *fusiform aneurysms*. The most frequent location is in the posterior fossa where the basilar artery or one or both VAs are involved.[57–61] Figure 11-9A shows a montage of six patients with vertebrobasilar dolichoectatic arteries. Figures 11-9B and C show ectatic basilar arteries with poor antegrade blood flow. The dolichoectatic anomaly is often recognized on CT as curvilinear calcified-enhancing channels that usually cross the cerebellopontine angle.[57,58] The MCAs are also often involved, and some patients have dolichoectatic abnormalities in both circulations.[57,59]

Extensive atherosclerotic plaques, often with calcification, encroachment on the lumen, and thrombus formation, are often found at necropsy. On microscopic examination, there are often fibrotic changes in the vessel wall with reduced muscularis and attenuated, fragmented, or absent elastica.[62] Clinically, the most common symptoms are caused by brain ischemia. Mass effect with compression or displacement of cranial nerves or brain parenchyma is also common. The aneurysmally dilatated arteries can compress the medullary pyramids and cerebral peduncles and may indent and deform the basis pontis. Some patients have had hydrocephalus, possibly related to the effects of the dolichoectatic aneurysms on the third ventricle.

Ischemia is most often found in the distribution of penetrating arteries to the brain stem and basal ganglia. Ischemia is related to the effects of the disease in the parent arteries on the branches. Plaques or clot may obliterate or obscure the orifices of branches or can embolize into the branches. Angiography may show thrombi within dolichoectatic aneurysms.[57,63] In other patients, distortion and elongation of the branches may reduce blood flow without obliteration of the branch ostia or lumens. Occasionally, clot within the aneurysm can embolize to the larger distal branches.[57,63,64] Rupture of these aneurysms with resulting subarachnoid bleeding is unusual but does occur.[57,62,63]

CT, MRI, and MRA[65] usually suffice to identify the aneurysmally dilatated ectatic arteries and may suggest the presence of clot within the vessels. TCD is helpful in diagnosis and may show reduced mean-flow velocities with relatively preserved

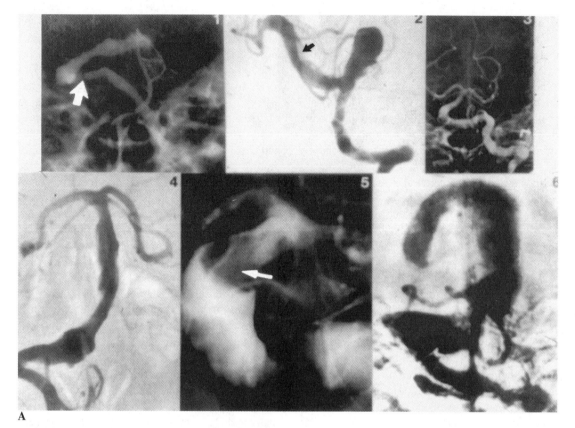

A

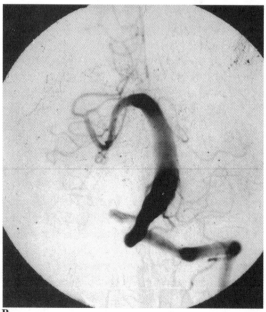

B

Figure 11-9. Dolichoectatic vertebrobasilar arteries.
(**A**) Vertebrobasilar fusiform aneurysms in six patients.
Patient 1 has marked tortuosity and ectasia of the basilar
artery with a proximal atheromatous stenosis (*arrow*).
Patient 2 has a filling defect (*arrow*) representing thrombus
in the mid-basilar artery. Patient 3 has a tortuous left vertebral and basilar artery. Patient 4 shows irregular plaques in a
dilatated basilar artery. Patient 5 has a markedly dilatated
basilar artery with a filling defect (*arrow*) representing
thrombus. The apparent lower filling defect (*arrowhead*) is
an artifact representing an aerated sinus. Patient 6 has a
dilatated ectatic artery with poor filling of the distal segment
and nonfilling of the posterior cerebral arteries because of
reduced antegrade flow. (Reprinted with permission from
MS Pessin, MI Chimowitz, SR Levine, et al. Stroke in
patients with fusiform vertebrobasilar aneurysms. Neurology 1989;39:16–21.) (**B**) Vertebral angiogram, anteroposterior view. The basilar artery is extremely dilatated, and the
distal portion and its branches are poorly opacified. (**C**)
Irregular ectatic basilar artery with extensive atheromatous
plaques. The branches of the rostral basilar artery are not
opacified because of reduced antegrade blood flow.

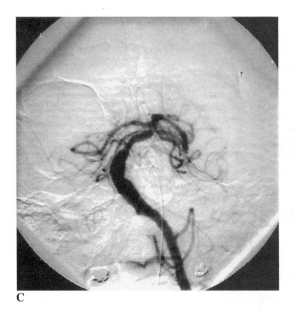

C

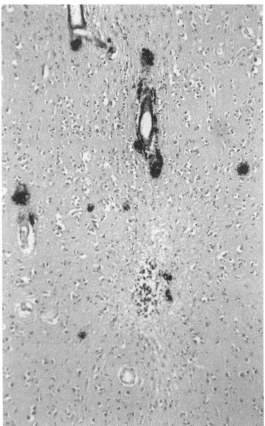

Figure 11-10. Photomicrograph of the occipital lobe cortex immunostained for beta-amyloid with a hematoxylin counterstain. Amyloid is seen in vessels and senile plaques. (Courtesy of Steven Greenberg, M.D., Department of Neurology, Massachusetts General Hospital.)

peak-flow velocities.[66] Blood flow may be to-and-fro within the dilatated artery, causing reduced antegrade flow. The reduced antegrade flow may lead to poor opacification on MRA, falsely suggesting occlusion of the dolichoectatic artery. CTA and standard angiography are able to image the artery in this circumstance. In patients with recurrent ischemia and thrombi within the dolichoectatic arteries, warfarin may prevent strokes. Intravenous thrombolytic agents also have been used in patients with large thrombi within dolichoectatic arteries.[63] Agents that modify platelet function have not been studied in patients with dilatative arteriopathy.

Cerebral Amyloid Angiopathy

Cerebral amyloid angiopathy (CAA), also called *congophilic angiopathy*, is also discussed in Chapter 13 because the major clinical feature is recurrent lobar ICH. The disorder is characterized by thickening of the walls of small- and medium-sized arteries by an amorphous eosinophilic-staining material with a smudged appearance on light microscopy.[67] The material within the vessel wall shows a yellow-green birefringence when stained with Congo red and viewed under a polarizing microscope—hence the term *congophilic*. Figure 11-10 is a photomicrograph of the occipital lobe cortex stained for beta-amyloid in a patient with CAA. The abnormalities usually involve many arteries, especially those in the leptomeninges and cerebral cortex of the cerebral lobes. The brain stem, basal gray nuclei, hippocampi, and subcortical white matter are spared.[67] The changes are most prevalent in the parietal and occipital lobes, but ICH is often frontal and central.[68–72] Affected arteries, especially those in the leptomeninges, have a distinctive double-barrel lumen with amyloid found in the outer or inner media.[67]

The most common clinical syndromes recognized are ICH, usually multiple and subcortical lobar, and SAH.[67–72] MRI susceptibility-weighted echo-planar images often show multiple, small, old hemorrhages

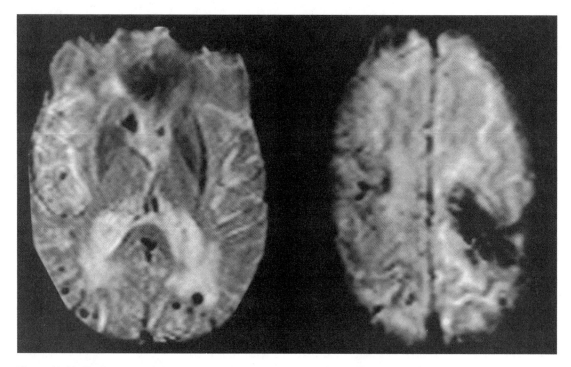

Figure 11-11. Gradient echo magnetic resonance imaging of a 71-year-old man with a recent left intracerebral hemorrhage. The black regions represent hemorrhages. Multiple old hemorrhages are shown. The specimen in Figure 11-10 is from this patient, who died after progressive intellectual deterioration. (Courtesy of Steven Greenberg, M.D., Department of Neurology, Massachusetts General Hospital.)

in patients with CAA who present with a stroke. Brain imaging shows a recent hemorrhage. Figure 11-11 shows a recent amyloid angiopathy–related hematoma along with multiple old hemorrhages that were clinically unsuspected. Senile plaques containing amyloid and Alzheimer's changes are also prevalent in brains of patients harboring CAA. Many patients with CAA are demented or develop intellectual deterioration with time caused by multiple strokes and Alzheimer's pathology.

Early studies also noted that scattered small infarcts were also prevalent in brains of patients with amyloid-related ICH.[69–71] TIAs can occur.[73] Some patients with CAA have multiple infarcts and a prominent leukoencephalopathy with periventricular, subcortical, and corona radiata lucency on CT and signal abnormalities on MRI.[72,74–77] The clinical picture is that of Binswanger's disease. In fact, CAA may be an important, often unrecognized, cause of this chronic ischemic microangiopathy.

The cause of CAA is unknown. Familial CAA has been identified, especially in Icelandic, Dutch, and German families, and is usually inherited as an autosomal-dominant trait with high penetrance. The Icelandic variety has been attributed to abnormal metabolism of a gamma-trace protein.[78,79]

At times, there are prominent inflammatory changes in relation to the amyloid-staining arteries,[67,79] and there have been reports of patients who had CAA and granulomatous arteritis (or the CAA evoked a granulomatous reaction in these patients).[67,80,81] Although it was formerly thought that drainage of CAA-related hematomas might be hazardous, data show that surgical results are not different from other causes of ICH.[82,83] Reducing the systemic blood pressure to the lowest levels tolerated is a strategy often used to reduce the frequency of ICH. Advances in recognition and understanding the pathogenesis of CAA should lead to more specific therapeutic strategies.[84]

Vasculitis and Other Possibly Inflammatory Vascular Disorders

Arteritis is mentioned as a cause of stroke in the differential diagnosis of nearly every medical student, non-neurologist, and some neurologists. Although often considered, documented arteritis is a rare cause of stroke. Most often, central nervous system (CNS) vasculitis presents as an encephalopathy with headache, seizures, decreased alertness, and cognitive and behavioral abnormalities, often with multifocal signs. Recognition of those rare instances in which arteritis is caused by a specific microbial infection is critical for effective treatment. Patients with allergic hypersensitivity and systemic vasculitis may respond to corticosteroids or other treatments used to control systemic autoimmune diseases.

Arteritis Caused by Infections

Bacterial and Fungal Infections

In patients with acute bacterial meningitis (e.g., pneumococcal or meningococcal), the pial arteries and veins are often surrounded by pus. Vascular occlusions and strokes may complicate the clinical picture, which is invariably dominated by headache, fever, stiff neck, and decreased alertness. *Listeria monocytogenes* may produce a characteristic inflammatory disorder involving predominantly the medulla and pontine tegmentum.[85–87] Multiple, lower cranial nerve palsies and vestibular and oculomotor signs develop. At times, the onset of symptoms is abrupt, and subsequent necropsy shows an arteritis with multiple infarcts as well as focal encephalitis. The cerebrospinal fluid (CSF) shows a pleocytosis. Occasionally, patients with cat-scratch disease, a disorder known to be caused by *Bartonella henselae*, have had intracranial stenoses and arteritis.[88]

In patients with syphilis, the spirochete probably invades cerebral arteries at the time of the meningitis of secondary lues. Meningovascular syphilis results and is characterized by apoplectic attacks of hemiplegia, headache, seizures, and CSF pleocytosis. The serology is always positive in patients with meningovascular syphilis. The spinal arterial circulation can also be affected. All forms of syphilis are more common and severe in patients with acquired immunodeficiency syndrome (AIDS).

Lyme borreliosis mimics syphilis in many ways.[89] Meningitis, multiple cranial nerve palsies, and root- and peripheral nerve syndromes predominate.[89–91] Strokes have been described but are unusual and not as common as a syndrome of headache, fatigue, and difficulty concentrating.[92] The CSF is invariably abnormal and specific antibodies to *Borrelia* are present in the blood and CSF.

Chronic basal meningitis, usually caused by the tubercle bacillus or particular fungi (i.e., *Cryptococcus, Histoplasma,* or *Coccidioides*) is frequently complicated by inflammation of the arteries within the exudate.[93,94] The proximal MCA and arteries in the posterior perforated substance are most often involved. The exudate surrounds the arteries, producing thickening and inflammation of the walls of the arteries, usually called *Heubner's arteritis* (Figure 11-12A). Infarcts in the basal ganglia and midbrain result and can develop even after sterilization of the microbial agent. Other fungi, especially *Mucor* and *Aspergillus*, cause a necrotizing arteritis with regions of brain infarction and necrosis. *Mucor* is usually spread from the paranasal sinuses and *Aspergillus* reaches the cerebral circulation by hematogenous spread usually without meningitis.[95] *Aspergillus* infections are especially common in patients who take corticosteroids or who are immunosuppressed.[95]

Viral Infections

Viruses may be responsible for many cases of vasculitis that are considered idiopathic. Hepatitis B surface antigen, immunoglobulin, and complement are found in the vessel walls of patients with polyarteritis nodosa who have hepatitis B antigenemia.[96] The varicella-zoster virus is also known to directly invade CNS vessels, sometimes without causing much visible inflammatory reaction. Viruses can cause vasculitis by direct invasion or by triggering an immune response to components of vessels.[97] Alternatively, immune complex deposition can injure arteries and cause inflammation. Evidence of herpes varicella-zoster virus (HZV) infection by polymerase chain reaction (PCR) analysis of biopsy or necropsy material may be found in patients with the typical clinical findings of polyarteritis nodosa.[97]

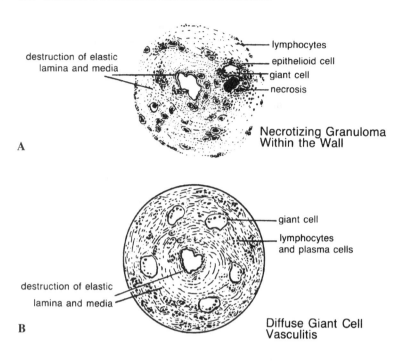

destruction of elastic lamina and media

lymphocytes
epithelioid cell
giant cell
necrosis

Necrotizing Granuloma Within the Wall

A

giant cell

lymphocytes and plasma cells

destruction of elastic lamina and media

Diffuse Giant Cell Vasculitis

B

Figure 11-12. Changes in the vessel wall in (**A**) tuberculosis and (**B**) giant cell arteritis.

HZV is the most well known and best documented of the viral arteritides. The most common clinical syndrome is delayed brain infarction, usually causing hemiplegia contralateral to herpes zoster ophthalmicus.[98–100] The symptoms begin days to weeks (average 6–8 weeks)[98,99] after onset of the painful rash. Infarctions are usually hemispheral and cause hemiparesis, hemisensory loss, and aphasia, or right-hemispheric types of cognitive and behavioral changes. Usually, the infarct is ipsilateral to the rash. Angiography has shown occlusion of the carotid siphon, MCA, or ACA and sometimes stenosis of these arteries.[98–100] At times, TIAs may precede the stroke but most often the onset is abrupt and the neurologic signs develop immediately. Some patients have an accompanying encephalitis. Recurrent ischemia and multiple infarcts have been reported. The mortality has been estimated at approximately 25%. This mortality rate is higher than comparable-sized infarcts caused by atherosclerosis.[99] The CSF usually shows a slight pleocytosis and immunoglobulins (Ig) and IgG indices may be elevated.[98,99] Rarely, the rash involves other divisions of the V nerve (maxillary or mandibular) and can occur in the back of the neck and upper cervical dermatomes.[101–103] The PCA and vertebrobasilar territory are rarely involved.[101–103]

Brain infarction and arterial narrowing and occlusion have occasionally been described after clinical chickenpox in children and young adults.[104–106] Angiography in these patients has shown stenosis of the proximal MCA and basilar artery,[106] occlusion of the supraclinoid ICA,[104] and irregularity and stenosis of the intracranial ICA and the proximal anterior and middle cerebral arteries.[105]

At necropsy, patients with HZV arteritis may show inflamed necrotic arteries, granulomatous changes,[97,98] or occluded arteries with scant inflammation. Doyle and colleagues were able to demonstrate virions that were characteristic of HZV in the nuclei and cytoplasm of smooth-muscle cells in the involved arteries.[100] Amplification of HZV viral DNA by PCR was obtained in the left anterior, middle, and posterior cerebral arteries of a patient who developed left cerebral hemisphere infarction after left herpes zoster opthalmicus.[107] Presumably, the virus spread from the infected gasserian ganglion through trigeminovascular connections to the proximal portions of the ipsilateral MCA and ACA.[107] Trigeminovascular projections also go from V[1] to the SCA, and the upper cervical ganglia probably project to the ICVAs, basilar artery, and the anterior inferior cerebellar artery (AICA) and

SCA.[108] Spread to the intima can activate the endothelium to release factors promoting thrombosis. As in other virus diseases, inflammation is not always visible under the microscope.

Patients with human immunodeficiency virus infection have an increased frequency of stroke. The mechanisms of stroke in AIDS patients vary. Some strokes are caused by hypercoagulability provoked by chronic infection, concomitant drug abuse, and infection with agents that can cause arteritis, such as fungi.[109,110] Children with AIDS may have a dilatative arteriopathy with fusiform aneurysms involving the intracranial arteries.[111] SAH may develop.[111]

Parasitic Infections

Cysticercosis may be associated with endarteritis and strokes.[112–117] Cysticercosis is caused by infection with the larvae (cysticerci) of *Taenia solium*, the pork tapeworm. Paracytic cysts containing cysticerci lodge within brain parenchyma in the subarachnoid space and within the brain ventricles. Stroke occurs predominantly in the subarachnoid form of the disease.[112–114] Meningitic inflammation can spread to the major basal intracranial arteries, leading to an endarteritis and brain infarction. Subcortical small infarcts and large cortical-subcortical infarcts may occur. The most common vessels involved are the MCAs, PCAs, and the ACAs, but the basilar artery may also be affected.[114,115] In one study among 28 patients with subarachnoid cysticercosis who had cerebral angiography, 15 patients (53%) had angiographic evidence of arteritis.[115] A clinical stroke syndrome was present in 12 of these patients, and eight patients had brain infarcts on MRI.[115] When patients with arterial narrowing caused by cysticercosis are followed sequentially using TCD, sometimes the stenosis improves with time.[116] Precipitation of brain infarction after praziquantel therapy has also been reported.[117] Destruction of the cysticercotic cysts within the subarachnoid space may cause an inflammatory response, which can cause or exacerbate an endarteritis.[117]

Plasmodium falciparum is the most frequent parasitic infection of the CNS. Cerebral malaria is characterized by coma and convulsions after a prodromal period of fever and headache.[118] Parasitized red blood cells distend capillaries and venules and lead to intracranial hypertension, brain edema, and petechial hemorrhages throughout the brain. In children, convulsions and hemiparesis are relatively common. Angiography and TCD in children with hemiparesis often show focal stenosis of the basal intracranial arteries.[119,120]

Systemic Vasculitides, Including Collagen Vascular Diseases

Systemic vasculitis syndromes can be conveniently divided into polyarteritis nodosa, allergic angiitis and granulomatosis (Churg-Strauss syndrome), hypersensitivity vasculitis, Wegener's granulomatosis, and overlap syndromes sharing features of other subtypes.[96,121–127] All of these syndromes have multisystem involvement in common.

Polyarteritis nodosa (PAN) affects small- and medium-sized arteries, especially at branch points.[125–128] Infiltration of polymorphonuclear leukocytes and monocytes is followed by intimal proliferation, fibrinoid necrosis, and thrombosis of arteries.[96] The most common neurologic signs probably relate to mononeuritis multiplex. CNS involvement occurs in 20–40% of patients and the onset occurs usually after systemic symptoms and signs and neuropathy.[122,128] Some patients have a diffuse encephalopathy and others have focal or multifocal abnormalities. Occasionally, hemispheral, spinal cord, and cerebellar and brain stem strokes occur. When strokes occur, it is usually late in the illness. Hypertension is common in patients with PAN and is responsible for many of the ischemic infarcts and hemorrhages. I have not seen or known of a report of PAN presenting initially as a stroke syndrome.

Patients with Churg-Strauss syndrome invariably have pulmonary involvement, including asthma, and eosinophilia.[122,129–132] A history of previous allergic disorders usually exist. The lesions tend to involve smaller vessels, especially capillaries and venules.[96,132,133] Encephalopathy and peripheral neuritis are common, but strokes are extremely rare.

The hypersensitivity vasculitides are a group of disorders in which the cause is usually known and a major finding is a rash, often with palpable purpuric skin lesions, especially on the legs. Some are drug induced, postinfectious, or related to known foreign antigens (e.g., serum sickness). Mixed cryoglobulinemia and Henoch-Schönlein purpura are other forms of hypersensitivity vasculitis. Neurologic involvement is not prominent in patients with the various hypersensitivity vasculitis syndromes, and when it occurs, neuropathies, plexopathies, and encephalopathies predominate.[96,133] Strokes rarely occur except occasionally because of bleeding related to systemic purpura.

Wegener's granulomatosis is a necrotizing, often fatal, granulomatous vasculitis that involves chiefly the lungs, sinuses, upper respiratory tract, and kidneys.[122,134] Orbital involvement, palsies of extraocular muscles, and retinal and optic nerve ischemia are often reported.[135–138] Brain infarcts and cerebral arteritis are occasionally described.[139,140] The diagnosis can be made by biopsy and by detection of anti-neutrophilic cytoplasmic antibody and is treatable with cyclophosphamide and other immune suppressants.[141]

Nervous system findings are quite common in patients with systemic lupus erythematosus (SLE). Headaches that often share features with migraine, seizures, psychosis with decreased cognition, chorea, and mono- and polyneuropathies are important features of SLE.[122,142] The usual assumption has been that vasculitis underlies these diverse neurologic syndromes. Necropsy and clinical studies, however, indicate that true arteritis is not a common cause of the CNS findings.[143,144] In a necropsy study, Johnson and Richardson found scant evidence of inflammation of brain arteries.[143] However, sudden-onset neurologic signs do occur in patients with SLE and can be a prominent clinical feature. MRI often shows discrete focal lesions in patients with SLE usually in the absence of a clinical history of stroke.[145] The infarcts are of diverse causes. Small vessel vasculopathy with small deep infarcts and hemorrhages is usually caused by hypertension, which accompanies the renal disease of SLE. Cortical and cortical-subcortical infarcts are most often caused by abnormalities of coagulation and cardiac-origin embolism. Angiography often shows occlusion of intracranial artery branches.[146]

Hematologic abnormalities are extremely common in SLE. The presence of lupus anticoagulant (LA) often correlates with clinical hypercoagulability, characterized by miscarriages, recurrent thrombophlebitis, and strokes.[147] Thrombocytopenia and other platelet abnormalities are also common, as is reduced prostacyclin activity.[148] In a 1988 clinicopathologic study of 50 patients dying with SLE, a syndrome clinically resembling thrombotic thrombocytopenic purpura (TTP) developed in 14 patients (28%).[144] Seven of these 14 patients had platelet-thrombi occluding their capillaries and arteries, segmental subendothelial hyalin deposits, and arteriolar microaneurysms at necropsy—findings typical for TTP.[144] In this same study, vasculitis was not seen in the brain or spinal cord in any of the 50 patients.

Echocardiography in patients with SLE shows a high frequency of valvular disease, especially Libman-Sacks endocarditis.[149] Other heart lesions are also common. Devinsky et al. in their clinicopathologic study found that 25 of 50 patients had cardiac lesions that were potentially emboligenic.[144] These included Libman-Sacks vegetations (eight patients), acute and chronic mitral valvulitis (12), marantic endocarditis (two), and bacterial endocarditis (one). Two patients had mural thrombi—one in the left atrium and one in the left ventricle.[144] Endocarditis in SLE is discussed in more length in Chapter 9. Myocarditis is also a feature of SLE. Evaluation of patients with SLE who have focal neurologic signs or focal lesions on MRI should include thorough hematologic and cardiac evaluation.

TPP is characterized clinically by fever, renal failure, thrombocytopenia, and microangiopathic hemolytic anemia.[150,151] Platelet-rich thrombi are found packing arterioles and capillaries, causing microinfarcts within the brain. Transient focal neurologic signs, which improve quickly, and a more diffuse encephalopathy are common clinical features.[150,152] Occasionally, reports document persistent neurologic deficits and even occlusion of large intracranial arteries and their branches.[153,154] Brain hemorrhages are also sometimes found.[155] Some patients with TTP develop an encephalopathy associated with headache, seizures, and vision loss, accompanied by reversible brain-imaging abnormalities predominantly located in the posterior portions of the cerebral hemispheres.[155] This reversible posterior leukoencephalopathy syndrome is related to altered renal function and probably represents a "capillary leak" syndrome that is potentially reversible.[156] Modern neuroimaging might show in the future that strokes are rather common in TTP but are usually minor and nondisabling. Plasma exchange can be an effective treatment, so this condition is important to recognize.[157]

Severe rheumatoid arthritis (RA) can be complicated by neuropathies, meningitis, and rheumatoid dural nodules. True arteritis with fibrinoid necrosis is occasionally seen and can cause an encephalopathy or multifocal small infarcts.[122,158–160] In patients with active RA, levels of fibrinogen, fibrinogen turnover, and fibrin degradation products are increased.[158–161] Also, high titers of circulating rheumatoid factor can cause a hyperviscosity syndrome.[162] Undoubtedly, these serologic changes contribute to brain infarcts in patients with RA.

Patients with Sjögren's syndrome have a high incidence of neuropathy, especially involving the trigeminal nerves.[163] These patients also often have cognitive and behavioral abnormalities.[164,165] In a neuroimaging study of 38 patients with Sjögren's syndrome, eight patients had focal neurologic deficits—most often hemiparesis, aphasia, and ataxia, as well as other cognitive and behavioral abnormalities.[165] MRI in this study showed CNS abnormalities in 75% of patients, most often in the white matter. Occasionally, discrete cortical lesions were seen that resembled infarcts.[165] Vasculitis has been found at necropsy in patients with Sjögren's syndrome, but many of the lesions clinically and on MRI resemble multiple sclerosis.[165,166]

Headache is common in patients with systemic sclerosis (scleroderma). Occasionally, brain infarcts and SAH are reported.[167,168] Hypertension is common in scleroderma, and some of the neurovascular symptoms are probably caused by high blood pressure and reversible vasoconstriction.

Sarcoidosis

Sarcoidosis causes a variety of CNS manifestations, including intraparenchymatous granulomas, meningitis, and myelopathy.[169,170] Sarcoidosis occasionally causes a cerebral vasculitis almost invariably accompanied by a CSF pleocytosis. Retinal inflammatory changes are also present.[171–174] The cerebrovascular abnormalities probably represent spread of inflammatory cells from the meninges through Virchow-Robin spaces to the smaller pial vessels. Veins are predominantly affected, so the vascular lesion is probably most accurately classified as a *phlebitis or venulitis*.[175] Periphlebitis can be noted on ophthalmoscopic examination of the fundus. The retinal lesions are characterized by a yellowish-white focal or diffuse sheathing of retinal veins. Figure 11-13 shows fundus photographs that illustrate the periphlebitis. Hard exudates, sometimes termed *taches de bougie* because of their resemblance to candle-wax drippings, are often related to the periphlebitis and can leave white chorioretinal scars.[172,176] TIAs, strokes, and evidence of meningeal, hypothalamic, and pituitary dysfunction are the clinical features of angiitic neurosarcoidosis, a disorder that can also affect the spinal cord, peripheral nervous system, and muscle. The periphlebitis and meningitis often respond to corticosteroids when given in substantial doses and over long periods (e.g., 60 mg of prednisone daily for 3–6 months or more). Immunosuppressant drugs, such as immuran, cyclosporine, and methotrexate, have been used with success in some patients.

Temporal (Giant Cell) Arteritis

Temporal (giant cell) arteritis usually affects elderly men and women. Although the branches of the ECA, especially the superficial temporal and occipital arteries, are most frequently involved, the ICA, ECVA, subclavian, coronary, femoral, and even intracranial arteries can be affected.[177–180] Blindness is caused by granulomatous arteritis in the arteries supplying the optic nerve and retina (Figure 11-12B). The lesions most often causing strokes are located in the distal extracranial ICAs as they enter the carotid siphon and in the distal ECVAs.[179,180] Rarely, patients have been described with encephalopathy and multifocal neurologic signs who have the findings of temporal arteritis in pial and brain arteries.[181] Occasionally, patients may present with multi-infarct dementia.[182]

Temporal arteritis usually presents as a systemic illness. Patients often develop headaches that differ from past headaches. Headaches are not pulsatile and are accompanied by aching in the proximal muscles, low-grade fever, weight loss, malaise, fatigue, and jaw claudication. Jaw claudication results from ischemia of the masseter muscles supplied by branches of the ECAs. The superficial temporal arteries may be tender, cord-like, and nonpulsatile, and the scalp may be diffusely tender. The best known and most feared complication is

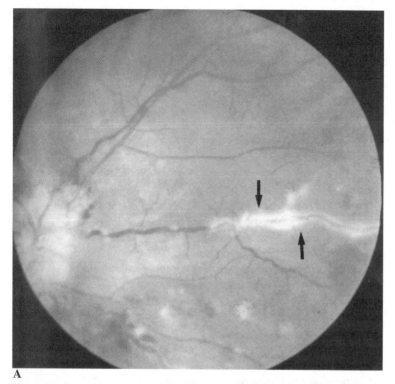

A

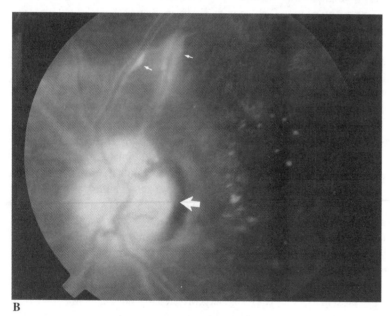

B

Figure 11-13. Retinal fundus photographs of patients with sarcoidosis that illustrate periphlebitis. **(A)** Extensive focal perivenous sheathing (*arrows*). (Reprinted with permission from CD Forbes, WF Jackson. A Color Atlas and Text of Clinical Medicine. London: Wolfe Publishing, 1993.) **(B)** Perivenous sheathing is prominent and involves the veins at the top of the fundus photograph (*small arrows*). The optic disk is pale and atrophic (*large arrow*). (Courtesy of Larry Frohman, M.D., UMDNJ—New Jersey Medical School.)

vision loss. An ischemic optic neuropathy results from occlusion of the posterior ciliary arteries. Additionally, occlusion of the central retinal artery can lead to an ischemic retina. If vision loss occurs, it is usually severe. Involvement of one eye is often followed by involvement of the other.

Laboratory findings that may be of help are an elevated erythrocyte sedimentation rate, mild anemia, and an elevated leukocyte count. Temporal arteritis may be present with a normal erythrocyte sedimentation rate. Color duplex ultrasonography of the superficial temporal arteries and their major branches may show stenoses, occlusions, or a diagnostic hypoechoic halo around the perfused lumen of the arteries.[183] Biopsy of the temporal artery is the most secure manner to make the diagnosis. Angiography with opacification of the ECA branches and the intracranial circulation can be suggestive. If possible, I choose to biopsy a smaller scalp branch of the superficial temporal artery. It is best to biopsy a segment of artery identified as abnormal by palpation, ultrasonography, or angiography. A long segment of the artery is taken to avoid possible skip lesions, but the major portion of this artery is preserved. It is important to look for the general features of temporal arteritis in elderly patients with stroke. Stroke, however, is rarely the first manifestation of temporal arteritis.

Treatment with prednisone (60–80 mg/day) is begun before biopsy in patients with clinically probable temporal arteritis. In such patients, rapid relief of headache and other systemic symptoms usually occurs. Steroids are tapered by titrating the dose against the symptoms and the erythrocyte sedimentation rate. Treatment does not reverse established central or ocular ischemia but helps prevent further involvement of blood vessels.

Isolated Central Nervous System Angiitis

In some patients, arteritis is limited to the CNS. This syndrome of isolated CNS angiitis, also called *granulomatous angiits* and *giant cell granulomatous angiitis of the CNS,* can be difficult to diagnose. Any age can be affected (mean age is approximately 49 years), and there is a male predominance (nearly 2 to 1).[184] The disorder can be acute, with symptoms developing within a few weeks, or it can evolve during a period of months to years.[122,184,185] Usually, the clinical picture is that of a diffuse or multifocal encephalopathy.[96,184–187] Cognitive and behavioral changes are found in more than 60% of patients, and headache, asymmetric motor signs, somnolence, and seizures are common findings.[184–187] Occasionally, TIAs or sudden strokes are described.[184–188] A myelopathy may also be present.[184,185] Focal signs may occur at onset but more often step-like worsen-

ing punctuates the course of a progressive multifocal encephalopathy. The erythrocyte sedimentation rate is elevated in approximately two-thirds of patients, but other serologic and systemic tests are not helpful.[184] The CSF usually has a slight-to-moderate pleocytosis, and the CSF protein is usually high (80%), often higher than 100 mg/dl.[184] CT and MRI may show small or large focal lesions, usually infarcts, but small hematomas and hemorrhagic infarcts have also been noted.[184,189] In approximately one-half of the patients, angiography is abnormal and shows segmental narrowing and sausage-shaped dilatation of arteries ("beading").[184,189,190] In some patients, however, angiography is completely normal or shows nonspecific abnormalities.[122,188,189] Segmental vascular narrowing is also found in patients who abuse drugs and in reversible vasoconstriction syndromes, so this angiographic finding is not specific for arteritis. Figure 11-14 is from a patient who had a reversible vasoconstriction syndrome and illustrates vascular narrowing and dilatation that is often misdiagnosed by radiologists as representing an arteritis.

Biopsy or necropsy shows a segmental, necrotizing granulomatous vasculitis affecting mostly the leptomeningeal, cortical, and spinal vessels. Any size artery or vein can be involved, but usually vessels 200–500 μ in diameter are most affected. In some patients, granulomatous changes have been predominantly venular.[184,185] The intima and adventitia of arteries are infiltrated with lymphocytes, giant cells, and granulomas. Granulomas can extend into the adjacent brain parenchyma. Specific diagnosis is important because treatment with prednisone and immunosuppressant agents, such as cyclophosphamide, may allow recovery from a disease that is nearly always fatal when untreated.[96,122,127,184,187] Biopsy should be pursued in patients with multifocal lesions and encephalopathy, especially if they have a CSF pleocytosis and a high-protein content. Moore urges biopsy of the nondominant hemisphere, especially the tip of the temporal lobe, choosing tissue that contains a longitudinally oriented surface vessel.[187]

Takayasu's Arteritis

Often called *pulseless disease,* Takayasu's arteritis was originally described in young Japanese girls and women.[191] The condition is well known in

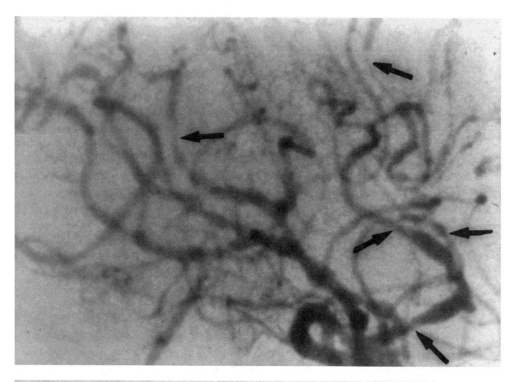

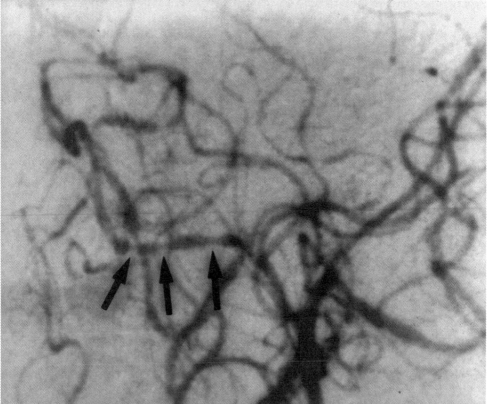

Figure 11-14. Carotid artery angiograms. Intracranial magnified views from a patient with a reversible vasoconstriction syndrome. The arrows point to focal regions of narrowing of arterial branches. Sausage-like dilatations are also present.

Asian countries but is still uncommon in North America.[192] Some patients have a prodromal phase of malaise, fever, and night sweats, and laboratory analysis reveals anemia and an increased sedimentation rate. Later, severe occlusive disease of the aortic arch and its branches develops, often leading to absent neck and limb pulses.[193,194] Surprisingly, strokes or focal neurologic signs are not the predominant clinical feature. Headache, dizziness, syncope, and visual blurring are more common. In some patients, neurologic function is well preserved despite striking radiologic signs of occlusion of vessels at their origin from the aortic arch.[195] Occlusions, stenosis, luminal irregularities, and ectasia or aneurysm formation are found. The most common sites of involvement are the midportion of the left CCA, left and right subclavian arteries, and the midportion of the innominate artery.[195–198] The inflammatory process involves the media and adventitia, which are infiltrated with plasma cells, lymphocytes, and histiocytes.[196–199] During the inflammatory stage, elastic fibers and smooth muscle cells are destroyed. After the inflammatory stage subsides, fibrosis replaces the damaged portions of the arterial intima, media, and adventitia.[199]

Diagnosis of Takayasu's arteritis can often be made by ultrasonography. Duplex scans invariably show bilateral involvement in the proximal portions of the CCAs, consisting of long segments of concentric thickening of the arterial walls.[200] The subclavian artery lesions are also readily shown by ultrasonography.[200] Ultrasound can also be used to monitor the lesions and their response to treatment.

Arm and leg claudication is commonly related to the subclavian, aortic, and iliofemoral disease. Hypertension is present in more than one-half of the patients and may be difficult to control. The chronic proximal occlusive disease often leads to retinal microaneurysms and arteriovenous anastomoses. Vision loss can result from the chronic eye ischemia.[201] The proximal occlusive disease leads to extensive collateral circulation. Hypertension and increased flow through collateral channels can cause SAHs and ICHs similar to that found in the moyamoya syndrome. Corticosteroids, immunosuppressive therapy, angioplasty, and surgical bypass treatment[199,202] have all been used. Moore[96] and others[199,203] are impressed that corticosteroids (prednisone 30 mg/day initially, then tapered to 5–

10 mg/day maintenance) may prevent or diminish vascular complications.

Behçet's Disease

Behçet's disease is a relapsing, remitting illness first described by a Turkish dermatologist who recognized the triad of oral ulcers, genital ulcers, and uveitis. The disease is most often found in Turkey, Saudi Arabia, Mediterranean countries, and Japan but does occur in North America, Europe, and worldwide. Behçet's disease is important for neurologists to recognize. The predominant clinical systemic findings are aphthous ulcers in the mouth and genital tissues, uveitis, synovitis, other skin findings (e.g., folliculitis and erythema nodosum), ulcerative lesions in the bowel mucosa (especially the colon), and thrombophlebitis.[204–207] The disorder affects mostly young adults in their 20s. The male to female ratio ranges from 2 to 1 to 4 to 1.[204–209] Neurologic involvement probably occurs in approximately 6–10% of patients. Among a large series containing 323 patients with Behçet's disease followed in a clinic in Turkey, only 46 patients were referred because of headache and neurologic signs and only 17 patients (5.3%) had neurologic abnormalities.[208]

The most common neurologic syndromes are (1) a meningitic form, in which headache is the major symptom; (2) an encephalitic form, with gradually evolving multifocal signs; (3) strokes, characterized by relatively acute-onset focal signs; and (4) headache, with papilledema caused by dural sinus thrombosis.[208–215] Characteristically, the neurologic signs come in attacks with remissions between, a course that closely mimics multiple sclerosis. CT and MRI show that the most frequent sites of involvement are the pons and midbrain, followed by the basal ganglia and thalamus. The lesions most often are small foci that have high signals on T2-weighted MRI images and are isointense or hypointense on T1-weighted images.[211,212] Some lesions are large. The brain stem lesions often do not conform to arterial territories and are larger than those found in arteritis.[210] The spinal cord is also frequently involved clinically and by MRI. The lesions often contain hemosiderin, and the distribution in gray and white matter separates the lesions from those found in multiple sclerosis. Usually, angiography does not show arterial abnormalities.

The CSF is almost always abnormal, including pleocytosis, high-protein content, and increased levels of immunoglobulins, which are produced intrathecally.[216] The CSF pressure is sometimes elevated. The levels of oligoclonal bands of IgA and IgM correlate well with neurologic disease activity and are useful to follow. At necropsy, there often is a diffuse meningoencephalitis with perivascular lymphocytic cuffing predominantly around veins, venules, and capillaries, with occasional arterial involvement.[209,212] The dural sinuses and large veins may be occluded.[210,213,215] Thromboses of leg veins and even the vena cava are important systemic features, and the pathology is predominantly venous. The brain shows areas of necrosis, demyelination, and scarring, especially in the rostral brain stem, internal capsule, and basal ganglia, as well as in the spinal cord. The lesions probably represent focal hemorrhagic venous infarcts and areas of encephalitic change. Corticosteroids may suppress ocular and brain symptoms.[96,210] Moore recommends "early and aggressive treatment of CNS involvement with corticosteroids."[96]

Cogan's Syndrome

Cogan described a syndrome of interstitial keratitis with vestibulo-auditory dysfunction.[217] The condition is probably an autoimmune vasculitic disorder that affects young adults. The earliest symptoms are photophobia, reduced vision, and redness of the eyes.[217,218] An interstitial keratitis is found on ophthalmologic examination, occasionally with uveitis. Blindness can result from corneal opacification. Tinnitus, reduced hearing, vertigo, and ataxia appear before, during, or after eye abnormalities.[219] Microscopic study shows a vasculitis of small- and medium-sized arteries. Some patients have fever, and the aortic valve and bowel may be involved.[218] The aorta is occasionally involved, causing aortitis and aortic aneurysm formation.[220] I am not aware of brain infarcts or CNS findings in patients with Cogan's syndrome.

Eales's Disease

Eales described an ocular disorder characterized by abnormal retinal vessels and recurrent vitreous hemorrhages.[221] The disease affects mostly young men

and is common in the Middle East and India. Visual symptoms include specks, floaters, cobwebs and curtains, and blurred vision.[222] The disease is characterized by retinal periphlebitis, nonperfusion of retinal capillaries, and vitreous hemorrhages.[223] Some patients have extensive retinal revascularization and fibrovascular proliferation.[223] Ophthalmologic examination shows prominent sheathing of veins and arteries, flame-shaped retinal hemorrhages, and vitreous hemorrhages. Although the symptoms usually begin in one eye, both eyes are invariably involved. The macular arteries are relatively spared, so that central vision is often preserved.[222] A vasculitis affecting both retinal arteries and veins causes the eye findings. Sometimes, the uvea is also involved. CNS involvement has been described in the form of meningitis, focal infarcts, and vascular occlusions.[43,224–227] In one patient, a left cerebral infarct was caused by MCA occlusion.[224] Spinal cord involvement is also common.[226] Usually, there are no systemic symptoms or characteristic laboratory abnormalities, although the CSF may show a pleocytosis.[224] Diagnosis is made on the basis of the characteristic ophthalmoscopic abnormalities.

Microangiopathy of the Brain, Ear, and Retina

An unusual, but distinct, occlusive vascular disorder was called *microangiopathy of the brain and retina* by Susac and colleagues.[228] Although this condition, which is also called *Susac's syndrome*[229,230] and *retinocochleocerebral vasculopathy*,[231] resembles granulomatous angiitis in some ways, there are important differences. In microangiopathy of the brain and retina, there is always obliteration of large retinal arteries, causing gradual, severe, bilateral vision loss.[228–234] The retinal vascular changes are easily observed through the ophthalmoscope. Some retinal arteries are amputated, whereas others are severely narrowed or attenuated, and light streaking characterizes their thickened arterial walls. Figure 11-15 shows photographs of the ocular fundus in a patient with this condition. Tinnitus and hearing loss are also prominent. The most important clinical neurologic signs are dementia, bilateral motor weakness with pyramidal signs, and cerebellar dysfunction. The disorder affects mostly young women in their second to fourth decade and progresses stepwise or gradually. The CSF protein is high, sometimes more than 1 g/dl, but

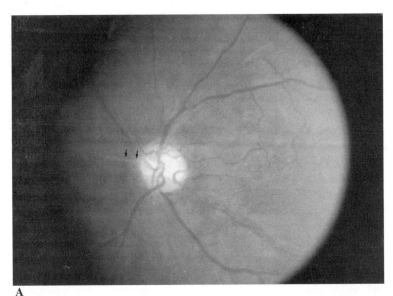

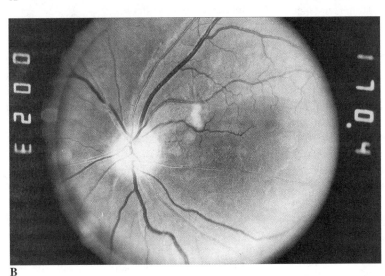

Figure 11-15. Retinal fundus photographs of a patient with microangiopathy of the brain and retina. **(A)** Arrows point to a white occluded retinal artery. The other arteries are also attenuated. The larger vessels are veins. The optic disk is pale and atrophic. **(B)** The other eye shows many occluded and attenuated retinal arteries. Fluffy exudates and pale regions of retina are also shown. The optic disk is chalky-white. The patient was blind because of the retinal arterial disease. (Courtesy of Thomas Hedges III, M.D., New England Medical Center.)

usually there is no major pleocytosis. Brain biopsy has shown obliteration of small arteries without prominent inflammation or granulomas, as well as multiple microinfarcts.[228–234] Some patients with this condition have improved at least temporarily after corticosteroids and immuno-suppressive therapy.[234]

Other Oculocerebral Arteriopathies

Acute posterior multifocal placoid pigment epitheliopathy is an acute chorioretinal disease that usually develops in young adults often after a flu-like febrile illness.[235–237] Usually, both eyes are affected simultaneously but sometimes sequentially. Symptoms include visual blurring, distortion, and scotomas. The optic fundus shows multiple, well-circumscribed, gray-white flat lesions at the level of the retinal pigment epithelium. Vision usually returns to normal during several weeks. Occasionally, however, patients develop progressive disease with significant loss of vision.[237] The condition is posited to be caused by a choroidal vasculitis. Headache, CSF pleocytosis, optic neuritis, and strokes have been described.[237–240] Cerebral angiography sometimes shows an arteritis.[237] In one patient, brain histopathology showed focal granulomatous inflammation of medium-sized arteries.[241]

Vogt-Koyanagi-Harada syndrome is an important differential diagnostic consideration in patients with ocular inflammatory lesions. The disorder is often called *uveomeningoencephalitis*. Patients with this syndrome have premature whitening of the hair and eyelashes, alopecia, vitiligo, iridocyclitis, choroiditis, and loss of hearing.[242] They may also have meningeal signs and a CSF pleocytosis. An inflammatory adhesive arachnoiditis develops and explains many of the symptoms. Fluorescein angiography shows leakage from retinal vessels. Papilledema and increased intracranial pressure can occur. Some patients have had prominent neurologic signs but whether these were a manifestation of vascular inflammation is not clear. The clinical findings are similar to Behçet's disease except for dermatologic abnormalities. Usually, the disorder remits after 6–12 months, but there may be recurrences.

I have seen a number of patients during the years with ocular inflammatory disorders with vascular abnormalities in the optic fundus who also had CSF pleocytosis, headache, neurologic signs, and MRI lesions that could represent infarcts. These patients did not have illnesses that correspond to the common recognized oculocerebral vasculopathies. Many other arteriopathies probably exist that have a predilection for the eye and nervous system among other organ involvement.

Sneddon's Syndrome

Sneddon's syndrome is characterized by a chronic skin lesion, livedo reticularis, and recurrent strokes. This syndrome is often found in young patients without risk factors for stroke.[243–246] The most important and diagnostic clinical feature is livedo reticularis, a grayish-pale mottling of the skin that usually involves the trunk and all limbs. The cutaneous findings are obvious by simply looking at the skin with the patient undressed. I have seen several patients with Sneddon's syndrome who had undergone multiple invasive tests but apparently had never been examined without clothes. Usually, the hands and feet are cold and peripheral pulses are reduced. Hand angiography shows dramatic occlu-

sions of digital arteries with areas of narrowing and dilatation.[246] Skin biopsy usually shows distinctive abnormalities. Small- to medium-sized arteries at the border between the dermis and subcutis show early inflammatory lesions followed by subendothelial proliferation and later, fibrosis.[246] The neurologic findings are multiple acute-onset strokes. CT and MRI often show multiple infarcts in the cerebral cortex and white matter.[246] Cerebral angiography often shows branch occlusions of intracranial arteries.[243,247] At times, the disorder is familial.[248] Some patients with Sneddon's syndrome have antiphospholipid antibodies.[249] Valvular cardiac abnormalities are also relatively common in patients with Sneddon's syndrome, and some of the brain infarcts may be caused by cardiac-origin embolism.[244,248,249]

Kohlmeier-Degos Syndrome

Kohlmeier-Degos syndrome, also called *malignant atrophic papulosis*, is a vascular occlusive disorder with characteristic skin changes. The skin lesions begin as small, yellow-pink raised lesions, usually on the trunk and arms.[250,251] The central part of the skin lesions becomes atrophic and looks porcelain-white, flat, and depressed, and each lesion is surrounded by a raised pink zone, often with telangiectasis.[250] Small- and medium-sized arteries in the skin undergo a progressive fibrosis with infarcts of the skin.[251,252] Biopsy shows fibrous proliferation between the intima and internal elastica with rare inflammatory changes.[250–252] The bowel is also commonly involved, causing ulcers, decreased motility, bowel dilatation, and, often, perforation.[251,252] Although the vessels in other visceral organs are often involved at necropsy, systemic symptoms are usually limited to the skin and gut. CNS symptoms occur in approximately one-fifth of patients with Kohlmeier-Degos syndrome.[250] Strokes do occur.[252] Brain-imaging tests show infarcts and small hemorrhages. Angiography may show occlusion and beading of distal branches of intracranial arteries.[250] Neuropathologic examination shows hyalinization or fibrous proliferation between the endothelium and internal elastic membrane, often with superimposed thrombosis.[250–252] Inflammatory abnormalities are slight or absent. Occasionally, SAH and dural sinus thrombosis are present.[250,252] At times, strokes precede skin and bowel involvement. Degos' disease is often fatal, but some patients may have remissions.[252]

Vasculopathy in Drug Abusers

Drug abuse has become an important cause of stroke in adolescents and young adults. ICH caused by drugs is considered in Chapter 13 and is most often caused by amphetamines and cocaine.[253] Ischemic stroke usually relates to one of five different situations: (1) heroin addiction, (2) amphetamine abuse, (3) intravenous use of drugs synthesized for oral use, (4) infection as a complication of an addictive lifestyle, and (5) cocaine use.

Heroin Addiction

In heroin addicts, strokes are invariably ischemic and may be cerebral or spinal. Stroke frequently follows the reintroduction of intravenous heroin after a period of abstention.[254–257] Brain ischemia may directly follow the heroin injection but is more often delayed by 6–24 hours. Heroin addicts also have serologic and systemic abnormalities, including eosinophilia, elevated immune globulins and gamma globulins, false-positive serology, Coombs-positive hemolysis, and lymph-node hypertrophy.[256] Increased binding of serum globulins by morphine has been found in rabbits with implanted morphine pellets. In some narcotic addicts, morphine also binds gamma globulins.[258] Illicitly available heroin is often adulterated with a host of fillers and foreign substances. These observations make it likely that immune-complex deposition or other hyperimmune mechanisms underlie the strokes in patients who are chronically exposed to many recurrently introduced antigens.[256] Definitive immunologic or pathologic studies of strokes in heroin addicts are wanting.

Amphetamine Abuse

In amphetamine abuse, necrotizing angiitis has been demonstrated pathologically. The lesions resemble polyarteritis nodosa and can affect the brain and other viscera.[259] In experimental animals[260] and humans[261] who have taken amphetamines orally or intravenously, angiography shows segmental changes in intracerebral vessels with prominent beading. The most common clinical syndrome is ICH, usually beginning shortly after amphetamine exposure, but ischemic infarcts have been found at necropsy.

Patients with SAH or ICH after amphetamine abuse have a relatively low frequency of harboring aneurysms and vascular malformations that are the source of intracranial bleeding.[253]

Abuse of Drugs Synthesized for Oral Use

A different pattern of disease affects patients who inject intravenous drugs that have been synthesized for oral use; methylphenidate (Ritalin) and pentazocine (Talwin) with pyribenzamine are the best-documented drugs. These compounds contain talc, microcrystalline cellulose, and other fillers designed to maintain the chemicals in pill form. Addicts mash the pills, dissolve them in tap water, and inject them intravenously or even directly into the carotid artery.[262] Particles of drugs and fillers still remain and are trapped by the lung arterioles and small arteries, causing an obliterative arteritis.[262,263] Pulmonary arteriovenous shunts develop and are probably responsible for crystals that reach the brain and eyes of addicts.[262–264] Strokes and seizures usually follow quickly after intravenous injection. Deep, small cerebral arteries, such as the lenticulostriate[262] and anterior spinal arteries, are most often affected.[265]

Infection as a Complication of an Addictive Lifestyle

Drug abusers seldom follow strict sterile precautions. Hepatitis, AIDS, infective endocarditis, and fungal infections are common complications of their habit and lifestyle. Endocarditis can cause embolic strokes. Fungal infections, especially *Nocardia* and *Aspergillus*, can cause focal necrotic infarcts or brain abscesses.[94,95]

Cocaine Use

Cocaine use has become the most common cause of drug-related strokes. Cocaine use is rampant. In a 1990 study among 214 patients ages 15–44 years admitted to the San Francisco General Hospital during a 10-year period, 34% were drug users and cocaine was the predominant drug used.[266] Cocaine can be snorted or injected as cocaine hydrochloride or can be smoked as the free-base alkaloidal form, usually called *crack cocaine*.[267–269] Crack cocaine is made by mixing aqueous cocaine hydrochloride with ammonia and sometimes baking soda. The free-base cocaine is usually smoked after the cocaine has become alkalinized and precipitated. Crack cocaine produces a more rapid high than does snorted or injected cocaine hydrochloride. Its use is associated with a higher frequency of brain infarcts.[270] The strokes usually begin shortly after cocaine use, irrespective of the portal of entry (snorted, inhaled, or injected). These strokes have a predilection for the brain stem.[271] Spinal cord infarcts also have been reported to develop soon after cocaine use.[272] The mechanism of ischemia is unknown. Bowel and myocardial ischemia and an eosinophilic myocarditis are also found after cocaine abuse.[273] Vasoconstriction, increased platelet aggregation, and apparent vasculitis are posited as potential causes of stroke in cocaine users. Arterial constrictions (predominantly MCAs and PCAs—focal and diffuse) were found on MRA studies taken 20 minutes after intravenous cocaine administration in healthy subjects who had used cocaine previously but were not addicts.[274]

Cocaine use is also associated with SAHs and ICHs. For unclear reasons, there is a higher incidence of aneurysms and vascular malformations in cocaine-related hemorrhages than in hemorrhages after amphetamine use.[253,275] Angiography should be performed unless the cocaine-related hemorrhage is in a characteristic location for hypertensive ICH. Cocaine users can also develop a picture that resembles hypertensive encephalopathy with multiple hemorrhages and brain edema. Figure 11-16 is a brain specimen that illustrates hypertensive encephalopathy with hemorrhages after cocaine use.

Migraine and Vasoconstriction

Vascular headaches are among the most common disorders treated by physicians and neurologists. Migraine is prevalent at all ages, including young children and the elderly. During migraine attacks, angiography, CBF studies, and TCD have clearly documented changes in intracranial vessel diameter, flow velocities, and CBF.[276] Reversible vasoconstriction has been shown to be an important cause of ischemia, especially in the coronary circulation and in the brain after subarachnoid bleeding. Migraine is a clinical diagnosis usually applied when there is a past history and family history of pulsating, usually unilateral headaches, with or without characteristic visual, somatosensory, or other migraine accompaniments and followed by nausea and vomiting. Although vasoconstriction and vasodilatation have been shown to occur during migraine attacks, not all vasoconstriction occurs in patients with migraine.

Neuroimaging in patients with migraine shows a more-frequent-than-expected incidence of infarcts. Migraine-related strokes have also been reported more often than in the past.[276–280] Infarction can be caused by prolonged intense vasoconstriction,[276,281] causing permanent ischemia or thrombosis of arteries. Intense vasoconstriction can impede flow, promoting thrombosis; platelets are activated during migraine, and the vasoconstrictive process itself may stimulate the endothelium to release factors that promote thrombosis. My own investigations on stroke within the PCA[276,282] and basilar-artery territories in patients with migraine[276,279] show that some patients develop thrombi within the basilar artery and the PCA.

Migrainous accompaniments can precede, accompany, or follow headache and can occur in the absence of headache. Transient vasoconstriction accounts for many examples of temporary spells of neurologic dysfunction in the elderly,[283–285] including transient global amnesia.[276,286,287] Fisher[283,284] and I[276] have tried to separate migraine accompaniments from atherosclerotic ischemia by analyzing the clinical features (Table 11-1). To complicate matters, atherosclerotic lesions in the coronary arteries of humans and in the extracranial and retinal arteries of experimental animals seem to predispose them to superimposed vasoconstriction. Thus, vasoconstriction can complicate atherostenosis. TCD shows promise in identification of vasoconstriction by showing high velocities that change with time and various pharmacologic treatments.

Call, Fleming, and colleagues called attention to a syndrome that they called *reversible cerebral segmental vasoconstriction*.[288] The syndrome most often affects young women, especially during the puerperium, but also occurs at menopause and is found at all ages. Some patients have developed this syndrome after carotid endarterectomy.[289] Vasoconstriction involves many large, medium, and small cerebral arteries. The clinical findings include severe headache, decreased alertness, seizures, and changing multifocal neurologic signs. Brain edema and death can occur. Angiography shows sausage-shaped focal regions of vasodilatation and multifo-

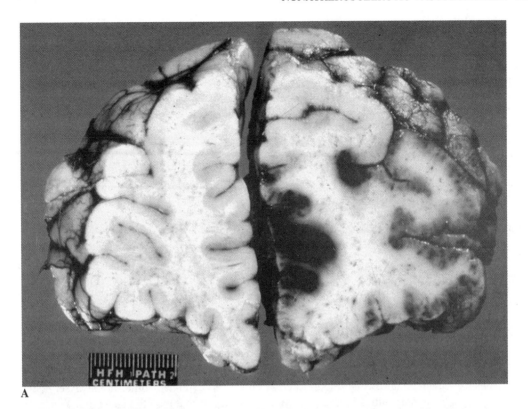

A

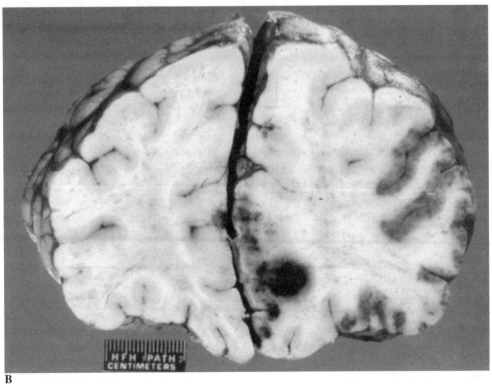

B

Figure 11-16. Brain specimen at necropsy in a patient who died after crack cocaine use. Multiple brain hemorrhages (**A**) and brain edema (**B**) are shown. (Courtesy of Steven Levine, M.D., Department of Neurology, Wayne State University School of Medicine.)

Table 11-1. Migraine Accompaniments versus Atherosclerotic Ischemia

Migraine	Atherosclerosis
Sensory modalities involved sequentially (e.g., vision, tactile, speech)	Modalities involved together (e.g., visual, somatosensory, and aphasic abnormalities noted at same time)
Within each modality, first symptoms are "positive" (e.g., visual brightness, shining, somatosensory paresthesias)	Usually negative symptoms (e.g., loss of vision, numbness)
Symptoms gradually progress within each modality; vision loss gradually affects field; paresthesias move from one finger to hand to body—often takes 20 mins to travel fully	Visual field or body involved at once
Within each modality, positive followed by negative (e.g., brightness leaves scotoma in its wake; paresthesias followed by numbness)	Usually negative effects only
One modality clears before the next is involved	Modalities are involved simultaneously
Headache most often followed after neurologic symptoms have cleared	Headache accompanies persistent deficits or is absent
Attacks usually last 15–30 mins (average, 20 mins)	Usually 1–2 mins; often 5 mins
Different attacks involve different sides and vascular territories	Usually always the same vascular territory
Spells may occur over years	Usually limited to days, weeks, or months
Stroke risk factors often absent	Risk factors present
Women predominate over men	Men predominate over women

cal regions of vascular narrowing. Figure 11-14 shows angiographic abnormalities in a patient with this syndrome. TCD shows high velocities in many intracranial arteries. CT and MRI may show brain edema and small areas of infarction and hemorrhage. Corticosteroids, calcium channel blockers, anticonvulsants, and treatments for increased intracranial pressure have been used to treat this disorder. Many of the patients had migraine in the past.

ICH has been shown to occasionally complicate a severe migraine attack.[290,291] Intense vasoconstriction leads to ischemia of a local brain region with edema and ischemia of the small vessels perfused by the constricted artery. When vasoconstriction abates, blood flow to the region is augmented and the reperfusion can cause hemorrhage from the damaged arteries and arterioles.[291,292] The mechanism is the same as that found in hemorrhage after carotid endarterectomy and in reperfusion after brain embolization.

I believe that vasoconstriction accounts for many more strokes than is currently recognized or appreciated. Surveys of strokes in the young attribute many infarcts to migraine. I take seriously the risk of stroke in patients with prolonged classic migraine attacks, especially if the deficits last for hours or more after the attack. In these patients and in those with migraine-related infarcts, I use prophylactic agents (most often phenytoin, calcium channel blockers, cyproheptadine, or methysergide), along with agents that modify platelet function and coagulation. Aspirin is used most often, but I sometimes use warfarin in patients with prior infarcts.

Moyamoya Syndrome

Moyamoya, although sometimes referred to as a disease, is probably better thought of as a syndrome defined by a characteristic angiographic appearance. The intracranial ICAs undergo progressive tapering and progressive occlusion at their intracranial bifurcations (the so-called T-portion of the ICAs). Basal penetrating branches of the ICAs, ACAs, and MCAs enlarge to provide collateral circulation. These vessels form large prominent anastomosing channels, basal telangiectasias, which appear on angiograms as a cloud of smoke; these arteries are especially prominent because of the paucity of MCA sylvian branches. The appearance of these basal telangiectasias led Japanese clinicians to use the term *moyamoya*, which means "something hazy like a puff of cigarette smoke drifting in the air." [293,294] Although first described in Japan,[294] the disease has been reported worldwide.[293,295,296]

Necropsy studies, although few, have shown severe vascular occlusive abnormalities characterized by endothelial hyperplasia and fibrosis, with intimal thickening and abnormalities of the internal elastic lamina.[297] In contrast, the intracerebral perforating arteries show microaneurysm formation, lipohyalinosis, focal fibrin deposition, and thinning of the elastic laminas and arterial walls.[298] These changes in the perforating arteries are probably the result of greatly increased flow through these small vessels.[293,294,298] Inflammatory changes have universally been absent. In 1991, Ikeda studied the extracranial arteries of 13 Japanese patients with spontaneous occlusions of the circle of Willis at necropsy who met the research definition of moyamoya syndrome.[299] Extracranial arteries showed the same intimal lesions as the intracranial arteries. Characteristically, the proximal pulmonary arteries had fibrous nodular intimal thickening without inflammatory abnormalities.[299] Moyamoya changes have been found in a variety of situations, including sickle cell disease, neurofibromatosis, Takayasu's disease, Down's syndrome, atherosclerosis, and fibromuscular dysplasia, and can be found in young women, especially those who smoke cigarettes and take oral contraceptives.[297] A variety of different conditions can probably cause intimal changes, which lead to fibrosis and luminal narrowing.

Moyamoya syndrome is approximately 50 times more common in girls and women than in boys and men.[300] Clinically, the disorder has an interesting bimodal distribution, presenting most often in children younger than 15 years and in adults in their third to fifth decades of life. Children usually present with transient episodes of hemiparesis or other focal neurologic signs often precipitated by physical exercise or hyperventilation. Several of my own young patients have had intermittent choreoathetosis. Other patients have sudden-onset deficits, such as hemiplegia, or the gradual development of intellectual deterioration. Headaches and seizures are common.[293,294] These symptoms are often accompanied by CT and MRI evidence of infarction and CBF studies that show regions of hypoperfusion. The abnormal vasculature is often visible on MRI.

Adults, in contrast, usually present with brain hemorrhages, usually in the thalamus, basal ganglia, or deep white matter. These hemorrhages are the result of degenerative changes (aneurysmal dilatation and thinning) in the anastomotic basal vessels, which are overtaxed and cannot accommodate the volume of blood needed for perfusion. At times, the hemorrhages are subarachnoid and intraventricular. Some patients with moyamoya syndrome develop aneu-

rysms involving arteries of the circle of Willis, especially the anterior cerebral- anterior communicating artery region and the basilar artery.[301] Angiography shows progressive changes that may be asymmetric initially but always involve the intracranial ICAs bilaterally and usually also involve the proximal portions of the MCAs and ACAs. As the intracranial arteries narrow, collaterals develop involving the basal penetrating arteries, orbital vessels (so-called ethmoidal moyamoya), and vessels over the vault derived from transdural anastomoses from the meningeal and superficial temporal arteries.[293] Later, the telangiectasias may regress and become less prominent. Suzuki and others have staged the severity of disease by the angiographic findings.[293,294]

Some patients with moyamoya syndrome stabilize clinically, often after they have developed disabilities. The best treatment is not known. A variety of different surgical revascularization procedures have been used. These usually involve anastomosing the superficial temporal artery to the MCA or placing the superficial temporal and middle meningeal arteries adjacent to the pia or both, or placing vascularized connective tissue elements and muscle on the surface of the pia mater.[300,302,303] The surgical revascularization created is often called *synangiosis*. Angiography after surgical revascularization shows improved collateral blood flow.[302,303] It is hoped that revascularization might prevent further ischemia and hemorrhage, but no systematic trials have investigated the effectiveness of revascularization procedures.

Hematologic Disorders, Including Abnormalities of Coagulation, Viscosity, and Serum Constituents

Since the 1980s, knowledge of blood constituents and their function in the coagulation process has dramatically advanced. Brain ischemia and hemorrhage often result from hematologic abnormalities rather than from primary diseases of the blood vessels.[304,305] In other patients with endothelial lesions in the aorta, heart, and vessels, activation of coagulation functions causes thrombi to form on the abnormal endothelial surfaces and often precipitates strokes. In turn, occlusion of arteries increases coagulation factors. The endothelia, blood vessels, and circulating blood are so intricately interwoven that it is often difficult to know which changes are primary and cause the disorder and which are secondary to the occlusive vascular process. I have already discussed most of the hematologic conditions in Chapters 4 and 5 regarding laboratory diagnosis and treatment. Only a brief cataloging of these disorders are presented here.

Cellular Abnormalities

Abnormalities in the formed cellular constituents of the blood may be quantitative or qualitative. Polycythemia has long been known to increase blood viscosity, decrease CBF, and increase thrombosis. Sickle cell disease and sickle cell–hemoglobin C disease are examples of qualitative red blood cell abnormalities that affect blood flow. Sickle cell disease is associated with occlusive changes in large intracranial arteries and small penetrating vessels.[306,307] Subcortical, cortical, and border-zone infarcts are often found on CT and MRI[307]; angiography has shown intracranial occlusions of the major basal arteries. The walls of intracranial arteries are thickened, and intimal and subintimal proliferation occurs. Arteries may become dilatated and ectatic even in childhood.[308] Occasionally, veins and dural sinuses may thrombose.[309] TCD offers a noninvasive method for detecting velocity changes related to intracranial large artery narrowing and allows monitoring of patients with sickle cell disease.[310] Blood transfusions for children whose TCD blood-flow velocities in the ICAs or MCAs or both exceed 200 cm per second have been shown in a trial to prevent stroke from developing.[311]

Paroxysmal nocturnal hemoglobinuria (PNH) is characterized by a qualitative abnormality of red blood cells that leads to hemolysis and life-threatening episodes of venous thromboses.[312] This condition is known to be caused by a mutation in hematopoietic stem cells that leads to clones of blood cells that are deficient in surface proteins that are normally attached to cell membranes.[312] Neutropenia and thrombocytopenia are also common. Patients with PNH may develop cerebral venous and dural sinus thromboses.[312,313] Systemic and intracranial hemorrhages can result from the thrombocytopenia, which may be severe.[312]

Increased platelet counts, especially those higher than 1 million, are also associated with hypercoagulability. The thrombocytosis can be primary, so-called essential thrombocythemia, and can be associated with other myeloproliferation, or, less

often, can be secondary to systemic disease. Essential thrombocythemia is associated with strokes and digital occlusions.[314–316] The lack of correlation between the platelet count and the thrombotic complications has led to the assumption that there are also qualitative abnormalities of platelet function.[304,314–317] In some patients, increased coagulability has been attributed to increased adhesion and aggregation of platelets (so-called sticky platelets) in the absence of thrombocytosis.[315–319]

Leukemia is complicated occasionally by brain hemorrhages and microinfarcts. When the white blood cell count is high (increased leukocrit), the white blood cells can pack capillaries, leading to microinfarcts and vascular rupture with small brain hemorrhages. Larger brain hemorrhages and SAHs are most often related to thrombocytopenia caused by replacement of the bone marrow with leukocyte precursors.

Serologic Abnormalities

Normally, natural inhibitors of coagulation circulate to discourage spontaneous blood clotting. The best known of these inhibitors, antithrombin III and proteins C and S, can be deficient on a hereditary basis or be reduced by disease.[304,305] Congenital deficiency of antithrombin III may be quantitative or qualitative and is most often an autosomal-dominant condition.[304,320] Reduced synthesis of antithrombin III, as in patients with liver disease or renal loss in the nephrotic syndrome, can lead to acquired deficiencies. Inherited deficiencies of proteins C and S can also contribute to or cause increased coagulability.[304,305,321] An inherited coagulation deficit referred to as *resistance to activated protein C* was described by Dutch investigators from Leiden and is the most common cause of abnormal protein C activity.[322,323] In most instances, resistance to activated protein C is caused by a point mutation in the gene that encodes for coagulation factor V.[323] The presence of this mutation, called *factor V Leiden*, is accompanied by a three- to fivefold increase in the frequency of venous thromboembolism in the lower extremities[324] and an increased frequency of cerebral venous and dural sinus thrombosis. Factor V Leiden is the most common genetic disorder that leads to hypercoagulability. The second most common genetic mutation that leads to a prothrombic state is a mutation in the gene encoding prothrombin.[325] This mutation involves a transition from guanine to adenine at position 20210 in the sequence of the 3' untranslated region of the prothrombin gene.[325] The frequency of cerebral and peripheral venous thrombosis is greatly increased in carriers of the prothrombin gene mutation, especially if they also take oral contraceptive pills.[325–327] Genetic analysis is warranted in patients with unexplained hypercoagulability, especially those with cerebral venous thrombosis and recurrent peripheral venous thromboembolism. Most often, clotting is venous, but arterial occlusions have also been described.

Systemic and inherited conditions can alter the levels of the serine protease coagulation factors. The best known of these disorders is hemophilia, which causes bleeding into the joints, skin, and cranium. In 1989, my colleagues and I measured factor VIII levels in a large number of patients with brain ischemia.[328] Some patients have chronically increased concentrations of factor VIII, with frequent episodes of thrombophlebitis, spontaneous abortion, and strokes.[329] In others, factor VIII levels are high, probably as an epiphenomenon to the initial thromboembolic event. Some patients with infectious and inflammatory diseases, such as Crohn's disease and ulcerative colitis, have increased factor VIII levels as a result of serologic changes induced by the primary disease.[330–332] Venous dural sinus occlusions, thrombophlebitis, and arterial occlusions may result. Hematologic changes in inflammatory bowel disease are complex because elevated levels of factors V and VIII, reduced levels of antithrombin III, and quantitative and qualitative platelet abnormalities have all been described.[331] Studies have also shown that infections of various types are often present in the days and weeks before stroke onset.[333,334] Infections and various inflammatory disorders provoke an increase in acute phase reactants and white blood cells, fibrinogen, and coagulation factors V, VII, and VIII, which induce thrombosis in patients with pre-existing endothelial lesions.[335,336]

Cancers are also often associated with hypercoagulability.[337,338] My colleagues and I studied patients with mucinous adenocarcinomas who had venous occlusions, large artery thrombi, and multiple small artery occlusions.[339] Mucin was seen inside and directly outside of small vessels, presumably contributing to the hypercoagulabil-

ity evident clinically. In some situations (e.g., during pregnancy, the puerperium, or use of oral contraceptives), the mechanism of hypercoagulability is not fully known.

The advent of thrombolytic and fibrinolytic treatment, especially with recombinant tissue plasminogen activator, has led to more detailed study of the body's normal fibrinolytic activity and abnormalities of the fibrinolytic system.[340,341] Plasminogen deficiencies, dysfibrinogenemias, and abnormalities of tissue plasminogen activator and its inhibitors can cause an increased tendency toward thrombosis.[304,305,342,343] Thrombin and fibrinolytic activity can be monitored during acute stroke by measuring a number of substances.[344,345] For example, the levels of fibrinopeptide A correlate with thrombin activity, and the levels of cross-linked D-dimer, a breakdown product of fibrin polymer, are a useful index of fibrinolytic activity.[344,345]

Immunologic Abnormalities

Attention has been drawn to the presence of circulating antibodies that react to various hematologic and vascular components. The best known of these disorders are the so-called LA and anticardiolipin antibodies. These substances react against phospholipids. The presence of LA or anticardiolipins has been referred to as the *antiphospholipid antibody (APLA) syndrome*. The LA (a misnomer because it is associated with increased coagulability, not bleeding) is a phospholipid antibody that interferes with the formation of the prothrombin activator.[346,347] In the laboratory, there is a prolonged activated partial thromboplastin time that does not correct when normal plasmin is added, indicating the presence of an inhibitor of clotting rather than a deficiency of a needed component.[346–348] Some patients with LA have SLE but most do not. When antiphospholipids of the IgG, IgM, or IgA classes are found in the absence of a known systemic illness, the disorder is referred to as a *primary APLA syndrome*.[347–352] Clinically, these patients have an increased incidence of spontaneous abortions, thrombophlebitis, pulmonary embolism, and large- and small-artery occlusions. In addition to the presence of LA or anticardiolipins or both, laboratory abnormalities include positive VDRL, thrombocytopenia, and antinuclear antibodies. Some patients have mitral and aortic valve abnormalities and ocular ischemia.[347,351,352] The mechanism of increased coagulability and valvular changes is not known, but these probably relate to immune-related endothelial and valve-surface injuries.[353] Patients with high-positive IgG and APLA have a high incidence of subsequent vascular occlusive lesions.[354,355] Angiography in patients with APLA syndrome shows a high frequency of intracranial occlusive disease, atypical extracranial occlusive arterial disease, and venous and dural sinus occlusions.[356] Some patients with APLA have a Binswanger type of leukoencephalopathy.

Disseminated intravascular coagulation (DIC) is a disorder that affects cellular and serologic factors. When a primary disorder leads to local or diffuse clotting, the coagulation cascade may be activated with generation of excess intravascular thrombin. The coagulation system then is further activated, fibrin is deposited into the microcirculation, hemostatic elements have a shortened survival, and the fibrinolytic system is activated.[357] The most common disorders inciting DIC are infections, obstetric and vascular emergencies, and cancer.[358,359] Head trauma, SAH, brain tumors, and vascular malformations can also cause DIC.[358,360,361] The laboratory findings usually include thrombocytopenia, reduced fibrinogen levels, prolongation of prothrombin time and partial thromboplastin time, and increased levels of fibrin split products. DIC can be associated with nonbacterial thrombotic endocarditis, especially in patients with cancer.[339,358,360] Neurologic findings are frequent and include an encephalopathy with multifocal signs and frank thrombotic and embolic infarcts. Bleeding can also occur.

Blood flow, especially in the brain microcirculation, depends heavily on the viscosity of the blood. Blood viscosity is most affected by the erythrocyte content of the blood and serum fibrinogen level.[362,363] Polycythemia and hyperfibrinogenemia can increase whole-blood viscosity and decrease CBF, especially in patients with cerebrovascular disease. High fibrinogen levels are an important risk factor for stroke and other large artery occlusive disease.[364] Less often, increased viscosity is caused by high levels of globulins (e.g., in Waldenström's macroglobulinemia or in other disorders with abnormal proteins or cryoglobulins, such as multiple myeloma).[365] Rarely, high levels of serum lipids cause significant hyperviscosity.[366]

Clinically, patients with hyperviscosity syndromes have an encephalopathy characterized by somnolence, stupor, headache, seizures, ataxia, and decreased vision.[365] A clue to the presence of hyperviscosity is the ophthalmoscopic appearance of the retina. Retinal veins are dilatated and tortuous and may show segmentations in the blood columns within retinal vessels. Serum viscosity is measured relative to water; the average normal level is approximately 1.8. Serum viscosity of 5 or 6 is usually associated with encephalopathy but lower levels may be important in patients with hypertensive microvasculopathy and atherosclerotic disease.

Neoplastic Conditions

Lymphomatoid granulomatosis is a neoplastic condition probably related to lymphoma in which granulomatous nodules can involve brain arteries and veins and produce stroke-like deficits.[367,368]

Lymphomas can present as a solely intravascular tumor. This entity, usually called *intravascular lymphoma,* was previously called *neoplastic angioendotheliosis.* Large pleomorphic mononuclear cells proliferate within the lumens of capillaries, venules, arterioles, and small arteries. Early authors posited that the neoplastic cells were of endothelial origin,[369–371] but recent studies show that the neoplastic intraluminal cells are lymphocytes that show either B-cell or T-cell markers or both.[372,373] The neoplastic cells occlude small arteries, leading to multiple microinfarcts. The disorder can be systemic, producing erythematous skin plaques and patches, subcutaneous nodules, high sedimentation rates, fever, and renal failure.[370,374] The disorder can affect the spinal cord.[375] Headache, multifocal neurologic signs, and a progressive course are typical. The brain lesions on MRI vary and range between white matter hyperintensity to large areas of signal abnormalities.[373] Meningeal enhancement can occur and is explained by microinfarcts within the meninges or slow flow through meningeal blood vessels. Angiography is usually normal because the blood vessels involved are too small to be seen during angiograms.

Hodgkin's disease in the meninges often causes occlusions of meningeal arteries and veins, with hemorrhagic infarction in the underlying cerebral cortex. I have already commented in this chapter on leukemic blockage of small arteries and on the coagulopathies associated with cancer, especially of the mucinous adenocarcinoma type.

Some Genetic Disorders That Cause Strokes

Many of the conditions already discussed in this chapter, such as hereditary disorders of connective tissue and familial CAA, are known to be genetically determined. Many others are probably influenced by genetic predispositions. Dyslipoproteinemias, hemoglobinopathies, diabetes, hypertension, and atherosclerosis are strongly governed by genetic factors. I close this chapter by briefly discussing a few other disorders with mendelian etiologies. Knowledge of the genetic factors in stroke is growing rapidly.[376–378]

MELAS syndrome (*m*itochondrial myopathy, *e*ncephalopathy, *l*actic *a*cidosis, and *s*troke-like episodes) is one form of mitochondrial encephalomyopathy.[379,380] Seizures, headaches, and intellectual deterioration are most prominent clinically.[381–383] Short stature and sensorineural deafness are also common features.[380] Affected patients often have abrupt episodes of visual deterioration, hemiparesis, and ataxia, often with seizures. Lactic and pyruvic acid levels in the blood are often high and muscle biopsy may show ragged red fibers.[380,381] CT and MRI show discrete multifocal abnormalities that are most often in the parieto-occipital and temporal lobes.[382–386] These lesions affect the cortex and underlying white matter. These lesions are caused by ischemia, but the arteries supplying these zones are normal. They are probably caused by the metabolic abnormality characterized by decreased cytochrome oxidase activity within mitochondria, leading to energy failure. Basal-ganglia calcifications are also prominent. The disorder is caused by a maternal mutation in mitochondrial DNA. Other mitochondrial disorders may also be associated with white matter abnormalities on MRI that resemble infarcts.

Strokes, renal failure, painful dysesthesias, and cutaneous angiokeratomas characterize Fabry's disease. The disorder is a sex-linked lysosomal storage disease. Most clinical cases involve homozygous men. Occasionally, heterozygous women are affected.[387–390] The diagnosis is suggested by finding the characteristic tiny, pinhead-size, dark-reddish-purple non-pruritic papules that are located predominantly along the inner thighs, perineum, and near the umbilicus in a so-called bathing trunk distribution. Because of a deficiency of a lysosomal enzyme (α-galactosidase), trihexosyl ceramide (a sphingolipid) accumulates and causes a diffuse vasculopathy.[390–392] Multiple vascular occlusions and strokes are common. Patients often have severe pain and syncope related to a small fiber and autonomic neuropathy. Sweating is also diminished or absent, so that heat and exercise intolerance are common. Angiography often shows occlusion of branch arteries. The endothelium is infiltrated with the sphingolipid. The myocardium is also often involved, and the condition presents in some patients as a cardiomyopathy. Death is most often caused by renal failure unless dialysis is performed. Renal transplantation may delay vascular complications and may improve the prognosis.[392] The enzyme has been synthesized and is involved in therapeutic trials.

Cerebral autosomal dominant arteriopathy with subcortical infarcts and leukoencephaly (CADASIL) is an important familial condition characterized by headache, multiple lacunar infarcts, and extensive white matter abnormalities of the Binswanger type.[393–397] The small arteries within the brain are thickened by eosinophilic, periodic acid–Schiff positive granular deposits, which have not been characterized fully biochemically.[397] The substance within the arteries is not amyloid. Skin biopsy, especially using electron microscopy, shows the same material within skin arteries. The clinical findings are strokes, progressive gait-disorder, and frontal lobe–type subcortical dementia.[393–397] Mood disorders, especially depression, are also common. Headache is a prominent symptom in some patients and in relatives of patients with this leukoencephalopathy. The MRI shows characteristic lesions.[398] White matter hyperintensities are sometimes found before clinical symptoms develop. CADASIL is caused by a mutation of the *notch 3* gene on chromosome 19.[399] A somewhat similar microangiopathic familial disorder has also been described in Japan. This condition affects predominantly young men and is characterized by a Binswanger type leukoencephalopathy, alopecia, and prominent back pain.[400] The small arteries are infiltrated by fibrous intimal proliferation and severe hyalinosis, with splitting of the intima and internal elastic membrane.[400]

Menkes' disease (trichopoliodystrophy or kinky-hair disease) is an X-linked recessive condition in which mitochondrial dysfunction is caused by impaired intestinal absorption of copper.[401–403] The delivery of copper to cells requires transporters, one of which is deficient in patients with Menkes' disease. The deficiency of copper leads to subnormal cytochrome oxidase function within mitochondria and widespread energy failure. The hair is abnormal and is course, stiff, and easily broken. Hypotonia, hypothermia, seizures, and failure to thrive are common.[401–403] Ragged red fibers may be seen on muscle biopsy. Electron microscopic studies of the brain can show abnormal mitochondria. MRI studies of the brain show rapidly developing cerebral atrophy. At necropsy, the brain contains multiple microinfarcts and intracranial branch arteries are often occluded. Most patients die in early childhood.

Patients with neurofibromatosis type 1 are known to develop renal artery and cerebrovascular abnormalities. Aneurysms and arterial stenoses occur. The most frequent cerebrovascular site of involvement is within the ICAs as they emerge from the cavernous sinus just after the ophthalmic artery branches.[404–406] A moyamoya picture can result. Hypertension may be caused by renal artery occlusion or pheochromocytomas, which occur at increased frequency in patients with this genetic condition.

Homocystinuria is probably the most common genetic disease that affects the brain vasculature and leads to premature atherosclerosis and strokes.[407,408] Severe hyperhomocystinemia and homocystinuria is a genetic disorder first described in children and known to be associated with premature strokes, mental retardation, and a Marfan-like syndrome. It has become clear that lesser degrees of hyperhomocystinemia are associated with premature atherosclerosis.

Classic homocystinuria is caused by a hereditary deficiency of the enzyme cystathione-beta-synthase, an enzyme that is required for the conversion of methionine-derived homocysteine to cystathione. In humans, approximately 15–20 mmol of homocysteine is formed each day by demethylation of the amino acid methionine.[408] Homocysteine is subsequently metabolized by one of two pathways, either remethylation or transulfuration. In the remethylation process, homcysteine is remethylated to methionine in a reaction catalyzed by methionine synthase.[408] Vitamin B_{12} is an essential cofactor for methionine synthase, and N^5-methyl-tetrahydrofolate is the methyl donor in this reaction. N^5,N^{10}-methylene-tetrahydrofolate reductase functions as the catalyst in this remethylation reaction.[408,409] Homocysteine can also be transulfurated when homocysteine condenses with serine to form cystathione, a reaction catalyzed by the vitamin B_6-dependent enzyme cystathione beta-synthase.[408–410]

Cystathione is then hydrolyzed to cysteine, which in turn can be incorporated into glutathione

or further metabolized to sulfate and excreted in the urine.[408,409,411]

Cystathione-beta-synthase deficiency is the most common genetic cause of severe hyperhomocystinemia. The homozygous form of this disorder is called *congenital homocystinuria* and is associated with plasma homocystine concentrations of up to 400 μmol/l during the fasting state.[408,409] This genetic disorder is rare (5 in 1 million births). Affected individuals have lens ectopias, skeletal deformities, a Marfan-like habitus, and severe premature atherosclerosis. Typically, a clinical thromboembolic event in the form of strokes or myocardial infarcts occurs before age 30 years.[412] A homozygous deficiency of N^5,N^{10}-methylenetetrahydrofolate reductase, the enzyme involved in the B_{12}-dependent remethylation of homocysteine, can also cause severe hyperhomocystinemia. Patients with this metabolic defect have an even worse prognosis than those with cystathione-beta-synthase deficiency.[408,409]

Milder forms of hyperhomocystinemia occur in heterozygotes with these enzyme deficiencies. Deficiencies in the cofactors, folate, and vitamins B_{12} and B_6, which are required for homocysteine metabolism, can also cause an elevated homocysteine level. In patients with nutritional deficiencies in these vitamin cofactors, prescribing these substances can reduce homocysteine levels. Increased levels of homocysteine also occur in patients being treated with methotrexate, theophylline, and phenytoin and in patients with (1) renal insufficiency; (2) hyperthyroidism; (3) breast, pancreatic, and ovarian cancers; (4) lymphatic leukemia; and (5) pernicious anemia.[408,409] Cigarette smoking has also been associated with elevated homocysteine levels, presumably because of interference with the synthesis of pyridoxal phosphate.[413]

Elevated levels of homocysteine have been unequivocally related to strokes, premature atherosclerosis, myocardial infarction, and venous thromboembolism.[408,409,414,415] Evidence from more than 20 case-controlled studies that included more than 2,000 individuals has validated the relationship between elevated homocysteine levels and accelerated atherosclerosis.[408,409] Patients with increased levels of homocysteine have more severe carotid artery disease than individuals with normal levels.[416] Experimental evidence shows that increased homocysteine levels injure the vascular endothelium. This injury leads to platelet activation and the formation of thrombi.[417,418] Homocysteine also stimulates vascular smooth muscle cells to proliferate.[419]

References

Arterial Dissections

1. Ojemann RG, Fisher CM, Rich JC. Spontaneous dissecting aneurysms of the internal carotid artery. Stroke 1972; 3:434–400.
2. Fisher CM, Ojemann RG, Roberson GH. Spontaneous dissection of cervicocerebral arteries. Can J Neurol Sci 1978;5:9–19.
3. Caplan LR, Zarins C, Hemmatti M. Spontaneous dissection of the extracranial vertebral artery. Stroke 1985;16:1030–1038.
4. Caplan LR, Tettenborn B. Vertebrobasilar occlusive disease: review of selected aspects: I. Spontaneous dissection of extracranial and intracranial posterior circulation arteries. Cerebrovasc Dis 1992;2:256–265.
5. Barbour PJ, Castaldo JE, Rae-Grant AD, et al. Internal carotid artery redundancy is significantly associated with dissection. Stroke 1994;25:1201–1206.
6. Brandt T, Hausser I, Orberk E, et al. Ultrastructural connective tissue abnormalities in patients with spontaneous cervicocerebral artery dissections. Ann Neurol 1998;44:281–285.
7. Ehrenfeld WK, Wylie EG. Spontaneous dissection of the internal carotid artery. Arch Surg 1976;111:294–330.
8. Hart RG, Easton JD. Dissection of Cervical and Cerebral Arteries. In HJM Barnett (ed), Eurologic Clinics, Vol 1. Philadelphia: Saunders, 1983;155–182.
9. Biller J, Hingtgen WL, Adams HP, et al. Cervico-cephalic arterial dissection. A 10 year experience. Arch Neurol 1986;43:1234–1238.
10. Friedman WA, Day AL, Quisling RG, et al. Cervical carotid dissecting aneurysms. Neurosurgery 1980;7:207–214.
11. Mokri B, Houser OW, Sandok BA, Piepgras DG. Spontaneous dissection of the vertebral arteries. Neurology 1988;38:880–885.
12. Bogousslavsky J, Despland PA, Regli F. Spontaneous carotid dissection with acute stroke. Arch Neurol 1987;44:137–140.
13. Biousse V, Schaison M, Touboul P-J, et al. Ischemic optic neuropathy associated with internal carotid artery dissection. Arch Neurol 1998;55:715–719.
14. Pozzali E, Giuliani G, Poppi M, Faenza A. Blunt traumatic carotid dissection with delayed symptoms. Stroke 1989;20:412–416.
15. Sturzenegger M. Ultrasound findings in spontaneous carotid artery dissection: the value of duplex sonography. Arch Neurol 1991;48:1057–1063.
16. Hennerici M, Steinke W, Rautenberg W. High-resistance Doppler flow pattern in extracranial ICA dissection. Arch Neurol 1989;46:670–672.
17. Touboul PJ, Mas JL, Bousser MG, Laplane D. Duplex scanning in extracranial vertebral artery dissection. Stroke 1987;18:116–121.
18. Krueger BR, Okazaki H. Vertebral-basilar distribution infarction following chiropractic cervical manipulation. Mayo Clin Proc 1980;55:322–332.
19. Sherman DG, Hart RG, Easton JD. Abrupt change in head position and cerebral infarction. Stroke 1981;12:2–6.
20. Caplan LR. Posterior Circulation Disease. Clinical Findings, Diagnosis, and Management. Boston: Blackwell, 1996.
21. Cook JW, Sanstead JK. Wallenberg's syndrome following self-induced manipulation. Neurology 1991;41:1695–1696.
22. Rothrock JF, Hesselink JR, Teacher TM. Vertebral artery occlusion and stroke from cervical self-manipulation. Neurology 1991;41:1696–1697.
23. Tramo MJ, Hainline B, Petito F, et al. Vertebral artery injury and cerebellar stroke while swimming: case report. Stroke 1985;16:1039–1042.
24. Hope EE, Bodensteiner JB, Barnes P. Cerebral infarction related to neck position in an adolescent. Pediatrics 1983;72:335–337.
25. Bostrom K, Liliequist B. Primary dissecting aneurysm of the extracranial part of the internal carotid and vertebral arteries. Neurology 1967;17:179–186.
26. Grossman FI, Davis KR. Positional occlusion of the vertebral artery: a rare cause of embolic stroke. Neuroradiology 1982;23:227–230.
27. Tettenborn B, Caplan LR, Sloan MA, et al. Postoperative brainstem and cerebellar infarcts. Neurology 1993;43:471–477.
28. Giroud M, Gras P, Dumas R, Becker F. Spontaneous vertebral artery dissection initially revealed by a pain in one upper arm. Stroke 1993;24:480–481.
29. Dubard T, Pouchot J, Lamy C, et al. Upper limb peripheral motor deficits due to extracranial vertebral artery dissection. Cerebrovasc Dis 1994;4:88–91.
30. Goldsmith P, Rowe D, Jager R, Kapoor R. Focal vertebral artery dissection causing Brown-Sequard syndrome. J Neurol Neurosurg Psychiatry 1998;64:416–417.
31. Yonas H, Agamanolis D, Takaoka Y, White RJ. Dissecting intracranial aneurysms. Surg Neurol 1977;8:407–415.
32. Caplan LR, Baquis G, Pessin MS, et al. Dissection of the intracranial vertebral artery. Neurology 1988;38:868–879.
33. Anson J, Crowell RM. Cervicocranial arterial dissection. Neurosurg 1991;29:89–96.
34. O'Connell B, Towfighi J, Brennan R, et al. Dissecting aneurysms of head and neck. Neurology 1985;35:993–997.
35. Kasner SE, Hankins LL, Bratina P, Morganstern LB. Magnetic resonance angiography demonstrates vascular healing of carotid and vertebral artery dissections. Stroke 1997;28:1993–1997.
36. Leclerc X, Lucas C, Godefroy O, et al. Helical CT for the follow-up of cervical internal carotid artery dissections. AJNR Am J Neuroradiol 1998;19:831–837.

Fibromuscular Dysplasia

37. So EL, Toole JF, Dalal P, et al. Cephalic fibromuscular dysplasia in 32 patients. Arch Neurol 1981;38:619–622.
38. Corrin LS, Sandok BA, Houser OW. Cerebral ischemic events in patients with carotid artery fibromuscular dysplasia. Arch Neurol 1981;38:616–618.
39. Sandok BA. Fibromuscular Dysplasia of the Internal Carotid Artery. In HJM Barnett (ed), Neurologic Clinics, Vol 1. Philadelphia: Saunders, 1983;17–26.

40. Luscher TF, Lie JT, Stanson AW, et al. Arterial fibromuscular dysplasia. Mayo Clin Proc 1987;62:931–952.
41. Kubis N, von Langsdorrff D, Petitjean C, et al. Thrombotic carotid megabulb: fibromuscular dysplasia, septae, and ischemic stroke. Neurology 1999;52:883–886.
42. Mettinger K, Ericson K. Fibromuscular dysplasia and the brain. Stroke 1982;13:46–52.

Heritable Disorders of Connective Tissue

43. Pessin MS, Chung C-S. Eales disease and Gröenblad-Strandberg disease (pseudoxanthoma elasticum). In J Bogousslavsky, LR Caplan (eds), Stroke Syndromes. Cambridge: Cambridge University Press, 1995;443–447.
44. Lebwohl MG, Distefano D, Prioleau PG, et al. Pseudoxanthoma elasticum and mitral-valve prolapse. N Engl J Med 1982;307:228–231.
45. Strole WE, Margolis R. Case records of the Massachusetts General Hospital: Case 10-1983. N Engl J Med 1983;308:579–585.
46. Altman LK, Fialkow PJ, Parker F, et al. Pseudoxanthoma elasticum: an underdiagnosed genetically heterogenous disorder with protean manifestations. Arch Intern Med 1974;134:1048–1054.
47. Rios-Montenegro E, Behrens MM, Hoyt WF. Pseudoxanthoma elasticum: association with bilateral carotid rete mirabile and unilateral carotid-cavernous sinus fistula. Arch Neurol 1972;26:151–155.
48. Roach ES, Zimmerman CF. Ehlers-Danlos Syndrome. In J Bogousslavsky, LR Caplan (eds), Stroke Syndromes. Cambridge: Cambridge University Press, 1995;491–496.
49. Leier CV, Call TD, Fulkerson PK, Wooley CF. The spectrum of cardiac defects in the Ehlers-Danlos syndrome types I and III. Ann Intern Med 1980;92:171–178.
50. Pretorius ME, Butler IJ. Neurologic manifestations of Ehlers-Danlos syndrome. Neurology 1983;33:1087–1089.
51. Lach B, Nair SG, Russell NA, Benoit BG. Spontaneous carotid-cavernous fistula and multiple arterial dissections in type IV Ehlers-Danlos syndrome. J Neurosurg 1987;66:462–467.
52. Pyeritz RE, McKusick VA. The Marfan syndrome: diagnosis and management. N Engl J Med 1979;300:772–777.

Dilatative Arteriopathy

53. Read D, Esiri MM. Fusiform basilar artery aneurysm in a child. Neurology 1979;29:1045–1049.
54. Hirsch CS, Roessmann U. Arterial dysplasia with ruptured basilar artery aneurysm: report of a case. Hum Pathol 1975;6:749–758.
55. Makos MM, McComb RD, Hart MN, Bennett DR. Alpha-glucosidase deficiency and basilar artery aneurysm: report of a sibship. Ann Neurol 1987;22:629–633.
56. Schwartz A, Rautenberg W, Hennerici M, Dolichoectatic intracranial arteries: review of selected aspects. Cerebrovasc Dis 1993;3:273–279.
57. Pessin MS, Chimowitz MI, Levine SR, et al. Stroke in patients with fusiform vertebrobasilar aneurysms. Neurology 1989;39:16–21.
58. Moseley IF, Holland IM. Ectasia of the basilar artery: the breadth of the clinical spectrum and the diagnostic value of computed tomography. Neuroradiology 1979;18:83–91.
59. Little JR, St Louis P, Weinstein M, et al. Giant fusiform aneurysms of the cerebral arteries. Stroke 1981;12:183–188.
60. Echiverri HC, Rubino FA, Gupta SR, Gujrati M. Fusiform aneurysm of the vertebrobasilar arterial system. Stroke 1989;20:1741–1747.
61. Nishizaki T, Tamaki N, Takeda N, et al. Dolichoectatic basilar artery: a review of 23 cases. Stroke 1986;17:1277–1281.
62. Shokunbi MT, Vinters HV, Kaufmann JC. Fusiform intracranial aneurysms: clinicopathologic features. Surg Neurol 1988;29:263–270.
63. DeGeorgia M, Belden J, Pao L, et al. Thrombus in vertebrobasilar dolichoectatic artery treated with intravenous urokinase. Cerebrovasc Dis 1999;9:28–33.
64. Cohen MM, Hemalatha CP, D'Addario RT, Goldman HW. Embolism from a fusiform middle cerebral artery aneurysm. Stroke 1980;11:158–161.
65. Aichner FT, Felber SR, Birhamer GG, Posch A, Magnetic resonance imaging and magnetic resonance angiography of vertebrobasilar dolichoectasia. Cerebrovasc Dis 1993;3:280–284.
66. Hennerici M, Rautenberg W, Schwartz A. Transcranial Doppler ultrasound for the assessment of intracranial arterial flow velocity: II. Evaluation of intracranial arterial disease. Surg Neurol 1987;27:523–532.

Cerebral Amyloid Angiopathy

67. Vinters HV. Cerebral amyloid angiopathy: a critical review. Stroke 1987;18:311–324.
68. Vinters HV, Gilbert JJ. Cerebral amyloid angiopathy: incidence and complications in the aging brain: II. The distribution of amyloid vascular changes. Stroke 1983;14:924–928.
69. Okazaki H, Reagan TJ, Campbell RJ. Clinicopathological studies of primary cerebral amyloid angiopathy. Mayo Clin Proc 1979;54:22–31.
70. Cosgrove G, Leblanc R, Meagher-Villemure K, et al. Cerebral amyloid angiopathy. Neurology 1985;34:625–631.
71. Gilbert JJ, Vinters HV. Cerebral amyloid angiopathy: incidence and complications in the aging brain: I. Cerebral hemorrhage. Stroke 1983;14:915–923.
72. Kase CS. Cerebral Amyloid Angiopathy. In CS Kase, LR Caplan, Intracerebral Hemorrhage. Boston: Butterworth–Heinemann, 1994;179–200.
73. Smith DB, Hitchcock M, Philpott PJ. Cerebral amyloid angiopathy presenting as transient ischemic attacks: case report. J Neurosurg 1985;63:963–964.
74. Gray F, Dubas F, Roullet E, Escourolle R. Leukoencephalopathy in diffuse hemorrhagic cerebral amyloid angiopathy. Ann Neurol 1985;18:54–59.
75. Loes DJ, Biller J, Yuh WTC, et al. Leukoencephalopathy in cerebral amyloid angiopathy: MR imaging in four cases. AJNR Am J Neuroradiol 1990;11:485–488.
76. DeWitt LD, Louis DN. Case records of the Massachusetts General Hospital: Case 27-1991. N Engl J Med 1991;325:42–54.
77. Greenberg SM, Vonsattel JPG, Stakes JW, Gruber M, Finkelstein SP. The clinical spectrum of cerebral amyloid angiopathy: presentations without lobar hemorrhage. Neurology 1993;43:2073–2079.

78. Grubb A, Jensson O. Gudmundsson G, et al. Abnormal metabolism of Y-trace alkaline microprotein: the basic defect in hereditary cerebral hemorrhage with amyloidosis. N Engl J Med 1984;311:1547–1549.

79. Stefansson K, Antel JP, Ojer J, et al. Autosomal dominant cerebrovascular amyloidosis: properties of peripheral blood lymphocytes. Ann Neurol 1980;7: 436–440.

80. Fountain NB, Eberhard DA. Primary angiitis of the central nervous system associated with cerebral amyloid angiopathy: report of two cases and review of the literature. Neurology 1996;46:190–197.

81. Caplan LR. Case records of the Massachusetts General Hospital. Case 10-2000. N Engl J Med 2000;(in press).

82. Greene GM, Godersky JC, Biller J, et al. Surgical experience with intracerebral hemorrhage secondary to cerebral amyloid angiopathy. Stroke 1990;21:170.

83. Izumihara A, Ishihara T, Iwamoto N, et al. Postoperative outcome of 37 patients with lobar intracerebral hemorrhage related to cerebral amyloid angiopathy. Stroke 1999;30: 29–33.

84. Greenberg SM. Cerebral amyloid angiopathy. Prospects for clinical diagnosis and treatment. Neurology 1998;51:690–694.

Listeria monocytogenes

85. Weinstein AJ, Schianone WA, Furlan AJ. *Listeria* rhomboencephalitis. Arch Neurol 1982;39:514–516.

86. Brown RH, Sobel RA. Case records of the Massachusetts General Hospital. N Engl J Med 1989;321:739–750.

87. Frayne J, Gates P. *Listeria* rhomboencephalitis. Clin Exp Neurol 1987;24:175–179.

Cat-Scratch Disease

88. Selby G, Walker GL. Cerebral arteritis in cat-scratch disease. Neurology 1979;29:1413–1418.

Lyme Disease

89. Rahn DW, Malawista SE. Lyme disease: recommendations for diagnosis and treatment. Ann Intern Med 1991; 114:472–481.

90. Halperin JJ, Luft BJ, Anand AK, et al. Lyme neuroborreliosis: central nervous system manifestations. Neurology 1989;39:753–759.

91. Pachner AR, Duray P, Steere AC. Cerebral nervous system manifestations of Lyme disease. Arch Neurol 1989;46: 790–795.

92. Uldry PA, Regli F, Bogousslavsky J. Cerebral angiopathy and recurrent strokes following *Borrelia burgdorferi* infection. J Neurol Neurosurg Psychiatry 1987;50:1703–1704.

Fungal Infections

93. Kobayashi RM, Coil M, Niwayama G, Trauner D. Cerebral vasculitis in coccidioidal meningitis. Ann Neurol 1977;1:281–284.

94. Walsh TJ, Hier DB, Caplan LR. Fungal infection of the central nervous system: comparative analysis of the risk factors and clinical signs in 57 patients. Neurology 1985; 35:1654–1657.

95. Walsh TJ, Hier DB, Caplan LR. Aspergillosis of the central nervous system: clinicopathological analysis of 17 patients. Ann Neurol 1985;18:574–582.

Virus-Related Vasculitis

96. Moore PM, Cupps TR. Neurologic complications of vasculitis. Ann Neurol 1983;14:155–167.

97. Gilden DH, Kleinschmidt-DeMasters BK, Wellish M, et al. Varicella-zoster virus, a cause of waxing and waning vasculitis: The *New England Journal of Medicine* case 5-1995 revisited. Neurology 1996;47:1441–1446.

98. Bourdette DN, Rosenberg NL, Yatsu FM. Herpes zoster ophthalmicus and delayed ipsilateral cerebral infarction. Neurology 1983;33:1428–1432.

99. Hilt DC, Buchholz D, Krumholz A, et al. Herpes zoster ophthalmicus and delayed contralateral hemiparesis caused by cerebral angiitis: diagnosis and management approaches. Ann Neurol 1983;14:543–553.

100. Doyle PW, Gibson G, Dolman C. Herpes zoster ophthalmicus with contralateral hemiplegia: identification of cause. Ann Neurol 1983;14:84–85.

101. Powers JM. Herpes zoster maxillaris with delayed occipital infarction. J Clin Neuroophthalmol 1986;2:113–115.

102. Snow BJ, Simcock JP. Brainstem infarction following cervical herpes zoster. Neurology 1988;38:1331.

103. Ross MH, Abend WK, Schwartz RB, Samuels MA. A case of C2 herpes zoster with delayed bilateral pontine infarction. Neurology 1991;41:1685–1686.

104. Leopold NA. Chickenpox stroke in an adult. Neurology 1993;43:1852–1853.

105. Silverstein FS, Brunberg JA. Postvaricella basal ganglia infarction in children. AJNR Am J Neuroradiol 1995;16: 449–452.

106. Caekebeke JFV, Peters ACB, Vandvik B, et al. Cerebral vasculopathy associated with primary varicella infection. Arch Neurol 1990;47:1033–1035.

107. Melanson M, Chalk C, Georgevich L, et al. Varicella-zoster virus DNA in CSF and arteries in delayed contralateral hemiplegia: evidence for viral invasion of cerebral arteries. Neurology 1996;47:569–570.

108. Saito K, Moskowitz MA. Contributions from the upper cervical dorsal roots and trigeminal ganglia to the feline circle of Willis. Stroke 1989;20:524–526.

Human Immunodeficiency Virus/ Acquired Immunodeficiency Syndrome

109. Pinto AN. AIDS and cerebrovascular disease. Stroke 1996;27:538–543.

110. Gillams AR, Allen E, Hrieb K, et al. Cerebral infarction in patients with AIDS. AJNR Am J Neuroradiol 1997;18: 1581–1585.

111. Dubrovsky T, Curless R, Scott G, et al. Cerebral aneurysmal arteriopathy in childhood IDS. Neurology 1998;51:5 60–565.

Cysticercosis

112. Caplan LR. How to manage patients with neurocysticercosis. Eur Neurol 1997;37:124–131.
113. Rodriguez-Carbajal J, del Brutto OH, Penagos P, et al. Occlusion of the middle cerebral artery due to cysticercotic angiitis. Stroke 1989;20:1095–1099.
114. Monteiro L, Almeida-Pinto J, Leite I, et al. Cerebral cysticercus arteritis: five angiographic cases. Cerebrovasc Dis 1994;4:125–133.
115. Barinagarrementaria F, Cantu C. Frequency of cerebral arteritis in subarachnoid cysticercosis. An angiographic study. Stroke 1998;29:123–125.
116. Cantu C, Villarreal J, Soto JL, Barinagarrementaria F. Cerebral cysticercotic arteritis: detection and follow-up by transcranial Doppler. Cerebrovasc Dis 1998;8:2–7.
117. Bang OY, Heo JH, Choi SA, Kim DI. Large cerebral infarction during praziquantel therapy in neurocysticercosis. Stroke 1997;28:211–213.

Malaria

118. Newton CR, Warrell DA. Neurological manifestations of falciparum malaria. Ann Neurol 1998;43:695–702.
119. Omanga U, Ntihinyurwa M, Shako D, Mashako M. Les hemiplegies au cours de l'acces pernicieux a Plasmodium falciparum de l'enfant. Ann Pediatr (Paris) 1983;30:294–296.
120. Newton CR, Marsh K, Peshu N, Kirkham FJ. Perturbations of cerebral hemodynamics in Kenyan children with cerebral malaria. Pediatr Neurol 1996;15:41–49.

Systemic Arteritis

121. Fauci AS, Haynes BF, Katz P. The spectrum of vasculitis: clinical, pathologic, immunologic and therapeutic considerations. Ann Intern Med 1978;89:660–676.
122. Moore PM, Richardson B. Neurology of the vasculitides and connective tissue disease. J Neurol Neurosurg Psychiatry 1998;65:10–22.
123. Scott DG. Classification and treatment of systemic vasculitis. Br J Rheumatol 1988;27:251–257.
124. Moore PM, Fauci AS. Neurologic manifestations of systemic vasculitis: a retrospective and prospective study of the clinico-pathologic features and responses to therapy in 25 patients. Am J Med 1981;71:517–524.
125. Kissel JT, Rammohan KW. Pathology and therapy of nervous system vasculitis. Clin Neuropharmacol 1991;14:28–48.
126. Moore PM, Richardson B. Neurology of the vasculitides and connective tissue diseases. J Neurol Neurosurg Psychiatry 1998;65:10–22.
127. Villringer A, Moore PM. Vasculitides and other Nonatherosclerotic Vasculopathies of the Nervous System. In T Brandt, LR Caplan, J Dichgans, et al (eds), Neurological Disorders. San Diego: Academic, 1996;305–327.
128. Caplan LR, Hedley-White ET. Case records of the Massachusetts General Hospital: Case 5-1995. N Engl J Med 1995;332:452–459.
129. Churg J, Strauss L. Allergic granulomatosis, allergic angiitis, and periarteritis nodosa. Am J Pathol 1951;27:277–301.
130. Chumbley LC, Harrison EG, DeRemee RA. Allergic granulomatosis and angiitis (Churg-Strauss syndrome): report and analysis of 30 cases. Mayo Clin Proc 1977;52:477–484.
131. Sehgal M, Swanson JW, DeRemee RA, Colby TV. Neurologic manifestations of Churg-Strauss syndrome. Mayo Clin Proc 1995;70:337–341.
132. Hauser SL, Shahani B, Hedley-White ET. Case records of the Massachusetts General Hospital: Case 38-1990. N Engl J Med 1990;323:812–822.
133. Jennette JC, Falk RJ. Small-vessel vasculitis. N Engl J Med 1997;337:1512–1523.

Wegener's Granulomatosis

134. Fauci AS, Haynes BF, Katz P, Wolff SM. Wegener's granulomatosis: prospective clinical and therapeutic experience with 85 patients for 21 years. Ann Intern Med 1983;98:76–85.
135. Haynes BF, Fishman ML, Fauci AS, Wolff SM. The ocular manifestations of Wegener's granulomatosis: fifteen years' experience and review of the literature. Am J Med 1977;63:131–141.
136. Lapresle J, Lasjaunias P. Cranial nerve ischemic arterial syndromes. Brain 1985;109:207–215.
137. Palaic M, Yeadon C, Moore S, Cashman N. Wegener's granulomatosis mimicking temporal arteritis. Neurology 1991;41:1694–1695.
138. Frohman LP, Lama P. Annual review of systemic diseases: 1995–1996, part l. J Neuroophthalmol 1998;18:67–79.
139. Satoh J, Miyasaka N, Yamada T, et al. Extensive cerebral infarction due to involvement of both anterior cerebral arteries by Wegener's granulomatosis. Ann Rheum Dis 1988;47:606–611.
140. Provenzale JM, Allen NB. Wegener granulomatosis: CT and MR findings. AJNR Am J Neuroradiol 1996;17:785–792.
141. Nölle B, Specks U, Lüdemann J, et al. Anticytoplasmic autoantibodies: their immunodiagnostic value in Wegener's granulomatosis. Ann Intern Med 1989;111:28–40.

Systemic Lupus Erythematosus

142. Feinglass EJ, Arnett SC, Dorsch CA, et al. Neuropsychiatric manifestations of systemic lupus erythematosus: diagnosis, clinical spectrum, and relationship to other features of the disease. Medicine (Baltimore) 1976;55:323–339.
143. Johnson RT, Richardson EP. The neurological manifestations of systemic lupus erythematosus: a clinical-pathological study of 24 cases and review of the literature. Medicine (Baltimore) 1968;47:337–369.
144. Devinsky O, Petito C, Alonso D. Clinical and neuropathological findings in systemic lupus erythematosus: the role of vasculitis, heart emboli, and thrombotic thrombocytopenic purpura. Ann Neurol 1988;23:380–384.
145. Alsen AM, Gabrulsen TO, McCune WJ. MR imaging of systemic lupus erythematosus involving the brain. AJNR Am J Neuroradiol 1985;6:197–201.
146. Trevor RF, Sondheimer FK, Fessel WJ, et al. Angiographic demonstration of major cerebral vessel occlusion in systemic lupus erythematosus. Neuroradiology 1972;4:202–207.

147. Hart R, Miller V, Coull B, et al. Cerebral infarction associated with lupus anticoagulants: preliminary report. Stroke 1984;15:114–118.

148. McVerry BA, Machin SJ, Parry H, et al. Reduced prostacycline activity in systemic lupus erythematosus. Ann Rheum Dis 1980;39:524–525.

149. Galve E, Candell-Riera J, Pigrau C, et al. Prevalence, morphological types, and evaluation of cardiac valvular disease in systemic lupus erythematosus. N Engl J Med 1988;319:817–823.

Thrombotic Thrombocytopenic Purpura

150. Petitt RM. Thrombotic thrombocytopenic purpura: a thirty year review. Semin Thromb Hemost 1980;6:350–355.

151. Kwaan HC. Clinicopathological features of thrombotic thrombocytopenic purpura. Semin Hematol 1987;24:71–81.

152. Silverstein A. Thrombotic thrombocytopenic purpura: the initial neurological manifestations. Arch Neurol 1968;18:358–362.

153. Rinkel G, Wijdicks E, Hene RJ. Stroke in relapsing thrombotic thrombocytopenic purpura. Stroke 1991;22:1087–1088.

154. Kelly PJ, McDonald CT, Neill GO, et al. Middle cerebral artery main stem thrombosis in two siblings with familial thrombocytopenic purpura. Neurology 1998;50:1157–1160.

155. Bakshi R, Shaikh ZA, Bates VE, Kinkel PR. Thrombotic thrombocytopenic purpura: brain CT and MRI findings in 12 patients. Neurology 1999;52:1285–1288.

156. Hinchey J, Chaves C, Apignani B, et al. A reversible posterio leukoencephalopathy syndrome. N Engl J Med 1996;334:494–500.

157. Shepard KV, Bukowski RM. The treatment of thrombotic thrombocytopenic purpura with exchange transfusions, plasma infusions and plasma exchange. Semin Hematol 1987;24:178–193.

Rheumatoid Arthritis

158. Ramos M, Mandybur TI. Cerebral vasculitis in rheumatoid arthritis. Arch Neurol 1975;32:271–275.

159. Watson P. Intracranial hemorrhage with vasculitis in rheumatoid arthritis. Arch Neurol 1979;36:58.

160. Watson P, Fekete J, Dick J. Central nervous system vasculitis in rheumatoid arthritis. Can J Neurol Sci 1977;4:269–271.

161. Takeda Y. Studies of the metabolism and distribution of fibrinogen in patients with rheumatoid arthritis. J Lab Clin Med 1967;69:624–633.

162. Jasin HE, LoSpalluto J, Ziff M. Rheumatoid hyperviscosity syndrome. Am J Med 1970;49:484–493.

Sjögren's Syndrome

163. Alexander EL, Provost TT, Stevens MB, Alexander GE. Neurologic complications of primary Sjögren's syndrome. Medicine (Baltimore) 1982;61:247–257.

164. Alexander GE, Provost TT, Stevens MB, Alexander EL. Sjögren syndrome: central nervous system manifestations. Neurology 1981;31:1391–1396.

165. Alexander EL, Beall S, Gordon B, et al. Magnetic resonance imaging of cerebral lesions in patients with the Sjögren syndrome. Ann Intern Med 1988;108:815–823.

166. Alexander EL, Malinow K, Lijewski JE, et al. Primary Sjögren syndrome with central nervous system disease mimicking multiple sclerosis. Ann Intern Med 1986;104:323–330.

Scleroderma

167. Estey E, Lieberman A, Pinto R, et al. Cerebral arteritis in scleroderma. Stroke 1979;10:595–597.

168. Pathak R, Gabor AJ. Scleroderma and central nervous system vasculitis. Stroke 1991;22:410–413.

Sarcoidosis

169. Newman LS, Rose CS, Maier LA. Sarcoidosis. N Engl J Med 1997;336:1224–1234.

170. Scott TF. Neurosarcoidosis: progress and clinical aspects. Neurology 1993;43:8–12.

171. Stern BJ, Krumholz A, Johns C, et al. Sarcoidosis and its neurological manifestations. Arch Neurol 1985;42:909–917.

172. Caplan LR, Corbett J, Goodwin J, et al. Neuro-ophthalmological signs in the angiitic form of neurosarcoidosis. Neurology 1983;33:1130–1135.

173. Meyer J, Foley J, Campagna-Pinto D. Granulomatous angiitis of the meninges in sarcoidosis. Arch Neurol Psychiatry 1953;69:587–600.

174. Alajouanine T, Bertrand J, Degos R, et al. Sarcoidose ganglionaire, cutanee et oculaire, avec atteinte secondaire diffuse, peripherique et centrale du système nerveux. Rev Neurol (Paris) 1958;99:421–447.

175. Urich H. Neurosarcoidosis or granulomatous angiitis: a problem of definition. Mt Sinai J Med 1977;44:718–725.

176. Karma A. Ophthalmic changes in sarcoidosis. Acta Ophthalmol 1979;141(Suppl):1–94.

Temporal (Giant Cell) Arteritis

177. Goodwin J. Temporal Arteritis. In P Vinken, G Bruyn (eds), Handbook of Clinical Neurology, Vol 39, Part 2. Amsterdam: North Holland, 1980;313–342.

178. Klein RG, Hunder GG, Stanson AW, et al. Large artery involvement in giant cell arteritis. Ann Intern Med 1975;83:806–812.

179. Wilkinson I, Russel R. Arteries of the head and neck in giant cell arteritis. Arch Neurol 1972;27:378–391.

180. Thielen KR, Wijdicks EFM, Nichols DA. Giant cell (temporal) arteritis: involvement of the vertebral and internal carotid arteries. Mayo Clin Proc 1998;73:444–446.

181. Enzmann D, Scott WR. Intracranial involvement of giant-cell arteritis. Neurology 1977;27:794–797.

182. Casselli RJ. Giant cell (temporal) arteritis: a treatable cause of multi-infarct dementia. Neurology 1990;40:753–755.

183. Schmidt WA, Kraft HE, Vorpahl K, et al. Color Duplex ultrasonography in the diagnosis of temporal arteritis. N Engl J Med 1997;337:1336–1342.

Granulomatous Angiitis Limited to the Central Nervous System

184. Hankey GJ. Isolated angiitis/angiopathy of the central nervous system. Cerebrovasc Dis 1991;1:2–15.
185. Kolodny EH, Rebeiz JJ, Caviness VS, Richardson EP. Granulomatous angiitis of the central nervous system. Arch Neurol 1968;19:510–524.
186. Vollmer TL, Guarnaccia J, Harrington W, et al. Idiopathic granulomatous angiitis of the central nervous system. Diagnostic challenges. Arch Neurol 1993;50: 925–930.
187. Moore PM. Diagnosis and management of isolated angiitis of the central nervous system. Neurology 1989;39:167–173.
188. Burger PC, Burch JG, Vogel FS. Granulomatous angiitis: an unusual etiology of stroke. Stroke 1977;8:29–35.
189. Harris KG, Tran DD, Sickels WJ, Cornell SH, Yuh WTC. Diagnosing intracranial vasculitis: the role of MR and angiography. AJNR Am J Neuroradiol 1994;15:317–330.
190. Alhalabi M, Moore PM. Serial angiography in isolated angiitis of the central nervous system. Neurology 1994; 44:1221–1226.

Takayasu's Disease

191. Shimizuki K, Sano K. Pulseless disease. J Neuropathol Clin Neurol 1951;1:37–47.
192. Ask-Upmark E. On the pulseless disease outside of Japan. Acta Med Scand 1954;149:161–178.
193. Lupi-Herrera E, Sanchez-Torres G, Marcushamer J, et al. Takayasu's arteritis: clinical study of 107 cases. Am Heart J 1977;93:94–103.
194. Ishikawa K. Natural history and classification of occlusive thromboaortopathy (Takayasu's disease). Circulation 1978; 57:27–35.
195. Sano K, Alga T, Saito I. Angiography in pulseless disease. Radiology 1970;94:69–74.
196. Hall S, Barr W, Lee JT, et al. Takayasu arteritis: a study of 32 North American patients. Medicine (Baltimore) 1985; 54:89–99.
197. Hargraves RW, Spetzler RF. Takayasu's arteritis: case report. Barrow Neurol Inst Q 1991;7:20–23.
198. Kerr GS, Hallahan CW, Giordano J, et al. Takayasu arteritis. Ann Intern Med 1994;120:919–929.
199. Naritomi H. Takayasu's Arteritis. In J Bogousslavsky, LR Caplan (eds), Stroke Syndromes. Cambridge: Cambridge University Press, 1995;437–442.
200. Sun Y, Yip P-K, Jeng J-S, et al. Ultrasonographic study and long-term follow-up of Takayasu's arteritis. Stroke 1996;27:2178–2182.
201. Ishikawa K, Uyama M, Asayama K. Occlusive thromboaortopathy (Takayasu's disease): cervical occlusive stenosis, retinal artery pressure, retinal microaneurysms and prognosis. Stroke 1983;14:730–735.
202. Takagi A, Tada Y, Sato O, et al. Surgical treatment for Takayasu's arteritis: a long-term follow-up study. J Cardiovasc Surg 1989;30:553–558.
203. Fraga A, Mintz G, Valle L, Flores-Izquierdo G. Takayasu's arteritis: frequency of systemic manifestations (study of 22 patients) and favorable response to maintenance steroid therapy with adrenocorticosteroids (12 patients). Arthritis Rheum 1972;15:617–624.

Behçet's Disease

204. Chajek T, Fainaro M. Behçet's disease: report of 41 cases and a review of the literature. Medicine (Baltimore) 1975; 54:179–195.
205. Shimizu T, Ehrlich GE, Inaba G, et al. Behçet's disease (Behçet's syndrome). Semin Arthritis Rheum 1979;8: 223–260.
206. Wechsler B, Davatchi F, Mizushima Y, et al. Criteria for diagnosis of Behçet's disease. Lancet 1990;335:1078–1080.
207. International Study Group for Behçet's disease. Evaluation of diagnostic ('classification') criteria in Behçet's disease: towards internationally agreed criteria. Br J Rheum 1992;31:299–308.
208. Serdaroglu P, Yazici H, Ozdemir C, et al. Neurologic involvement in Behçet's syndrome: a prospective study. Arch Neurol 1989;46:265–269.
209. Herskovitz S, Lipton RB, Lantos G. Neuro-Behçet's disease: CT and clinical correlates. Neurology 1988;38: 1714–1720.
210. Bousser, M-G, Wechsler B. Behçet's Disease. In J Bogousslavsky, LR Caplan (eds), Stroke Syndromes. Cambridge: Cambridge University Press, 1995;460–465.
211. Al Kawi MZ, Bohlega S, Banna M. MRI findings in neuro-Behçet's disease. Neurology 1991;41:405–408.
212. Banna M, El-Ramahi K. Neurologic involvement in Behçet disease: imaging findings in 16 patients. AJNR Am J Neuroradiol 1991;12:791–796.
213. Pamir MN, Kansu T, Erbengi A, Zileli T. Papilledema in Behçet's syndrome. Arch Neurol 1981;38:643–645.
214. Bousser MG, Chiras J, Bories J, Castaigne P. Cerebral venous thrombosis: a review of 38 cases. Stroke 1985;16:199–213.
215. Wechsler B, Vidailhet M, Piette JC, et al. Cerebral venous thrombosis in Behçet's disease: clinical study and long-term follow-up of 25 cases. Neurology 1992; 42:614–618.
216. Sharief MK, Hentges R, Thomas E. Significance of CSF immunoglobulins in monitoring neurologic disease in Behçet's disease. Neurology 1991;41:1398–1401.

Cogan's Syndrome

217. Cogan DG. Syndrome of nonsyphilitic interstitial keratitis and vestibulo-auditory symptoms. Arch Ophthalmol 1945; 33:144–149.
218. Cheson BD, Bluming AZ, Alroy J. Cogan's syndrome: a systemic vasculitis. Am J Med 1976;60:549–555.
219. Peeters GJ, Pinckers AJ, Cremers CW, Hoefnagels WH. Atypical Cogan's syndrome: an autoimmune disease. Ann Otol Rhinol Laryngol 1986;95:173–175.
220. Romain PL, Aretz HT. Case records of the Massachusetts General Hospital: case 6-1999. N Engl J Med 1999;340: 635–641.

Eales's Disease

221. Eales H. Case of retinal hemorrhage, associated with epistaxis and constipation. Birmingham Med Rev 1880;9:262–273.
222. Miller NR. Walsh and Hoyt's Clinical Neuroophthalmology, Vol 4 (4th ed). Baltimore: Williams & Wilkins, 1991; 2575–2729.
223. Raizman MB, Haas JJ. Case records of the Massachusetts General Hospital: Case 4-1998. N Engl J Med 1998;338: 313–319.
224. Gordon MF, Coyle PK, Golub B. Eales disease presenting as stroke in the young adult. Ann Neurol 1988;24:264–266.
225. Herson RN, Squier M. Retinal perivasculitis with neurological involvement. J Neurol Sci 1978;36:111–117.
226. Singhal BS, Dastur DK. Eales disease with neurological involvement. J Neurol Sci 1976;27:312–321, 323–345.
227. White RH. The etiology and neurological complications of retinal vasculitis. Brain 1961;84:262–273.

Microangiopathy of the Brain, Ear, and Retina

228. Susac J, Hardman J, Selhorst J. Microangiopathy of the brain and retina. Neurology 1979;29:313–316.
229. Susac JO. Susac's syndrome: the triad of microangiopathy of the brain and retina with hearing loss in young women. Neurology 1994;44:591–593.
230. Papo T, Biousse V, Lehoang P, et al. Susac syndrome. Medicine (Baltimore) 1998;77:3–11.
231. Petty G, Engel A, Younge BR, et al. Retinocochleocerebral vasculopathy. Medicine (Baltimore) 1998;77:122–40.
232. Coppeto J, Currie J, Monteiro M, et al. A syndrome of arterial-occlusive retinopathy and encephalopathy. Am J Ophthalmol 1984;98:189–202.
233. Swanson R, Mario L, Monteiro M, et al. A microangiopathic syndrome of encephalopathy, hearing loss and retinal artery occlusion. Neurology 1985;35(Suppl 1):145.
234. Bogousslavsky J, Gaio JM, Caplan LR, et al. Encephalopathy, deafness, and blindness in young women: a distinct retino-cochleo-cerebral arteriolopathy. J Neurol Neurosurg Psychiatry 1989;52:43–46.

Acute Posterior Multifocal Placoid Pigment Epitheliopathy

235. Gass JDM. Acute posterior multifocal placoid pigment epitheliopathy. Arch Ophthalmol 1968;80:177–185.
236. Jones NP. Acute posterior multifocal placoid pigment epitheliopathy. Br J Ophthalmol 1995;79:384–389.
237. Comu S, Verstraeten T, Rinkoff JS, Busis NA. Neurological manifestations of acute posterior multifocal placoid pigment epitheliopathy. Stroke 1996;27:996–1001.
238. Smith CH, Savino PJ, Beck RW, et al. Acute posterior multifocal placoid pigment epitheliopathy and cerebral vasculitis. Arch Neurol 1983;40:48–50.
239. Weinstein JM, Bresnick GH, Bell CL, et al. Acute posterior multifocal placoid pigment epitheliopathy with cerebral vasculitis. J Clin Neuroophthalmol 1988;8: 195–201.

240. Bewermeyer H, Nelles G, Huber M, et al. Pontine infarction in acute posterior multifocal placoid pigment epitheliopathy. J Neurol 1993;241:22–26.
241. Wilson CA, Choromokos EA, Sheppard R. Acute posterior multifocal placoid pigment epitheliopathy and cerebral vasculitis. Arch Ophthalmol 1988;106:796–800.

Vogt-Koyanagi-Harada Syndrome

242. Manor RS. Vogt-Koyanagi-Harada Syndrome and Related Diseases. In P Vinken, G Bruyn, H Klawans (eds), Handbook of Clinical Neurology, Vol 34, Part 2. Amsterdam: North Holland, 1978;513–544.

Sneddon's Syndrome

243. Sneddon B. Cerebro-vascular lesions and livedo reticularis. Br J Dermatol 1965;77:180–185.
244. Tourbah A, Piette JC, Iba-Zizen MT, et al. The natural course of cerebral lesions in Sneddon syndrome. Arch Neurol 1997;54:53–60.
245. Thomas DJ, Kirby JD, Britton KE, Galton DJ. Livedo reticularis and neurological lesions. Br J Dermatol 1982; 106:711–712.
246. Rebollo M, Val JF, Garijo F, et al. Livedo reticularis and cerebrovascular lesions (Sneddon's syndrome). Brain 1983;106:965–979.
247. Stockhammer G, Felber SR, Zelger B, et al. Sneddon syndrome: diagnosis by skin biopsy and MRI in 17 patients. Stroke 1993;24:685–690.
248. Pettee AD, Wasserman BA, Adams NL, et al. Familial Sneddon's syndrome: clinical, hematologic, and radiographic findings in two brothers. Neurology 1994;44:399–405.
249. Levine SR, Langer SL, Albers JW, Welch KMA. Sneddon's syndrome: an antiphospholipid antibody syndrome? Neurology 1988;38:798–800.

Kohlmeier-Degos Syndrome

250. Petit WA, Soso MJ, Higman H. Degos disease: neurologic complications and cerebral angiography. Neurology 1982; 32:1305–1309.
251. Strole WE, Clark WH, Isselbacher KJ. Progressive arterial occlusive disease (Kohlmeier-Degos). N Engl J Med 1967;276:195–201.
252. Subbiah P, Wijdicks E, Muenter M, et al. Skin lesion with a fatal neurologic outcome (Degos' disease). Neurology 1996;46:636–640.

Strokes and Vasculopathy in Drug Abusers

253. Caplan LR. Drugs. In CS Kase, LR Caplan (eds), Intracerebral Hemorrhage. Boston: Butterworth–Heinemann, 1994;201–220.

254. Brust J, Richter R. Stroke associated with addiction to heroin. J Neurol Neurosurg Psychiatry 1978;39:194–199.

255. Woods B, Strewler G. Hemiparesis occurring six hours after intravenous heroin injection. Neurology 1972;22: 863–866.

256. Caplan LR, Hier DB, Banks G. Current concepts in cerebrovascular disease—stroke: stroke and drug abuse. Stroke 1982;13:869–872.

257. Brust JC. Stroke and Drugs. In P Vinker, G Bruyn, H Klawans (eds), Handbook of Clinical Neurology, Vol 11. Amsterdam: Elsevier, 1989;517–531.

258. Pearson J, Richter R. Addiction to Opiates: Neurologic Aspects. In P Vinken, G Bruyn (eds), Handbook of Clinical Neurology, Vol 37. Amsterdam: North Holland, 1979;365–400.

259. Citron B, Halpern M, McCarron M, et al. Necrotizing angiitis associated with drug abuse. N Engl J Med 1970; 283:1003–1011.

260. Rumbaugh C, Bergeron R, Gang H, et al. Cerebral vascular changes secondary to amphetamine abuse in the experimental animal. Radiology 1971;101:345–351.

261. Rumbaugh C, Bergeron R, Gang H, et al. Cerebral angiographic changes in the drug abuse patient. Radiology 1971;101:335–344.

262. Caplan LR, Thomas C, Banks G. Central nervous system complications of "T's and Blues" addiction. Neurology 1982;32:623–628.

263. Szwed JJ. Pulmonary angiothrombosis caused by "blue velvet" addiction. Ann Intern Med 1970;73:771–774.

264. Atlee W. Talc and cornstarch emboli in the eyes of drug abusers. JAMA 1972;219:49–51.

265. Mizutami T, Lewis R, Gonatas N. Medial medullary syndrome in a drug abuser. Arch Neurol 1980;37:425–428.

266. Kaku D, Lowenstein DH. Emergence of recreational drug abuse as a major risk factor for stroke in young adults. Ann Intern Med 1990;133:821–827.

267. Levine SR, Welch KM. Cocaine and stroke: current concepts of cardiovascular disease. Stroke 1988;19:779–783.

268. Daras M, Tuchman AJ, Marks S. Central nervous system infarction related to cocaine abuse. Stroke 1991;22:1320–1325.

269. Levine SR, Washington JM, Jefferson ME, et al. "Crack" cocaine-associated stroke. Neurology 1987;37:1849–1853.

270. Levine SR, Brust JC, Futrell N, et al. A comparative study of the cerebrovascular complications of cocaine—alkaloidal versus hydrochloride—a review. Neurology 1991;41:1173–1177.

271. Rowley HA, Lowenstein DH, Rowbotham MC, Simon RP. Thalamomesencephalic strokes after cocaine abuse. Neurology 1989;39:428–430.

272. Di Lazzaro V, Restuccia D, Oliviero A, et al. Ischaemic myelopathy associated with cocaine: clinical, neurophysiological, and neuroradiological features. J Neurol Neurosurg Psychiatry 1997;63:531–533.

273. Isner JM, Estes NA, Thompson PD, et al. Acute cardiac events temporally related to cocaine. N Engl J Med 1986; 315:1438–1443.

274. Kaufman MJ, Levin JM, Ross MH, et al. Cocaine-induced cerebral vasoconstriction detected in humans with magnetic resonance angiography. JAMA 1998;279:376–380.

275. Nolte KB, Brass LM, Fletterick CF. Intracranial hemorrhage associated with cocaine abuse: a prospective study. Neurology 1996;46:1291–1296.

Migraine

276. Caplan LR. Migraine in Posterior Circulation Disease: Diagnosis, Clinical Findings, and Management. Boston: Blackwell, 1996.

277. Rothrock JF, Walicke P, Swendon M, et al. Migrainous stroke. Arch Neurol 1988;45:63–67.

278. Bogousslavsky J, Regli F, Van Melle G, et al. Migraine stroke. Neurology 1988;38:223–227.

279. Caplan LR. Migraine and vertebrobasilar ischemia. Neurology 1991;41:55–61.

280. Rothrock J, North J, Madden K, et al. Migraine and migrainous stroke: risk factors and prognosis. Neurology 1993;43:2473–2476.

281. Solomon S, Lipton RB, Harris PY. Arterial stenosis in migraine: spasm or arteriopathy? Headache 1990;30:52–61.

282. Pessin MS, Lathi ES, Cohen MB, et al. Clinical features and mechanisms of occipital infarction in the posterior cerebral artery territory. Ann Neurol 1987;21:290–299.

283. Fisher CM. Late-life migraine accompaniments as a cause of unexplained transient ischemic attacks. Can J Neurol Sci 1980;7:9–17.

284. Fisher CM. Late-life migraine accompaniments: further experience. Stroke 1986;17:1033–1042.

285. Wijman CAC, Wolf PA, Kase CS, et al. Migrainous visual accompaniments are not rare in late life. The Framingham Study. Stroke 1998;29:1539–1543.

286. Caplan LR, Chedru F, Lhermitte F, Mayman C. Transient global amnesia and migraine. Neurology 1981;31:1167–1170.

287. Caplan LR. Transient Global Amnesia: Characteristic Features and Overview. In HJ Markowitsch (ed), Transient Global Amnesia and Related Disorders. Toronto: Hogrife and Huber, 1990;15–27.

288. Call GK, Fleming MC, Sealfon S, et al. Reversible cerebral segmental vasoconstriction. Stroke 1988;19:1159–1170.

289. Lopez-Valdes E, Chang H-M, Pessin MS, Caplan LR. Cerebral vasoconstriction after carotid surgery. Neurology 1997;49:303–304.

290. Cole AJ, Aube M. Migraine with vasospasm and delayed intracerebral hemorrhage. Arch Neurol 1990;47:53–56.

291. Gautier JC, Majdalani A, Juillard JB, et al. Hemorragies cerebrales au cours de la migraine. Rev Neurol (Paris) 1993;149:407–410.

292. Caplan LR. Intracerebral hemorrhage revisited. Neurology 1988;38:624–627.

Moyamoya Syndrome

293. Suzuki J, Kodama N. Moyamoya disease—a review. Stroke 1983;14:104–109.

294. Suzuki J. Moyamoya Disease. Berlin: Springer, 1986.

295. Chiu D, Shedden P, Bratina P, Grotta JC. Clinical features of Moyamoya disease in the United States. Stroke 1998; 29:1347–1351.

296. Taveras JM. Multiple progressive intracranial arterial occlusions: a syndrome of children and young adults. AJR Am J Roentgenol 1969;106:235–268.

297. Bruno A, Adams HOP, Bilbe J, et al. Cerebral infarction due to moyamoya disease in young adults. Stroke 1988; 19:826–833.
298. Mauro AJ, Johnson ES, Chikos PM, Alvord EC. Lipohyalinosis and miliary microaneurysms causing cerebral hemorrhage in a patient with Moyamoya. A clinicopathological study. Stroke 1980;11:405–412.
299. Ikeda E. Systemic vascular changes in spontaneous occlusion of the circle of Willis. Stroke 1991;22:1358–1362.
300. Ueki K, Meyer FB, Mellinger JF. Moyamoya disease: the disorder and surgical treatment. Mayo Clin Proc 1994; 69:749–757.
301. Herreman F, Nathal E, Yasui N, Yonekawa Y. Intracranial aneurysms in moyamoya disease: report of ten cases and review of the literature. Cerebrovasc Dis 1994;4:329–336.
302. Robertson RL, Burrows PE, Barnes PD, et al. Angiographic changes after pial synangiosis in childhood moyamoya disease. AJNR Am J Neuroradiol 1997;18:837–845.
303. Houkin K, Kamiyama H, Abe H, et al. Surgical therapy for adult Moyamoya disease. Can surgical revascularization prevent the recurrence of intracerebral hemorrhage? Stroke 1996;27:1342–1346.

Hematological Disorders and Stroke

304. Hart RG, Kanter MC. Hematologic disorders and ischemic stroke: a selective review. Stroke 1990;21:1111–1121.
305. Markus HS, Hambley H. Neurology and the blood: haematological abnormalities in ischaemic stroke. J Neurol Neurosurg Psychiatry 1998;64:150–159.

Sickle Cell Disease

306. Rothman SM, Fulling KH, Nelson JS. Sickle cell anemia and central nervous system infarction: a neuropathological study. Ann Neurol 1986;20:684–690.
307. Adams RJ, Nichols FT, McKie V, et al. Cerebral infarction in sickle cell anemia: mechanisms based on CT and MRI. Neurology 1988;38:1012–1017.
308. Steen RG, Langston JW, Ogg RJ, et al. Ectasia of the basilar artery in children with sickle cell disease: relationship to hematocrit and psychometric measures. J Stroke Cerebrovasc Dis 1998;7:32–43.
309. Oguz M, Aksungur EH, Soyupak SK, Yildirim AU. Vein of Galen and sinus thrombosis with bilateral thalamic infarcts in sickle cell anemia: CT follow-up and angiographic demonstration. Neuroradiology 1994; 36:155–156.
310. Adans RJ, McKie VC, Nichols F, et al. The use of transcranial ultrasonography to predict stroke in sickle cell disease. N Engl J Med 1992;326:605–610.
311. Adams RJ, McKie VC, Hsu L, et al. Prevention of a first stroke by transfusions in children with sickle cell anemia and abnormal results on transcranial Doppler ultrasonography. N Engl J Med 1998;339:5–11.

Paroxysmal Nocturnal Hemoglobinuria

312. Hillmen P, Lewis SM, Bessler M, et al. Natural history of paroxysmal nocturnal hemoglobinuria. N Engl J Med 1995;333:1253–1258.
313. Al-Hakim M, Katirji B, Osorio I, Weisman R. Cerebral venous thrombosis in paroxysmal nocturnal hemoglobinuria: report of two cases. Neurology 1993;43:742–746.

Platelet Disorders

314. Murphy S, Iland H, Rosenthal D, Laszlo J. Essential thrombocythemia: an interim report from the Polycythemia Vera Study Group. Semin Hematol 1986;23:177–182.
315. Jabaily J, Iland HJ, Laszlo J, et al. Neurologic manifestations of essential thrombocythemia. Ann Intern Med 1983;99:513–518.
316. Hehlmann R, Jahn M, Baumann B, Kopcke W. Essential thrombocythemia. Clinical characteristics and course of 61 cases. Cancer 1988;61:2487–2496.
317. Wu K. Platelet hyperaggregability and thrombosis in patients with thrombocythemia. Ann Intern Med 1978;88:7–11.
318. Al-Mefty O, Marano G, Rajaraman S, et al. Transient ischemic attacks due to increased platelet aggregation and adhesiveness. J Neurosurg 1979;50:449–453.
319. Trip MD, Cats VM, van Capelle FJL, Vreeken J. Platelet hyperreactivity and prognosis in survivors of myocardial infarction. N Engl J Med 1990;322:1549–1554.

Coagulopathies

320. Thaler E, Lechner K. Antithrombin III deficiency and thromboembolism. Clin Haematol 1981;10:369–390.
321. Camerlingo M, Finazzi G, Casto L, et al. Inherited protein C deficiency and nonhemorrhagic arterial stroke in young adults. Neurology 1991;41:1371–1373.
322. Dahlback B, Carlsson M, Svensson PJ. Familial thrombophilia due to a previously unrecognized mechanism characterized by poor anticoagulant response to activated protein C: prediction of a cofactor to activated protein C. Proc Natl Acad Sci U S A 1993;90:1004–1008.
323. Zoller B, Dahlback B. Linkage between inherited resistance to activated protein C and factor V gene mutation in venous thrombosis. Lancet 1994;343:1536–1538.
324. Ridker PM, Miletich JP, Stampfer MJ, et al. Factor V Leiden and risks of recurrent idiopathic venous thromboembolism. Circulation 1997;95:1777–1782.
325. Poort SR, Rosendaal FR, Reitsma PH, Bertina RM. A common genetic variation in the 3' untranslated region of the prothrombin gene is associated with elevated prothrombin levels and an increase in venous thrombosis. Blood 1996;88:3698–3703.
326. Huberfeld G, Kubis N, Lot G, et al. G20210A Prothrombin gene mutation in two siblings with cerebral venous thrombosis. Neurology 1998;51:316–317.
327. Martinelli I, Sacchi E, Landi G, et al. High risk of cere-

bral-vein thrombosis in carriers of a prothrombin-gene mutation and in users of oral contraceptives. N Engl J Med 1998;338:1793–1797.

328. Estol C, Pessin MS, DeWitt LD, Caplan LR. Stroke and increased factor VIII activity. Neurology 1989;39(Suppl 1): 1159.

329. Kosik KS, Furie B. Thrombotic stroke associated with elevated factor VIII. Arch Neurol 1980;8:435–437.

330. Talbot RW, Heppell J, Dozois RR, Beart RW. Vascular complications of inflammatory bowel disease. Mayo Clin Proc 1986;61:140–145.

331. Johns DR. Cerebrovascular complications of inflammatory bowel disease. Am J Gastroenterol 1991;86:367–370.

332. Sigsbee B, Rottenberg DA. Sagittal sinus thrombosis as a complication of regional enteritis. Ann Neurol 1978;3: 450–452.

333. Grau A, Buggle F, Heindl S, et al. Recent infection as a risk factor for cerebrovascular ischemia. Stroke 1995;26: 373–379.

334. Syrjanen J, Valtonen VV, Iivanainen M, et al. Preceding infection as an important risk factor for ischaemic brain infarction in young and middle aged patients. BMJ 1988; 296:1156–1160.

335. Grau A, Buggle F, Steichen-Wiehn C, et al. Clinical and histochemical analysis in infection-associated stroke. Stroke 1995;26:1520–1526.

336. Grau A. Infection, inflammation, and cerebrovascular ischemia. Neurology 1997;49(Suppl 4):S47–S51.

337. Sack GH, Levin J, Bell WR. Trousseau's syndrome and other manifestations of chronic disseminated coagulopathy in patients with neoplasms. Medicine (Baltimore) 1977;56:1–37.

338. Graus F, Rodgers LR, Posner JB. Cerebrovascular complications in patients with cancer. Medicine (Baltimore) 1985;64:16–35.

339. Amico L, Caplan LR, Thomas C. Cerebrovascular complications of mucinous cancers. Neurology 1989;39:523–526.

340. Sloane MA. Thrombolysis and stroke—past and future. Arch Neurol 1986;44:748–768.

341. Del Zoppo GH, Zeumer H, Harker LA. Thrombolytic therapy in stroke: possibilities and hazards. Stroke 1986;17: 595–607.

342. Francis RB. Clinical disorders of fibrinolysis. Blut 1989; 59:1–14.

343. Nagayama T, Shinohara Y, Nagayama M, et al. Congenitally abnormal plasminogen in juvenile ischemic cerebrovascular disease. Stroke 1993;24:2104–2107.

344. Hunt FA, Rylatt DB, Hart R, Bundesen PG. Serum cross-linked fibrin (XDP) and fibrinogen/fibrin degradation products (FDP) in disorders associated with activation of the coagulation or fibrinolytic systems. Br J Haematol 1985;60:715–722.

345. Feinberg WM, Bruck DC, Ring ME, Corrigan JJ. Hemostatic markers in acute stroke. Stroke 1989;20:582–587.

Antiphospholipid Antibodies

346. Levine SR, Welch KMA. Cerebrovascular ischemia associated with lupus anticoagulant. Stroke 1987;18:257–263.

347. DeWitt LD, Caplan LR. Antiphospholipid antibodies and stroke. AJNR Am J Neuroradiol 1991;12:454–456.

348. Coull BM, Goodnight SH. Antiphospholipid antibodies, prothrombotic states, and stroke. Stroke 1990;21:1370–1374.

349. Levine SR, Kim S, Deegan MI, Welch KMA. Ischemic stroke associated with anticardiolipin antibodies. Stroke 1987;18:1101–1106.

350. Montalban J, Codina A, Ordi J, et al. Antiphospholipid antibodies in cerebral ischemia. Stroke 1991;22:750–753.

351. Pope JM, Canny CL, Bell DA. Cerebral ischemic events associated with endocarditis, etinal vascular disease, and lupus anticoagulant. Am J Med 1991;90:299–309.

352. The Antiphospholipid Antibodies in Stroke Study (APASS) Group. Clinical and laboratory findings in patients with antiphospholipid antibodies and cerebral ischemia. Stroke 1990;21:1268–1273.

353. Feldmann E, Levine SR. Cerebrovascular disease with antiphospholipid antibodies: immune mechanisms, significance, and therapeutic options. Ann Neurol 1995;37 (Suppl 1):S114–S130.

354. Levine SR, Salowich-Palm L, Sawaya KL, et al. IgG anticardiolipin antibody titer >40 GPL and the risk of subsequent thrombo-occlusive events and death. A prospective cohort study. Stroke 1997;28:1660–1665.

355. Verro P, Levine SR, Tietjen GE. Cerebrovascular ischemic events with high positive anticardiolipin antibodies. Stroke 1998;29:2245–2253.

356. Provenzale JM, Barboriak DP, Allen NB, Ortel TL. Antiphospholipid antibodies: findings at arteriography. AJNR Am J Neuroradiol 1998;19:611–616.

Disseminated Intravascular Coagulation

357. Bick RL. Disseminated intravascular coagulation and related syndromes: a clinical review. Semin Thromb Hemost 1988;14:299–338.

358. Wen PY, Sobel RA. Case records of the Massachusetts General Hospital: Case 36-1991. N Engl J Med 1991;325: 714–726.

359. Colman RW, Rubin RN. Disseminated intravascular coagulation due to malignancy. Semin Oncol 1990;17:172–186.

360. Schwartzman RJ, Hill JB. Neurologic complications of disseminated intravascular coagulation. Neurology 1982; 32:791–797.

361. Schwartzman RJ. Disseminated Intravascular Coagulation. In J Bogousslavsky, LR Caplan (eds), Stroke Syndromes. Cambridge: Cambridge University Press, 1995; 470–475.

Hyperviscosity

362. Grotta J, Ackerman R, Correia J, et al. Whole blood viscosity parameters and cerebral blood flow. Stroke 1982; 13:296–301.

363. Coull BM, Beamer N, de Garmo P, et al. Chronic blood hyperviscosity in subjects with acute stroke, transient ischemic attack, and risk factors for stroke. Stroke 1991; 22:162–168.

364. Ernst E, Resch KL. Fibrinogen as a cardiovascular risk factor: a meta-analysis and review of the literature. Ann Intern Med 1993;118:956–963.

365. Fahey JL, Barth WF, Solomon A. Serum hyperviscosity syndrome. JAMA 1965;192:464–467.

366. Rosenson RS, Baker AL, Chow M, Hay R. Hyperviscosity syndrome in a hypercholesterolemic patient with primary biliary cirrhosis. Gastroenterology 1990;98:1351–1357.

Neoplastic Conditions

367. Fauci A, Haynes BF, Costa J, et al. Lymphatoid granulomatosis: prospective clinical and therapeutic experience over 10 years. N Engl J Med 1982;306:68–74.

368. Hogan PJ, Greenberg MK, McCarty GE. Neurologic complications of lymphomatoid granulomatosis. Neurology 1981;31:619–620.

369. Petito CK, Gottlieb GJ, Dougherty JH, Petito FA. Neoplastic angioendotheliosis: ultrastructural study and review of the literature. Ann Neurol 1978;3:393–399.

370. Beal MF, Fisher CM. Neoplastic angioendotheliosis. J Neurol Sci 1982;53:359–375.

371. Reinglass JL, Miller J, Wissman S. Central nervous system angioendotheliosis. Stroke 1977;8:218–221.

372. Raroque HG, Mandler RN, Griffey MS, et al. Neoplastic angioendotheliomatosis. Arch Neurol 1990;47:929–930.

373. Williams RL, Meltzer CC, Smirniotopoulos JG, et al. Cerebral MR imaging in intravascular lymphomatosis. AJNR Am J Neuroradiol 1998;19:427–431.

374. LeWitt PA, Forno LS, Brant-Zawadzki M. Neoplastic angioendotheliosis: a case with spontaneous regression and radiographic appearance of cerebral arteritis. Neurology 1983;33:39–44.

375. Hamada K, Hamada T, Satoh M, et al. Two cases of neoplastic angioendotheliomatosis presenting with myelopathy. Neurology 1991;41:1139–1140.

Genetic Disorders

376. Natowicz M, Kelley RI. Mendelian etiologies of stroke. Ann Neurol 1987;22:175–192.

377. Massa SM. An update on genetic influences on stroke. J Neurovasc Dis 1998;3:109–116.

378. Albert M. Genetics of Cerebrovascular Disease. Mt. Kisco, Armonk, New York: Futura, 1999.

Mitochondrial Myopathy, Encephalopathy, Lactic Acidosis, and Stroke-Like Episodes

379. Pavlakis SG, Phillips PC, DiMauro S, et al. Mitochondrial myopathy, encephalopathy, lactic acidosis, and stroke-like episodes: a distinctive clinical syndrome. Ann Neurol 1984;16:481–488.

380. Morgan-Hughes JA. Mitochondrial Diseases. In AG Engel, C Franzini-Armstrong (eds), Myology, Vol 2, (2nd ed). New York: McGraw-Hill, 1994;1610–1660.

381. Kuriyama M, Umezaki H, Fukuda Y, et al. Mitochondrial encephalomyopathy with lactate-pyruvate elevation and brain infarctions. Neurology 1984;34:72–77.

382. Allard JC, Tilak S, Carter AP. CT and MR of MELAS syndrome. AJNR Am J Neuroradiol 1988;9:1234–1238.

383. Koo B, Becker LE, Chuang S, et al. Mitochondrial encephalomyopathy, lactic acidosis, stroke like episodes (MELAS): clinical, radiological, and genetic observations. Ann Neurol 1993;34:25–32.

384. Matthews PM, Tampieri D, Berkovic SF, et al. Magnetic resonance imaging shows specific abnormalities in the MELAS syndrome. Neurology 1991;41:1043–1046.

385. Clark JM, Marks MP, Adalsteinsson E, et al. MELAS: clinical and pathological correlations with MRI, xenon/CT, and MR spectroscopy. Neurology 1996;46:223–227.

386. Sue CM, Crimmins DS, Soo YS, et al. Neuroradiological features of six kindreds with MELAS tRNALeu A3243G point mutation: implications for pathogenesis. J Neurol Neurosurg Psychiatry 1998;65:233–240.

Fabry's Disease

387. Brady RO, Gal AE, Bradley RM, et al. Enzymatic defect in Fabry's disease: ceramide trihexosidase deficiency. N Engl J Med 1967;276:1163–1167.

388. Dawson DM, Miller DC. Case records of the Massachusetts General Hospital: Case 2-1984. N Engl J Med 1984;310:106–114.

389. Kolodny E. Fabry Disease. In J Bogousslavsky, LR Caplan (eds), Stroke Syndromes. Cambridge: Cambridge University Press, 1995;453–459.

390. Mitsias P, Levine SR. Cerebrovascular complications of Fabry's disease. Ann Neurol 1996;40:8–17.

391. Kint JA. Fabry's disease: alpha-galactosidase deficiency. Science 1970;167:1268–1269.

392. Philippart M, Franklin SS, Gordon A. Reversal of an inborn sphingolipidosis (Fabry's disease) by kidney transplantation. Ann Intern Med 1972;77:195–200.

Cerebral Autosomal Dominant Arteriopathy with Subcortical Infarcts and Leukoencephaly (CADASIL)

393. Tournier-Lasserve E, Iba-Zizen M-T, Romero N, Bousser M-G. Autosomal dominant syndrome with stroke-like episodes and leukoencephalopathy. Stroke 1991;22:1297–1302.

394. Mas JL, Dilouya A, de Recondo J. A familial disorder with subcortical ischemic strokes, dementia, and leukoencephalopathy. Neurology 1992;42:1015–1019.

395. Hutchinson M, O'Riordan J, Javed M, et al. Familial hemiplegic migraine and autosomal dominant arteriopa-

thy with leukoencephalopathy (CADASIL). Ann Neurol 1995;38:817–824.

396. Ragno M, Tournier-Lasserve E, Fiori MG, et al. An Italian kindred with cerebral autosmal dominant arteriopathy with subcortical infarcts and leukoencephalopathy (CADASIL). Ann Neurol 1995;38:231–236.

397. Dichgans M, Mayer M, Uttner I, et al. The phenotypic spectrum of CADASIL: clinical findings in 102 cases. Ann Neurol 1998;44:731–739.

398. Chabriat H, Levy C, Taillia H, et al. Patterns of MRI lesions in CADASIL. Neurology 1998;51:452–457.

399. Joutel A, Corpechot C, Ducros A, et al. Notch 3 mutations in CADASIL, a hereditary adult-onset condition causing stroke and dementia. Nature 1996;383:707–710.

400. Fukutake T, Hirayama K. Familial young-adult-onset arteriosclerotic leukoencephalopathy with alopecia and lumbago without arterial hypertension. Eur Neurol 1995;35: 69–79.

Menkes' Disease

401. Menkes J, Alter M, Steigleder G, et al. A sex-linked recessive disorder with retardation of growth, peculiar hair and focal cerebral and cerebellar degeneration. Pediatrics 1962;29:764–779.

402. Iannaccone ST, Rosenberg RN. Menkes Disease. In B Berg (ed), Principles of Child Neurology. New York: McGraw-Hill, 1995;473–475.

403. Morgello S, Peterson HD, Kahn LJ, Laufer H. Menkes kinky hair disease with 'ragged red fibers.' Dev Med Child Neurol 1988;30:812–816.

Neurofibromatosis

404. Taboada D, Alonso A, Moreno J. Occlusion of the cerebral arteries in Recklinghausen's disease. Neuroradiology 1979;18:281–284.

405. Levinsohn PM, Mikhael MA, Rothman SM. Cerebrovascular changes in neurofibromatosis. Dev Med Child Neurol 1978;20:789–793.

406. Rizzo JF, Lessell S. Cerebrovascular abnormalities in neurofibromatosis type l. Neurology 1994;44:1000–1002.

Homocystinuria and Homocysteinemia

407. Boers GH, Smals AG, Trijbels FJ, et al. Heterozygosity for homocystinuria in premature peripheral and cerebral occlusive disease. N Engl J Med 1985;313:709–715.

408. Welch GN, Loscalzo J. Homocysteine and atherothrombosis. N Engl J Med 1998;338:1042–1050.

409. Caplan LR, Hurst JW. Homocysteinemia and Homocystinuria. In LR Caplan, JW Hurst, M Chimowitz (eds), Clinical Neurocardiology. New York: Marcel Dekker, 1999;431–432.

410. Ueland PM, Refsum H, Stabler SP, et al. Total homocysteine in plasma or serum; methods and clinical applications. Clin Chem 1993;39:1764–1769.

411. Finkelstein JD, Martin JJ, Harris BJ. Methionine metabolism in mammals: the methionine-sparing effect of cystine. J Biol Chem 1988;263:11750–11754.

412. Mudd SH, Skovby F, Levy HL, et al. The natural history of homocystinuria due to cystathione-beta-synthase deficiency. Am J Hum Genet 1985;37:1–31.

413. Vermaak WJ, Ubbink JB, Barnard HC, et al. Vitamin B6 nutrition status and cigarette smoking. Am J Clin Nutr 1990;51:1058–1061.

414. Clarke R, Daly L, Robinson K, et al. Hyperhomocysteinemia: an independent risk factor for vascular disease. N Engl J Med 1991;324:1149–1155.

415. Evers S, Koch H-G, Grotemeyer K-H, et al. Features, symptoms, and neurophysiological findings in stroke associated with hyperhomocysteinemia. Arch Neurol 1997;54:1276–1282.

416. Selhub J, Jacques PF, Bostom AG, et al. Association between plasma homocysteine concentrations and extracranial carotid-artery stenosis. N Engl J Med 1995;332: 286–291.

417. Harker LA, Slichter SJ, Scott CR. Homocystinemia: vascular injury and arterial thrombosis. N Engl J Med 1974; 291:537–543.

418. Harker LA, Ross R, Slichter SJ, Scott CR. Homocystine-induced arteriosclerosis: the role of endothelial cell injury and platelet response in its genesis. J Clin Invest 1976; 58:731–741.

419. Tsai J-C, Perrella MA, Yoshizumi M, et al. Promotion of vascular smooth muscle cell growth by homocysteine: a link to atherosclerosis. Proc Natl Acad Sci U S A 1994;91: 6369–6373.

Chapter 12

Subarachnoid Hemorrhage, Aneurysms, and Vascular Malformations

As with those hectic fevers, as doctors say, which at their beginning are easy to cure but difficult to recognise, but in the course of time when they have not at first been recognised and treated, become easy to recognise and difficult to cure.

—Niccolo Machiavelli

Intracranial hemorrhages involve the brain parenchyma or subarachnoid space, or both. Approximately 20% of strokes are hemorrhagic, with subarachnoid hemorrhage (SAH) and intracerebral hemorrhage (ICH) accounting for approximately 10%. SAH occurs when a blood vessel near the brain surface leaks, causing extravasation of blood into the subarachnoid space. SAH is most often caused by rupture of a saccular aneurysm or hemorrhage from an arteriovenous malformation (AVM). Less common causes include head injury, use of illicit drugs, especially amphetamines and cocaine, amyloid angiopathy, venous-sinus thrombosis, and bleeding disorders.

Symptoms depend on the rapidity and duration of the bleeding and the volume of blood. Rupture of an arterial aneurysm causes the abrupt introduction of blood under arterial pressure into the subarachnoid space. This increases intracranial pressure and leads to transient cessation of activity, severe headache, and vomiting. Slower leakage of blood does not increase intracranial pressure as rapidly. Blood in the subarachnoid space acts as a meningeal irritant and incites headache, photophobia, and stiff neck. Confusion, restlessness, and transient or persistent decreased levels of consciousness are common in patients with SAH and are caused by the increased intracranial pressure.

Aneurysms

Ruptured saccular aneurysms are a common and serious medical problem. According to necropsy and angiography series, approximately 5–6% of individuals have intracranial aneurysms.[1,2] The prevalence of aneurysms is low during the first two decades of life and increases steadily after the third decade.[1] The annual incidence of rupture of saccular aneurysms is less, approximately 10–12 per 100,000.[2–5] Overall, ruptured aneurysms are more common in women. Although ruptured aneurysms are more common in men younger than 40 years, women prevail after age 40.[6,7] The average age at rupture is approximately 50 years.[8]

Despite the low frequency of rupture, the high prevalence of aneurysms and the poor prognosis of patients with SAH result in considerable social and economic consequences. Among 100 typical patients with SAH caused by ruptured aneurysms, it is estimated that 33 will die before receiving medical attention. Another 20 will die while in the hospital or will remain incapacitated from the original hemorrhage. Seventeen patients who survive the initial hemorrhage will deteriorate later, with eight patients recovering and nine patients left with severe neurologic sequelae.[9] Only 30 of the original 100 patients will do well, surviving without major disability. If the ruptured aneurysm remains surgically untreated and the patient does not have recurrent hemorrhage during the first 6 months, approximately 3% of the remaining patients will rebleed each year.[10] Even among patients admitted to the hospital in good condition, the prognosis is poor. In one series, 29% of these patients died and only 55% made a good recovery at 90 days.[11] A delay often occurs in referring patients with SAH to neurologic and neurosurgical centers for treatment. In one series among 150 consecutive patients with aneurysmal SAH, only 36% were referred within 48 hours. The median time to referral was 3.6 days.[12] Tragically, delayed diagnosis by physicians and logistic and policy issues accounted for more than 70% of the delays.[12]

Dolichoectatic aneurysms and dissecting aneurysms can also rupture, causing SAH. These lesions are discussed in Chapters 2 and 11.

Pathogenesis

Saccular aneurysms typically form at arterial bifurcations (see Figure 2-21). Approximately 90% of aneurysms involve anterior circulation arteries.[13] Common sites in the anterior circulation include (1) the junction between the anterior communicating artery (AComA) and the anterior cerebral artery (ACA); (2) bifurcation of the middle cerebral artery (MCA); and (3) the internal carotid artery (ICA) junction with the ophthalmic artery, posterior communicating artery (PComA), anterior choroidal artery (AChA), and MCAs.[8] In the posterior circulation, the apex of the basilar artery and the intracranial vertebral artery, especially at the origins of the posterior inferior cerebellar arteries (PICAs), are the most common sites.[8,13] Approximately 25% of patients have more than one aneurysm. Saccular aneurysms are more common in patients with polycystic kidney disease, coarctation of the aorta, fibromuscular dysplasia, pseudoxanthoma elasticum, and Marfan's syndrome.

No completely satisfactory explanation of the origin, growth, and rupture of saccular aneurysms exists. Intracerebral arteries are normally composed of an outer collagenous adventitia, a prominent muscular media, an internal elastic lamina, and an intima lined by endothelial cells. An external elastic lamina does not exist. Intracranial arteries are more susceptible than extracranial arteries to aneurysm formation because intracranially, the arterial walls are thin, less elastin exists, an external elastic lamina

is not present, and vessels lying in the subarachnoid space lack surrounding supporting tissue. Various theories cite congenital and genetic abnormalities that cause defects in the arterial media, hypertensive and atherosclerotic degenerative changes in the vessel walls, inflammatory proliferative arteritis, and focal degeneration of the internal elastic lamina. Some investigators emphasize that aneurysms form because of congenital defects in the media of arteries. The most common defect in the arterial media is a localized loss of muscular elements. These focal deficits are often located at arterial bifurcations. Some patients with intracranial aneurysms have reduced production of type III collagen.[14]

A plausible and inclusive hypothesis was proposed by Ferguson.[15] Ferguson suggested that cerebral aneurysms result from mechanically induced degeneration of arteries. Maximal hemodynamic stress at the apices and bifurcations of arteries exist. Imbalance between the strength of an artery at a particular bifurcation and the hemodynamic stresses applied to it lead to degeneration of the internal elastic lamina and aneurysmal outpouching. Turbulent flow in and around aneurysms produces vibration in vessel walls, further weakening the vessel's structural integrity and allows aneurysm growth.[15] The observation that aneurysms may form at sites of increased flow, in arteries feeding AVMs or in vessels providing collateral blood flow, supports the contention that increased pressure and flow contribute to aneurysm formation. Stress of the vessel wall increases as aneurysms become thinner, the radius of the aneurysm enlarges, or the intra-aneurysmal pressure increases because of elevated blood pressure. When the wall stress exceeds the wall strength, aneurysms rupture.

Aneurysms may rupture at any time, but especially when blood pressure or blood flow is increased. Rupture often occurs during strenuous activity, such as weight lifting, exercise, coition, defecation, and heavy work. Many aneurysms, however, leak during relatively inactive periods. One-third of the aneurysms in the Cooperative Study of Intracranial Aneurysms and Subarachnoid Hemorrhage[7,9] ruptured while patients were asleep, and another one-third ruptured during ordinary daily activities.[16] Size also plays a major role; up to a point, the larger the aneurysm, the more likely it is to rupture. In different autopsy series, the critical size for rupture has varied from 7 to 10 mm.[17–19] Aneurysms larger than

10 mm in diameter are more likely to rupture during follow-up than smaller aneurysms.[2]

Aneurysms larger than 2.5 cm in size are usually referred to as *giant aneurysms*. The notion that they rarely rupture and produce SAH is erroneous. Drake reported that 33% of giant aneurysms present with bleeding and another 10% have a history of remote hemorrhage.[20] Giant aneurysms often contain intra-aneurysmal thrombi.

Once an intracranial aneurysm has ruptured, the course is often stormy and the outcome poor. It is estimated that of the 28,000 patients with ruptured aneurysms each year in the United States and Canada, 7,000 are misdiagnosed, never referred, or referred too late for definitive therapy.[12,21] The greatest impact improving morbidity and mortality from SAH is not through the efforts of neurologists or neurosurgeons, but rather through early recognition of SAH by primary care physicians. Diagnosed early, these patients can be referred while still relatively intact to centers with appropriate neurologic, neurosurgical, neuroradiologic, and neuroanesthetic capabilities. Neurologic intensive care units are also important for definitive treatment of patients with ruptured aneurysms and their complications.

Clinical Findings

A 32-year-old woman, PN, came to the emergency ward because of a headache that had been unremitting for 48 hours. She had migraine headaches as an adolescent. One month ago, she awakened at night with moderately severe headache and vomiting. After the headache persisted for 3 days, she consulted her physician, who diagnosed her with the flu. Although she had no fever, she felt too ill to do her daily chores and stayed in bed for 1 week, after which the headache gradually cleared. Two days ago, she developed a severe headache that came on suddenly. She was taking heavy trash cans out for garbage collection when the pain struck her in the left temple and top of the head and quickly radiated to her neck and back. Her knees buckled with the pain and she vomited. She stumbled into the house and was in bed and rather sleepy when her husband returned from work and insisted that she go to the hospital.

Headache

Intracranial saccular aneurysms often present with a warning leak or so-called sentinel hemorrhage—a minute rent in the aneurysm leaks for only seconds, spilling blood into the subarachnoid space under high pressure. The patient has sudden, severe headache, often occipital or nuchal in location, and constant. The headache generally resolves in 48 hours but can last longer. It is best distinguished from migraine by its rapidity of onset and longer duration. Only seconds elapse before it reaches maximum intensity. Vomiting and cessation of activity (e.g., the knees buckling in patient PN) and decrease in alertness often accompany the headache. Migraine headaches, on the other hand, are usually more throbbing and build in intensity over minutes. Nausea and vomiting usually develop after migraine headache has been present for minutes to hours. Sentinel headaches usually last from days to a week, during which time patients are seldom able to continue normal activities. Sentinel hemorrhages are often misdiagnosed as migraine, flu, hypertensive encephalopathy, aseptic meningitis, cervical neck strain, or even gastroenteritis.[22] Headache, restlessness, and vomiting are often falsely attributed to food poisoning or an acute gastrointestinal disorder.

In patient PN, the headache she had 1 month before her episode was probably a warning leak. The duration was too long for migraine and inability to carry out daily activities should have alerted her physician to evaluate her further. In the Michael Reese Stroke Registry and the University of Illinois Stroke Registry, 31% of patients with SAH had sentinel headaches.[23] In the Danish Aneurysm Study, a warning leak was present in 166 of 1,076 patients (15.4%).[24] In 99 of the 166 patients (54%) with warning leaks, the headache episode was evaluated by a doctor but misdiagnosed.[24] Ostergaard emphasized that as many as 50–60% of patients with SAH have headache or other warning signs before presenting with major bleeds.[25] In patients with headaches of acute onset, the index of suspicion for SAH should be high and the threshold for lumbar puncture (LP) low. In patients with sudden, severe headache without focal neurologic signs, the only absolute contraindications to LP are no back or no needle. If

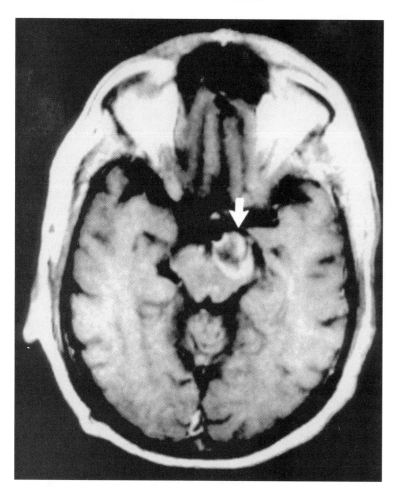

Figure 12-1. Magnetic resonance imaging shows a large aneurysm (*arrow*) compressing the cerebral peduncle on one side, associated with a third nerve palsy and contralateral hemiparesis (Weber's syndrome). (Reprinted with permission from LR Caplan. Subarachnoid Hemorrhage, Aneurysms, and Vascular Malformations. In LR Caplan, Posterior Circulation Disease: Clinical Findings, Diagnosis, and Management. Boston: Blackwell, 1996;633–685.)

series of LPs for headache contain only taps positive for blood, then too few LPs are being performed, and sentinel hemorrhages are being missed.

PN's headache, which began 2 days before her episode, is typical of that found in SAH. Sudden onset with rapid radiation, especially to the neck and back or sciatic region, suggests meningeal irritation. The focal asymmetric headache is a fairly reliable sign that the bleeding lesion was on the left side—the site of the head pain.

Neurologic Symptoms and Signs

Examination of PN showed a restless but sleepy woman with a stiff neck. The left eyelid was droopy. When the lid was lifted, the left eye rested down and out. The left pupil was dilated and unreactive to light. Plantar responses were bilaterally extensor.

Aneurysms may present by compressing adjacent brain tissue or cranial nerves. Giant aneurysms are particularly noted for their tendency to cause focal symptoms and signs related to mass effect. Giant MCA aneurysms can cause seizures, hemiparesis, or dysphasia. The third nerve can be compressed by aneurysms of the ICA and posterior cerebral artery (PCA) junction or by SCA aneurysms. A giant SCA aneurysm can cause contralateral hemiplegia (Weber's syndrome) by compressing the pyramidal tracts in the midbrain. Figure 12-1 shows a large aneurysm compressing the cerebral peduncle on one side. An isolated sixth-nerve paresis can be caused by mass effect. In the cavernous sinus, an aneurysm may compress the sixth, fourth, or third cranial nerves, producing ophthalmoplegia. Basilar bifurcation aneurysms that point forward can mimic pituitary tumors and cause visual field defects and hypopituitarism. Basilar bifurcation aneurysms that point vertically can cause an amnesic syndrome combined with third-nerve paresis, bulbar signs, and quadriparesis.[13,26] In PN, the left third-nerve palsy suggested a left PComA aneurysm.

Occasionally, aneurysms present with transient neurologic deficits. These transient ischemic attacks may be secondary to ischemia or seizures. Stewart et al. reported short, recurrent, stereotyped episodes in three patients with ischemia and in a fourth patient with transient spells secondary to partial complex seizures.[27] Computed tomography (CT) of the brain, LP, and electroencephalogram were normal. No cardiac source of embolism could be identified. Cerebral arteriography showed aneurysms in appropriate locations to explain the symptoms in all cases. Thrombi may form within aneurysms, dislodge, and then embolize distally, causing stroke. Sutherland et al. confirmed this hypothesis, showing deposition of platelets within giant aneurysms.[28] In three of the six patients in their series with active platelet deposition, episodes of recurrent transient neurologic dysfunction occurred. Identification of aneurysms presenting in this manner is another indication for performing arteriography in patients with recurrent transient neurologic deficits, particularly those in whom no cardiac source has been identified and those younger than 45 years of age. Magnetic resonance imaging (MRI) scans also often show heterogeneous signals, indicating thrombi within aneurysms. Figure 12-2 is an MRI that shows heterogeneous signals, indicating thrombus within a large basilar artery aneurysm that compresses the pons. Figure 12-3 is an angiogram that shows a filling defect caused by thrombus within an aneurysm.

Patients with SAH usually report sudden-onset, constant headaches that reach maximal intensity within seconds. Nausea, vomiting, stiff neck, and transient loss of consciousness are common accompaniments. The patient is often quite agitated and restless. The headache is of such note that the patient is sometimes later able to describe in minute detail the circumstances surrounding the episode. SAH is rarely present without headache. Occasionally, I have cared for patients in whom the initial manifestation of the subarachnoid bleed was neck pain or backache with sciatic radiation. Patients may not report headache if they have confusion, lethargy, aphasia, or amnesia for the event. Transient loss of consciousness is caused by the sudden increase of intracranial pressure (ICP) that occurs as arterial blood suddenly enters the subarachnoid space. The increased ICP, dissection of blood into the optic-nerve sheath, and increased pressure in central retinal veins can cause retinal hemorrhages, usually subhyaloid in location. These hemorrhages appear as large red masses of blood spreading outward from the optic disk into the retina. Papilledema may develop later. Unilateral or bilateral sixth-nerve paresis is also common and is a reflection of increased ICP. Some focal signs that suggest the sites of aneurysmal rupture have already been mentioned. Additional signs include:

1. Leg weakness, confusion, and bilateral Babinski signs in patients with AComA aneurysms [29]
2. Homonymous hemianopia in PCA aneurysms
3. Aphasia, hemiparesis, and anosognosia in MCA aneurysms
4. Monocular visual disturbances in ophthalmic-artery aneurysms

Because aneurysms that have previously bled may become adherent to the adjacent brain, recurrent rupture is often characterized by intracerebral and subarachnoid bleeding, so-called meningocerebral hemorrhage.

The patient's clinical state has traditionally been graded according to the scale of Hunt and Hess (Table 12-1),[30] which is useful for predicting short- and long-term prognosis.[31] In general, the higher the grade, the worse the prognosis. I classified patient PN's status as Hunt and Hess Grade II.

Diagnostic Procedures

Cranial CT in PN was suboptimal because of motion. Diffuse opacification of the cortical gyri occurred and blood was visible in the basal cisterns. LP revealed bloody fluid with an opening pressure of 420 mm Hg. She was placed at bed rest and observed carefully.

Computed Tomography

CT of the brain is most often the first diagnostic test in the evaluation of patients with suspected SAH. CT often verifies the presence of blood in the

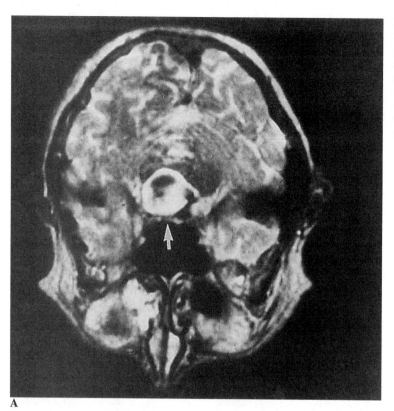

A

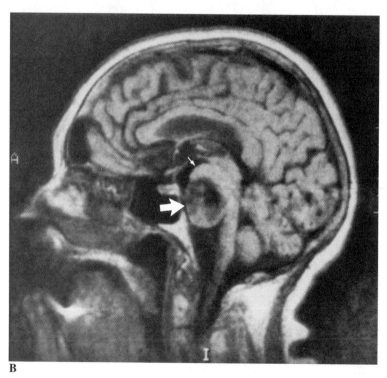

B

Figure 12-2. (**A**) T2-weighted magnetic resonance imaging: Arrow points to large basilar artery aneurysm that contains heterogeneous signals and represents thrombus formation. (**B**) Sagittal magnetic resonance imaging shows aneurysm with clot (*large arrow*) compressing the pons (*small arrow*).

Figure 12-3. Vertebral arteriogram, intracranial Towne view: Arrow points to a filling defect in a vertebral artery aneurysm, representing thrombus.

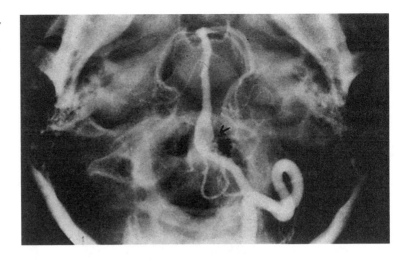

subarachnoid space and demonstrates associated intraparenchymal blood. The location of the blood may suggest the site of rupture, especially if there is a parenchymatous hematoma or the bleeding is from an AComA aneurysm.[29,32–34] A temporal-lobe hematoma or collection of blood in the sylvian fissure suggests an MCA aneurysm. Figure 12-4 is a CT scan that shows blood in the subarachnoid space and basal cisterns with the major collection occurring in the left sylvian fissure region. This patient has a large ruptured left MCA aneurysm. In AComA aneurysms, blood fills the subfrontal region, anterior interhemispheric fissure, pericallosal cistern, and septum.[29] Large aneurysms (larger than 10 mm) are occasionally also shown. In a contrast-infused CT scan, aneurysms appear as small, round densities on arteries located along the circle of Willis. Giant aneurysms may also be shown as contrast-enhancing masses. The amount of blood helps predict the likelihood of subsequent vasoconstriction.[35,36] CT may show a dilated ventricular system with hydrocephalus caused by disturbance of cerebrospinal fluid (CSF) dynamics by blood clogging the basal cisterns and pacchionian granulations. A normal CT scan does not exclude SAH; a normal scan occurs if the hemorrhage is small, especially if the scan is delayed 24–72 hours. Computed tomography angiography (CTA) can most often image intracranial aneurysms on the arteries of the circle of Willis.[37] In PN, SAH was confirmed by CT (Figure 12-5); the amount of blood was moderate and most of the blood was located in the basal cisterns, more on the left side.

Table 12-1. Hunt and Hess Classification of Subarachnoid Hemorrhage

Classification	Symptoms
Grade I	Asymptomatic or minimal headache and slight nuchal rigidity
Grade II	Moderate to severe headache, nuchal rigidity, no neurologic deficit other than cranial nerve palsy
Grade III	Drowsiness, confusion, or mild focal deficit
Grade IV	Stupor, moderate to severe hemiparesis, possible early decerebrate rigidity and vegetative disturbance
Grade V	Deep coma, decerebrate rigidity, moribund appearance

Source: Reprinted with permission from W Hunt, R Hess. Surgical risk as related to time of intervention in the repair of intracranial aneurysms. J Neurosurg 1968;28:14–20.

Magnetic Resonance Imaging

MRI is probably less sensitive than CT in showing acute subarachnoid blood. Vascular malformations, especially cavernous angiomas, however, are seen well on MRI as well-circumscribed structures with heterogeneous signals. Magnetic resonance angiography (MRA) is proving quite accurate in imaging aneurysms and showing the relationship of the aneurysm to adjacent brain structures. In one series, aneurysms as small as 3–4 mm were usually reliably detected by MRA,

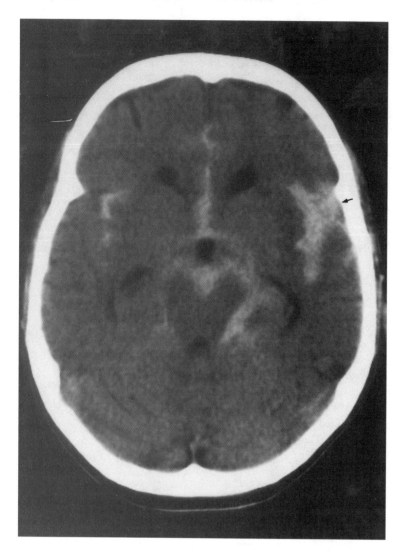

Figure 12-4. Computed tomography scan shows blood in the subarachnoid space and basal cisterns. The most blood is pooled in the left sylvian fissure (*arrow*). This patient had an aneurysm of the left middle cerebral artery that is shown in Figure 12-7B.

but some lesions (3 among 21 aneurysms) were missed.[38] Some arteries and aneurysms were not well imaged, and details were often insufficient for surgeons to define the neck and the extent of the aneurysms. At present, CTA and MRA are best used as screening tests for asymptomatic or large aneurysms, but not as definitive tests in patients with SAH who are potential surgical candidates.

Lumbar Puncture

I advocate LP as an important diagnostic step, especially if CT is normal and clinical suspicion of SAH is still present.[39] The spinal fluid usually shows:

1. Large numbers of red blood cells, without clearing of cells, between the first and last tubes
2. A faint pink color of supernatant fluid if examined within 4–5 hours of hemorrhage
3. A deep yellow (xanthochromic) color of the centrifuged supernatant fluid, secondary to breakdown of heme pigments; hemoglobin is first formed and is later transformed to bilirubin
4. Elevated protein
5. Pleocytosis, usually mononuclear
6. Increased pressure
7. Normal glucose

Spinal fluid obtained after 72 hours may show only an elevated pressure, xanthochromia, and

Figure 12-5. Computed tomography scan of patient PN shows blood in the subarachnoid space, predominantly in the basal cisterns. More blood is present on the left side.

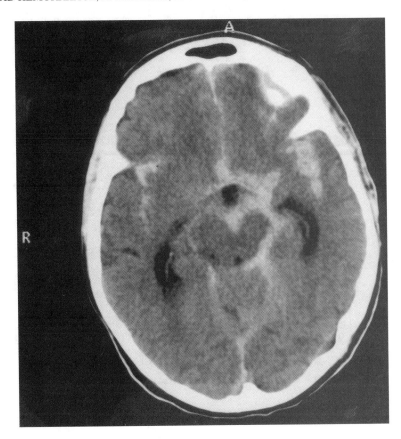

increased protein. Spectrophotometry, by quantifying the amounts of hemoglobin and bilirubin, gives information regarding the approximate age of the hemorrhage.[39]

Controversy exists as to the advisability of LP in confirmed SAH. Some argue that sudden lowering of pressure may provoke bleeding. I advocate LP, even in CT-confirmed SAH. The initial LP gives a baseline pressure and quantification of the number of red blood cells. This information may be useful later if the patient deteriorates and a second hemorrhage is suspected. The level of CSF pressure is an important parameter to follow. Spinal tap also helps remove blood and CSF. Also, by lowering the CSF pressure, spinal tap often relieves headache. Subsequent LPs help document the pressure and blood contents. Surgical complications are more common when the CSF pressure is greater than 180 mm Hg at the time of operation.

Angiography

PN gradually became more alert and her headache waned. By the third hospital day (5 days after onset of SAH), the plantar responses were flexor. Angiography showed an 8-mm by 12-mm large irregular aneurysm at the junction of the left ICA and PComA (Figure 12-6). No important focal or generalized vascular narrowing existed. On the next day, repeat LP showed an opening pressure of 160 mm Hg and no fresh blood. Surgical clipping of the aneurysm was accomplished on the following day.

Cerebral angiography remains the definitive method of showing intracranial aneurysms. Arterial digital subtraction angiography is the preferred technique, allowing excellent arterial opacification and rapid filming with less dye. In patients with con-

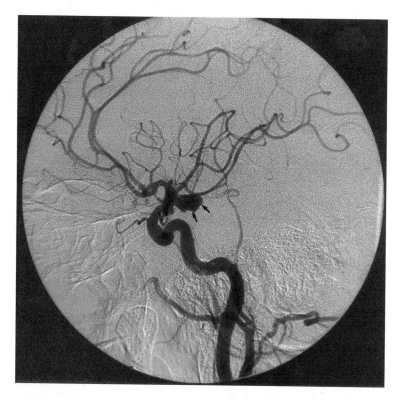

Figure 12-6. Large left posterior communicating artery aneurysm (*arrows*) 8 × 12 mm in size. (Submitted by Drs. Galen Henderson, Brigham and Women's Hospital and Rafael Llinas, Beth Israel Deaconess Hospital.)

firmed SAH, I delay angiography until the patient is considered operable. If the diagnosis is uncertain, however, I often pursue early angiography. Some physicians always obtain immediate arteriograms to define the bleeding aneurysm. If the patient is quite sick, definitive angiography is often difficult to perform early, so I prefer to wait. Figure 12-7 shows angiograms of aneurysms at the most common sites.

Vasoconstriction may also be potentiated by angiography, making complete studies difficult. In patient PN, I waited to perform angiography until she could be classified as Hunt and Hess Grade I. Because aneurysms may be multiple, all four intracranial arteries should be studied, with antero-posterior, lateral, and oblique views if needed. If multiple aneurysms are identified, the bleeding aneurysm is usually:

1. The largest aneurysm
2. The most irregularly shaped aneurysm
3. The aneurysm with the most associated focal spasm, as discussed later in this chapter
4. The aneurysm in the vascular territory, explaining the focal signs
5. The aneurysm that best correlates with the collection of blood on CT

At times, despite well-documented SAH, no aneurysm is identified angiographically. In general, the prognosis of these patients is better than when an aneurysm is demonstrated, but the etiologies of such bleeds are diverse.[40,41]

Other Diagnostic Techniques

Transcranial Doppler (TCD) is a useful technology for detecting AVMs [42–45] and monitoring the intra-cranial circulation for vasoconstriction.[42,46–49] Serial TCD measurements of flow velocities in the basal arteries after moderate- and large-volume SAHs often show an increase in velocities during days 3–10 and maximum velocities between days 11 and 20. Time-averaged maximum velocities in the MCA greater than 140 cm per second accurately predict vascular narrowing at angiography. Velocities greater than 200 cm per second predict severe vasoconstriction.[42] Doppler-measured velocities in the MCA have an inverse relationship to vascular diameter.

Single-photon emission computed tomography (SPECT) is also a useful test for monitoring the presence of vasoconstriction. Regional hypoperfusion correlates well with vasoconstriction and delayed brain infarcts in patients with SAH.[49,50]

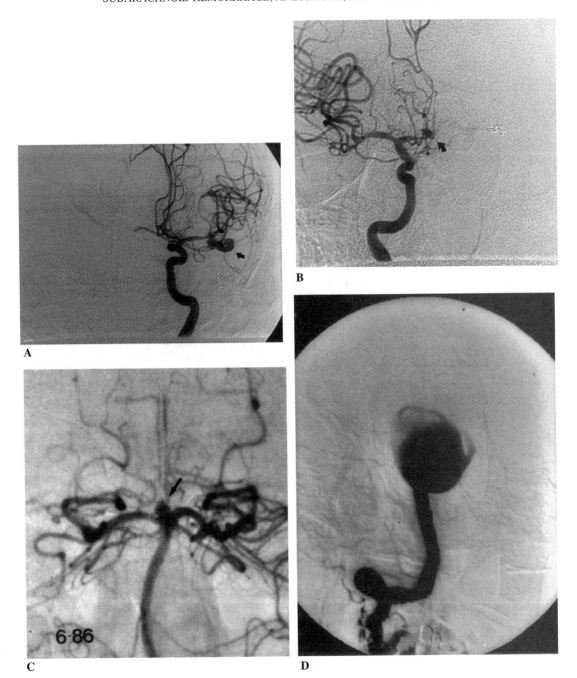

Figure 12-7. Angiograms show aneurysms at other common sites. **(A)** Large middle cerebral artery aneurysm (*arrow*). (Submitted by Drs. Galen Henderson, and Rafael Llinas, Brigham and Women's Hospital, Beth Israel Deaconess Hospital.) **(B)** Anterior communicating artery aneurysm (*arrow*). (Submitted by Drs. Galen Henderson and Rafael Llinas.) **(C)** Small basilar bifurcation aneurysm (*arrow*). **(D)** Large basilar bifurcation aneurysm.

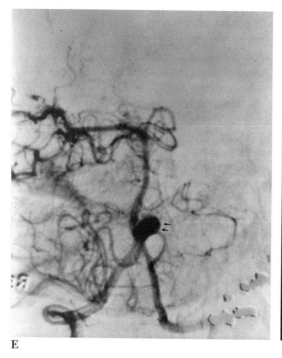
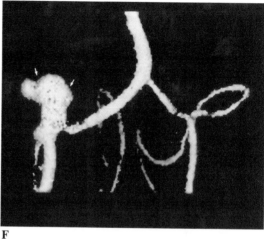

E

F

Figure 12-7 *continued.* Angiograms show aneurysms at other common sites. **(E)** Aneurysm (*arrows*) at the vertebral-basilar artery junction. **(F)** Aneurysm at the vertebral-posterior inferior cerebellar artery junction (*arrows*) shown on computed tomography angiography.

Differential Diagnosis

Van Gijn and colleagues noted that a high proportion of patients with SAHs located predominantly in the perimesencephalic cisterns by CT had normal cerebral angiography.[51,52] Newer-generation CT scans and MRI have shown that these hemorrhages are often centered around the prepontine cistern.[53] Because these hemorrhages are concentrated around the brain stem, Schievink, Wijdicks, and colleagues suggest that they be called *pretruncal subarachnoid hemorrhages* (*truncus cerebri* is another term for the brain stem), rather than *perimesencephalic hemorrhages.*[53,54] The clinical course in patients with pretruncal hemorrhage is different from aneurysmal SAH because few patients die, rebleed acutely, or develop delayed cerebral infarction or hydrocephalus.[52,55] The outcome is much more benign than in patients with aneurysms shown by angiography.[52,55] The etiology of these hemorrhages around the brain stem is unknown, but a venous or capillary leak is often posited. In one patient with a pretruncal hemorrhage, a capillary telangiectasia was shown in the

ventral pons by MRI.[56] Because SAH resulting from rupture of a posterior circulation aneurysm can also cause bleeding centered around the brain stem, an angiogram is always warranted in such patients. If the initial angiogram is technically adequate and negative, however, a repeat angiogram has a low yield of showing an aneurysm.

Patients with SAH and normal angiography have a variety of different etiologies.[41] I have seen a number of patients who had hemorrhage into the caudate nucleus with extension into the ventricular system, which simulates SAH.[57] AVMs may also involve the subependymal region and may bleed directly into the ventricles and CSF. Before the era of CT scans, these intraventricular hemorrhages and other brain hemorrhages may have accounted for some examples of SAH with normal arteriography. Other explanations include:

1. SAH secondary to trauma
2. Blood dyscrasias and sickle cell disease
3. Nonvisualizing angioma or an unseen small aneurysm
4. Thrombosis of a ruptured aneurysm

5. Leakage from a small nonaneurysmal artery on the brain surface[58]
6. Dural AVMs [41,59]
7. Intracranial arterial dissections
8. Cocaine abuse
9. Pituitary apoplexy
10. Spinal AVMs

The possibility of an erroneous diagnosis of SAH should also be considered. Other conditions, such as cerebral venous thrombosis, tumor, infection, or traumatic LP, can mimic SAH. If the clinical picture is characterized by back pain, radicular signs, or myelopathic signs, I order a spinal MRI and prone and supine myelograms and look for a spinal AVM. In situations in which vasoconstriction is prominent but no aneurysm is seen, I repeat angiography to better visualize the intracranial arteries after the clinical state improves.

Complications of Aneurysmal Subarachnoid Hemorrhage and Their Management

Rebleeding

Management of patients with SAH is one of the most difficult problems in clinical medicine. The complications are myriad and management trends change almost yearly. Table 12-2 lists common complications of SAH during the acute and later periods. For ease of recall, I think of the "nine Hs."

The most feared complication in patients with SAH is recurrent aneurysmal rupture. The initial bleed and rehemorrhage are the major causes of death in patients with aneurysmal SAH.[60] In one study, which had a 45% (36/80) mortality, 64% (23/36) of deaths were attributable to the initial SAH and eight of the remaining 13 deaths were caused by recurrent hemorrhages.[60] Rebleeding is heralded by sudden, abrupt, severe, headache; meningismus; focal signs associated with intraparenchymal hemorrhage; and rapid development of coma. Among aneurysms that rebleed, approximately 20% do so in the first 2 weeks, 30% by the end of the first month, and 40% by the end of 6 months. Beyond 6 months, rerupture occurs at a rate of approximately 3% per year.[3,7] Rebleeding is associated with 40% mortality.[7] No infallible rules predict which patients will have recurrent hemorrhage.

Table 12-2. Complications of Subarachnoid Hemorrhage (The Nine Hs)

Early
Hypertension (intracranial)
Hypertension (systemic)
Heart failure and arrhythmia
Hematoma
Delayed
Hemorrhage (rebleed)
Hypoperfusion (vasospasm)
Hydrocephalus
Hypovolemia
Hyponatremia

Efforts are directed to reduce those factors that may promote rebleeding. Patients are placed at bed rest with minimal stimuli. Pain is controlled with analgesics. Sedatives are used. Patients are kept from straining at stool by regular use of laxatives and stool softeners. These measures are attempts to avoid elevations in blood pressure, which could increase intra-aneurysmal pressure and increase the risk of rebleeding. When feasible, early surgery is the best measure to prevent a second bleed.

Delayed Cerebral Ischemia (Vasoconstriction)

Second only to rebleeding as a cause of significant morbidity and mortality is vasoconstriction. *Vasoconstriction* is defined as abnormal narrowing of intracranial arteries. The narrowing of intracranial arteries found in patients with SAH has customarily been called *vasospasm*. Purists argue that *vasoconstriction* is a more accurate designation because it is a structural term that does not imply mechanism, whereas *spasm* usually refers to functional reversible changes. The narrowing of arteries in SAH often persists, and chronic morphologic changes develop. Therefore, *vasospasm* is an inaccurate designation.

The pathogenesis of vasoconstriction is unknown but is probably related to the release of substances into the CSF from the subarachnoid blood and the interaction of these substances within the arteries in the subarachnoid space. Erythrocytes and their subsequent hemolysis are necessary for vasospasm to develop.[61,62] The most likely putative substance is oxyhemoglobin, which affects the function of platelet-derived growth factor, released from platelets adherent to the arterial wall; endothelial factors, especially endothelial-derived relaxing factor, and components of the coagulation cascade, especially thrombin, plasmin, and fibrinogen.[61] An abnormal contraction or failure of relaxation of the arterial smooth muscle occurs. Patients who die from SAH with vasoconstriction less than 3 weeks after the initial hemorrhage show necrosis of the media, whereas patients who live longer than 3 weeks show marked concentric intimal thickening, subendothelial fibrosis, and medial atrophy.[62–65] The adventitia shows adherent clot with inflammatory cell infiltrates and degeneration of perivascular nerve terminals.[62] The media shows smooth muscle contraction with varying degrees of fibrosis and necrosis.[62] The intima develops longitudinal furrows, and endothelial cells often desquamate, necrose, and have abnormalities of intercellular tight junctions.[62] Intracranial arteries in experimental animals subjected to SAH show severe subintimal proliferation, fibrosis of medial smooth muscle, and interruption of the internal elastic membrane.[65,66]

SAH probably induces vasoconstriction, which is then followed by arterial wall necrosis. Vasoconstriction usually has its onset 3–5 days after the hemorrhage. The peak timing for vasoconstriction is 5–9 days. Most vasospasm resolves after the second week.[62,67–69] Vasoconstriction also occurs postoperatively, probably because of the handling of arteries and, at times, is caused by intraoperative bleeding. Vasoconstriction has been detected arteriographically in 30–70% of SAH patients.[70] Approximately two-thirds of patients undergoing angiography during the second week after SAH show vasoconstriction.[62] Angiographic diagnosis is based on the narrowed appearance of the intracranial arteries. Severe vasoconstriction is associated with a lumen smaller than 0.5 mm with delayed forward flow and evidence of collateral artery blood flow from anastomotic circulation. Some arteries are diffusely narrowed, whereas others show focal constrictions. Only approximately one-half of the patients with arteriographically demonstrable vasoconstriction are symptomatic. Increased blood flow velocities detected by TCD correlate well with angiographically documented vasoconstriction.[47–49]

Early signs of vasoconstriction include tachycardia, hypertension, electrocardiographic abnormalities, and decreased level of consciousness. Some patients, especially those with diffuse vasoconstriction, develop signs of diffuse brain dysfunction, including headache, stupor, and confusion. Focal neurologic signs often accompany these global signs and depend on the artery involved. Often, the most severe vasoconstriction is in the artery harboring the aneurysm or lying within the surrounding blood clot. Occasionally, maximal vasoconstriction occurs at a distance from the aneurysm. Patients with MCA vasoconstriction develop hemiparesis, hemisensory loss, aphasia, anosognosia, and confusion. With ACA vasoconstriction, there may be weakness in one or both lower extremities, abulia, and apraxia. PCA territory ischemia causes hemianopia and hemisensory loss. CT scan of the brain provides confirmatory data, ruling out intraparenchymal hemorrhage and hydrocephalus as a cause of the delayed deterioration. Focal hypodensity representing infarction is often seen. SPECT and perfusion MRI may document decreased perfusion of brain supplied by the constricted arteries.

The following clinical and neuroimaging findings correlate with the development of significant vasoconstriction:

1. Thick blood clots localized in the subarachnoid cisterns[67] and the amount of subarachnoid blood[35,36,71]
2. Arterial lumen size smaller than 0.5 mm, with low distal perfusion
3. Aneurysms located on the circle of Willis[72]
4. Decreased level of consciousness[35]
5. Intraventricular blood[35]
6. Treatment with antifibrinolytic agents (treatment increases likelihood of vasoconstriction)[35]

The ideal treatment of vasoconstriction is prevention. Prevention has taken various directions, including early surgery, volume expansion, clot removal or lysis, and prophylactic drug regimens.[62,73] Blood can be washed from the subarachnoid space during early surgery, and some authors report a low incidence of symptomatic vasospasm in those patients in whom postoperative CT scans showed removal of blood.[74–76] Another approach has been to use urokinase or tissue plasminogen-activator to lyse clots after aneurysm clipping.[77,78] Another popular therapy to counteract vasoconstriction is expansion of intravascular volume, sometimes with elevation of blood pressure.[73,78–80] Blood and serum volumes are often low in patients with SAH.[81] Patients with normal blood volumes seldom have symptomatic ischemia, despite angiographically shown vasoconstriction.[81] Volume expansion, induced hypervolemia, hypertension, and hemodilution have no known effects on the vascular narrowing but help maintain CBF above ischemic thresholds by increasing cardiac output and improving blood rheology.[80–82] Aggressive volume expansion requires intensive care, and substantial risk of complications exists.[62] Many neurologists and neurosurgeons advocate avoidance of hypotension, hyponatremia, hypovolemia, and administration of at least 3 liters of fluid a day rather than aggressive volume expansion.[62] Elevation of arterial pressure pharmacologically is only advisable after aneurysms are clipped or when patients are hypotensive.

The results of preliminary British[83] and American[84] trials reported during the early 1980s suggested that nimodipine, a calcium channel blocker, might decrease the incidence and severity of vasoconstriction and could improve outcome. Potential mechanisms of action of nimodipine, nicardipine, and other calcium channel blockers include a decrease in vasospasm, improved blood flow by dilation of collateral arteries, neuronal protection by decreasing entry of calcium into cells, and improvement of blood rheology.[62] A number of trials have shown that nimodipine does improve outcome and decreases the frequency of delayed cerebral infarction. A systematic review of 10 trials (including 2,756 patients) of calcium channel blockers in patients with SAH reported a 33% relative risk reduction in the frequency of ischemic neurologic deficits and a 20% relative risk reduction in the development of infarcts on CT scans.[85] The relative risk reduction of poor outcome (death or dependence) was 16% and 10% for death alone.[85] Administration of nimodipine, nicardipine, and other calcium channel–blocking agents can cause decreased blood pressure and renal function, especially when the drugs are given intravenously, so that blood pressure, urinary output, and renal function must be carefully monitored. Nimodipine is the drug of choice and is given 15–30 g/kg per hour intravenously or 30–90 mg enterally every 4 hours.

Since 1989, patients with vasoconstriction demonstrated angiographically, with related neurologic symptoms, have been treated by interventional radiologists with transluminal angioplasty using various catheter devices.[86–88] The technology is quite new and changes frequently. Intra-arterial papaverine (a vasodilator) is often used as an adjunct to angioplasty.[88] Few physicians are trained and experienced in these intravascular interventions. Clearly, this treatment shows great promise for the future.

It seems prudent to prevent hypovolemia by liberal use of fluids orally and intravenously in patients with SAH. Nimodipine is given intravenously or enterally for the first 10 days. In those with vasoconstriction shown angiographically, volume expansion and maintenance of blood pressure should be pursued. This is best supervised in an intensive care unit, and, usually, measurement of pulmonary wedge pressures are needed during aggressive volume expansion. ICP monitoring is also often helpful in following the effects of osmotic diuretics, steroids, and fluid removal on ICP and CBF. TCD and SPECT are also useful in monitoring blood-flow velocities in the basal arteries and hemispheric blood flow. Diffusion and perfusion-weighted MRI is also helpful in detecting and quantifying vasoconstriction-related regions of hypoperfusion.[89] Small, often multiple regions of ischemia shown by diffusion-weighted imaging are surrounded by larger regions of decreased perfusion.[89] Angioplasty performed by a trained and experienced interventionist is used when available in patients with symptomatic vasospasm who have not responded to medical therapy. Surgery should be performed as early as possible when patients are in good condition.[90,91]

Hydrocephalus

In addition to rebleeding and vasospasm, other complications can lead to deterioration of patients with ruptured aneurysms. Acute hydrocephalus is caused by alteration in normal CSF dynamics. CSF flow is blocked by blood in the cisterns around the brain stem and reabsorption is impaired when blood attaches to the pacchionian granulations. The syndrome can be recognized by increasing headache, lethargy, incontinence, and decreased spontaneity. Diagnosis is readily confirmed by noncontrast CT scans. In a large study of the timing of aneurysm surgery, the authors analyzed factors that predicted hydrocephalus among 3,521 patients with SAH admitted within 3 days of bleeding.[92] The factors that increased the likelihood of hydrocephalus were older age, hypertension (by history, admission blood pressure, and postoperative measurements), thick local or diffuse blood on CT, intraventricular hemorrhage, use of antifibrinolytic drugs, and reduced level of consciousness.[92] Often, repeat LPs are adequate to treat ventricular enlargement, which often becomes obvious early after SAH. A few patients will need ventricular drainage shunts. In the months to years that follow SAH, normal-pressure hydrocephalus may develop as the arachnoid becomes fibrotic and adhesions prevent normal CSF flow.

Cardiac and Pulmonary Abnormalities

Cardiopulmonary complications often occur in patients with SAH. Careful surveillance for arrhythmias, heart failure, and myocardial infarction is required. I monitor cardiac rhythm, obtain baseline and follow-up electrocardiograms (ECGs) and cardiac enzymes, and carefully watch for clinical signs of congestive heart failure. Severe SAHs can be accompanied by ECG abnormalities,[93,94] enzyme elevations mimicking myocardial infarction,[95] and arrhythmias.[96–99] The most striking ECG changes are so-called waterfall T waves, which are seen across the endocardium. ECG abnormalities include alterations in QRS configuration, Q-T interval prolongation, T-wave abnormalities, and S-T segment elevation or depression.[93,94] Subendocardial hemorrhages and myofibrillar degeneration have been noted at necropsy in patients dying after SAH and other strokes.[100–102] The pathologic abnormalities of cardiac muscle cells have usually been referred to as *myocytolysis*. Striations within myocardial muscle cells are lost, and the cytoplasm often becomes hyalinized. Measurements show that some enzymes are lost from the muscle cells.[102] The number of muscle cells decrease, but the sarcolemma, stroma, and nuclei usually remain. Lipofuchsin is found within myofibrils. Often, there is a coagulative type of myocytolysis in which cardiac muscle cells die in a hypercontracted state with early myofibrillar damage and anomalous irregular cross-band formation.[102] This type of pathologic change have also been called *myofibrillar degeneration* and *contraction band necrosis*. Early calcium entry with calcifications are seen in regions of myocytolysis.[100–102]

Elevated circulating serum catecholamines or sympathetic discharges that originate from the hypothalamus and affect the myocardium may be responsible for these myocardial cell abnormalities.[101,102] Cardiac lesions probably represent excitotoxin-induced injury. Although ECG changes are common, myocardial infarction is rare.

Cardiac abnormalities are occasionally accompanied by clinical and necropsy evidence of pulmonary edema. In one series of 178 fatal SAHs, 71% had necropsy evidence of pulmonary edema, recognized clinically in only 31%.[103] Pulmonary edema is neurogenic in origin. It is characterized by rapid onset, high protein in the edema fluid, and acutely elevated ICP. Weir suggested that pulmonary edema is caused by an acute rise in ICP, which triggers a massive autonomic discharge that results in increased cerebral perfusion and accumulation of fluid within the lungs and hypoxemia.[103] Treatment is directed at lowering ICP and eliminating excess fluid. Intubation, controlled ventilation, positive end-expiratory pressure, osmotic and loop diuretics, and drainage of spinal fluid may be needed.

Fluid and Electrolyte Abnormalities

Less common, but still an important cause of neurologic worsening, are fluid and electrolyte abnormalities. Slight sodium and potassium shifts without clinical consequence occurred among 25% in one series of aneurysm patients.[104] Sodium levels were in the range of 130–135 mEq/liter. Potassium levels were in the range of 4.5–5 mEq/liter. In another 14% of patients, more severe abnormalities included five patients with diabetes insipidus, two abnormalities of thirst regulation, one instance of inappropriate secretion of antidiuretic hormone, and nine patients with serious sodium and potassium shifts.[104] In these patients, the serum sodium was less than 130 mEq/liter and the potassium was greater than 5 mEq/liter. Hyponatremia is associated with a poor prognosis. Water and electrolyte disturbances are most frequent with aneurysms of the AComA.

In postmortem studies, severe fluid and electrolyte abnormalities are associated with hemorrhage or ischemic changes in the hypothalamus.[105] In the past, hyponatremia has been attributed to inappropriate secretion of antidiuretic hormone, but in 1991, it was shown that the plasma concentration of atrial natriuretic factor is elevated and higher in those patients with suprasellar and intraventricular blood.[106,107] Peerless identified 30 additional, less common causes of neurologic deterioration after SAH, including enlargement of the aneurysm, seizures, pulmonary emboli, infection, medication side effects, renal failure, and hepatic failure.[108]

Other Treatment Considerations

Blood Pressure Control

Care must be taken in managing blood pressure. Elevated ICP causes an increase in venous pressure inside the cranium. To perfuse the brain, an arteriovenous pressure gradient must be maintained for systemic blood pressure to rise. Ordinarily, if the blood pressure is not excessively high, I do not routinely lower it, especially if vasoconstriction is present. If the blood pressure is excessive (i.e., above 160/100 mm Hg), I do attempt to reduce it while carefully monitoring the patient's level of alertness and neurologic signs to ensure that hypoperfusion does not develop as the pressure is lowered. If blood pressure remains excessive, I prescribe hydrochlorothiazide, low doses of propranolol, labetalol, nifedepine, angiotensin-converting-enzyme inhibitors, such as captopril or enalapril, or sodium nitroprusside. I prefer sodium nitroprusside because of its rapid and easily titratable effects.[109] No absolute levels of blood pressure to aim for exist; rather, the patient's clinical state should be observed to ensure that there is adequate blood flow and cerebral perfusion.

Antifibrinolytic Agents

Antifibrinolytic agents have been used in patients with SAH to prevent rebleeding.[110,111] The most common antifibrinolytic drug used was ε-aminocaproic acid (Amicar), which was usually given in a dose of 24 g per day intravenously for 3 days, followed by oral administration for 3 weeks or until surgery. Kassell and colleagues reviewed the experience of the Cooperative Study of Intracranial Aneurysms and Subarachnoid Hemorrhage with respect to antifibrinolytic drugs.[112] Although ε-aminocaproic acid decreased the rate of rebleeding, it did not improve morbidity or mortality. Vasoconstriction, thrombophlebitis with pulmonary embolism, and hydrocephalus were more common in patients given antifibrinolytic agents.[112] Although they may be useful in selected patients with high potential for rebleeding, antifibrinolytic agents have too many adverse effects to be recommended for general use in patients with SAH.

Surgery

The definitive treatment of an aneurysm is surgical obliteration. The patient is anesthetized using hypotensive anesthesia. The brain is made slack by using dehydrating agents and controlled removal of CSF, and the neurosurgeon uses a dissecting microscope to approach the aneurysm. Ideally, the aneurysm is clipped at its origin from the parent artery at its neck. If this is not possible, the aneurysm may be trapped between two clips and wrapped in supportive material, or the feeding arteries may be obliterated. During operations to obliterate aneurysms, rebleeding and ischemic infarction may occur. Infarction is secondary to arterial injury during retraction of the brain or from injury to penetrating arteries as aneurysms are approached and treated. Amnesic syndromes are common after surgery for AComA aneurysms, particularly if the aneurysms are trapped rather than ligated at their neck.[113,114] Trapping leads to disruption of the perforators that originate from the ACA and AComA, with resultant ischemia in the area of the anterior wall of the third ventricle and the orbital frontal lobes and basal forebrain nuclei.[113,114] Similarly, surgery on basilar artery bifurcation aneurysms can be followed by infarction in the paramedian midbrain and thalamus, causing a "top of the basilar syndrome."

Patients with surgical obliteration of aneurysms, if they survive surgery, do better in the long term than those who are treated only medically. The best timing for surgery remains controversial. Proponents of late surgery suggest that operations should be delayed until at least 10–14 days after the hemorrhage. The patient's medical condition should be optimal after medical complications have been treated. This technically difficult surgery is easier to perform as the brain edema resolves and the clot and blood in the subarachnoid space are diminished. Rebleeding at the time of surgery is also minimized, because the clot in the aneurysm is better organized.

In contrast, proponents of early surgery suggest operation during the first 72 hours. Although the surgery may be technically more difficult, early operation affords two advantages. First, if the aneurysm is successfully clipped, the possibility of rebleeding is eliminated. Second, early surgery may also afford a better outcome with regard to vasoconstriction. If a clot can be removed from the subarachnoid space at the time of surgery, vasoconstriction may be less likely to occur. If it does occur because the aneurysm has been clipped, more aggressive medical treatment can be given.

I favor early surgery in Hunt and Hess grade I or II patients. For these individuals, I order an early arteriogram, followed by prompt mobilization of the surgical team. For patients in higher grades, I favor the later time frame. I monitor the clinical signs, blood pressure, spinal fluid pressure, and blood-flow velocities as shown with TCD. Surgery is performed when the patient becomes alert and in Hunt and Hess grade I or II, when spinal fluid pressure is below 180 mm Hg on spinal puncture, and when blood-flow velocities do not indicate severe vasoconstriction.

Treatment of Unruptured Aneurysms

Management of patients with unruptured aneurysms presents a challenging problem in risk-factor analysis.[18] Unruptured aneurysms are discovered as part of the evaluation of another ruptured aneurysm, during investigation of a mass lesion, or during evaluation of another neurologic problem, such as ischemic vascular disease. Unruptured aneurysms that are not compressing neural structures are thought to bleed at a rate of 2–3% per year.[115] Aneurysms that cause neurologic symptoms rupture at a higher rate, with 15% bleeding within 6 months of onset of symptoms.[19] The operative mortality in patients with aneurysms and normal neurologic function is quite low (1.6% or less) when performed by some neurosurgeons.[116] Therefore, I recommend surgical therapy in selected patients with unruptured aneurysms.

The rate of aneurysm rupture is related to size. The International Study of Unruptured Intracranial Aneurysms showed that aneurysms 10 mm in size or larger ruptured much more frequently than smaller aneurysms.[2] In other studies, the critical size for aneurysmal rupture has been 7–10 mm[9] and 8 mm.[17] Surgery on unruptured aneurysms has a relatively high morbidity and mortality that is highly dependent on age. In a meta-analysis that included 2,460 patients (in 61 studies), the mortality of surgery was 2.6%, and the permanent morbidity was 10.9%.[117] In a study of 1,172 patients operated on for newly diagnosed unruptured intracranial aneurysms, the combined surgery related morbidity and mortality at 1 year was 6.5% for patients younger than 45 years old, 14.4% for those between 45–64 years, and 32% for those older than

64 years.[2] I concur with Kassell and Drake that the data support the idea that aneurysms 5–10 mm in size bleed more often than smaller lesions,[21] and aneurysms larger than 10 mm probably rupture at an even higher rate.[2] In good-risk young patients, aneurysms larger than 5 mm should most often be surgically treated by neurosurgeons experienced in aneurysm surgery. Lesions smaller than 5 mm should be followed using vascular imaging. If these smaller aneurysms show growth, then surgical therapy can be considered. CTA and MRA allow recognition and monitoring of unruptured aneurysms because patients can be studied noninvasively as outpatients. The decision with regard to surgery or interventional obliteration, or both, of unruptured aneurysms is complex, especially in older patients, and many factors must be carefully considered in each patient. Blood pressure control is important in patients with unruptured aneurysms.

Once a cerebral aneurysm has ruptured, the course is stormy, and the prognosis may be grim, even in the best of hands. To make a major impact on the morbidity and mortality of cerebral aneurysms, there must be early recognition of this serious disease, so that appropriate therapy can be undertaken while the patient is still in good condition. I stress the need for a high index of suspicion of SAH and a low threshold for use of LP in suspected cases.

Endovascular Treatment

The endovascular treatment of aneurysms by introducing various foreign materials to thrombose and obliterate aneurysms began in the 1960s. Luessenhop and Velasquez were probably the first to catheterize intracranial arteries and to introduce an inflatable catheter tip into aneurysms.[13] Fedor Serbinenko during the early 1970s devised microballoons and catheters containing detachable balloons and introduced the technique of artificial occlusion of intracranial vessels to treat aneurysms.[13] Endovascular techniques are rapidly being introduced and new technologies continue to emerge. Now various materials, including coils, balloons, and glues, have been used to obliterate aneurysms, even including giant aneurysms. Endovascular treatment promises to develop even more in the future, especially for large aneurysms and aneurysms that are not readily accessible for direct surgical clipping.

Figure 12-8. Unruptured parietal lobe arteriovenous malformation. (Reprinted with permission from JG Golfinos, TM Wachsler, JM Zabramski, et al. The management of unruptured intracranial vascular malformations. BNI Q 1992;8: 2–11.)

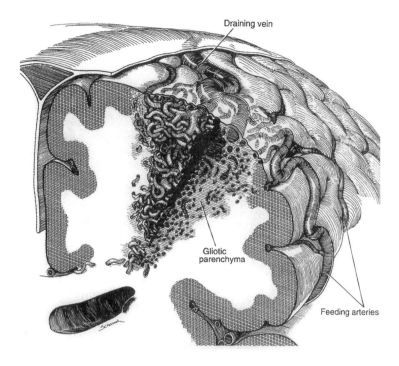

Draining vein

Gliotic parenchyma

Feeding arteries

Vascular Malformations

AVMs are the second most common cause of non-traumatic SAH. AVMs are one-tenth as common as aneurysms; an estimated 1,000 new cases are identified each year in the United States.[118] Cerebral aneurysms have a peak incidence of rupture beyond the age of 30 years: AVMs, however, rupture more commonly in the second and third decades of life.[119] Hemorrhage from an AVM is not strictly limited to the subarachnoid space. Often, there is a large parenchymatous component. Hemorrhages from other types of vascular malformations are predominantly intracerebral.

Classification and Distribution

Vascular malformations, often also called *angiomas*, usually arise from the failure of normal development of embryonic vascular networks. Some malformations, such as some arteriovenous fistulas, especially dural AVMs, are acquired during life. Because dural arteriovenous fistulas represent different clinical problems, they are discussed separately at the end of this chapter. McCormick wrote extensively about his experience with vascular malformations and classified them into five subtypes based on the predominant vasculature.[13,120–124]

Arteriovenous Malformations

AVMs contain arteries, arterialized veins, and veins. The size of the component vessels vary greatly, but the largest vessels are always venous. Sometimes the arterial supply is small and "cryptic." These lesions contain no recognizable normal capillary bed[123]; abnormal gliotic parenchyma usually is found between the component vessels. The small arteries within the malformation often have a deficient muscularis.[125] Thrombosis and inflammation are often found within AVMs. Arteriograms usually show shunting directly from the arteries to the venous components of the malformations. Figure 12-8 is a cartoon that illustrates the appearance of an unruptured AVM.

Venous Angiomas

The most common type of vascular malformation found in the brain at necropsy are venous angiomas, which are composed of anomalous veins; there is no direct arterial input. These lesions are most appropriately referred to as *developmental venous anomalies* (DVAs), rather than angiomas. They are composed of a group of anomalous veins usually separated by morphologically normal brain parenchyma. One or more large central draining veins are usually conspicuous and may be dilatated into a varix or varices. The

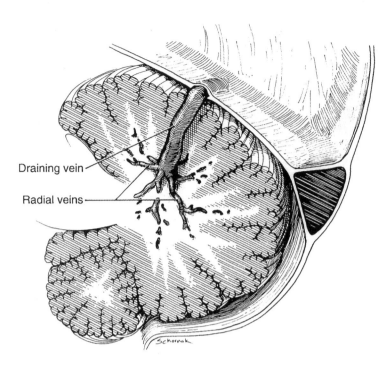

Figure 12-9. Illustration of a cerebellar developmental venous anomaly (venous angioma). (Reprinted with permission from JG Golfinos, TM Wachsler, JM Zabramski, et al. The management of unruptured intracranial vascular malformations. BNI Q 1992;8:2–11.)

walls of the veins can become thick and hyalinized. These angiomas do not opacify during the arterial phase of cerebral angiography. Figure 12-9 illustrates a DVA. Figure 12-10 shows the lesion in a brain specimen and Figure 12-11 is an MRI that shows a DVA.

Cavernous Angiomas

Cavernous angiomas consist of a relatively compact mass of sinusoidal vessels close together without intervening brain parenchyma. The lesions are well encapsulated, especially those that are superficial and large. Hyalinization and thickening of the component vessels, especially on the periphery of the angiomas, is common. These angiomas are not visualized well, if at all, on angiography because they have no direct arterial input. Cavernous angiomas are often multiple and can be familial.[126–128] Figure 12-12 is a cartoon that illustrates the gross appearance of a cavernous angioma in the brain. Figure 12-13 shows cavernous angiomas located in the pons and lateral cerebral ventricles.

Patients with DVAs have a much higher-than-expected co-occurrence of cavernous angiomas, especially in the posterior fossa. These two congenital lesions often occur close together, so that these lesions probably share etiologic features during their development.[129,130]

Telangiectasis

Telangiectasis (also called *telangiectasias*) are small lesions in which the component capillaries are separated from each other by normal brain parenchyma. They appear as small, pink, spongy areas most often located in the pons. These lesions are not shown by angiography.

Pathogenesis of Arteriovenous Malformations

AVMs are composed of clusters of abnormal vessels comprised of arteries and veins of varying size. The arteries within the cluster are large, thin-walled vessels with poorly developed internal elastic lamina and media, whereas the arteries feeding this abnormality have hypertrophy of the media and endothelial thickening.[120] The hypertrophic media and endothelial thickening sometimes lead to thrombosis of feeding arteries. Deep malformations are usually fed by penetrating arteries and drain into the deep venous system, whereas superficial cortical malformations usually drain into cortical veins.[125] In some patients, the afferent vessels of the malformation can become stenotic and even occluded.[131,132] Some patients with AVMs have more diffuse occlusive arterial disease, despite the fact that they have no atherosclerotic risk factors.[132] Blood circulates rapidly through the central core of AVMs and is quickly shunted into large, dilatated, draining veins. The increased flow can promote the formation of aneurysms, and, occasionally, aneurysms are found associated with AVMs, especially along major feeding arteries.[133,134] The aneurysms and afferent vascular stenoses are related to altered vascular hemodynamic factors involving the inflow channels. Occlusive changes can also be found in the draining venous channels and contribute to changes in pressures and flow within the malformations.[135,136]

Location of Malformations

Any part of the brain and spinal cord can harbor a vascular malformation. Cavernous angiomas and AVMs are often larger than the other types of malformations and more commonly cause symptoms. Telangiectases are usually asymptomatic but can be a source of repeated small bleeds. Some extensive malformations extend from the cortical surface to abut on the ventricular surface. Cavernous angiomas may be limited to the brain, spinal cord, subarachnoid space, or dura, or they may involve more than one of these regions. Table 12-3 shows the locations of cavernous angiomas in one large series.[13,137] Bleeding from cavernous angiomas is predominantly into brain parenchyma, but angiomas that abut on the ventricular or meningeal surface may also leak into the CSF.

AVMs can be predominantly within brain parenchyma or within the subarachnoid space, but most AVMs have parenchymatous and subarachnoid components so bleeding can be intracerebral, subarachnoid, or meningocerebral. Table 12-4 shows the location of AVMs in three large series of patients.[13,138–141] The blood supply of large AVMs is usually extensive, originating from the anterior and posterior intracranial circulations, as well as from extracranial components. AVMs are believed to arise in early fetal life as a result of the failure of primitive vessels to differentiate into normal arteries, veins, and capillaries. Despite their congenital origin, AVMs rarely produce symptoms during the first decade of life. The asymptomatic nature of

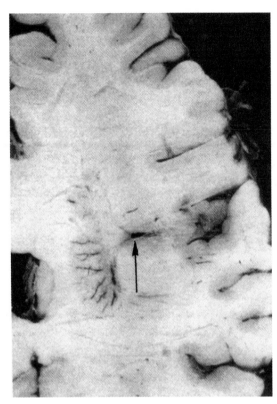

Figure 12-10. Brain specimen shows a venous malformation located mostly in the cerebral periventricular white matter. A radial array of dilatated medullary veins drain into a dilatated central vein (*arrow*), which then drains toward the cerebral cortex. (Reprinted with permission from PC Johnson, TM Wachser, J Golfinos, RF Spetzler. Definition and Pathological Features. In: LI Awad, DL Barrow [eds], Cavernous Malformations. Park Ridge, IL: American Association of Neurological Surgeons, 1993;1–11.)

lesions in early life is probably related to their small size and the inherent plasticity of the developing brain, which allows the function of one area of the brain to be assumed by another. AVMs often enlarge as individuals age. The feeding arteries and draining veins grow, and additional vasculature is recruited. Malformations may enlarge for multiple reasons. Hook suggested that undifferentiated arteries and veins might not tolerate arterial pressure well and therefore would enlarge.[142] Small recurrent ICHs cause loss of brain substance as clot and necrotic brain are reabsorbed. The decrease in supporting tissue around malformations might allow growth of the vascular anomaly.[143] Decreased strength of supporting tissue may also be caused by pulsation of arteries, which can damage the surrounding brain.

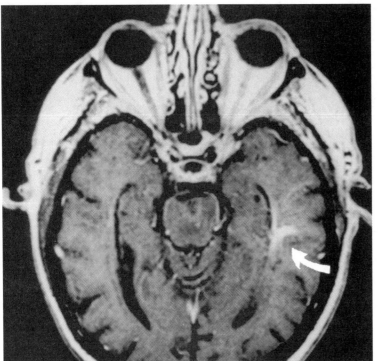

Figure 12-11. Magnetic resonance imaging shows a developmental venous anomaly located in the temporal lobe. The arrow points to an abnormal venous structure. (Reprinted with permission from LR Caplan. Subarachnoid Hemorrhage, Aneurysms, and Vascular Malformations. In LR Caplan, Posterior Circulation Disease: Clinical Findings, Diagnosis, and Management. Boston: Blackwell, 1996;633–685.)

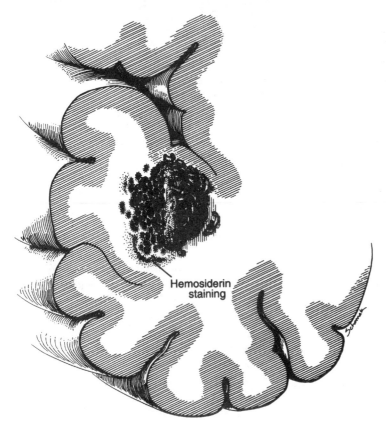

Hemosiderin staining

Figure 12-12. Unruptured cavernous malformation. Smooth muscle or intervening brain parenchyma do not exist within the interstices of the thin-walled vascular channels. Surrounding hemosiderin indicates prior bleeding. (Reprinted with permission from JG Golfinos, TM Wachsler, JM Zabramski, et al. The management of unruptured intracranial vascular malformations. BNI Q 1992;8:2–11.)

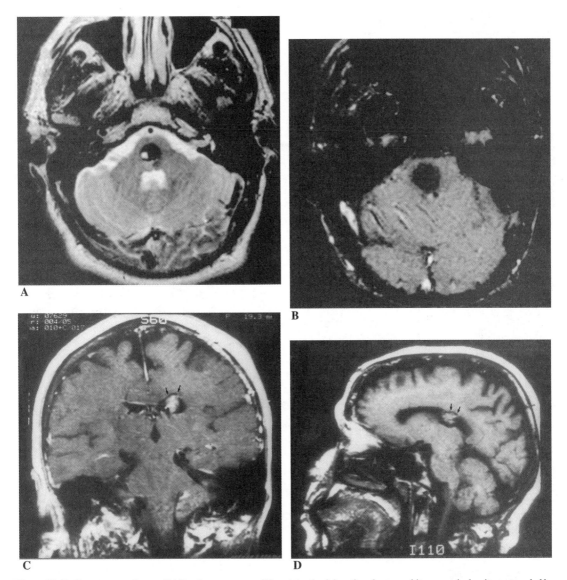

Figure 12-13. Cavernous angiomas. (**A**) Pontine cavernoma. T2-weighted axial section shows a white eccentric density surrounded by a dark hemosiderin ring. (**B**) Gradient echo magnetic resonance imaging section shows the hemosiderin ring around the lesion quite well. (Reprinted with permission from LR Caplan. Subarachnoid Hemorrhage, Aneurysms, and Vascular Malformations. In LR Caplan, Posterior Circulation Disease: Clinical Findings, Diagnosis, and Management. Boston: Blackwell, 1996;633−685.) (**C, D**) An intraventricular cavernoma. The lesion appears as a white hyperintensity (*arrows*) within the lateral ventricle.

Clinical Symptoms and Signs

As vascular malformations enlarge, symptoms are related to a number of mechanisms. Consider the following patient:

> At 15 years of age, AG began to have spells in which she saw sparkling lights off to her left. Some spells were followed by loss of consciousness and a generalized seizure. By age 21 years, she noted progressive loss of vision toward her left. Four years later during the first trimester of her first pregnancy while shopping, she fell to the ground with a severe headache, nausea, vomiting, and a stiff neck. Examination showed a left homonymous hemianopia.

Table 12-3. Distribution of Cavernous Angiomas

Distribution	Number (%)
Supratentorial	455 (74)
Lobar	256 (41)
Frontal lobe	99
Temporal lobe	68
Parietal lobe	72
Occipital lobe	16
Deep	31 (5)
Basal ganglia	22
Thalamus	7
Hypothalamus	2
Ventricular	20 (3)
Lateral ventricles	13
Paraventricular	2
Third ventricle	5
Extra-axial	4 (0.5)
Infratentorial	163 (26)
Cerebellum	28 (4.5)
Brain stem	82 (13)
Midbrain	20
Pons	43
Medulla	13
Pontomedullary	6
Fourth ventricle	3 (0.5)
Cerebellopontine angle	6 (1)
Spinal cord	2 (0.3)
Unspecified	58 (9)

Source: Reprinted with permission from LR Caplan. Subarachnoid Hemorrhage, Aneurysms, and Vascular Malformations. In LR Caplan, Posterior Circulation Disease: Clinical Findings, Diagnosis, and Management. Boston: Blackwell, 1996;633–685.

The most frequent and dramatic presentation of vascular malformations is bleeding. Fifty percent of symptomatic AVMs present in this manner,[142] as in the patient described. The immediate cause of the rupture is unknown, but probably relates to fragility of the abnormal vessels. Vessels on the cortical or ventricular surfaces are more prone to rupture, because they lack the support offered by the surrounding brain parenchyma. Symptoms and signs depend on the location of the hemorrhage. With CSF extension of blood, there are signs of meningeal irritation similar to those accompanying aneurysmal rupture. Not all ruptures are symptomatic. Frequently, patients with no clinical history of hemorrhage show evidence of bleeding at surgery or necropsy. In one surgical series, 6 of 55 patients with AVMs had evidence of hemorrhage without recognized symptoms.[118]

In the years before the hemorrhage, AG had partial seizures with secondary generalization and progressive neurologic signs. An estimated 46% of patients with AVMs present with epilepsy and 21% have progressive neurologic deficits.[144] Supratentorial cavernous angiomas often present because of seizures. Progressive symptoms are probably caused by two mechanisms:

1. Large volumes of blood may be shunted or stolen through the malformation to the venous circulation; this shunt could deprive adjacent brain tissue of blood, causing relative ischemia.
2. The ischemic process is aggravated by the pulsatile nature of the malformation; the pulsating blood vessels compress adjacent brain tissue and can lead to local atrophy. Also, partially ischemic tissue is prone to electrical instability and seizures.

Chronic headaches are also a frequent complaint in patients with AVMs. The headaches are often migrainous in nature, sometimes closely mimicking classic migraine. No good rules exist to distinguish migrainous headaches related to vascular malformations. Migraine accompaniments that are always stereotyped and occur on the same side or headaches always localized to the same side should lead doctors to suspect an AVM. Even patients with unruptured AVMs can have increased ICP and papilledema.[145] The increased pressure may contribute to headaches.

In the brain stem, AVMs and cavernous angiomas may present with serious bleeding or gradually progressive neurologic deficits. Depending on location, there may be cranial nerve, cerebellar, pyramidal, or sensory dysfunction. Some have a fluctuating course of neurologic dysfunction, which may simulate multiple sclerosis.[13,146,147] Distinction between these two processes is possible. With cavernous angiomas, the neurologic dysfunction can be localized to one site. CT or MRI shows hemorrhage or cystic changes at the site of prior bleeding.

AVMs rarely present with hydrocephalus. In such cases, the mass of blood vessels can compress the ventricular system, disrupting the normal flow of CSF. Aneurysms of the vein of Galen are the most common cause of this rare presentation. Prior small bleeds can also block absorption of CSF, leading to hydrocephalus. Rarely, patients with

Table 12-4. Location of Arteriovenous Malformations (AVMs) Diagnosed during Life

Location of AVMs	Perret and Nishioka[138] Number (%)	Crawford et al.[139] Number (%)	Graf et al.[140] Number (%)
Frontal lobe	102 (23)	85 (21)	33 (25)
Temporal lobe	82 (18)	41 (10)	25 (19)
Parietal lobe	122 (27)	145 (36)	41 (30)
Occipital lobe	23 (5)	69 (17)	7 (5)
Brain stem	11 (2)		5 (4)
Cerebellum	21 (4)	36* (9)	6 (4.5)
Basal ganglia		27	14 (10)
Other	92 (20)		3 (2.5)
Total	**453**	**403**	**134**

*Brain stem and cerebellar lesions grouped together.
Source: Reprinted with permission from LR Caplan. Subarachnoid Hemorrhage, Aneurysms, and Vascular Malformations. In LR Caplan, Posterior Circulation Disease: Clinical Findings, Diagnosis, and Management. Boston: Blackwell, 1996;633–685.

large AVMs can present because of a bruit that is audible to the patient or doctor. In children, large AVMs can produce enough shunting of blood to cause high-output congestive heart failure.

In the spinal cord, vascular malformations typically present with back pain, myelopathic symptoms, and root dysfunction. These lesions are discussed in Chapter 15. Because headache so often accompanies spinal AVM rupture, cerebral sources of hemorrhage are often sought, and the spinal origin can be missed. In one series, 80% of patients with spinal malformations had intracranial symptoms, including headache, mental status changes, loss of consciousness, papilledema, decreased vision, nystagmus, diplopia, seizures, sixth nerve paresis, and oculomotor paresis.[148]

Imaging Findings

Diagnosis of vascular malformations can often be suspected clinically. Typical features include:

1. History of a seizure disorder or progressive neurologic deficit
2. Throbbing headaches or migraine-like auras, or both, always localized to one side of the cranium
3. A patient in the second or third decade of life
4. SAH in a pregnant woman (pregnancy is said to be a particularly hazardous time for women with AVMs; peak time for hemorrhages is when the cardiac output is increased, particularly early in pregnancy and during labor and delivery)[149]
5. Clinical signs and symptoms of intraparenchymal and subarachnoid blood
6. Cranial bruit

Brain imaging in nearly all patients shows vascular malformations. MRI is able to define the lesions better than CT. Serpiginous channels sometimes can be seen on plain CT scans and may be enhanced after intravenous contrast administration.[150] Brain atrophy and dilatation of ventricles adjacent to malformations may exist. Small calcifications may be seen within malformations. Sometimes, frank cysts are also found adjacent to AVMs.[151] If there has been a recent hemorrhage, these recent findings may be obscured by the intraparenchymal, subarachnoid, and intraventricular blood.

MRI has definitely improved the diagnosis of vascular malformations. AVMs usually appear as a region of honeycomb-like spaces with flow voids that contrast with the surrounding brain tissue on T1- and T2-weighted images. Cavernous angiomas usually appear as well-circumscribed, well-defined lesions, with a central core of mixed heterogenous signal intensity surrounded by a rim of signal void.[152–156] Figures 12-13A and B are MRIs that show this appearance. The heterogeneous center is caused by blood and blood metabolites in various stages of evolution, and the dark rim is caused by hemosiderin. The typical MRI appearance of DVAs is a linear or globular hypointense region on T1-weighted images and hypo- or hyperintensity on T2-weighted images.[157–159] DVAs can usually be seen to join deep or superficial veins, or both.[159]

Figure 12-11 illustrates the MRI findings in a patient with a DVA. Recent hemorrhages in all types of malformations have the same imaging characteristics as other causes of ICH. MRI can also be helpful by showing hemosiderin resulting from old hemorrhage in the lesions and adjacent meninges. MRA may help noninvasively to identify large AVM feeding arteries and veins.

TCD is also useful in the initial diagnosis and monitoring of AVMs.[42–45] The increased flow to the AVMs is associated with increased flow velocities in arteries feeding the malformations. At times, musical-type murmurs can be heard, and unusual unmodulated high- or middle-frequency bands are seen on the Doppler spectrum.[44] Abnormal collateralization and steal effects can be found with reduction of mean and peak flow velocities in some arteries.[44] Changes in velocities can be monitored during therapeutic embolization and after surgical or radiation therapy.[45] Vasomotor reactivity to CO_2 inhalation also gives information about AVMs. Relatively normal vasomotor reactivity in arteries ipsilateral to AVMs suggests a high-pressure AVM with a high risk of bleeding, whereas abnormal vasomotor reactivity in ipsilateral and contralateral arteries is most often found in low-pressure AVMs that show hemodynamically-induced neurologic signs.[160]

A detailed angiogram is needed to identify all possible arterial feeders when surgery is considered in patients. Angiographic features typical of AVMs include (1) large feeding arteries; (2) a central tangle of vessels; (3) enlarged, tortuous draining veins; and (4) rapid arterial-to-venous shunting of blood. Some angiographic findings, such as large size, presence of multiple feeding arteries, and drainage into peripheral cortical veins, correlate with the development of progressive neurologic signs that have been attributed by some to stealing of blood from normal vessels to the malformations.[161] Four circumstances may arise in which the clinical syndrome appears to be a hemorrhage secondary to a vascular malformation, but arteriography is normal:

1. There may have been spontaneous thrombosis of the malformation; this represents a self-cure.
2. With rupture, there may have been obliteration of the malformation, representing another cure.
3. Alternatively, the malformation may be a cavernous angioma or a DVA, without a direct arterial feeder, and therefore not visualized on angiography.

4. Finally, when a malformation or aneurysm is not found during the investigation of an SAH, a spinal malformation must be considered; the history and physical examination should be repeated, looking closely for a history of back pain and myelopathic or radicular symptoms and signs.

Prognosis

In the short term, the prognosis of ruptured AVMs is much better than that of aneurysms. The rebleeding rate is low during the first months. Only 6% rebleed during the first year, [162] and vasoconstriction occurs only rarely. Mortality from the first hemorrhage is low, only approximately 10%. In the long term, however, the prognosis of vascular malformations is not as good. Estimates of recurrent hemorrhage during subsequent years vary from 1% in 4–7 years[143] to 2% per year after the first year.[162] With subsequent hemorrhages, the mortality rate is higher, approximately 20%.[161]

With each recurrence, the chances of additional hemorrhages increase.[143] In one large series of 137 patients with AVMs treated conservatively between 1942 and 1967, 10% died from AVMs, 24% were disabled, and only 40% were well at the time of the 1970 report[162]; 7 years later, only 19% of the initial group were well.[163,164] Because AVMs tend to occur in younger patients, the probability that recurrent hemorrhage with disability or death will occur is substantial. The authors of one study estimated that almost 50% of patients with recurrent hemorrhage will have some deterioration in working capacity or become invalid during the 20–40 years after the first hemorrhage.[165] One study noted a better outcome for patients with hemorrhage from AVMs than prior reports. Among 119 AVM patients followed at Columbia Presbyterian Medical Center, 115 had a bleed as the diagnostic event, and 27 of these patients had subsequent hemorrhages.[166] Four other patients had symptoms other than hemorrhage that prompted diagnosis, but had subsequent bleeds during follow-up. The incident hemorrhage resulted in no clinical deficit in 47%, and another 37% were independent in daily activities. During follow-up, 20 of 27 patients (74%) with more than one hemorrhage were still normal or independent.[166]

Parietal, central, and infratentorial malformations may be more likely to bleed than frontal, temporal, or occipital malformations.[164] Morbidity from hemorrhages depends on the location of the malformation. Occurrence in an "eloquent" brain region poses a higher risk for morbidity from a bleed, but also from surgical intervention. High arterial input pressures and restriction of venous outflow to only deep venous drainage are risk factors that increase the likelihood of hemorrhage in AVMs.[167]

Patients who present with seizures alone have a better prognosis than those that present with hemorrhage. Only a 25% chance exists of a clinically symptomatic hemorrhage in 15 years.[165] In one long-term series of patients with seizures, there was only a 12% mortality and an additional 16% overall disability.[162] A more conservative approach, prescribing only anticonvulsant therapy for patients with seizures alone, is reasonable. Seizures can be well controlled by anticonvulsants, and surgical removal of malformations often does not improve seizure control.[168] Patients presenting with progressive neurologic deficits have a poor prognosis, but these patients also often have the largest malformations, which are difficult to treat.[161]

Data are not available regarding long-term prognosis in patients with asymptomatic AVMs. These are usually discovered during the evaluation of other problems. With the advent of CT and MRI, it is possible to collect information regarding the fate of these malformations and the outcome of patients who harbor them. Aminoff has argued convincingly for conservative management of most unruptured AVMs.[168]

The most common presentation of cavernous angiomas is seizures, which occur in approximately one-half of the patients.[169] Focal neurologic deficits and hemorrhages are the next most common presentations. Although almost all cavernous malformations show some surrounding blood on MRI or when examined pathologically, clinically significant hemorrhage is not common. Hemorrhage is more common in patients who have already bled than in patients whose lesions have never bled. Robinson and colleagues prospectively followed 76 cavernomas detected by MRI among 66 patients.[170] Only one hemorrhage occurred during a 26-month period, for a rate of 0.7% per lesion per year.[170] In another study, follow-up information was available for 122 patients with cavernous malformations.[171] Multiple lesions were present in one-fifth of patients. Cavernomas were located in the brain stem (35%), basal ganglia and thalamus (17%), and cerebral hemispheres (48%). In retrospect, one-half of the patients had one bleed, 7% had two hemorrhages, and 2% had had three bleeds.[171] The retrospective annual hemorrhage rate was 1.3%. Prospective follow-up of these patients for an average of 34 months showed a prospective annual rate of hemorrhage of only 0.6% for those lesions that had never previously bled. Patients with prior bleeds had a 4.5% per year rate of recurrent hemorrhage.[171] In this study, location of the cavernomas did not affect the rate of bleeding.[171] Hemorrhages are more common in women, especially if they are pregnant.[172] Hemorrhages are often difficult to document clinically or on MRI because part of the natural history of cavernous angiomas is slow oozing of blood into surrounding brain tissue, forming a hemosiderin-laden ring around the angioma.[172]

Moran et al. performed a systematic review of the literature and analyzed the findings among supratentorial cavenous angiomas.[173] Figure 12-14 from this report diagrams the clinical manifestations among 296 patients and shows overlapping of symptoms. Seizures were by far the most common presentation, followed by hemorrhage and focal neurologic deficits.[173] Subsequent to diagnosis, only six patients developed a hemorrhage during a mean of 5.6 years of follow-up, yielding a hemorrhage rate of 0.7% per year.[173]

Prognosis for Developmental Venous Anomalies

In the majority of patients, venous malformations have a benign course.[174–176] Garner et al. observed 100 patients with DVAs; only one of which was associated with hemorrhage.[174] Naff et al. followed 92 patients with DVAs for an average of 4.2 years.[176] The most common locations of the lesions were the frontal lobes (56%) and the cerebellum (27%). The most frequent presenting symptoms were headache (51%), focal neurologic deficits (40%), and seizures (30%). The prevalence of headache and seizures decreased over time, even without treatment. Only two patients developed a symptomatic hemorrhage during follow-up, giving an annual risk of hemorrhage of 0.15%.[176]

Treatment of Vascular Malformations

A 33-year-old, right-handed schoolteacher, BC, had occasional left-sided throbbing headaches while in college. At age 27 years, he had his first epileptic seizure, which began with a warm feeling in his

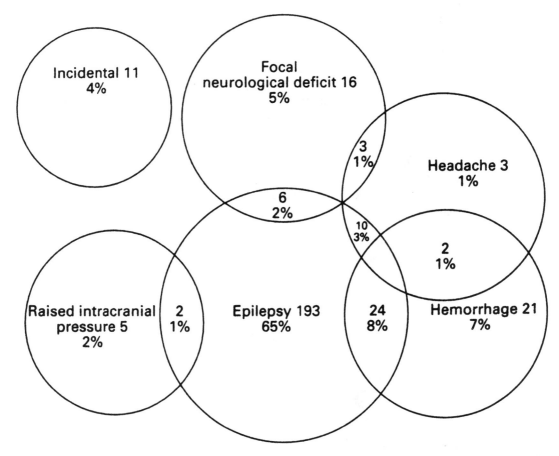

Figure 12-14. Clinical findings among 296 patients with supratentorial cavernous malformations. (Reprinted with permission from NF Moran, DR Fish, N Kitchen, et al. Supratentorial cavernous hemangiomas and epilepsy: a review of the literature and case series. J Neurol Neurosurg Psychiatry 1999;66:561–568.)

right lip and tongue. The feeling rapidly spread to his hand, and then he lost consciousness. At age 33 years while shoveling snow, he developed a severe diffuse headache and vomited. On examination, he was restless and complained of headache, but had no abnormal neurologic signs except a right extensor plantar response. LP showed blood-tinged CSF at a pressure of 210 mm Hg. CT showed a thin layer of subarachnoid blood and contrast injection opacified a large sylvian group of tortuous veins. Angiography revealed a large parasylvian central AVM fed primarily from the left MCA.

How should this patient be treated? In this case, the diagnosis of AVM is certain. The prodromal history of headaches and seizures was typical. The present bleed was subarachnoid, arising from the surface of the lesion. No intraparenchymatous hematoma was evident, either clinically or by CT. In this patient, surgery or embolization carries the risk of aphasia or right hemiparesis, each possibly disabling. Because there were no important neurologic signs, I chose to watch the patient during the next years to see the natural history of the lesion. If he had presented with an intracerebral hematoma and had aphasia and right hemiplegia, the situation would have been quite different and surgery might have been indicated.

Four therapeutic options are available that can be used in combination or alone to treat vascular malformations: (1) surgery; (2) interventional radiology, including embolization; (3) radiotherapy; and (4) a strictly medical approach. Interventional radiologic treatment is only used for AVMs because the other lesions do not have important arterial feeders. Because venous anomalies are developmental abnormalities with a benign natural history and resection carries a substantial risk of venous infarction, hemorrhage, and brain edema, lesions should be managed only medically.[176]

Surgery

A surgical approach is the oldest method of treatment. Initially, neurosurgeons ligated the major feeding vessels to the malformation. This method of treatment has been largely abandoned because of its failure to obliterate the lesion and the hazards inherent in the procedure. Stroke often occurs as blood flow to normal brain is interrupted. Malformations continue to draw blood from nonligated, deep, inaccessible vessels.

Direct surgical excision of lesions has been improved with the use of the operating microscope. Lesions are meticulously approached, avoiding critical cerebral vessels and vital neurologic structures. Operations may be performed using local anesthesia and evoked response monitoring, so that the exact location of vital areas can be accurately determined. Dissection is done, if possible, in the gliotic plane that surrounds the tangle of vessels, so malformations can be removed en bloc. Surgical excision can be carried out in appropriate patients with a low morbidity and mortality.[163, 164]

The major complications of surgical excision are loss of normal brain tissue, with additional loss of neurologic function, bleeding, and the so-called breakthrough phenomenon.[177] This term is used to describe massive brain swelling and ICH occurring postoperatively, which is caused by redirection of the large volume of blood that previously flowed into the malformation into the small vessels surrounding the malformation. These vessels are unable to handle the large volume of blood, and cerebral edema or hemorrhage can result.[177]

The advent of microsurgical techniques also makes it possible to remove deep-seated cavernous angiomas, including those in the brain stem. Surgical treatment of cavernomas is appropriate only for lesions that have caused intractable seizures and serious neurologic signs or have rebled.

Interventional Radiology Approaches,
Including Embolization

Embolization of AVMs can be used alone, before surgery, or at the time of surgery. Initially, small pellets were used to fill the abnormal vessels within the central nidus. Because flow to malformations is increased, pellets released into feeding arteries tend to travel to the malformations. There, they occlude the lumens of vessels, it is hoped, in sufficient quantity to thrombose the vascular malformation. The particle embolization technique, however, has many problems. Emboli rarely enter arteries with acute or right angles. Furthermore, as vessels within malformations become occluded, flow to the malformations equals the flow to the normal brain and particles stray into the normal circulation, causing ischemia. Advances have greatly improved the embolization technique.[178]

Since the early 1980s, calibrated-leak balloon catheters have been advanced into feeding arteries close to the malformation. Various kinds of "glues," rapidly setting tissue adhesives, such as isobutyl-2-cyanoacrylate, can then be administered.[179] These adhesives form clots in the segments of the lesion irrigated predominantly by that artery. Several feeding arteries are then injected. This technique often reduced the size of the lesion, but rarely obliterated the abnormality.

Embolization can also be done at the time of surgery when materials can be injected into cannulized blood vessels. Complications of this technique, in addition to postembolization hemorrhage related to altered blood flow, include hemorrhage or ischemic stroke induced by the balloon catheter, gluing of the balloon catheter complex in place by the tissue adhesive, or occlusion of normal arteries by the plastic material. Also, some substances, such as bucrylate, can be toxic to tissues and cause angionecrosis and escape into the extravascular spaces.[180]

Endovascular techniques are especially important in treating lesions that are not surgically accessible and as an adjunct to surgical removal. Newer imaging technology has clearly facilitated the use of various interventional techniques.

Radiotherapy

Attempts have been made to use radiotherapy to obliterate AVMs. High energy from conventional x-rays, gamma rays, or protons induces subendothelial deposition of collagen and hyaline substances, which narrow the lumen of small vessels and shrink the nidus of the malformation by progressive occlusion of vessels during the months after treatment.[181] Newer techniques focus the radiation beam on small regions. An example is the so-called gamma knife, a system that uses a cobalt source to generate highly collimated gamma rays that converge on a focal point.[182] Modified linear accelerators can deliver radiation to a defined volume of tissue with good accuracy. Radiation necrosis occurs in approximately 9% of patients.[182] Approximately 40% of AVMs are obliterated in 1 year, 84% after 2 years, and 97% after 3 years.[183] Small volume, deep location, and plexiform angioarchitecture correlate with successful obliteration of AVMs by radiotherapy.[183,184] Bleeding has occurred after treatment, especially during the period of obliteration. Reports on the use of Bragg-peak proton-beam radiotherapy[180] and stereotactic helium-ion Bragg-peak radiation[185] are encouraging. Complications include radionecrosis of normal brain, hydrocephalus, immediate post-therapy seizures, loss of body temperature regulation, and possibly long-term cognitive-function deficits. Further data are needed before the frequency of these complications and the therapeutic use of focused radiotherapy in patients with AVMs is known. Focused radiotherapy is probably best reserved for small deep lesions not easily amenable to surgery that have bled.

Because cavernous angiomatous lesions have only been well defined since the advent of MRI, there is less information about the use of radiotherapy in treating cavernomas as compared to AVMs. Gamma knife radiosurgery aiming the treatment precisely at the lesions using a stereotaxic three-dimensional frame has made it possible to treat small, deep lesions in the brain stem, basal ganglia, and thalamus with preliminary success.[186]

Medical Approach

The most conservative therapeutic option for AVMs is a medical approach. Blood pressure is strictly controlled within the normal range. Anticoagulants and platelet-antiaggregant drugs are avoided. Because the rate of hemorrhage in pregnant women with AVMs is relatively high, I discuss the risk of pregnancy with fertile women and suggest appropriate contraception if desired.

Vascular malformations, if left untreated, are hazardous. No one therapeutic option is entirely successful or without risk. Treatment of the malformations is often complicated by numerous feeding arteries, extensive size, or location within the brain parenchyma in areas vital to normal neurologic function. Decisions regarding therapy must con-

sider these factors. Of additional importance is the age of the patient and mode of presentation. These two factors are major determinants of the natural history of the disease.

For the most common mode of presentation in patients with AVMs and ICH, I recommend an aggressive approach, including surgery or surgery combined with embolization if the following criteria are met:

1. The patient is relatively young (younger than 55 years and has a life expectancy of more than 15 years).
2. Recovery of neurologic function after the hemorrhage is moderately good, so that a reasonable lifestyle can be anticipated.
3. The malformation is superficial in location and does not extensively involve vital neurologic structures—so-called eloquent brain.

Because the rate of early rebleeding is low, I wait until the patient is in good medical condition before suggesting surgery. Because surgery can cause neurologic signs, the presence of a remaining neurologic deficit related to the bleeding is a factor favoring surgery, whereas postbleed return to complete normality argues against surgery.

I adopt a more conservative approach, using embolization, radiotherapy if available, or strictly medical management if the following criteria are met:

1. The patient is older than 55–60 years, and life expectancy is less than 10 years.
2. The deficit from the initial hemorrhage is severe.
3. The malformation is extensive and deep within the dominant hemisphere, in the brain stem or other vital eloquent areas.

I use these same criteria for patients who present with progressive neurologic deficits. I treat patients who present with seizures medically. Anticonvulsants are given to control the spells, blood pressure is regulated, and anticoagulants and platelet antiaggregating drugs are avoided. If seizures remain intractable despite medical therapy, a more aggressive plan using surgical excision might be considered.

In asymptomatic patients, including those with only headache, I follow a conservative medical approach. Because the natural history of asymptomatic lesions is unknown, it is unwise to undertake therapy that may be more hazardous than the

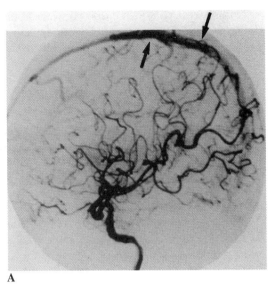 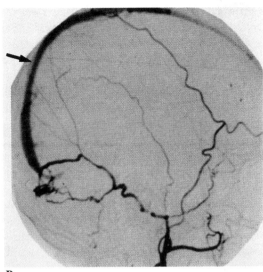

A   **B**

Figure 12-15. Dural arteriovenous malformation of the superior sagittal sinus and torcula. (**A**) Internal carotid artery angiogram, lateral view, shows that multiple branches of the middle cerebral artery drain directly into the superior sagittal sinus (*arrows*). (**B**) External carotid injection shows that internal maxillary branches also fill the sagittal sinus (*arrow*). (Reprinted with permission from J Dion. Dural Arteriovenous Malformations: Definition, Classification, and Diagnostic Imaging. In IA Awad, DL Barrow [eds], Dural Arteriovenous Malformations. Park Ridge, IL: American Association of Neurological Surgeons, 1993;1–19.)

lesion itself. Furthermore, initial hemorrhages are rarely fatal; if a hemorrhage does occur, the opportunity for more aggressive therapy is then available.

Dural Arteriovenous Malformations

Dural arteriovenous malformations (DAVMs) are lesions that contain abnormal arteriovenous shunts within the leaflets of the dura mater, usually within or near the walls of dural venous sinuses.[13,187] Figure 12-15 shows angiograms in a patient who has a DAVM with filling from arterial branches of the MCAs and external carotid arteries that drain into the superior sagittal sinus and torcula herophili. DAVMs have different etiologies, pathophysiologies, and clinical symptoms when compared with parenchymal and pial AVMs. DAVMs represent 10–15% of all AVMs.

DAVMs may drain only into dural sinuses or there may be prominent drainage into the cortical and deep veinous systems. DAVMs with prominent cortical venous drainage have a higher incidence of bleeding then those without.[188,189] The cause of most of the complications and symptoms and signs in patients with DAVMs is thought to be venous hypertension.[190,191] The two major mechanisms of increased

pressure within the venous drainage system are (1) increased blood flow through draining veins (e.g., related to increased arterial inputs); and (2) restriction or obstruction of the draining system, causing an increase in pressure in the tributary veins. Venous hypertension probably promotes cortical venous drainage and increases the risk of brain hemorrhage.

Some DAVMs are probably congenital, especially those that involve the vein of Galen. Retention of an embryonic median porencephalic vein, which normally drains the choroid plexus of the fetus, is the explanation usually given for vein of Galen malformations.[192] When this vein persists, it becomes the sac for the aneurysmally enlarged vein of Galen. These lesions should probably be classified as AVMs rather than true DAVMs. Most DAVMs are probably acquired.[13,191] Well-documented instances exist of adult patients who had normal angiograms and later, angiography showed that DAVMs had formed, proving these lesions were acquired in these patients.[193,194] Trauma is undoubtedly an important cause in some patients. Hormonal factors may also be important because female hormones are known to influence placental and uterine vascular growth and increase angiomas at many body sites. Dural sinus thrombosis, an important cause of DAVMS is more common in women. Approximately twice as many women as men have the most common form of DAVM with drainage into the lateral sinuses.[194,195] DAVMs may first become symptomatic during pregnancy. Some DAVMs have been reported to regress after delivery.[193] Occlusion of a dural sinus is probably also an important cause of DAVMs.[194] Houser and colleagues reported two patients in whom dural sinus thrombosis was documented years before development of DAVMs.[194] One patient had previous angiography because of transient bilateral limb weakness that showed sigmoid sinus occlusion but no fistula; a year later after the development of pulsatile tinnitus, a repeat angiogram showed a DAVM of the transverse sinus adjacent to the occluded sigmoid sinus. Another patient with a history of thrombophlebitis and thromboembolism developed headache, drowsiness, leg weakness, and papilledema. Angiography showed a transverse sinus occlusion. When he developed an increase in his symptoms, a repeat angiogram 2.5 years later showed a transverse sinus DAVM.[194] Thrombosis or stenosis within the draining dural sinus often causes enlargement of the DAVMs and augments venous hypertension. Several reports document progressive obstruction and occlusion of dural sinuses in patients known to have DAVMs.[13,196]

The clinical problems that develop in patients with DAVMs, such as headaches, papilledema, hydrocephalus, and hemorrhages, are probably explained by venous hypertension.[196] The focal symptoms and signs that develop depend heavily on the anatomic location of the DAVMs and whether the lesions are solely dural or have a prominent drainage pattern into the brain's cortical and deep veins.[197] Hemorrhages are most often intraparenchymatous or subdural, but occasionally are subarachnoid. First hemorrhages from DAVMs have approximately a 30% mortality. An especially high mortality and severe disabling morbidity rate occurs in patients with hemorrhages from DAVMs who are taking anticoagulants. Veinous infarcts, which are often hemorrhagic, and brain edema can also result from the venous hypertension. Seizures, headache, and signs of increased intracranial pressure develop, often with papilledema. Brain edema is an important sequel in some patients with DAVMs, especially those with venous hypertension and sinus occlusions.[13,198] Pulsatile tinnitus is another frequent and annoying symptom. Some patients only have headaches, either generalized or localized to the side of the DAVM. I have seen several patients with DAVMs who had positionally sensitive headache with worsening in the supine position and improvement when sitting or standing.[13] The erect position may have allowed better venous drainage toward the heart.

The most common location of DAVMs is in relation to the lateral sinuses, involving the transverse or sigmoid portion of the lateral sinus. Lateral sinus malformations account for five-eighths of DAVMs.[13,199] Potential feeding arteries to these lateral sinus fistulas include (1) external carotid artery branches, such as the occipital, middle meningeal, accessory meningeal, and ascending pharyngeal arteries; (2) dural branches of the ICA, especially the meningo-hypophyseal trunk (the artery of Bernasconi and Casaneri); and (3) dural branches of the vertebral arteries, such as posterior meningeal, cerebellar falcine, and cervical muscular anastomotic arteries. Venous drainage of lateral sinus DAVMs can be into a normal transverse or sigmoid sinus, or the wall of the sinus may be irregular and partially or completely thrombosed.

Cavernous sinus fistulae are the next most common lesion and are found in approximately one-eighth of patients with DAVMs.[199] These lesions are characterized by abnormal shunting of blood from the internal or external carotid arteries into the cavernous sinus. Blood often drains into the orbital veins, causing increased venous pressure in the eye and orbital contents leading to proptosis, chemosis caused by conjunctival edema, scleral injection, conjunctival hemorrhages, glaucoma, and papilledema.[200,201] These lesions can drain into the petrosal veins and sinuses and the basal vein of Rosenthal, and cause venous hypertension within the brain stem.[202,203] Trauma and rupture of infraclinoid carotid artery aneurysms into the cavernous sinus are important causes of these fistulae.

Tentorial-incisural DAVMs account for approximately one-twelfth of all DAVMs.[204] Less common locations include the cerebral convexity-sagittal sinus region, orbital-anterior falx region, sylvian-middle fossa region, and those that drain into the torcula herophili. Some DAVMs drain into deep structures, such as the vein of Galen, straight sinus, or dural venous structures in the posterior falx region. The vein of Galen is an unusual structure, both anatomically and embryologically. It is a bridge between the subarachnoid veinous system and the dural straight sinus. The vein of Galen can be the site of shunting or can be recruited into the venous drainage pattern in cases of high-flow lesions or when distal outlets are stenosed or thrombosed. The two distinct types of vein of Galen malformations are[192]:

1. A congenital lesion that develops in utero in which the arterial input is into a persistent medial porencephalic vein, which can become aneurysmally dilatated. These patients present with congestive heart failure. These lesions are probably true AVMs and the dural sinuses are patent.

2. A DAVM in which the shunt is into the wall of the vein of Galen. These are acquired in adulthood usually in relation to dural sinus occlusions in a similar fashion to other DAVMs. True vein of Galen DAVMs presenting in adulthood are supplied from the middle meningeal and vertebral artery, PCA, and meningo-hypophyseal artery branches. Occasionally, a vein of Galen aneurysm can be associated with DAVMs.

DAVMs are difficult to diagnose without angiography. In my experience, the angiographic results often come as a surprise and were not suspected from the clinical or imaging data. CT does not show the DAVM but can show related abnormalities, such as hemorrhages, thrombosed sinuses, hydrocephalus, and dilatated pial veins or varices. Contrast enhancement aids recognition of the abnormal veins and thrombosed sinuses. Similarly, MRI may show the abnormal veins and sinuses, suggesting the diagnosis, but does not show the arterial input. Although MRI and MRA can undoubtedly be helpful in suggesting the diagnosis, catheter angiography using high-resolution digital arterial subtraction angiography is still needed to identify the arterial feeders and draining veinous patterns.

The natural history of DAVMs is variable. Some close spontaneously. In others, symptoms are slight and include mostly headache and pulsatile tinnitus. The nature of the venous drainage pattern is considered by many to be important in predicting the prognosis.[13] Drainage into subarachnoid and parenchymal veins with retrograde flow away from the lesion seems to correlate with dural sinus outflow obstruction and venous hypertension.[199] This predicts an aggressive course, often with brain hemorrhages, intraventricular hemorrhages, subdural hemorrhages, and SAHs.[199]

Endovascular treatment of DAVMs has been limited, although technology is rapidly changing.[205,206] The plethora of arterial feeders from multiple major arterial systems, and the small size of many of the feeders, especially pial arteries, limit the effectiveness of embolization strategies. Transvenous endovascular treatment is promising. In some patients, a combined approach using transarterial embolization, transvenous ablation, and microneurosurgery has been effective.[206]

Surgical treatment of DAVMs is often quite difficult. Mullan emphasized that surgeons should attempt to obliterate the fistulous communication, which appears as "multiple watering can spouts into the sinus lumen."[207] Some fistulas drain into an isolated vein in the wall of a dural sinus. Effective obliteration involves occluding the vein flush with the external wall of the sinus.[207] Obliteration or ligation of feeders often does not result in effective ablation of the DAVMs because new feeders are recruited. Packing the sinus in the region of the fistula is usually effective but is difficult and requires considerable surgical experience. The high flow in DAVMs makes blood loss and a bloody surgical field important problems in effective ablation. A conservative nonsurgical approach to DAVMs is probably best in fistulas that do not have prominent leptomeningeal venous drainage or variceal or aneurysmal abnormalities within the draining venous system.[208] Clinical observation, repeat neuroimaging, and angiography are advised for those patients not treated surgically.[208]

Modern neuroimaging technology greatly facilitates diagnosis and should allow physicians to learn more about the natural history of DAVMs and other cranio-cerebral vascular malformations. Modern technology facilitates logical treatment.

References

1. Rinkel GJE, Djibuti M, Algra A, van Gijn J. Prevalence and risk of rupture of intracranial aneurysms. A systematic review. Stroke 1998;29:251–256.
2. The International Study of Unruptured Intracranial Aneurysms Investigators. Unruptured intracranial aneurysms—risk of rupture and risks of surgical intervention. N Engl J Med 1998;339:1725–1733.
3. Parkarinen S. Incidence, etiology, and prognosis of primary subarachnoid hemorrhage: a study based on 589 cases diagnosed in a defined urban population during a defined period. Acta Neurol Scand 1967;43(Suppl 29):1–128.
4. Phillips LH, Whisnant JP, O'Fallan W, et al. The unchanging pattern of subarachnoid hemorrhage in a community. Neurology 1980;30:1034–1040.
5. Ingall TJ, Whisnant JP, Wiebers DO, O'Fallon WM. Has there been a decline in subarachnoid hemorrhage mortality? Stroke 1989;20:718–724.
6. Garraway WM, Whisnant JP, Furlan AJ, et al. The declining incidence of stroke. N Engl J Med 1979;300:449–452.

7. Locksley HB. Report of the Cooperative Study of Intracranial Aneurysms and Subarachnoid Hemorrhage: sec V, part I. Natural history of subarachnoid hemorrhage, intracranial aneurysms, and arteriovenous malformation—based on 6,368 cases in the cooperative study. J Neurosurg 1966; 25:219–239.

8. Weir B. Aneurysms Affecting the Nervous System. Baltimore: Williams & Wilkins, 1987.

9. Locksley HB. Report of the Cooperative Study of Intracranial Aneurysms and Subarachnoid Hemorrhage: sec V, part II. Natural history of subarachnoid hemorrhage, intracranial aneurysms, and arteriovenous malformation. J Neurosurg 1966;25:321–368.

10. Heros RC, Kistler JP. Intracranial arterial aneurysms—an update. Stroke 1983;14:628–631.

11. Winn WR, Richardson AE, Jane JA. The long-term prognosis in untreated cerebral aneurysms: I. The incidence of late hemorrhage in cerebral aneurysms—a ten year evaluation of 364 patients. Ann Neurol 1977;1:358–370.

12. Kassell NF, Kongable GL, Torner JC, et al. Delay in referral of patients with ruptured aneurysms to neurosurgical attention. Stroke 1985;16:587–590.

13. Caplan LR. Subarachnoid Hemorrhage, Aneurysms, and Vascular Malformations. In LR Caplan. Posterior Circulation Disease. Clinical Findings, Diagnosis, and Management. Boston: Blackwell, 1996;633–685.

14. van den Berg JSP, Limburg M, Pais G, et al. Some patients with intracranial aneurysms have a reduced type III/type I collagen ratio. Neurology 1997;49:1546–1551.

15. Ferguson GG. Physical factors in the initiation, growth, and rupture of human intracranial saccular aneurysms. J Neurosurg 1972;37:666–677.

16. Adams HP, Kassell N, Torner JC, et al. Early management of aneurysmal subarachnoid hemorrhage. J Neurosurg 1981;54:141–145.

17. Ferguson GG, Peerless SJ, Drake CG. Natural history of intracranial aneurysms. N Engl J Med 1981;305:99.

18. Caplan LR. Should intracranial aneurysms be treated before they rupture? N Engl J Med 1998;339:1774–1775.

19. Wiebers DO, Whisnant JP, O'Fallon WM. The natural history of unruptured intracranial aneurysms. N Engl J Med 1981;304:696–698.

20. Drake CG. Giant Intracranial Aneurysm: Experience with Surgical Treatment in 174 Patients. In PW Carmel (ed), Clinical Neurosurgery. Baltimore: Williams & Wilkins, 1979;12–95.

21. Kassell N, Drake CG. Review of the management of saccular aneurysms. In HJM Barnett (ed), Neurological Clinics, Vol 1. Philadelphia: Saunders, 1983;73–86.

22. Adams HP, Jergenson DD, Kassell NF, Sahs AL. Pitfalls in the recognition of subarachnoid hemorrhage. JAMA 1980;244:794–796.

23. Gorelick PB, Hier DB, Caplan LR, Langenberg P. Headache in acute cerebrovascular disease. Neurology 1986; 36:1445–1450.

24. Hauerberg J, Andersen BB, Eskesen V, et al. Importance of the recognition of a warning leak as a sign of a ruptured intracranial aneurysm. Acta Neurol Scand 1971;83:61–64.

25. Ostergaard JR. Warning leak in subarachnoid haemorrhage. BMJ 1990;301:190–191.

26. Drake CG. The Treatment of Aneurysms of the Posterior Circulation. In PW Carmel (ed), Clinical Neurosurgery. Baltimore: Williams & Wilkins, 1979;96–144.

27. Stewart RM, Samsom D, Diehl J, et al. Unruptured cerebral aneurysms presenting as recurrent transient neurological deficits. Neurology 1980;30:47–51.

28. Sutherland GR, King ME, Peerless SJ, et al. Platelet interaction within giant intracranial aneurysms. J Neurosurg 1982;56:53–61.

29. Weisberg LA. Ruptured aneurysms of anterior cerebral or anterior communicating arteries. Neurology 1985;35: 1562–1566.

30. Hunt WE, Hess RM. Surgical risk as related to time of intervention in the repair of intracranial aneurysms. J Neurosurg 1968;28:14–20.

31. Alvord EC, Loeser JD, Bailey WL, et al. Subarachnoid hemorrhage due to ruptured aneurysm: a simple method of estimating prognosis. Arch Neurol 1972;27:273–284.

32. Weisberg L. Computed tomography in aneurysmal subarachnoid hemorrhage. Neurology 1979;29:802–808.

33. Liliequist B, Lindquist M. Computer tomography in the evaluation of subarachnoid hemorrhage. Acta Radiol Diagn (Stockh) 1980;21:327–331.

34. van der Jagt M, Hasan D, Bijvoet HWC, et al. Validity of prediction of the site of ruptured intracranial aneurysm with CT. Neurology 1999;52:34–39.

35. Hijdra A, van Gijn J, Nagelkerke N, et al. Prediction of delayed cerebral ischemia, rebleeding, and outcome after aneurysmal subarachnoid hemorrhage. Stroke 1988;19: 1250–1256.

36. Brouwers PJ, Dippel DW, Vermeulen M, et al. Amount of blood on computed tomography as an independent predictor after aneurysm rupture. Stroke 1993;24:809–814.

37. Alberico RA, Patel M, Casey S, et al. Evaluation of the circle of Willis with three-dimensional CT angiography in patients with suspected intracranial aneurysms. AJNR Am J Neuroradiol 1995;16:1571–1578.

38. Ross J, Masaryk T, Modic M, et al. Intracranial aneurysms: evaluation by MR angiography. AJNR Am J Neuroradiol 1990;11:449–456.

39. Caplan LR, Flamm ES, Mohr JP, et al. Lumbar puncture and stroke. Stroke 1987;18:540A–544A.

40. Hayward RS. Subarachnoid hemorrhage of unknown etiology. J Neurol Neurosurg Psychiatry 1977;40:926–931.

41. Rinkel GJE, van Gijn J, Wijdicks EFM. Subarachnoid hemorrhage without detectable aneurysm: a review of the causes. Stroke 1993;24:1403–1409.

42. Caplan LR, Brass LM, DeWitt LD, et al. Transcranial Doppler ultrasound: present status. Neurology 1990;40: 696–700.

43. Lindegaard K, Grolemund P, Aaslid R, Normes H. Evaluation of cerebral AVMs using transcranial Doppler ultrasound. J Neurosurg 1986;65:335–344.

44. Schwartz A, Hennerici M. Noninvasive transcranial Doppler ultrasound in intracranial angiomas. Neurology 1986; 36:626–635.

45. Petty GW, Massaro AR, Tatemichi TK, et al. Transcranial Doppler ultrasonographic changes after treatment for arteriovenous malformations. Stroke 1990;21:260–266.

46. Harders AG, Gilsbach JM. Time course of blood velocity changes related to vasospasm in the circle of Willis measured by transcranial Doppler ultrasound. J Neurosurg 1987;66:718–728.

47. Sloan MA, Haley EC, Kassell NF, et al. Sensitivity and specificity of transcranial Doppler ultrasonography in the diagnosis of vasospasm following subarachnoid hemorrhage. Neurology 1989;391:1514–1518.

48. Sekhar L, Wechsler L, Yonas H, et al. Value of transcranial Doppler examination in the diagnosis of cerebral vasospasm after subarachnoid hemorrhage. Neurosurgery 1988; 22: 813–821.

49. Davis SM, Andrews JT, Lichtenstein M, et al. Correlations between cerebral arterial velocities, blood flow, and delayed ischemia after subarachnoid hemorrhage. Stroke 1992; 23:492–497.

50. Davis S, Andrews J, Lichtenstein M, et al. A single-photon emission computed tomography study of hyperperfusion after subarachnoid hemorrhage. Stroke 1990;21:252–259.

51. Van Gijn J, van Dongen KJ, Vermeulan M, et al. Perimesencephalic hemorrhage: a nonaneurysmal and benign form of subarachnoid hemorrhage. Neurology 1985;35: 483–487.

52. Rinkel GJ, Wijdicks E, Vermeulen M, et al. The clinical course of perimesencephalic nonaneurysmal subarachnoid hemorrhage. Ann Neurol 1991;29:463–468.

53. Schievink WI, Wijdicks EFM. Pretruncal subarachnoid hemorrhage: an anatomically correct description of the perimesencephalic subarachnoid hemorrhage. Stroke 1997;28:2572.

54. Wijdicks EFM, Schievink W, Miller GM. Pretruncal subarachnoid hemorrhage. Mayo Clin Proc 1998;73:745–752.

55. Rinkel GJ, Wijdicks E, Vermeulen M, et al. Outcome in perimesencephalic (nonaneurysmal) subarachnoid hemorrhage: a follow-up study in 37 patients. Neurology 1990; 40:1130–1132.

56. Wijdicks EFM, Schievink WI. Perimesencephalic nonaneurysmal subarachnoid hemorrhage: first hint of a cause? Neurology 1997;49:634–636.

57. Stein RW, Kase CS, Hier DB, et al. Caudate hemorrhage. Neurology 1984;34:1549–1554.

58. Hochberg F, Fisher CM, Roberson G. Subarachnoid hemorrhage caused by rupture of a small superficial artery. Neurology 1974;24:309–311.

59. Lasjaunias P, Chiu M, ter Brugge K, et al. Neurological manifestations of intracranial dural arteriovenous malformations. J Neurosurg 1986;64:724–730.

60. Broderick JP, Brott TG, Duldner JE, et al. Initial and recurrent bleeding are the major causes of death following subarachnoid hemorrhage. Stroke 1994;25:1342–1347.

61. Macdonald RL, Weir BKA. A review of hemoglobin and the pathogenesis of cerebral vasospasm. Stroke 1991;22: 971–982.

62. Macdonald RL. Cerebral Vasospasm. In KMA Welch, LR Caplan, DJ Reis, et al (eds), Primer on Cerebrovascular Diseases. San Diego: Academic, 1997;490–497.

63. Hughes JT, Schianchi PM. Cerebral artery spasm: a histological study at necropsy of the blood vessels in cases of subarachnoid hemorrhage. J Neurosurg 1978;48:515–525.

64. Conway LW, McDonald LW. Structural changes of the intradural arteries following subarachnoid hemorrhage. J Neurosurg 1972;37:715–723.

65. Wellum GR, Peterson JW, Zervas NT. The relevance of in vivo smooth muscle experiments to cerebral vasospasm. Stroke 1985;16:573–581.

66. Clower BR, Smith RR, Haining JL, Lockard J. Constrictive endarteropathy following experimental subarachnoid hemorrhage. Stroke 1981;12:501–508.

67. Kassell NF, Sasaki T, Colohan AR, Nazar G. Cerebral vasospasm following aneurysmal subarachnoid hemorrhage. Stroke 1985;16:562–572.

68. Kwak R, Niizuma H, Ohi J, et al. Angiography study of cerebral vasospasm following rupture of intracranial aneurysms: I. Time of the appearance. Surg Neurol 1979; 11:257–262.

69. Weir B, Grace M, Hansen J, et al. Time course of vasospasm in man. J Neurosurg 1978;48:173–178.

70. Heros RC, Zervas NT, Varsos V. Cerebral vasospasm after subarachnoid hemorrhage: an update. Ann Neurol 1983; 14:599–608.

71. Fisher CM, Kistler JP, Davis JM. Relation of cerebral vasospasm to subarachnoid hemorrhage visualized by computed tomographic scanning. Neurosurgery 1980; 6:1–9.

72. Graf CJ, Nibbelink DW. Cooperative Study of Intracranial Aneurysms and Subarachnoid Hemorrhage: report on randomized treatment study: III. Intracranial surgery. Stroke 1974;5:559–601.

73. Wilkins RH. Attempts at prevention or treatment of intracranial arterial spasm: an update. Neurosurgery 1986;18: 808–825.

74. Auer LM. Acute operation and preventive nimodipine improve outcome in patients with ruptured cerebral aneurysms. Neurosurgery 1984;15:57–66.

75. Mizukami M, Kawase T, Usami T, et al. Prevention of vasospasm by early operation with removal of subarachnoid blood. Neurosurgery 1982;10:301–307.

76. Taneda M. Effect of early operation for ruptured aneurysm in prevention of delayed ischemic symptoms. J Neurosurg 1982;5:622–628.

77. Findlay JM, Kassell NF, Weir BKA, et al. A randomized trial of intraoperative, intracisternal tissue plasminogen activator for prevention of vasospasm. Neurosurgery 1995;37:168–178.

78. Macdonald RL. Cerebral vasospasm. Neurosurg Q 1995;5: 73–97.

79. Kassell NF, Peerless SJ, Durward QJ, et al. Treatment of ischemic deficits from vasospasm with hypervolemia and induced arterial hypertension. Neurosurgery 1982;11: 337–343.

80. Solomon RA, Fink ME, Lennihan L. Prophylactic volume expansion therapy for the prevention of delayed cerebral

ischemia after early aneurysm surgery. Arch Neurol 1988; 45:325–332.

81. Solomon RA, Post KD, McMurty JG. Depression of circulating blood volume in patients after subarachnoid hemorrhage: implications for the management of symptomatic vasospasm. Neurosurgery 1984;15:354–361.

82. Wood JH, Simeone FA, Kron RE, et al. Rheological aspects of experimental hypervolemic hemodilation with low molecular weight dextran. Neurosurgery 1982;11:739–753.

83. Pickard JD, Murray GD, Illingworth R, et al. Effect of oral nimodipine in cerebral infarction and outcome after subarachnoid hemorrhage: British aneurysm nimodipine trial. BMJ 1981;298:636–642.

84. Allen GS. Cerebral arterial spasm: a controlled trial of nimodipine in subarachnoid hemorrhage patients—the nimodipine cerebral arterial spasm study group. Stroke 1983;14:122.

85. Feigin VL, Rinkel GJE, Algra A, et al. Calcium antagonists in patients with aneurysmal subarachnoid hemorrhage. A systematic review. Neurology 1998;50:876–883.

86. Higashida RT, Halbach VV, Cahan LD, et al. Transluminal angioplasty for treatment of intracranial arterial vasospasm. J Neurosurg 1989;71:648–653.

87. Newell DW, Eskridge JM, Mayberg M, et al. Angioplasty for the treatment of symptomatic vasospasm following subarachnoid hemorrhage. J Neurosurg 1989;91:654–660.

88. Eskridge JM. A practical approach to the treatment of vasospasm. AJNR Am J Neuroradiol 1997;18:1653–1660.

89. Rordorf G, Koroshetz WJ, Copen W, et al. Diffusion- and perfusion-weighted imaging in vasospasm after subarachnoid hemorrhage. Stroke 1999;30:599–605.

90. Haley EC, Kassell NF, Torner JC. The International Cooperative Study on the Timing of Aneurysm Surgery. The North American experience. Stroke 1992;23:205–214.

91. Leroux PD, Winn HR. Timing of Surgery and Special Features of Ruptured Anterior Circulation Aneurysms. In KMA Welch, LR Caplan, DJ Reis, et al (eds), Primer on Cerebrovascular Diseases. San Diego: Academic, 1997; 450–454.

92. Graff-Radford NR, Torner J, Adams HP, Kassell NF. Factors associated with hydrocephalus after subarachnoid hemorrhage. Arch Neurol 1989;46:744–752.

93. Samuels MA. Electrocardiographic manifestations of neurologic disease. Semin Neurol 1984;4:453–460.

94. Brouwers PJ, Wijdicks EF, Hasan D, et al. Serial electrocardiographic recording in aneurysmal subarachnoid hemorrhage. Stroke 1989;20:1162–1167.

95. Fabinyi G, Hunt D, McKinley L. Myocardial creatine kinase isoenzyme in serum after subarachnoid hemorrhage. J Neurol Neurosurg Psychiatry 1977;40:818–820.

96. Norris JW, Frogatt GM, Hachinski VC. Cardiac arrythmias in acute stroke. Stroke 1978;9:392–396.

97. Oppenheimer SM, Cechetto DF, Hachinski VC. Cerebrogenic cardiac arrythmias. Cerebral electrocardiographic influences and their role in sudden death. Arch Neurol 1990;47:513–519.

98. Di Pasquale G, Pinelli G, Andreoli A, et al. Holter detection of cardiac arrythmias in intracranial subarachnoid hemorrhage. Am J Cardiol 1987;59:596–600.

99. Di Pasquale G, Pinelli G, Andreoli A, et al. Torsade de pointes and ventricular flutter-fibrillation following spontaneous cerebral subarachnoid hemorrhage. Int J Cardiol 1988;18:163–172.

100. Kolin A, Norris JW. Myocardial damage from acute cerebral lesions. Stroke 1984;15:990–993.

101. Samuels M. "Voodoo" death revisited: the modern lessons of neurocardiology. The Neurologist 1997;3:293–304.

102. Caplan LR, Hurst JW, Chimowitz M. Clinical Neurocardiology. New York: Marcel Dekker, 1999;303–312.

103. Weir BK. Pulmonary edema following fatal aneurysmal rupture. J Neurosurg 1978;49:502–507.

104. Landolt AM, Yasargil MG, Krayenbuhl H. Disturbances of the serum electrolytes after surgery of intracranial arterial aneurysm. J Neurosurg 1972;37:210–218.

105. Takaku A, Shindo K, Tanaki S, et al. Fluid and electrolyte disturbances in patients with intracranial aneurysms. Surg Neurol 1979;11:349–356.

106. Diringer MN, Lim JS, Kirsch JR, Hawley DF. Suprasellar and intraventricular blood predict elevated plasma atrial natriuretic factor in subarachnoid hemorrhage. Stroke 1991;22:572–581.

107. Wijdicks EFM, Ropper AH, Hunnicutt EJ, et al. Atrial natriuretic factor and salt wasting after aneurysmal subarachnoid hemorrhage. Stroke 1991;22:1519–1524.

108. Peerless SJ. Pre- and postoperative management of cerebral aneurysm. Clin Neurosurg 1979;26:209–231.

109. Calhoun DA, Oparil S. Treatment of hypertensive crises. N Engl J Med 1990;323:1177–1183.

110. Adams HP. Current status of antifibrinolytic therapy for treatment of patients with aneurysmal subarachnoid hemorrhage. Stroke 1982;13:256–259.

111. Ramirez-Laseppas M. Antifibrinolytic therapy in subarachnoid hemorrhage caused by ruptured intracranial aneurysm. Neurology 1981;31:316–322.

112. Kassell N, Torner D, Adams H. Antifibrinolytic therapy in the acute period following aneurysmal subarachnoid hemorrhage. J Neurosurg 1984;61:225–230.

113. Garde A. Amnesia after operations on aneurysms of the anterior communicating artery. Surg Neurol 1982;18:46–49.

114. Damasio AR, Graff-Radford N, Eslinger P, et al. Amnesia following basal forebrain lesions. Arch Neurol 1985;42: 263–271.

115. Winn HR, Berga SL, Richardson AE, et al. Long-term evaluation of patients with cerebral aneurysms. Ann Neurol 1981;10:106.

116. Sundt TM, Whisnant JP. Subarachnoid hemorrhage from intracranial aneurysm. N Engl J Med 1978:299:116–122.

117. Raaymakers TWM, Rinkel GJE, Limburg M, Algra A. Mortality and morbidity of surgery for unruptured intracranial aneurysms. A meta-analysis. Stroke 1998;29:1531–1538.

118. Stein BM, Wolpert SM. Arteriovenous malformations of the brain: I. Current concepts and treatment. Arch Neurol 1980:37:1–5.

119. Tonnis W, Schiefer W, Walter W. Signs and symptoms of supratentorial arteriovenous aneurysms. J Neurosurg 1953; 15:471–480.

120. McCormick WF. The pathology of vascular ("arteriovenous") malformations. J Neurosurg 1966;24:807–816.

121. McCormick WF. Pathology of Vascular Malformations of the Brain. In CB Wilson, BM Stein (eds), Intracranial Arteriovenous Malformations: Current Neurosurgical Practice. Baltimore: Williams & Wilkins, 1984.

122. McCormick WF, Boulter TR. Vascular malformations ("angiomas") of the dura mater. J Neurosurg 1966; 25: 309–311.

123. McCormick WF. The Pathology of Angiomas. In JM Fein, ES Flamm (eds), Cerebrovascular Surgery, Vol IV. New York: Springer, 1985;1073–1095.

124. McCormick WF, Hardman JM, Boulter TR. Vascular malformations ("angiomas") of the brain, with special reference to those occurring in the posterior fossa. J Neurosurg 1968;28:241–251.

125. The Arteriovenous Malformations Study Group. Arteriovenous Malformations of the brain in adults. N Engl J Med 1999;340:1812–1818.

126. Rigamonti D, Hadley MN, Drayer BP, et al. Cerebral cavernous malformations: incidence and familial occurrence. N Engl J Med 1988;319:343–347.

127. Savoiardo M, Strada L, Passerini A. Intracranial cavernous hemangiomas: neuroradiologic review of 36 operated cases. AJNR Am J Neuroradiol 1983;4:945–950.

128. Mason I, Aase JM, Orrison WW, et al. Familial cavernous angiomas of the brain in an Hispanic family. Neurology 1988;38:324–326.

129. Wilms G, Bleus E, Demaerel P, et al. Simultaneous occurrence of deveopmental venous anomalies and cavernous angiomas. AJNR Am J Neuroradiol 1994;15:1247–1254.

130. Abe T, Singer RJ, Marks MP, et al. Coexistence of occult vascular malformations and developmental venous anomalies in the central nervous system: MR evaluation. AJNR Am J Neuroradiol 1998;19:51–57.

131. Omojola M, Fox A, Vinuela F, Debrun G. Stenosis of afferent vessels of intracranmial arteriovenous malformations. AJNR Am J Neuroradiol 1985;6:791–793.

132. Mawad ME, Hilal SK, Michelson J, et al. Occlusive vascular disease associated with cerebral arteriovenous malformations. Radiology 1984;153:401–408.

133. Marks MP, Lane B, Steinberg GK, Snipes GJ. Intranidal aneurysms in cerebral arteriovenous malformations: evaluation and endovascular treatment. Radiology 1992;183: 355–360.

134. Kondziolka D, Nixon BJ, Lasjaunias P, et al. Cerebral arteriovenous malformations with associated arterial aneurysms: hemodynamic and therapeutic considerations. Can J Neurol Sci 1988;15:130–134.

135. Miyasaka Y, Yada K, Ohwada T, et al. An analysis of the venous drainage system as a factor in hemorrhage from arteriovenous malformations. J Neurosurg 1992; 76:239–243.

136. Vinuela F, Nombela L, Roach MR, et al. Stenotic and occlusive disease of the draining venous system of deep brain AVMs. J Neurosurg 1985;63:180–184.

137. Hsu FPK, Rigamonti D, Huhn SL. Epidemiology of Cavernous Malformations. In IA Awad, DL Barrows (eds), Cavernous Malformations. Park Ridge, IL: American Association of Neurological Surgeons, 1993;13–23.

138. Kase CS. Aneurysms and Vascular Malformations. In CS Kase, LR Caplan (eds), Intracerebral Hemorrhage. Boston: Butterworth–Heinemann, 1995;153–178.

139. Perret G, Nishioka H. Report on the Cooperative Study of Intracranial Aneurysms and Subarachnoid Hemorrhage. Section VI. Arteriovenous malformations. An analysis of 545 cases of cranio-cerebral arteriovenous malformations and fistulae reported to the Cooperative Study. J Neurosurg 1966;25:467–490.

140. Crawford PM, West CR, Chadwick DW, et al. Arteriovenous malformations of the brain: natural history in unoperated patients. J Neurol Neurosurg Psychiatry 1986;49:1–10.

141. Graf CJ, Perret GE, Torner JC. Bleeding from cerebral arteriovenous malformations as part of their natural history. J Neurosurg 1983;58:331–337.

142. Hook C, Johanson C. Intracranial arteriovenous aneurysms: a follow-up study with particular attention to their growth. Arch Neurol Psych 1958;80:39–54.

143. Patterson JH, McKissock W. A clinical survey of intracranial angiomas with special reference to their mode of progression and surgical treatment: a report of 110 cases. Brain 1965;79:233–266.

144. Svien J, McRae JA. Arteriovenous anomalies of the brain. J Neurosurg 1965;23:23–28.

145. Chimowitz MI, Little JR, Awad IA, et al. Intracranial hypertension associated with unruptured cerebral arteriovenous malformations. Ann Neurol 1990;27:474–479.

146. DeJong RN, Hicks SP. Vascular malformation of the brainstem: report of a case with long duration and fluctuating course. Neurology 1980;30:995–997.

147. Stahl SM, Johnson KP, Malamud N. The clinical and pathological spectrum of brainstem vascular malformations. Arch Neurol 1980;37:25–29.

148. Caroscio JT, Brannan T, Budabin M, et al. Subarachnoid hemorrhage secondary to spinal arteriovenous malformation and aneurysm. Arch Neurol 1980;37:101–103.

149. Robinson JC, Hall CS, Sedzimir CB. Arteriovenous malformations, aneurysms, and pregnancy. J Neurosurg 1974; 41:63–70.

150. Jensen H, Klinge H, Lemke J, et al. Computerized tomography in vascular malformations of the brain. Neurosurg Rev 1980;3:119–127.

151. Daniels D, Houghton V, Williams A, et al. Arteriovenous malformation simulating a cyst on computed tomography. Radiology 1979;133:393–394.

152. Rigamonti D, Drayer B, Johnson PC, et al. The MRI appearance of cavernous malformations (angiomas). J Neurosurg 1987;67:518–524.

153. Gomori JM, Grossman RI, Hackney DB, et al. Variable appearances of subacute intracranial hematomas on high-field spin-echo MR. AJR Am J Roentgenol 1988;150: 171–178.

154. Farmer J-P, Cosgrove GR, Villemure FG, et al. Intracerebral cavernous angiomas. Neurology 1988;38:1699–1704.

155. Requena I, Arias M, Lopez-Iber L. Cavernomas of the cerebral nervous system in clinical and neuroimaging manifestations in 47 patients. J Neurol Neurosurg Psychiatry 1991;54:590–594.

156. Perl J, Ross JS. Diagnostic Imaging of Cavernous Malformations. In IA Awad, DL Barrow (eds), Cavernous Malformations. Park Ridge, IL: American Association of Neurological Surgeons, 1993;37–48.

157. Hardjasudarma M. Cavernous and venous angiomas of the central nervous system. Neuroimaging and clinical controversies. J Neuroimaging 1991;1:191–196.

158. Rigamonti D, Spetzler RF, Drayer BP, et al. Appearance of venous malformations on magnetic resonance imaging. J Neurosurg 1988;69:535–539.

159. Lee C, Pennington MA, Kenney CM. MR evaluation of developmental venous anomalies: medullary venous anatomy of venous angiomas. AJNR Am J Neuroradiol 1996;17:61–70.

160. Diehl RR, Henkes H, Nahser H-C, et al. Blood flow velocity and vasomotor reactivity in patients with arteriovenous malformations. A transcranial Doppler study. Stroke 1994;25:1574–1580.

161. Marks M, Lane B, Steinberg G, Chang P. Vascular characteristics of intracerebral arteriovenous malformations in patients with clinical steal. AJNR Am J Neuroradiol 1991;12:489–496.

162. Drake CG. Arteriovenous malformations of the brain: the options for management. N Engl J Med 1983;309:308–310.

163. Heros RC, Tu Y-K. Is surgical therapy needed for unruptured arteriovenous malformations? Neurology 1987;37:279–286.

164. Drake CG. Cerebral arteriovenous malformations: considerations for and experience with surgical treatment in 166 cases. Clin Neurosurg 1979;26:145–208.

165. Forster DMC, Steiner L, Hakanson S. Arteriovenous malformations of the brain: a long-term clinical study. J Neurosurg 1972;37:562–570.

166. Hartmann A, Mast H, Mohr JP, et al. Morbidity of intracranial hemorrhage in patients with cerebral arteriovenous malformation. Stroke 1998;29:931–934.

167. Duong DH, Young WL, Vang MC, et al. Feeding artery pressure and venous drainage pattern are primary determinants of hemorrhage from arteriovenous malformations. Stroke 1998;29:1167–1176.

168. Aminoff MJ. Treatment of unruptured cerebral arteriovenous malformations. Neurology 1987;37:815–819.

169. Barrow DL. Classification and natural history of cerebral vascular malformations: arteriovenous, cavernous, and venous. J Stroke Cerebrovasc Dis 1997;6:264–267.

170. Robinson JR, Awad IA, Little JR. Natural history of the cavernous angioma. J Neurosurg 1991;75:709–714.

171. Kondziolka D, Lundsford LD, Kestle JRW. The natural history of cerebral cavernous malformations. J Neurosurg 1995;83:820–824.

172. Robinson JR, Awad IA. Clinical Spectrum and Natural Course. In IA Awad, DL Barrows (eds), Cavernous Malformations. Park Ridge, IL: American Association of Neurological Surgeons, 1993;25–36.

173. Moran NF, Fish DR, Kitchen N, et al. Supratentorial cavernous haemangiomas and epilepsy: a review of the literature and case series. J Neurol Neurosurg Psychiatry 1999; 66:561–568.

174. Garner TB, Curling OD Jr, Kelly DL Jr, et al. The natural history of intracranial venous angiomas. J Neurosurg 1991;75:715–722.

175. Rigamonti D, Spetzler RF, Medina M, et al. Cerebral venous malformations. J Neurosurg 1990;73:560–564.

176. Naff NJ, Wemmer J, Hoenig-Rigamonti K, Rigamonti DR. A longitudinal study of patients with venous malformations: documentation of a negligible hemorrhage risk and benign natural history. Neurology 1998;50:1709–1714.

177. Spetzler RF, Wilson CB, Weinstein P, et al. Normal perfusion pressure breakthrough theory. Clin Neurosurg 1978; 25:651–672.

178. Fournier D, TerBrugge KG, Willinsky R, et al. Endovascular treatment of intracerebral arteriovenous malformations: experience in 49 cases. J Neurosurg 1991;75:228–233.

179. Vinuela F, Fox AJ, Debrun G, et al. Progressive thrombosis of brain arteriovenous malformations after embolization with isobutyl-2-cyanoacrylate. AJNR Am J Neuroradiol 1983;4: 959–966.

180. Vinters HV, Lundie MJ, Kaufmann JC. Long-term pathological follow-up of cerebral arteriovenous malformations treated by embolization with buccylate. N Engl J Med 1986;314:477–483.

181. Kjellberg RN, Hanamura T, Davis KR, et al. Bragg-peak proton beam therapy for arteriovenous malformations of the brain. N Engl J Med 1983;309:269–274.

182. Lunsford LD, Flickinger J, Coffey RJ. Stereotactic gamma knife radiosurgery. Initial North American experience in 207 patients. Arch Neurol 1990;47:169–175.

183. Heros R, Korosue K. Radiation treatment of cerebral arteriovenous malformations. N Engl J Med 1990;323:127–129.

184. Meder JF, Oppenheim C, Blustajn J, et al. Cerebral arteriovenous malformations: the value of radiologic parameters in predicting response to radiosurgery. AJNR Am J Neuroradiol 1997;18:1473–1483.

185. Steinberg G, Fabrikant J, Marks MP, et al. Stereotactic heavy-charged-particle Bragg-peak radiation for intracerebral arteriovenous malformations. N Engl J Med 1990; 323:96–101.

186. Coffey RJ, Lunsford LD. Radiosurgery of Cavernous Malformations and Other Angiographically Occult Vascular Malformations. In IA Awad, DL Barrow (eds), Cavernous Malformations. Park Ridge, IL: American Association of Neurological Surgeons, 1993;187–200.

187. Dion J. Dural Arteriovenous Malformations: Definition, Classification, and Diagnostic Imaging. In IA Awad, DL Barrow (eds), Dural Arteriovenous Malformations. Park Ridge, IL: American Association of Neurological Surgeons, 1993;1–19.

188. Castaigne P, Bories J, Brunet P, et al. Les fistules arterioveineuse meningees pures a drainage veineux cortical. Rev Neurol (Paris) 1976;132:169–181.

189. Gaston A, Chiras J, Bourbotte G, et al. Meningeal arteriovenous fistulae draining into cortical veins: 31 cases. J Neuroradiol 1984;11:161–177.

190. Bederson JB. Pathophysiology and Animal Models of Dural Arteriovenous Malformations. In IA Awad, DL Barrow (eds), Dural Arteriovenous Malformations. Park Ridge, IL: American Association of Neurological Surgeons, 1993;23–33.

191. Friedman AH. Etiologic Factors in Intracranial Dural Arteriovenous Malformations. In IA Awad, DL Barrow (eds), Dural Arteriovenous Malformations. Park Ridge, IL: American Association of Neurological Surgeons, 1993;35–47.

192. Raybaud CA, Hald JK, Strother CM, et al. Aneurysms of the vein of Galen. Angiographic study and morphogenetic considerations. Neurochirurgie 1987;33:302–314.

193. Hansen JH, Segaard I. Spontaneous regression of an extra- and intracranial arteriovenous malformation: case report. J Neurosurg 1976 45:338–341.

194. Houser OW, Campbell JK, Campbell RJ. Arteriovenous malformation affecting the transverse dural venous sinus: an acquired lesion. Mayo Clin Proc 1979;54:651–661.

195. Fermand M, Reizine D, Melki JP, et al. Long term follow-up of 43 pure dural arteriovenous fistulae (AVF) of the lateral sinus. Neuroradiology 1987;29:348–353.

196. Lasjaunias PL, Rodesch G. Lesion Types, Hemodynamics, and Clinical Spectrum. In IA Awad, DL Barrow (eds), Dural Arteriovenous Malformations. Park Ridge, IL: American Association of Neurological Surgeons, 1993; 49–79.

197. Awad IA, Little JR, Akrawi WP, et al. Intracranial dural arteriovenous malformations: factors predisposing to an aggressive neurological course. J Neurosurg 1990;72: 839–850.

198. Zeidman SM, Monsein LH, Arosarena O, et al. Reversibility of white matter changes and dementia after treatment of dural fistulas. AJNR Am J Neuroradiol 1995; 16:1080–1083.

199. Awad IA. Dural Arteriovenous Malformations with Aggressive Clinical Course. In IA Awad, DL Barrow (eds), Dural Arteriovenous Malformations. Park Ridge, IL: American Association of Neurological Surgeons, 1993;93–104.

200. Wecht DA, Awad IA. Carotid Cavernous and Other Dural Arteriovenous Fistulas. In KMA Welch, LR Caplan, DJ Reis, et al (eds), Primer on Cerebrovascular Diseases. San Diego: Academic, 1997;541–548.

201. Purdy PD. Management of Carotid Cavernous Fistula. In HH Batjer, LR Caplan, L Friberg, et al (eds), Cerebrovascular Disease. Philadelphia: Lippincott-Raven,1997; 1159–1168.

202. Takahashi S, Tomura N, Watarai J, et al. Dural arteriovenous fistula of the cavernous sinus with venous congestion of the brain stem: report of two cases. AJNR Am J Neuroradiol 1999;20:886–888.

203. Halbach VV, Higashida RT, Hieshima GB, et al. Treatment of dural fistulas involving the deep cerebral venous system. AJNR Am J Neuroradiol 1989;10:393–399.

204. Awad IA. Tentorial Incisura and Brain Stem Dural Arteriovenous Malformations. In IA Awad, DL Barrow (eds), Dural Arteriovenous Malformations. Park Ridge, IL: American Association of Neurological Surgeons, 1993;131–146.

205. Halbach VV, Higashida RT, Hieshima GB, et al. Transvenous embolization of dural fistulas involving the transverse and sigmoid sinuses. AJNR Am J Neuroradiol 1989; 10:385–392.

206. Barnwell S. Endovascular Therapy of Dural Arteriovenous Malformations. In IA Awad, DL Barrow (eds), Dural Arteriovenous Malformations. Park Ridge, IL: American Association of Neurological Surgeons, 1993; 193–211.

207. Mullan S. Surgical Therapy: Indications and General Principles. In IA Awad, DL Barrow (eds), Dural Arteriovenous Malformations. Park Ridge, IL: American Association of Neurological Surgeons, 1993;213–229.

208. Awad IA, Barrow DL. Conceptual Overview and Management Strategies. In IA Awad, DL Barrow (eds), Dural Arteriovenous Malformations. Park Ridge, IL: American Association of Neurological Surgeons, 1993;131–241.

Chapter 13
Intracerebral Hemorrhage

Bleeding into the substance of the brain was recognized as a cause of stroke by Morgagni in 1761.[1] Cheyne wrote a treatise on apoplexy and coma in 1812, in which he included examples of intracerebral hemorrhage (ICH).[2] Clinicians of the nineteenth and twentieth centuries considered ICH invariably lethal. Postmortem examples were usually studied because the tests available could not identify ICH during life. Clinicians correlated the clinical findings with the size and location of hemorrhages found in brains at necropsy. Gowers[3] and Osler,[4] writing at the turn of the twentieth century, included long and detailed chapters on the usual locations of ICH, and accompanying clinical signs and symptoms in their respective textbooks. In 1935, Aring and Merritt[5] correlated the clinical and pathologic findings of 245 patients with stroke who came to necropsy at the Boston City Hospital. Aring and Merritt emphasized the features that separated hemorrhage from infarction. The major teachings emanating from these works are summarized in the following general rules:

1. ICH occurred at a younger age than brain infarction.
2. The major cause of ICH was hypertension, often severe.
3. Symptoms of ICH began abruptly.
4. Loss of consciousness was a nearly constant feature.
5. Headache always accompanied ICH, and was usually severe.
6. The most common locations for ICH were the putamen, internal capsule, thalamus, pons, and cerebellum.

7. ICH was invariably fatal or devastating, with few, if any, intact survivors.

This work, however, was published long before computed tomography (CT) scanning. Aring and Merritt's teachings evolved from correlation with fatal cases. Technology did not exist to diagnose less severe hemorrhages during life, especially if the lesions did not communicate with the cerebrospinal fluid (CSF). CT now allows accurate localization of small- and medium-sized hemorrhages. CT not only shows clinicians whether a lesion is a hemorrhage, but also accurately shows the location, size, spread within the brain, drainage into the ventricles and spaces around the brain, and presence of edema and mass effect. Magnetic resonance imaging (MRI), by its capability of showing the presence of hemosiderin, can help define whether lesions are old hemorrhages. Old infarcts and hemorrhages can look similar on CT. When the subject of ICH is reviewed in light of results with newer imaging techniques, the old rules are found to apply to larger hemorrhages, which is only a small fraction of ICHs. I begin this chapter by reviewing the general rules and findings applicable to ICH at any site. I then review the etiologies of ICH and the findings in hemorrhages at their common locations in the brain.

Incidence and Epidemiology

Approximately 10% of strokes are caused by ICH. The pilot Stroke Data Bank (SDB),[6] Michael Reese Stroke Registry (MRSR),[7] and Harvard Stroke Reg-

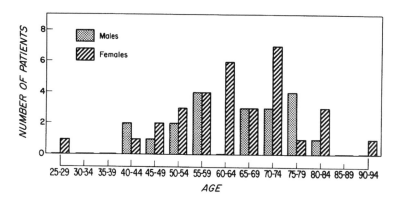

Figure 13-1. Age distribution in patients with intracerebral hemorrhage. (Reprinted with permission from LR Caplan, JP Mohr. The Harvard Cooperative Stroke Registry. Intracerebral hemorrhage: an update. Geriatrics 1978;33:42–52. Copyright © Advanstar Comm. Inc.)

istry (HSR)[8] found that approximately 1 stroke in 10 was caused by parenchymatous brain hemorrhage; the same figure was reached in studies of stroke at the Mayo Clinic in Rochester, Minnesota.[9,10] Populations that have a high frequency of hypertension, such as African-Americans and individuals of Chinese, Japanese, and Thai ancestry, have higher frequencies of ICH. ICH affects a wide age range, with many examples in the seventh, eighth, and ninth decades of life. Figure 13-1 displays the age and sex distribution of ICH in the HSR.[11] Figure 13-2 is a graph of age distribution in the combined MRSR and SDB. Although it is probably accurate to say that a higher percentage of strokes in patients younger than 40 years are hemorrhagic, ICH is also common during the later years of life.

Clinical Course and Accompanying Symptoms

JT, a 44-year-old African-American schoolteacher, rushed to arrive at an important job interview. While being stressfully interrogated, he noted tingling in his left hand, which gradually spread to his arm. He excused himself to go to the washroom, and then noted a similar feeling in his left leg. As he washed his hands, he realized his left hand and arm were clumsy and weak. He tripped on his left foot as he walked back. The interviewer was alarmed by slurring of words and a droop of the left face, which he noticed when JT returned. An ambulance was called. JT began to feel

a headache over his right scalp. After 10 minutes, the emergency team arrived. JT could no longer move his left arm and leg, but seemed unaware and unconcerned with his handicap. He now had a severe headache and was sleepy. While being placed on a stretcher, he began to vomit. He had no history of hypertension or drug use. Blood pressure was 175/110 mm Hg when he was first examined by the emergency personnel.

The course of illness in this patient was the gradual accumulation of focal neurologic signs, during a period of approximately 20 minutes. As the neurologic symptoms and disability worsened, headache, decreased alertness, and vomiting developed.

ICH develops gradually. Bleeding into the brain tissues from small, deep, penetrating vessels is usually under arteriolar or capillary pressure. This situation contrasts with subarachnoid hemorrhage (SAH), in which arteries on the brain surface leak blood under systemic arterial pressure. Symptoms in patients with SAH begin instantaneously and consist of headache, loss of concentration and alertness, and vomiting. These symptoms are caused by sudden increase in intracranial pressure (ICP), resulting from blood rapidly disseminating through the CSF around the brain substance. In contrast, ICH develops gradually during minutes or sometimes hours.

Fisher examined serial sections of ICH studied at necropsy.[12] At the center of the lesions was a large mass of blood. At the periphery were many of what he called *fibrin globes*, representing little caps of fibrinous material that plugged small vessels, which had broken and leaked during life. As ICH develops, pressure within the central core increases and compresses small vessels at the periphery of the hematoma. These peripheral arterioles and capillaries in turn break, and blood escapes, enlarging the lesion. The hematoma grows like a snowball rolling downhill, accumulating more snow on its outer circumference as it rolls. ICP rises as the lesion enlarges, and tissue pressure around the lesion also mounts. Eventually, an equilibrium is reached between the pressure within the hematoma and surrounding pressure, and bleeding stops. If the hematoma reaches the ventricle or brain surface, it may communicate with the CSF, discharge part of its contents at the same time, and, in doing so, decompress the pressure within the lesion.

Visualizing the pathology of the lesion and its development helps predict the pace of the symptoms. Bleeding is directly into brain parenchyma, rather than the CSF, as occurs in SAH. The brain is devoid of pain fibers, so the initial release of blood does not cause headaches. Instead, blood disrupts the function of that particular local brain region. If the hematoma began in the left putamen, the patient might note right-limb weakness. As the hemorrhage grows during the next few minutes, the weakness becomes more severe. Sensory symptoms, loss of speech, and conjugate eye deviation to the side of the hemorrhage might ensue. In JT, the combination of sensory (tingling) and motor symptoms in the left side of his face, and left arm and leg, suggests a process in the deep structures of the right cerebral hemisphere, affecting the internal capsule region. If the hemorrhage grew to a size that increased ICP and distorted adjacent meningeal structures, the patient would develop headache, vomiting, and reduced alertness. In JT, headaches, sleepiness, and vomiting started and evolved after he became hemiplegic and his lesion expanded. If the hematoma continued to grow, coma and death might result from compression of vital brain stem centers.

Sometimes, clinical symptoms and signs evolve over a period of days, rather than minutes or hours. Herbstein and Schaumburg studied a group of patients with ICH to determine whether progressive clinical decline was caused by continued bleeding or edema around the lesion.[13] They tagged red blood

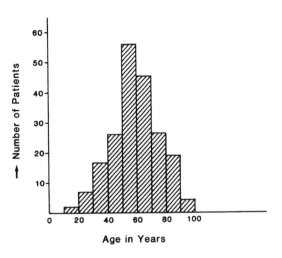

Figure 13-2. Age distribution by decade of 111 patients with intracerebral hemorrhage from the Michael Reese Stroke Registry and the Stroke Data Bank.

cells with chromium 51 and injected these erythrocytes into the circulation 1–5 hours after their initial examination. Counts of radioactivity were made from the hematoma cavities at necropsies performed from 1 to 15 days later. Radioactivity within the hematomas did not increase, but patients who developed secondary (Düret lesion) brain stem hemorrhages after the injection had increased activity within the brain stem lesions, but not within the primary hemorrhages. Hematomas were often surrounded by edema.[13] Although this study showed that hematomas usually do not expand after the initial hours, studies of patients with acute ICHs using sequential CT studies show that hematomas can, at times, expand dramatically.[14–17] Repeat CT may show dramatic enlargement of hematoma mass and ventricular drainage, developing within hours after the first CT scan. Invariably, clinical worsening was also present and was an indication for repeat scanning in some patients. In one study, 41 out of 204 patients with ICH had expansion of ICHs on repeat CT scans.[17] Expansion in this study was most often detected during the first 6 hours, but 5 out of 33 hematomas (15%) expanded between 6 and 12 hour scans, and 2 out of 34 hematomas (6%) enlarged between 12 and 24 hour scans.[17] Patients with ICH who have a bleeding diathesis are especially prone to hematomas that expand gradually and enlarge over a period of days.[18,19]

Analysis of the course of illness in 54 well-documented patients with ICH studied in the HSR showed that 37 had gradual development of symptoms during a period of minutes or a few hours.[11] In the 17 remaining patients, progression of symptoms did not seem to occur after the patients were first found by others. In many of this latter group, an accurate account of the earliest development of symptoms was not available because of aphasia, lack of awareness of the deficit, or stupor. A smooth, gradual worsening of function during minutes, followed by headache and vomiting, was the rule in larger lesions. Some patients who had stabilized during the first 24–48 hours later developed progressively decreased alertness and increasing focal signs within 48–72 hours, probably caused by edema around the hematomas.

I find an early description of the gradual evolution of symptoms in a fatal case of ICH memorable.[20] This patient, seen in 1937, developed and evolved his hematoma while entirely under observation. He was sent to the hospital because of "malignant hypertension." While his history was taken, he noted weakness and dizziness. He stated that he noted numbness and tingling of the hands just before he left the admitting area, at which time his heart had been examined. He became extremely restless and apprehensive while his history was taken. He complained of inability to hear, difficulty in swallowing, and dyspnea. The patient was placed on the examining table, and his blood pressure was found to be 245 systolic and 170 diastolic. Under the eyes of several examiners, complete bilateral palsy of the sixth nerve developed; both pupils dilated, and the corneal reflexes disappeared. The patient was still able to talk, but with a typical bulbar speech, and he appeared almost completely deaf. His left leg became paretic, and rapid clonic movements were observed. Babinski's sign was present bilaterally. Within an hour, the patient was completely stuporous and his blood pressure had risen to 280 systolic and 170 diastolic. This rapidly progressive chain of events was most unpleasant to witness and produced a depressing effect on the nurses and physicians.[20]

I had a similar experience during my first week as a medical intern at the Boston City Hospital. An elderly hypertensive Chinese man came to the emergency room with slight weakness of his right limbs. He spoke normally. He was placed on the danger list, and a porter and I pushed his stretcher through the underground hospital tunnels toward the ward. As we pushed the stretcher, his right limbs became weaker, and he stopped talking. Soon, his eyes and head deviated to the left, and I could not arouse him. By the time we reached the ward, he was comatose and decerebrate. He died within hours.

Like Kornyey and his colleagues,[20] I felt helpless watching brain function inexorably vanish. When a detailed history is possible, nearly all patients with ICH have had a gradual evolution of symptoms and signs—some more rapidly evolving than others.[21]

Headache

Headache was not an invariable symptom in the 60 HSR patients with ICH. Headache was described in only 17 patients (28%) near the outset of neurologic symptoms.[11] Another seven patients (12%) noted headache later. Twenty-four patients (40%) had no headache at any time during their ICH. The 12 stuporous or comatose patients (20%) could not provide data regarding headache.[11] Headache was much more frequent with larger lesions, and was often absent or minimal in patients with small lesions.

Among 289 patients with ICH studied at one Portuguese hospital, 165 patients (57%) had a headache near the onset of their ICHs.[22] Headache was most common in patients with lobar and cerebellar hematomas, locations near the meningeal surface, and was common in patients with meningeal signs.[22] Patients with small, deep hematomas often never develop headache during their course of illness. In many patients, headache occurs as the hematoma enlarges and is accompanied by vomiting and decreased alertness.[21]

Decreased Level of Consciousness

Loss of consciousness accompanies only large hematomas and those found in the brain stem. Diminished alertness in patients with ICH is caused by mass effect and increased ICP, or direct involvement of the brain stem reticular activating system. In the HSR, 30 of 60 patients were alert when first seen.

Fourteen patients (23%) were lethargic, and 16 patients (27%) were stuporous or comatose.[11] In SDB patients with ICH, decreased level of consciousness was the most important adverse prognostic sign. Decreased level of consciousness predicts poor outcome in nearly all studies of prognosis in patients with ICH.[21,23–25] All patients with ICH who had severely reduced levels of consciousness in the SDB died.[23] Early reduction of consciousness is not an invariable accompaniment of ICH. When it occurs, however, it has an ominous prognosis. The sleepiness that developed in JT was a serious finding and should have triggered urgent evaluation and treatment when he arrived at the hospital.

Vomiting

JT started to vomit while he was taken to the hospital, and continued to vomit in the emergency room. Vomiting is an especially important sign in patients with ICH. In ICH and SAH, vomiting is usually caused by increased ICP or local distortion of the fourth ventricle. Few patients with ischemic lesions within the cerebral hemispheres vomit, but nearly one-half of patients with hemispheral hemorrhages vomit. In the posterior circulation, vomiting usually reflects dysfunction of the vestibular nuclei, or the so-called vomiting center, in the floor of the fourth ventricle.[26] Vomiting occurs in approximately one-third of patients with occlusive posterior circulation disease. Vomiting also occurs in more than one-half of patients with posterior circulation hemorrhages. Patients with cerebellar hemorrhage almost always vomit early in their clinical course.

Seizures

Seizures are not common during the acute phase of a stroke, but are slightly more frequent in ICH than other stroke types, except embolism.[8,21] Among three series of patients with spontaneous nontraumatic ICH, 12.5%,[27] 15.4%,[28] and 17%[29] of patients had seizures during their early course. Lobar hemorrhages, slit-like hemorrhages situated near the gray-white junction of the cortex, and putaminal hemorrhages that undercut the cerebral cortex[29] are especially epileptogenic.

Other Symptoms and Signs

Neck stiffness is uncommon in putaminal hemorrhage,[30] but is often found in patients with caudate, thalamic, and cerebellar hemorrhages.[30–32] Fever is relatively common, but is often related to infectious complications, such as pulmonary and urinary tract infections. Subhyaloid retinal hemorrhages, common in SAH, are rare in ICH, unless the hematoma has developed rapidly and is large.[33] Cardiac arrhythmias and pulmonary edema develop in some patients with ICH, and are usually attributed to changes in ICP and catecholamine release, a similar pathogenesis to that used to explain cardiac findings in patients with SAH.[21]

Etiologies

Although aneurysms and vascular malformations are important causes of ICH, I discuss these vascular lesions in Chapter 12 and do not repeat the discussions here.

Hypertension

The most common cause of ICH is hypertension, but the blood pressure does not need to be elevated to malignant ranges. Figure 13-3 shows the distribution of blood pressure in the MRSR and SDB. Many patients present to the hospital with ICH and have no prior history of hypertension, but have high blood pressure on admission. In this circumstance, it is difficult to know how much, if any, of the blood pressure elevation is secondary to raised ICP (the Cushing response), and what the level of blood pressure was before the bleed.

When hypertension first develops, the small arteries and capillaries are exposed to a high head of pressure and could leak. This situation is comparable to the hemodynamics found in patients with mitral valve stenosis. Left atrial failure develops because of mitral valve obstruction. The left atrial failure causes increased pressure in the pulmonary veins. To perfuse the lungs, pulmonary artery pressure rises to maintain an arteriovenous pressure gradient. The pulmonary capillaries and arterioles are exposed to the increased head of pressure and break, causing hemoptysis. Later,

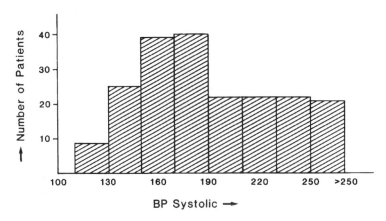

Figure 13-3. Systolic blood pressure (BP) distribution in 110 patients with intracerebral hemorrhage in the Michael Reese Stroke Registry and the Stroke Data Bank.

small arteries and arterioles hypertrophy, protecting the capillary bed from high central pressure. Hemoptysis becomes less frequent when arterioles hypertrophy, but the heart bears the brunt of the increased arterial resistance. In this instance, right heart failure may develop. Similarly, increased arterial pressure, early in the course of development of systemic hypertension, causes arteriolar and capillary rupture. Later in the course of hypertension, degenerative changes in the form of lipohyalinosis and miliary Charcot-Bouchard aneurysms develop, caused by long-standing pressure elevations. ICH occurs when these and related degenerative abnormalities cause arterial and arteriolar rupture. The occurrence of ICH is biphasic, with patients presenting both at the onset of hypertension and later, after developing considerable wear and tear on penetrating brain arteries.[34,35]

Some hypertensive hemorrhages arise from degenerative changes, such as fibrinoid degeneration and microaneurysms, which develop in patients with hypertension. Cole and Yates examined the brains of 100 hypertensive patients and 100 normotensive controls.[36] All 13 patients with ICH had microaneurysms and were hypertensive. Among 63 patients with microaneurysms, 46 patients had hypertension recognized during life. The age distribution of microaneurysms is also interesting. Among 21 hypertensive patients younger than 50 years, only two patients had microaneurysms, whereas 71% of hypertensive patients in the 65- to 69-year age range had microaneurysms.[36]

Rosenblum analyzed the morphology of aneurysms and their parent vessels.[37] Some arteries bore early aneurysmal dilatations, whereas others had sclerosed aneurysms with flask-shaped collections of collagen joined to a small artery by a narrow neck. Microaneurysms are often surrounded by hemosiderin-laden macrophages, indicating previous leakage. The lesions are most common in penetrating arteries that supply the basal ganglia, thalamus, pons and cerebellum, and arteries supplying the gray–white matter cortical junctions of the hemispheres. Figure 13-4 shows a section through a microaneurysm that was found associated with a hemorrhage in the pons. The same arteries that bear microaneurysms also contain foci of lipohyalinosis and fibrinoid degeneration, which explains the dictum that ischemic lacunes have the same relative distribution as hypertensive ICH.

Fisher described the results from examination of serial sections of patients with ICH. Fibrin globes, meshes of platelets encircled by a thin layer of fibrin, protruded from ruptured sites and clearly marked vessels that had bled.[12] A relationship between iris aneurysms and cerebral microaneurysms exists because rabbits with experimentally induced hypertension develop iris aneurysms approximately proportional to their development of cerebral microaneurysms.[38] Studies from Japan regarding surgical specimens of acute ICH show that penetrating arteries frequently break, but often not in relation to microaneurysms.[39,40] Degenerative lipohyalinotic changes were present in the broken and adjacent arteries. Degenerative changes caused by aging and hypertension can predispose to ICH, but it is not certain that microaneurysms represent the bleeding lesion.[35,39,40]

Figure 13-4. Section of a pontine aneurysm stained with hematoxylin, eosin, and Sudan III. The sac is partially occluded by organizing blood clot. Recent hemorrhage is seen around the aneurysm. (Reprinted with permission from FHK Green. Miliary aneurysms in the brain. J Pathol Bacteriol 1930;33:71–77.)

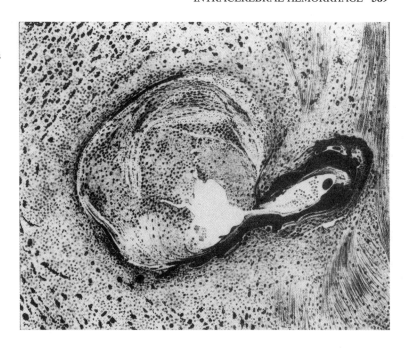

Considerable evidence has accumulated that shows acute changes in blood pressure and blood flow can precipitate rupture of penetrating arteries in the absence of prior hypertension.[34,35] In a large necropsy study of patients who died from ICH, Bahemuka used heart weights to estimate the frequency of hypertension; only 46% of fatal cases of spontaneous ICH had moderate to severe chronic hypertension or left ventricular hypertrophy.[41] Brott and colleagues reviewed the records of 154 patients with spontaneous ICH in Cincinnati, Ohio, during 1 year, to determine the frequency of hypertension.[42] Only 45% had a history of hypertension; another 12% without a history of hypertension had left ventricular hypertrophy. The authors judged that approximately 50% of cases were not attributable to chronic hypertension.[42]

In these two series,[41,42] the location of the hemorrhages, increased blood pressure on admission, and absence of other etiologies makes it highly probable that these hematomas were, in fact, satisfactorily classified as hypertensive ICH. Probably, hypertension was acute and led to bleeding from unprotected capillaries and arterioles. My own observations and those of others have documented ICH in situations in which blood pressure probably increased abruptly.[34,35]

My first experience with patients who had acute hypertension-related ICH was with patients who developed ICH after exposure to severe cold weather.[43] While outdoors in temperatures below −10°F, three patients developed putaminal, thalamic, and cerebellar hematomas, respectively. One patient was in the midst of alcohol withdrawal, one was removing ice from his car window, and the third patient was waiting in line to pay rent. All had increased blood pressure on admission, but their pressures normalized soon thereafter. Immersion in cold is known to be a strong sympathetic nervous system stimulus. Formerly, the cold-pressor test[44] (immersion of hands in ice water) was used clinically to induce transient hypertension, a phenomenon said to be more common in patients with essential hypertension. Sympathetic stimulation caused by alcohol withdrawal and stress may have added to the effects of cold exposure in these patients.

Dental procedures,[45,46] surgery directly involving or placing traction on the trigeminal nerve,[47,48] and stimulation of the trigeminal nerve[49] have also been associated with ICH. In one patient known to have been previously normotensive, dental pain after irrigation of the mouth was followed immediately by a fatal temporal lobe hemorrhage.[45] Blood pressure was elevated acutely. Necropsy showed no evidence of hypertensive vascular damage in any organ and no other cause of brain hemorrhage.[45] In a series of patients operated on intracranially for trigeminal neuralgia, hematomas developed at locations typical for hypertensive ICH.[47] Other procedures involving manipulation of the trigeminal nerve for treatment of trigeminal neuralgia have also been complicated by ICH.[35,49] Monitoring of blood pressure and heart rate during trigeminal stimulation often shows important fluctuations in blood pressure and pulse rate.[50,51] The blood vessels of the brains of animals and humans have important trigeminal innervation.[52,53]

ICH has been frequently associated with the use of illicit drugs, especially cocaine and methamphetamine, which are known to have sympatheticomimetic effects. I discuss drug-induced ICH in more detail later in this chapter because of its growing frequency as an important cause of stroke and ICH. Patients have also developed ICH after sudden augmentation of cerebral blood flow, either locally to one hemisphere, as in the circumstance of ICH after carotid endarterectomy,[54–56] or systemically, after correction of congenital heart defects or cardiac transplantation in the young.[57,58] ICH has also been reported to develop during recovery from migraine.[34,59] Intense vasoconstriction leads to diminished flow and, perhaps, ischemia to local blood vessels. Reperfusion then leads to ICH in the zone of prior vascular damage. A similar mechanism probably underlies most examples of hemorrhagic infarction caused by cerebral embolism.[60] This mechanism of brain hemorrhage is discussed in Chapter 9.

Probably more important than the unusual circumstances just cited are events of everyday life that can raise blood pressure. Wilson was quite aware of this concept. He wrote in his neurology text, "Emotional experience, joy, anger, fear, or apprehension may disturb the action of the heart, trivial though the incident may be—an address at a public meeting, trouble with a cook, and so on."[61]

A patient of mine, LF, presented a vivid example of the possible interrelationship between daily activities and stresses, and the triggering of ICH. He was a retired university professor who came to ask my opinion about what he called a "strange stroke" he had a few years previously. Because he never had high blood pressure before or after the stroke, he was puzzled that his physicians attributed his condition to a hypertensive ICH. The events of his day are as follows:

> LF had an active teaching day, with more than the usual responsibilities. He hurried to finish his work so he could be on time for an engagement that night. His wife had symphony tickets. They planned to go with a couple (whom he considered to be unpleasant bores) to hear Mahler (whom he found tedious). He arrived late at the restaurant, and had a hurried and unpleasant meal. The two couples had to run to the symphony hall nearby to arrive in time to be seated, and they rushed to their seats in front. As he hustled toward his seat, he recalled thinking how wonderful it would have been to remain at work. He got to his seat in a sweat and noticed a gradually developing left hemiparesis.

I reviewed LF's CT and hospital records. A typical small right putaminal hemorrhage was present. His blood pressure was transiently elevated on admission, but soon normalized. Acute fluctuations in blood pressure and flow, and chronic degenerative changes are important in the etiology of so-called hypertensive ICH. In either case, bleeding is into the territories of penetrating arteries. It is not known whether the size, location, and clinical picture in these two types of hypertensive ICH differ.[35]

In the case of JT, he was hypertensive when first examined, but had no history of hypertension. Could the stressful interview have contributed to an acute blood pressure rise, or had he developed hypertension recently? His blood pressure stayed elevated during hospitalization, and he required antihypertensive treatment at the time of hospital discharge.

Older patients, often in their 70s or 80s, may present with ICH. Is this because of degenerative changes in these patients' arterial system? Does ICH occur because of coexistent amyloid angiop-

Table 13-1. Causes of Intracerebral Hemorrhage in Large Series of Patients

	Russell,[101] Number (%)	Mutlu,[102] Number (%)	McCormick,[103] Number (%)	Schutz,[104] Number (%)	Jellinger,[105] Number (%)	Weisbeg,[106] Number (%)	Qureshi,[107] Number (%)
Hypertension	232 (50)	135 (60)	37 (26)	140 (56)	80 (47)	197 (66)	311 (77)
Vascular malfor-mations[a]	117 (25)	50 (22)	35 (24)	30 (12)	53 (31)	28 (9)	11 (3)
Bleeding disorder[b]	36 (8)	30 (13)	28 (20)	21 (8)	5 (3)	14 (5)	8 (2)
Tumor	9 (2)	2 (1)	13 (9)	8 (3)	12 (7)	5 (2)	—
Arteritis	13 (3)	2 (1)	5 (3)	2 (1)	2 (1)	—	—
Other	38 (8)	6 (3)	14 (10)	—	13 (8)	2 (1)	—
Unknown	16 (4)	—	12 (8)	49 (20)	5 (3)	50 (17)	73 (18)
Totals	**461**	**225**	**144**	**250**	**170**	**296**	**403**

[a]Including aneurysms.
[b]Including thrombolysis/anticoagulation.
Source: Modified from LR Caplan, CS Kase. Mechanisms of Intracerebral Hemorrhage. In CS Kase, LR Caplan (eds), Intracerebral Hemorrhage. Boston: Butterworth–Heinemann, 1994;95–98.

athy, which is recognized with increasing frequency when sought in elderly patients with lobar hemorrhages? Older patients seem to develop ICH at relatively lower blood pressures than younger patients. Probably because of atrophy, symptoms of increased ICP, such as headache, vomiting, and reduced alertness, are less common in older patients, even with sizable lesions. This observation makes differentiation between hemorrhage and infarction more difficult in geriatric patients.

Bleeding Diathesis

A variety of coagulopathies can lead to bleeding into the brain substance, sometimes accompanied by systemic bleeding. Anticoagulation with heparin or warfarin accounts for an all-too-high percentage of this type of ICH. Considering the large number of patients treated with anticoagulants, the number that develop ICH is small. Among a series of 1,626 patients treated with long-term anticoagulants, 30 had ICH, of which two-thirds were fatal.[62] The most consistent risk factor for intracranial or systemic bleeding was prolongation of the prothrombin time beyond the therapeutic range.

Some hemorrhages occur even when the international normalized ratio is in the therapeutic range.[18,19] As with other etiologies of ICH, hypertension aggravates the tendency to bleed intracranially. The three features that characterize anticoagulant-induced ICH as distinct from other causes are as follows:

1. Hemorrhage often develops gradually and insidiously during many hours, or even days (6 of 14 patients with anticoagulant-related ICH had an insidious clinical course).[18]
2. The cerebellum and cerebral lobes are involved more frequently than in hypertensive ICH.[18,19]
3. A high morbidity and mortality rate exists (15 of 24 patients died,[18,19] and only patients with smaller hematomas [less than 30-cc volume] had a favorable chance for survival; only 1 of 24 patients with ICH had bleeding elsewhere).

Anticoagulant-related ICH is a particularly difficult situation to treat because many patients take warfarin to prevent ischemic stroke. Patients with prosthetic heart valves, rheumatic mitral stenosis, or atrial fibrillation have a high risk for cerebral emboli without warfarin therapy. Especially when the indication for anticoagulants is strong and the early presenting symptoms are slight, treating physicians might be inclined to continue anticoagulant therapy. Treating physicians may not reverse the hypoprothrombinemia with vitamin K or fresh frozen plasma. In my experience, this tactic is a mistake because many anticoagulant-related hemorrhages insidiously progress. Because of their size and location in the surgically accessible cerebellum and cerebral lobes, many eventually require lifesaving surgery.

The initial clinical diagnosis may also be difficult in the group on warfarin for stroke prophylaxis because the first reaction to the neurologic symptoms is to predict that the patient had an ischemic stroke despite the treatment. I have found two useful axioms:

1. If a patient on anticoagulants develops neurologic symptoms, the cause is anticoagulant-related hemorrhage until proven otherwise.
2. If anticoagulant hemorrhage is verified, immediately give vitamin K and fresh frozen plasma.

Pursue all measures aggressively to stop the bleeding. Although no formal prospective studies clarify the optimal time for restarting anticoagulants after ICH in patients who require long-term treatment, a retrospective analysis found that after 10–14 days, recurrent ICH did not develop.[63] I believe it is safe to restart heparin or warfarin 2–3 weeks after ICH when indicated. When the indication for anticoagulation is relative or questionable, it is probably best to discontinue anticoagulants, perhaps using platelet antiaggregants instead. When the risk of embolism is high, heparin can be used after a few days.

Leukemia, hemophilia, thrombocytopenia, and disseminated intravascular coagulation are other important causes of ICH, although it is unusual in these disorders for bleeding to be confined only to the brain. Patients given recombinant tissue plasminogen activator to treat coronary artery thrombosis sometime develop ICH, most often in the cerebral lobes or cerebellum.[64] The frequency is rather low, but the brain hematomas are usually devastating or fatal.[64] ICH also occurs after recombinant tissue plasminogen activator infusion to treat occlusive cerebrovascular lesions. In this circumstance, hematomas usually begin within the region of brain infarction.

Drugs

A variety of commonly abused substances are known to cause ICH.[65] Alert clinicians should always think of the possibility of drug-related hemorrhage in young patients, in whom other causes of ICH, except trauma and arteriovenous malformations (AVMs), are rare. Perhaps best known are amphetamine ("speed") hemorrhages. Hemorrhage often develops within a few minutes of drug use. The most frequent presenting symptoms are headache, confusion, and seizures.[65,66] Despite large-volume ICHs, few focal signs are present in such patients. This phenomenon is perhaps explained by the frequent coexistence of brain edema, infarcts, and a diffuse vasculopathy, in addition to the focal ICH. In some patients, acute hypertension follows amphetamine use and can potentiate ICH. When first examined by physicians, most patients with amphetamine hemorrhage do not have signs of sympathetic overactivity, such as hypertension, tachycardia, or fever.[65–67]

Citron et al. studied 14 drug abusers, almost all admitting use of methamphetamine, among other drugs.[68] At necropsy, a fibrinoid necrosis of the media and intima of small- and medium-sized arteries existed, resembling polyarteritis nodosa.[68] Rumbaugh and colleagues studied the angiographic features of a group of methamphetamine abusers and noted beaded arteries with segmental constriction and dilatation of intracranial arteries.[69] In monkeys given intravenous amphetamines, angiography showed similar changes as found in human patients. Necropsy showed small brain hemorrhages, zones of infarction, microaneurysms, and a vasculitis similar to that described by Citron.[70]

I reviewed 30 reported, well-documented examples of intracranial hemorrhage after amphetamine use.[65] Twenty-four patients were known drug abusers; some patients also used other drugs, and many often used alcohol. Amphetamine, methamphetamine, and dextroamphetamine were the most frequently used drugs. Seventeen individuals (57%) took oral amphetamines, 12 (40%) administered the drug intravenously, and one person inhaled amphetamine nasally. Amphetamine (14% of patients) and methamphetamine use were more often responsible for hemorrhage than dextroamphetamine (4%) use in causing intracranial bleeding. The dose used was often unknown or unstated, but hemorrhage followed doses as small as 20 mg of oral amphetamine.[65,67] Age among the 22 men and eight women ranged from 19 to 51 years, with an average age of 25.4 years.[65] In 23 individuals, the bleeding was intracerebral and most often lobar. In contrast to cocaine-related hemorrhage, only 1 of the 30 individuals (3%) had an underlying vascular lesion in the form of an aneurysm or AVM.[65,71] Amphetamine-related hemorrhage can be serious; seven patients with hemorrhage died (23%), and nine required surgical drainage (30%).[65] A potent solid form of D-methamphetamine base that can be smoked has appeared in the streets under the name *ice*. This form is more potent and rapid acting. The ice-amphetamine relation has the potential to prove similar to the crack-cocaine-hydrochloride relationship in terms of complications and potency.

Angiography has often shown striking abnormalities in chronic amphetamine users and other patients with amphetamine-related ICH. Most common are segmental areas of constriction, irregularity, and occasionally fusiform dilatation.[65,67,72,73] The focal vascular abnormalities usually emphasize superficial cortical arterial branches and are often referred to as *beading*. At times, the changes disappear on subsequent angiography.[72] Customarily, these arteriographic changes have been attributed to arteritis. Immunologic phenomena are common in drug users.[65,66] Amphetamines are known to be potent vasoconstrictors. Vasoconstriction can become chronic and produce chronic morphologic changes in the media of involved arteries. Segmental changes and beading in some amphetamine users is probably caused by pharmacologic effects of the drugs used, and does not represent a true arteritis.

Since the early 1980s, cocaine has far surpassed amphetamines as a public health problem and cause of stroke and drug-related ICH. Cocaine hydrochloride is usually snorted nasally. During the 1980s, addicts turned to crack cocaine, a substance made by mixing aqueous cocaine hydrochloride with ammonia and sometimes baking soda. Crack cocaine is smoked or inhaled after the cocaine is mixed in the alkaline solution and is precipitated as alkaloidal cocaine. Crack cocaine is absorbed quickly, reaching the brain in less than 10 seconds.[65] Cocaine hydrochloride can be taken in a variety of ways—orally, vaginally, rectally, sublingually, nasally, and by subcutaneous, intramuscular, or intravenous injection. Cardiovascular effects

begin immediately after use and consist of an increase in pulse, blood pressure, temperature, and metabolism. The pressor effects of cocaine are similar to those of amphetamine and are probably mediated through a peripheral catecholamine mechanism.[65,74,75]

In a 1994 text, I reviewed 45 examples of cocaine-related ICH.[65] The series included 28 men and 17 women, with ages ranging from 22 to 57 years (average age, 33.6 years). Headache, focal neurologic signs, and sudden loss of consciousness were the most frequent symptoms and usually began immediately or shortly after the episode of drug use.[65,75] Concurrent use of alcohol was common. ICH followed use of cocaine by any route. Fifteen individuals used crack, 14 snorted cocaine nasally, and 11 injected the drug intravenously. The acute mortality was relatively high (14 out of 45, 31%).[65]

The most common location of cocaine-related ICH was lobar (57%). In others, the bleeding often involved deep structures known as frequent sites of hypertensive ICH. These included one caudate, three thalamic, and eight putaminal hematomas. Of great interest and importance was the frequent presence of an underlying vascular lesion. Twelve patients had AVMs, three had aneurysms, and one had a glioma with recurrent hemorrhage.[65] Similarly, among 31 patients who developed SAH after cocaine use, 15 (48%) had aneurysms. Among 29 patients with adequate angiographic or necropsy study, or both, 25 (86%) had aneurysms.[65] Cocaine-related ICH has a high mortality and high frequency of underlying aneurysms and AVMs. Clearly, cocaine-related intracranial bleeding is an indication for angiography, especially when the bleeding is subarachnoid or lobar. Underlying vascular lesions are less common when the ICH is deep. Most authors have attributed cocaine-related hemorrhage to the sympatheticomimetic effects of the drug. In some reported cases, the blood pressure is high after admission (i.e., 240/140 mm Hg, 220/110 mm Hg, or 210/120 mm Hg).[65] Some patients have had a hypertensive encephalopathy with multiple ICHs and brain edema. An example of these changes is shown in Figure 11-15.

Another drug known to have sympatheticomimetic capabilities is phencyclidine, known as *PCP* or *angel dust*, which has also been occasionally implicated as a cause of ICH[76,77] and hypertensive encephalopathy.[78] Two other hallucinogens, lysergic acid diethylamide (known as *LSD*) and mescaline, are also known to raise blood pressure and cause vasoconstriction. To my knowledge, however, no reports document ICH after use of these drugs.

More controversial is the issue of ICH after use of amphetamine-like drugs that are mostly used as anorexic agents to lose weight. These drugs are usually sold over the counter as diet suppressants or stimulants. The most commonly cited agent is phenylpropanolamine (PPA), which is often combined with an antihistamine and caffeine. PPA is primarily a partial α-adrenergic agonist and has little, if any, β-adrenergic agonist activity.[79] PPA was used by individuals who developed ICH, but the numbers are relatively small, considering the frequency of use. Among 19 patients, only four were men.[65] Ten of the 19 patients were younger than 30 years old. In some, the PPA compounds were taken in high doses in suicidal attempts. Two patients had SAH only, and 17 patients had ICH (two of which were multiple).[80,81] Twelve PPA-related hematomas were lobar, seven were putaminal-capsular, and two were thalamic.[65] Blood pressures recorded on initial examination were usually within the normal range, but some were high (i.e., 210/130 mm Hg, 160/104 mm Hg, and 210/110 mm Hg).

Segmental vascular changes on angiography, similar to those found after amphetamine use, have been described.[82] In one patient, the angiographic changes cleared after abstinence from PPA for 1 month.[82] In four patients, histologic analysis of tissue removed at surgical drainage of hematomas was available. Three patients had no indication of vascular lesion on light microscopy, but the fourth patient did have a necrotizing vasculitis.[83]

Examples of putative PPA-related hemorrhages are difficult to evaluate. In some cases, use of diet pills was surely incidental, and in other patients, other multiple drugs and risk factors coexisted.[65] In several patients, ICH occurred a few weeks postpartum, a time of vulnerability for spontaneous vascular complications. Although PPA has been shown to be associated with ICH in experimental animals[84] and humans,[65,79–85] reactions to PPA compounds are often idiosyncratic. A risk of ICH clearly exists for those who use PPA in a higher-than-suggested dose. Prior hypertension; additional use of alcohol, coffee, or caffeine; concomitant use of monoamine oxidase inhibitors;

and use during the postpartum period increase the risk of hemorrhage after PPA ingestion.

Occasionally, ICH develops after the intravenous use of drugs that are manufactured for oral consumption, such as pentazocine and pyribenzamine ("T's and blues") or methylphenidate.[65,86] Talc, methylcellulose crystals, and cornstarch obliterate the lung arterioles, allowing the injected particles to reach the systemic circulation after intravenous use. The damage to brain arterioles then predisposes users to develop ICH.[86]

Amyloid Angiopathy

Congophilic or cerebral amyloid angiopathy (CAA) was recognized by Zenkevich as a potential cause of ICH,[87] but Jellinger is probably most responsible for bringing this disorder to the attention of the neurologic community.[88,89] I discuss this condition in Chapter 11.

Awareness of CAA has led to wider use of special stains and recognition that an ever-increasing percentage of ICH, especially in the elderly, is related to CAA. The disorder usually affects small arteries and arterioles in the leptomeninges and cerebral cortex; involved arteries are thickened by an acellular hyaline material that stains positively with periodic acid–Schiff stains, and has an apple-green birefringence with polarized Congo red stain.[90] Figure 11-10 shows a brain section that contains amyloid-staining arterioles. Sometimes, the vessel wall seems to be reduplicated or split. CAA predominantly affects persons older than 65 years and increases in frequency in the eighth and ninth decades[90]; in some series of patients, a striking female predilection exists.[91,92] At necropsy, most patients have senile plaques, and many patients have been diagnosed clinically with Alzheimer's disease.

Amyloid-laden arteries are most often found in the occipital and parietal regions, less often in the other cerebral lobes; rarely, if ever, are these arteries found in the deep basal gray matter, brain stem, or cerebellum. Hemorrhages may be quite large and are often multiple.[92–95] Some patients have recurrent ICH or SAH in different lobar sites, a finding in an elderly person that is virtually diagnostic of CAA. At necropsy, small scattered cerebral infarcts and Alzheimer's-related changes are found, along with evidence of old slit-like lobar hemorrhages. Echo planar MRI scans may show many small old hemorrhages (Figure 11-11). Some patients have a Binswanger-like picture, with chronic white matter gliosis and atrophy. Like anticoagulant-related hemorrhages, CAA-related hemorrhages may develop insidiously. Perhaps because of coexisting atrophy, pressure symptoms, such as headache and vomiting, are less frequent than in younger patients with hypertensive or AVM-related hemorrhages.

Trauma

Trauma is an important cause of intracerebral bleeding. In some patients, a traumatic etiology is not clear from the history. I have seen several patients who were rendered aphasic or stuporous by head blows delivered by others and who could give no history of the trauma; assailants and others did not disclose their complicity. In other patients, retrograde amnesia developed after the head injury, and patients had no recollection of a fall or other injury. A search for superficial head bruises or lacerations is worthwhile when the etiology of ICH is not obvious. Traumatic ICH is most often accompanied by contusions in the basal frontal and temporal lobes, which may be multiple.[96] Occasionally, a late or delayed hemorrhage, referred to as a *spät hemorrhage*, develops into an area of traumatic brain edema when the local swelling subsides.[96,97]

Other Causes and Frequency of Various Etiologies

Brain tumors[98] and vasculitis and vasculopathies of various types [99] are occasionally complicated by ICH. Dural sinus and cerebral venous thrombosis is another important cause of ICH and is discussed in Chapter 14. Table 13-1 lists the frequencies of common etiologies among six large series of ICH patients.[100–107] These series predated recognition of amyloid angiopathy as an important cause of ICH. Table 13-2 shows the frequency of various causes of ICH in a series of 200 Mexican patients younger than 40 years. This table illustrates the locations of

hemorrhages in patients with these etiologies according to age.[108]

Signs and Symptoms of Intracerebral Hemorrhage at Common Locations

Just as there are physicians who believe the introduction of chest x-rays made the stethoscope obsolete, some doctors believe that detailed knowledge of the findings on neurologic examination of patients with central nervous system lesions is no longer necessary since the advent of CT and MRI scans. Because hemorrhages are so well imaged by CT, why bother to learn the physical findings? In the future, physicians will probably not have an inexpensive pocket or portable CT or MRI to replace the examination of patients. Prognosis and treatment of ICH often depends on the locale of the hemorrhage. Particular locations (i.e., cerebral lobes, right putamen, and cerebellum) are relatively accessible to surgical drainage, whereas others (i.e., thalami and brain stem) are not accessible. Clinical distinction between ICH and superficial cerebral infarction caused by large vessel occlusive disease or cerebral embolism depends on localization of the lesion to deep (ICH) or superficial (infarct) location. Knowledge of findings in patients with hemorrhages at various locations teaches clinicians to search for tumors, abscesses, demyelinating lesions, and other disorders in the same locations in other patients. Historically, hemorrhages in the cerebellum, thalami, and caudate nucleus were recognized before cerebellar, thalamic, or caudate infarction. Awareness of the clinical syndromes associated with ICH in these locations made it possible to later recognize infarcts in these regions. For these and many other regions, it is still important for clinicians to know the common clinical syndromes in ICH and be able to localize clinically the lesion in most patients with intracranial hemorrhages.[109]

Keys to localization of ICH are as follows:

1. Motor signs—quadriparesis, hemiparesis, or no paresis
2. Pupillary function—asymmetry, size, and light reaction
3. Extraocular movements—supranuclear, nuclear, internuclear gaze palsies

Table 13-2. Frequency of Location of Intracerebral Hemorrhage by Cause in Patients Younger Than 40 Years

Cause (Number)	Lobar (n = 110)	Ganglionic (n = 43)	Brain Stem (n = 26)	Cerebellum (n = 10)	Intraventricular (n = 8)	Mixed (n = 3)
Hypertension (22)	2	16	3	0	0	1
AVM (67)	45	7	6	6	3	0
Cavernous angioma (32)	15	3	11	2	1	0
CVT (10)	9	1	0	0	0	0
Drugs (7)	3	4	0	0	0	0
Toxemia (7)	3	4	0	0	0	0
Other (14)	9	1	0	1	2	1
Unknown (41)	24	7	6	1	2	1

AVM = arteriovenous malformation; CVT = cerebral venous thrombosis.
Source: Reprinted with permission from JL Ruiz-Sandoval, C Cantu, F Barinagarrementeria. Intracerebral hemorrhage in young people: analysis of risk factors, locations, causes, and prognosis. Stroke 1999;30:537–541.

4. Gait abnormalities—especially ataxia

Figure 13-5 and Table 13-3 summarize the usual abnormalities of these functions in patients with hemorrhages at the most common locations of ICH.

Hemorrhages of the Lateral Basal Ganglia, Putamen, and Internal Capsule

The most common location of hypertensive ICH is the lateral basal ganglionic capsular region.[110] These lesions are usually referred to as *putaminal hemorrhage* because they most often begin in the putamen. The usual findings include contralateral hemiparesis, contralateral hemisensory loss, and conjugate deviation of the eyes toward the side of the hematoma. The pupils are generally normal and gait is hemiparetic. Patients with a left putaminal hemorrhage usually have a nonfluent aphasia with relative preservation of ability to repeat spoken language. Right-sided lesions are associated with left visual neglect, motor impersistence, and constructional dyspraxia. These abnormalities of higher cortical function are probably caused by disconnection and undercutting of cortical zones, and are usually more transient than in patients with cortical infarcts of equal size. Some patients develop ipsilateral adventitious movements that the family or observers call "tremor"; these movements are probably caused by involvement of ipsilateral descending projections of the extrapyramidal system.

In patients with large putaminal hemorrhages, stupor increases as the lesion enlarges; the ipsilateral pupil at first becomes smaller, and later, larger than the opposite pupil; the ipsilateral plantar response becomes extensor; and a bilateral horizontal gaze palsy develops. The presence of any of these signs—ipsilateral Babinski's sign, abnormal ipsilateral pupil, or ipsilateral gaze paresis—has a grim prognosis.[11,23,110] These additional findings are caused by midline shift or compression of the rostral brain stem by the expanding hematoma. Figure 13-6 shows necropsy brain specimens of large putaminal hemorrhages.

The findings described are those found in patients with large hematomas, which involve the medial and most anterior portions of the posterior putamen, and the anterior two-thirds of the posterior limb of the internal capsule.[110–112] This location is the most common site for putaminal hemorrhage because it is supplied by the largest of the lateral lenticulostriate arteries. Some lesions affect the anterior limb of the internal capsule and anterior putamen and produce a milder, more transient hemiparesis without sensory abnormalities.[110,111] When hematomas are in the posterior third of the internal capsule and far posterior extreme of the putamen, sensory abnormalities predominate, with little or no hemiparesis. An inferior quadrantanopia or hemianopia may be present. Patients with lesions in the far posterior left putamen

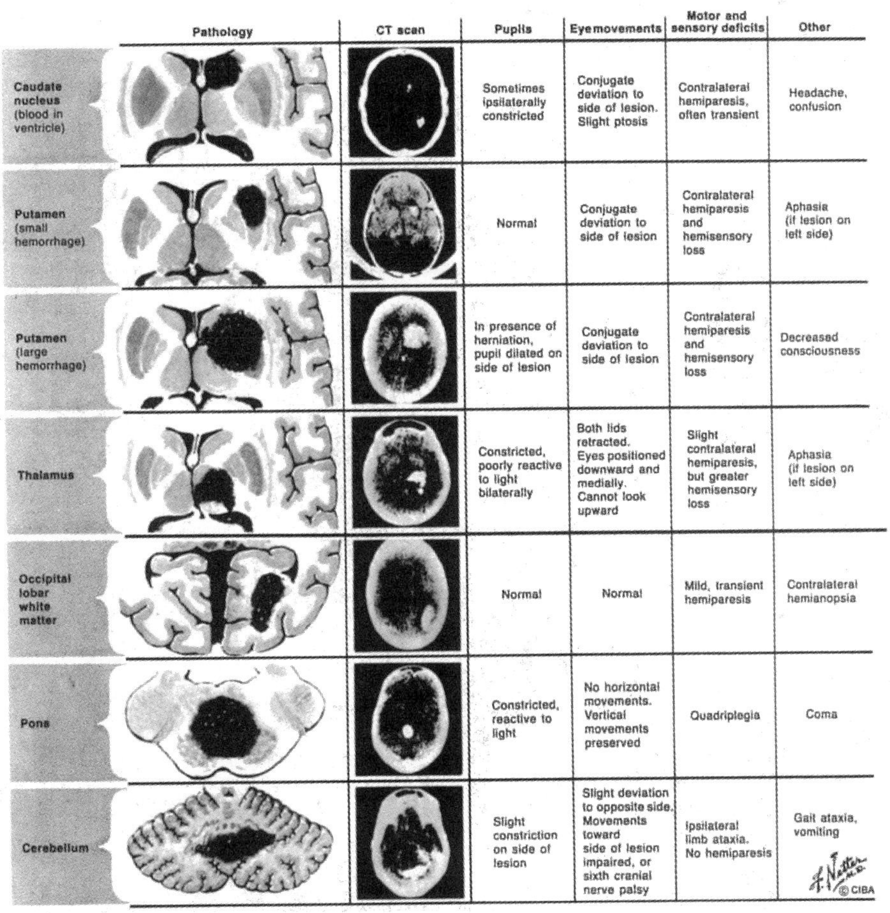

Pathology	CT scan	Pupils	Eye movements	Motor and sensory deficits	Other
Caudate nucleus (blood in ventricle)		Sometimes ipsilaterally constricted	Conjugate deviation to side of lesion. Slight ptosis	Contralateral hemiparesis, often transient	Headache, confusion
Putamen (small hemorrhage)		Normal	Conjugate deviation to side of lesion	Contralateral hemiparesis and hemisensory loss	Aphasia (if lesion on left side)
Putamen (large hemorrhage)		In presence of herniation, pupil dilated on side of lesion	Conjugate deviation to side of lesion	Contralateral hemiparesis and hemisensory loss	Decreased consciousness
Thalamus		Constricted, poorly reactive to light bilaterally	Both lids retracted. Eyes positioned downward and medially. Cannot look upward	Slight contralateral hemiparesis, but greater hemisensory loss	Aphasia (if lesion on left side)
Occipital lobar white matter		Normal	Normal	Mild, transient hemiparesis	Contralateral hemianopsia
Pons		Constricted, reactive to light	No horizontal movements. Vertical movements preserved	Quadriplegia	Coma
Cerebellum		Slight constriction on side of lesion	Slight deviation to opposite side. Movements toward side of lesion impaired, or sixth cranial nerve palsy	Ipsilateral limb ataxia. No hemiparesis	Gait ataxia, vomiting

Figure 13-5. Clinical manifestations related to site in intracerebral hemorrhage. (Reprinted with permission from The Ciba Collection of Medical Illustrations. Illustrated by Frank H. Netter, M.D. All rights reserved. Copyright ©1986 CIBA Pharmaceutical Company, division of CIBA-GEIGY Corporation.)

may have fluent Wernicke-like aphasia because of undercutting of the temporal lobe or extension of the lesion into the temporal isthmus, giving the hematoma a hockey stick–like configuration. Figure 13-7 shows the anatomic distribution of lesions within the lateral basal ganglionic region on horizontal brain section. The most common and largest lesions affecting the anterior part of the posterior limb of the internal capsule are often referred to as the *middle type,* whereas the others are termed *anterior* or *posterior* types of putaminal hematomas.[110] Figure 13-8 shows the lateral lenticulostriate arteries that supply the lateral ganglionic region. Figure 13-9 shows various typical putaminal hematomas.

Putaminal hemorrhages vary greatly in size. In one series of 24 patients,[30] the smallest hematoma volume was 20 mm^2, whereas the largest was 225 mm^2. Patients with small hematomas, as shown in Figure 13-10, have a good outcome. Larger hemorrhages are more likely to rupture into the ventricle, and have a much higher mortality than small putaminal hematomas.[30,110,113] Most often, bleeding extends along the anteroposterior axis of the brain, but some lesions are globoid, and others extend laterally toward the cortical surface along white matter tracts.[30,110] Analysis of CT scans at the level of the body of the lateral ventricles can help prognosticate the likelihood of recovery from

Table 13-3. Neurologic Findings in Patients with Intracerebral Hemorrhage at Common Sites

Locale	Motor Weakness	Sensory Loss	Hemiano-pia	Pupils	Eye Movements	Other
Caudate	Hemiparesis +	–	–	Normal	– or transient conjugate gaze palsy contralateral	Confusion
Putamen						
Small	Hemiparesis ++	+	–	Normal	–	–
Large	Hemiparesis ++++	++	++	± Ipsilateral fixed, dilated	Conjugate gaze, palsy contralateral	L: aphasia R: left-sided, neglect; constructional apraxia
Thalamus	Hemiparesis +	+++	±	Small, nonreactive	Eyes down, or down and in; vertical gaze palsy; conjugate gaze palsy ipsilateral or contralateral; pseudo sixth nerve palsy	Confusion L: aphasia
Lobar	Hemiparesis ±					Abular
Frontal		–	–	Normal	–	L: aphasia
Parietal		+++	++	Normal	–	R: left-sided neglect; constructional apraxia
Temporal	–	–	++	Normal	–	L: aphasia; agitation
Occipital (pontine)	– or transient	– or transient	++++	Normal	–	–
Median (large)	Quadraparesis ++++	±	–	Small reaction	Bilateral horizontal conjugate gaze palsy; bobbing	Hyperventilation
Lateral (tegmental)	– or transient	Contralateral hemisensory +++	–	Ipsilateral small reaction	1¹/₂ syndrome	Limb ataxia
Cerebellar	–	–	–	Small reaction	Ipsilateral sixth nerve palsy or ipsilateral conjugate gaze palsy	Gait ataxia

L = left; R = right; + to ++++ = increasing severity of finding; ± = may be present or absent; – = absent.

hemiplegia.[111] When the hematoma occupies CT sections containing the bodies of the lateral ventricles, then the middle type of hematoma is usually present and hemiplegia is likely to persist. When this region is free of bleeding, hemiparesis is more often absent, slight, or transient.[111]

Cerebral angiography may be helpful in studying patients with putaminal hemorrhage. Using microangiography, Mizukami and colleagues studied 60 postmortem specimens from patients with ICH.[114] They identified the source of bleeding as lateral lenticulostriate arteries, analyzed the postmortem dis-

Figure 13-6. Large putaminal hemorrhages. (**A**) A coronal section of the brain at necropsy shows a large hemorrhage on the left of the figure. The insular cortex is displaced laterally, and the basal ganglia are displaced medially. The hemorrhage has drained into the lateral ventricles. The midline is shifted to the right. (**B**) Axial section (in usual computed tomography plane) of the brain at necropsy shows a large putaminal hemorrhage that displaces the midline and drains into the lateral ventricles. (Reprinted with permission from LR Caplan. Putaminal Hemorrhage. In CS Kase, LR Caplan [eds], Intracerebral Hemorrhage. Boston: Butterworth–Heinemann, 1994;309–327.)

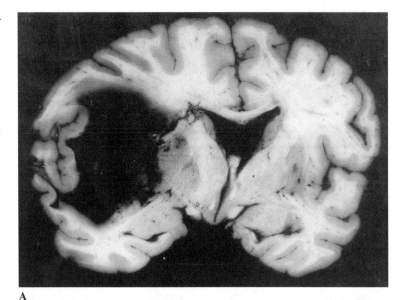

A

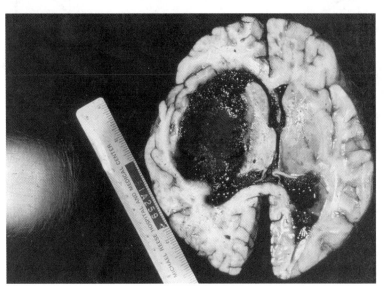

B

placement of these vessels, and correlated their findings with the angiographic anatomy in 100 other patients with autopsy or surgically confirmed ICH.[114] In large putaminal hemorrhages, the most lateral lenticulostriate arteries are displaced medially, increasing the distance between the most lateral lenticulostriate arteries and the insular artery. Anterior and posterior lesions have different patterns of displacement of lenticulostriate arteries.[114]

Since the mid-1980s, positron emission tomography and single-photon emission computed tomography have yielded insights into the clinical findings in patients with putaminal hemorrhage.[115] Anterior lesions show depression of frontal lobe function ipsilaterally, whereas posterior lesions more often affect the temporal and parietal lobes. The pattern of cortical depression helps predict aphasia type and recovery.[115]

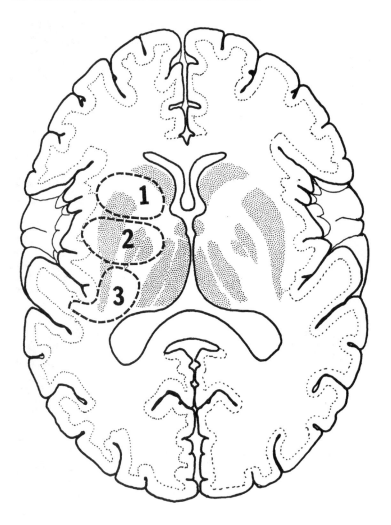

Figure 13-7. Axial brain section shows the loci of putaminal hemorrhages. (1) Anterior type, involving anterior putamen and anterior limb of the internal capsule. (2) Middle type, involving the capsular genus, globus pallidus, and middle portion of the putamen. (3) Posterior type, involving the far posterior limb of the internal capsule, often affecting the optic radiations, and spreading into the temporal lobe isthmus. (Reprinted with permission from LR Caplan. Putaminal Hemorrhage. In CS Kase, LR Caplan [eds], Intracerebral Hemorrhage. Boston: Butterworth–Heinemann, 1994;309–327. Drawn by Harriet Greenfield.)

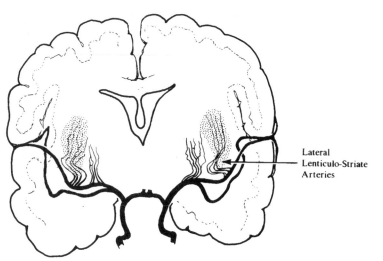

Lateral Lenticulo-Striate Arteries

Figure 13-8. Lenticulostriate arteries that supply the lateral ganglionic region. The medial lenticulostriate arteries are shown just medial to the lateral lenticulostriate group. (Reprinted with permission from Caplan LR. Putaminal hemorrhage. In Kase CS, Caplan LR [eds], Intracerebral Hemorrhage. Boston: Butterworth–Heinemann, 1994;309–327. Drawn by Harriet Greenfield.)

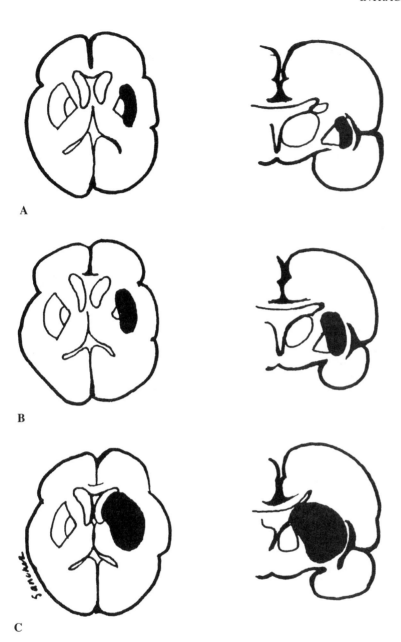

Figure 13-9. Examples of putaminal hemorrhage. (**A**) Hemorrhage within the boundaries of the putamen. (**B**) Encroachment on the internal capsule. (**C**) Hematoma progressing into the body of the lateral ventricle.

A

B

C

Caudate Hemorrhage

Hemorrhage into the caudate nucleus accounts for approximately 7% of ICH.[116–118] Hematomas at this site frequently discharge quickly into the adjacent lateral ventricle, or may spread laterally toward the internal capsule or inferiorly toward the hypothalamus. Early ventricular dilatation by blood probably accounts for the most common symptoms of caudate hemorrhage—headache, vomiting, decreased alertness, and stiff neck.[116–119] Some patients also are confused, disoriented, and have poor memory.[116–119] The larger parenchymatous hematomas cause a contralateral hemiparesis, conjugate deviation of the eyes to the side of the lesion, conjugate gaze palsy to the opposite side, and an ipsilateral small pupil or Horner's syndrome.[116,118] Sensory findings are usually absent or minimal. The usual cause of caudate hemorrhage is hypertension, but AVMs are also common, especially in the young. Caudate hematomas have a better prognosis than comparable-sized putaminal hemorrhages.

Symptoms and signs of caudate hemorrhage closely mimic SAH, but the CT appearance of blood in the caudate and lateral ventricles is distinctive.

Thalamic Hemorrhage

Neurologic signs in patients with thalamic hemorrhages differ greatly depending on the size, location within the thalamus of the hematoma, and dissection into and pressure effects on the third ventricle and adjacent brain structures.[120,121] The largest hemorrhages are located in the ventrolateral and posteromedial portions of the thalamus in the territories of the thalamogeniculate and thalamic-subthalamic arteries.[121] Other hemorrhages are located anteriorly in the territory of the tuberothalamic (polar) arteries and dorsally in the territory of the lateral posterior choroidal arteries.[121]

Most thalamic hematomas are posterior to the pyramidal-tract fibers in the internal capsule, so that contralateral sensory abnormalities are usually more prominent than contralateral hemiparesis. Some large thalamic hematomas dissect rostrally and involve the anterior portion of the posterior limb of the internal capsule, causing a hemiplegia. Sometimes, limbs contralateral to hematomas are slightly ataxic or have choreic movements. The contralateral hand may rest in a fisted or dystonic posture. The key neurologic findings that separate thalamic from caudate or putaminal hemorrhages are the eye signs. Patients with caudate or putaminal hemorrhages have conjugate deviation of the eyes toward the side of the lesion and paresis of conjugate gaze to the opposite side. The characteristic oculomotor abnormalities in patients with thalamic hematomas are as follows:

1. Paralysis of upward gaze, often with one or both eyes resting downward
2. Hyperconvergence of one or both eyes,[33,120,122] with a combination of these findings giving patients the appearance of peering downward and inward at the tops of their noses

3. Ocular skewing, in which one eye rests below the other, with this divergence in vertical eye position remaining constant in gaze in all directions
4. Eyes gazing the wrong way resting toward the opposite side[33,120]
5. Disconjugate gaze, with limited abduction of one or both eyes (so-called pseudo sixth-nerve paresis[120,123]), failure of ocular abduction caused by visual fixation from the adducted eye, and increased convergence vectors neutralizing abduction—not caused by involvement of the sixth nerve[123]

These oculomotor abnormalities are caused by direct extension of the hematoma to the diencephalic-mesencephalic junction or compression of the quadrigeminal plate region by the thalamic hematoma. In thalamic hemorrhage, the pupils are usually small and react poorly to light because of interruption of the afferent limb of the pupillary reflex arc.

Patients with large left thalamic hemorrhages often have an unusual aphasia.[120,124–126] After beginning a conversation almost normally, patients may lapse into a remarkable fluent aphasia, with many jargon or nonexistent words and poor communication of ideas. In contrast to patients with Wernicke's aphasia, comprehension of spoken language is good. Patients with thalamic ICH may repeat and duplicate words or syllables at the ends of words in spoken and written language. Paraphasic errors and poor naming are also common. Patients with right thalamic hematomas often have left visual neglect, anosognosia, and visuospatial abnormalities.[120,127]

Decreased levels of alertness, consciousness, and hypersomnolence are common at the onset of thalamic hemorrhage because of involvement of the rostral reticular activating system. The prognosis for recovery from thalamic hemorrhages is not as good as caudate or putaminal hemorrhages of comparable size, but coma is not as dire a prognostic sign in thalamic lesions as it is in other supratentorial sites. Also, unlike putaminal hemorrhage, the severity of the deficit and mortality do not correlate with ventricular extension in patients with thalamic hematomas.[128] Figure 13-11 shows a CT scan from a patient with an anterior-thalamic hematoma, which spread into the ventricles. She made an excellent recovery. Thalamic hemor-

Figure 13-10. Computed tomography shows a small left putaminal hemorrhage.

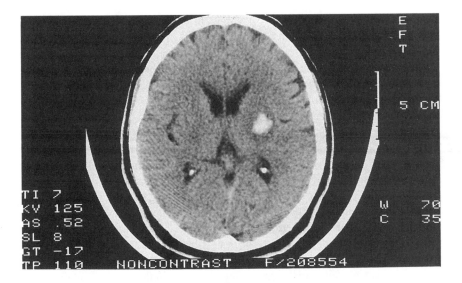

Figure 13-11. Computed tomography shows a small left anterior thalamic hematoma, which drained into the lateral ventricles; blood casts are seen within the ventricle.

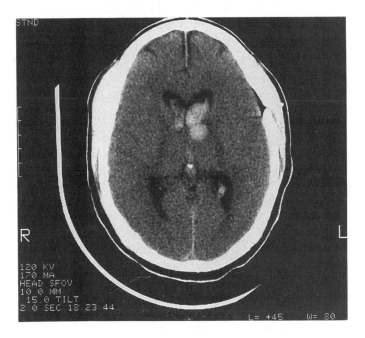

rhages are not accessible surgically unless they extend far laterally. Most studies have not differentiated medial from lateral or posterior thalamic hematomas, although lesions at these various sites yield different clinical syndromes and have different prognoses for recovery.[121]

Since the mid-1980s, it is possible to distinguish syndromes related to small discrete hemorrhages in the thalamus using MRI and CT.[121,129,130] The posterolateral type in the territory of the thalamogeniculate arteries are the most common and largest type of thalamic hematoma. These lesions often spill out of the thalamus laterally and may cause motor paralysis by involving the internal capsule. Sensorimotor signs predominate, and pupillary and eye-movement abnormalities are slight or absent, unless the hematoma is quite large and spreads to or compresses the medial thalamus.[120,121] Anterior or anterolateral thalamic hematomas are in the distribution of the tuberothalamic (polar) artery; behavioral abnormalities predominate, especially apathy and abulia.[120,121] Posteromedial hematomas are in the distribution of the thalamic-subthalamic thalamoperforating arteries; abnormalities of consciousness, pupillary function, and vertical gaze predominate. The hematoma often spreads to the third ventricle and can compress the diencephalic-mesencephalic junction and obstruct the third ventricle, causing hydrocephalus.[121,131,132] Oculomotor abnormalities found in patients with posteromedial hematomas may improve after ventricular drainage, indicating these abnormalities were caused by downward pressure on the midbrain.[131,132] Far posterior and dorsal lesions predominantly involve the pulvinar in the distribution of the posterior choroidal arteries; slight sensorimotor signs may be found but are usually transient, and aphasia and behavioral abnormalities are common.[121] Figure 13-12 shows MRIs of a large thalamic hematoma that likely originated in the pulvinar region in a patient with a prior brain hemorrhage.

Lobar Hemorrhages

ICH may develop beneath the region of the gray-white junction of the cerebral cortex. These subcortical hemorrhages usually spread in a linear direction along white matter pathways. When the hematomas absorb, linear cavities remain, giving the lesions the name *slit hemorrhage*. The lesions undercut cortex and often do not obey the strict divisions of cerebral lobes; hence, the term *lobar hemorrhage* actually is inaccurate. Nonetheless, I use this term because of its widespread acceptance. Undercutting of the cortex can be epileptogenic, causing repeated focal seizures of limited duration.[133-135]

Subcortical hemorrhages are important to diagnose because the symptoms and signs are often erroneously attributed to cerebral infarction. Inappropriate therapy might be prescribed unless brain imaging shows the hematomas. Also, if subcortical hemorrhages are large, they are relatively superficial and are more accessible to surgical drainage than deeper hematomas. In the past, subcortical hemorrhages were rarely diagnosed antemortem, but CT and MRI greatly enhance recognition of these lesions. Many lobar hemorrhages are caused by AVMs, cavernous angiomas, and amyloid angiopathy, each of which has a predilection for corti-cal and subcortical regions. Hypertension is also an important cause of lobar hematomas. The parietal and occipital lobes are affected more often than the frontal and parietal regions. Symptoms and signs depend on the lobes affected, as follows[133-135]:

1. Frontal hematomas: Far anterior lesions usually cause abulia. Patients appear apathetic and have reduced spontaneity, prolonged latency in responding, and short, terse replies. If the lesions extend deeply or toward the precentral gyrus, conjugate eye deviation toward the side of the hematoma and contralateral hemiparesis are found.

2. Paracentral hematomas: Lesions near the central sulcus produce contralateral motor and sensory signs, sometimes with aphasia if the lesion is in the left hemisphere.

3. Parietal hemorrhages: Parietal hemorrhages are usually accompanied by contralateral hemisensory loss, with neglect of the contralateral visual field. The limbs contralateral to the hemorrhage are often uncoordinated. Aphasia and disorders of reading, writing, and arithmetic functions are present when the lesions involve the left inferior parietal lobule. Patients with right inferior parietal hematomas have defective drawing and copying and may have difficulty with visual-spatial functions.

4. Occipital hematomas: Occipital hemorrhages cause a severe contralateral hemianopia, often with slight contralateral hemisensory or motor signs and visual neglect.

5. Temporal-lobe lesions: Temporal-lobe lesions often cause agitation and delirium. Wernicke-type aphasia accompanies left temporal lesions. Temporal-lobe hematomas are particularly likely to swell and may cause herniation without preceding hemiparesis. Brain stem compression may develop insidiously, with deepening stupor. An ipsilaterally dilated pupil follows.

Lobar hematomas are usually smaller in volume than deep lesions and have a lower mortality rate.[133-135] The functional outcome in patients with lobar ICH is also generally better than other forms of ICH. The diagnosis is often quite difficult without CT or MRI. Because of the higher incidence of vascular malformations and other bleeding lesions in patients with lobar hematomas, angiography is often indicated, especially in patients who are young and not hypertensive.[136]

Figure 13-12. Magnetic resonance imaging T2-weighted axial (**A**) and sagittal (**B**) sections show a large thalamic hematoma. A healed old slit hemorrhage cavity is visible lateral to the hemorrhage.

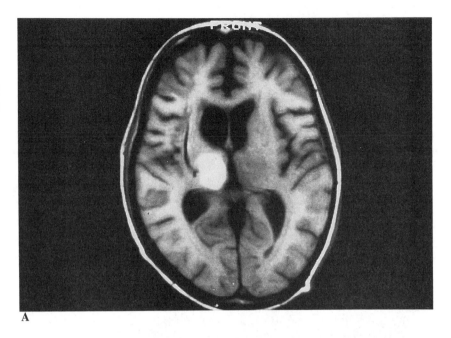

A

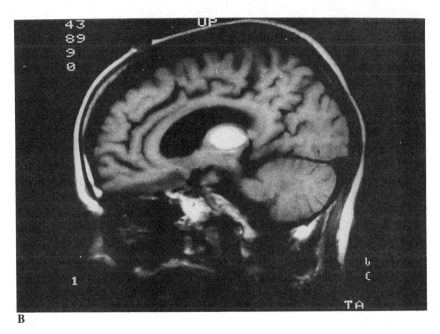

B

Primary Intraventricular Hemorrhages

In some patients, the principal locus of bleeding is into the ventricular cavities.[137–139] Ventricular bleeding usually arises from small subependymal AVMs or cavernous angiomas, or from hemorrhage into the caudate nucleus just adjacent to the ventricles. The clinical syndrome closely mimics SAH, with sudden headache, stiff neck, vomiting, and lethargy. At times, bilateral, usually symmet-

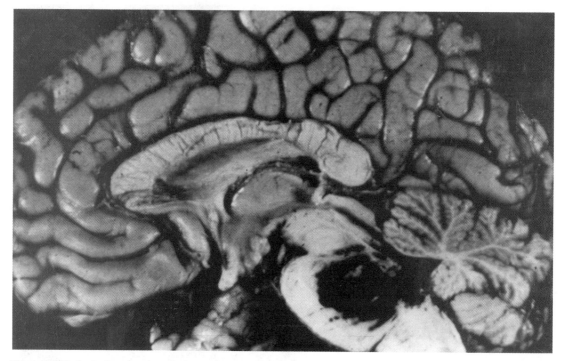

Figure 13-13. Sagittal section through the pons at necropsy shows a large hematoma. (Reprinted with permission from LR Caplan. Pontine Hemorrhage. In CS Kase, LR Caplan [eds], Intracerebral Hemorrhage. Boston: Butterworth–Heinemann, 1994;403–423.)

ric hyperreflexia and extensor plantar responses occur. Decreased consciousness is almost an invariable sign. CT shows blood distending the lateral ventricles and third ventricle, and some blood density within the subarachnoid space. In childhood, the most common cause is an AVM, which can destroy itself as it ruptures. Small angiomas may arise in the choroid plexus[137] (see Figure 12-13 C,D). In adults, most intraventricular hemorrhages are caused by ventricular spread of primary hypertensive bleeds into periventricular structures.[137–139]

Pontine Hemorrhage

Primary brain stem hemorrhages are located most often in the pons. Midbrain and medullary hemorrhages are rare and, when present, are usually caused by blood dyscrasias and vascular malformations.[140] Raised ICP, especially if it develops quickly, frequently causes secondary lesions, so-called Düret hemorrhages, in the median or paramedian zones of the thalamus, midbrain, and pons caused by stretching of paramedian vascular structures.[96,140–142] Primary pontine hemorrhages usually begin in the center of the pons at the tegmental-basal junction. Figure 13-13 is a sagittal section of a large pontine hematoma found at necropsy. These hematomas grow quickly and assume a round or oval shape, usually destroying the center of the tegmentum and base of the pons. Blood may dissect rostrally into the midbrain, but rarely extends caudally into the medulla. Hematomas frequently dissect into the fourth ventricle. Figure 13-14 shows a large paramedian pontine hematoma. These large pontine hemorrhages arise from the larger median pontine penetrating vessels that originate from the basilar artery. Figure 13-15 shows various pontine arteries. Bleeding from these arteries causes various syndromes, depending on the location and size of the pontine hematomas.

Signs accompanying large medial pontine hematomas include (1) quadriparesis, often with limb stiffness and rigidity; (2) coma; (3) absent horizontal eye movements; (4) small but reactive

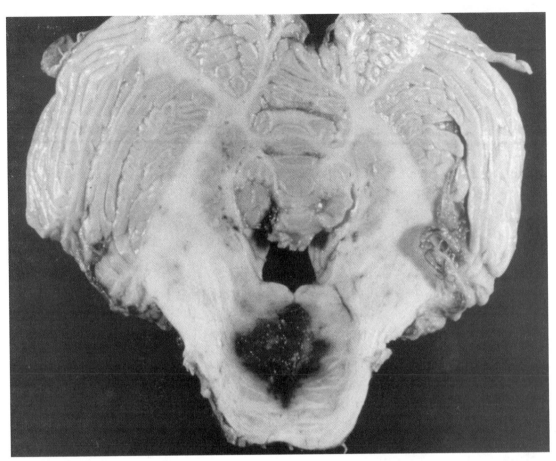

Fig 13-14. Section of the pons and cerebellum at necropsy shows a large paramedian pontine hematoma. (Reprinted with permission from LR Caplan. Pontine Hemorrhage. In CS Kase, LR Caplan [eds], Intracerebral Hemorrhage. Boston: Butterworth–Heinemann, 1994;403–423.)

pupils; and (5) rapid or irregular respirations.[141,143,144] Headache and vomiting occasionally occur. Some pontine hemorrhages develop gradually,[20] and early findings may be asymmetric. A hemiparesis is common early in the course. Deafness, dysarthria, facial numbness, asymmetric facial or limb weakness, and dizziness occasionally precede the development of coma. Some patients have twitching, shivering, or spasmodic movements of the limbs, usually culminating in decerebrate rigidity. Vertical reflex eye movements are preserved unless the lesion extends rostrally into the midbrain. In some patients, the eyes spontaneously and repeatedly bob downward.[141] Massive pontine hemorrhages are invariably fatal, but not usually instantaneously. Death usually occurs 24–48 hours after onset. Survival for 7–10 days,

however, is not rare. Some patients with large medial pontine hematomas survive with quadriplegia. Hyperthermia is sometimes noted.

MRI allows documentation of two other types of pontine hemorrhage–lateral tegmental pontine hematomas[141,145–150] and small basal hematomas.[141,151–155] These sites correspond to the usual distribution of penetrating pontine arteries (see Figure 13-15). In Silverstein's series of 50 necropsy-proven pontine hemorrhages found during autopsy at the Philadelphia General Hospital, 28 were massive central hematomas. Eleven were located in the lateral basis pontis, and 11 were tegmental.[144] Nakajima reported 24 patients with pontine hematomas who came to necropsy; among these, 21 patients had large central hematomas, two had bilateral tegmental lesions, and one had a

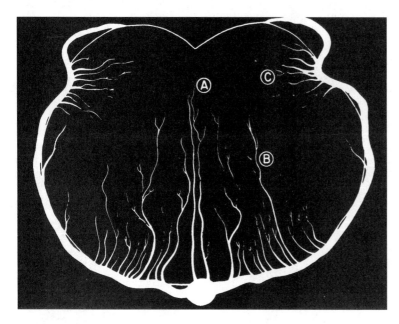

Figure 13-15. The distribution of pontine penetrating and circumferential arteries. Large paramedian penetrators (A); short circumferential arteries (B); and penetrators from long circumferential arteries (C). (Reprinted with permission from LR Caplan. Pontine Hemorrhage. In CS Kase, LR Caplan [eds], Intracerebral Hemorrhage. Boston: Butterworth–Heinemann, 1994;403–423. Drawn by Harriet Greenfield.)

unilateral basal-tegmental hematoma.[156] Undoubtedly, series of cases involving pontine hematomas identified by neuroimaging scans would contain a higher frequency of unilateral basal, tegmental, and basal-tegmental lesions.

Lateral basal hematomas can cause pure motor hemiparesis,[151,152] ataxic hemiparesis,[153,154] or dysarthria-clumsy hand syndrome,[155] thus mimicking the findings in lacunar infarction involving the pons. Lateral basal lesions can spread into the adjacent tegmentum, causing unilateral cranial nerve signs and contralateral hemiparesis. Lateral tegmental hematomas arise from penetrating vessels that course from lateral to medial after branching from the lateral circumferential pontine arteries (see C in Figure 13-15). These lesions involve the rostral pons. Findings on neurologic examination are those of a predominantly unilateral tegmental lesion.

Most distinctive and diagnostic of lateral tegmental pontine hematomas are the oculomotor abnormalities, which include ipsilateral conjugate gaze paresis, ipsilateral internuclear ophthalmoplegia, or a combination of ipsilateral internuclear ophthalmoplegia and gaze palsy (a "one and one-half syndrome"[33,141,145]), in which the only preserved eye motion is abduction of the contralateral eye. Because the sensory lemniscus (joining of the medial lemniscus and spinothalamic tracts) is lateral tegmental, accompanying loss of pinprick, temperature, and position sense on the opposite side of the body is common. Limb and truncal ataxia is usually present and may be bilateral or predominantly ipsilateral. Unilateral facial numbness or weakness, ipsilateral miosis, and transient deafness may also be present. When contralateral hemiparesis occurs, it is usually slight and transient. Patients with small pontine hematomas generally survive with slight to moderate clinical neurologic deficits. Small tegmental hematomas may cause only sensory abnormalities, involving the contralateral limbs and trunk (a pure sensory stroke syndrome)[147,148] or sensory findings limited to the ipsilateral face.[149,150]

Cerebellar Hemorrhages

Hemorrhage into the cerebellum probably accounts for approximately 10% of ICH, approximating the relative percentage of weight of the cerebellum in reference to the entire brain. Although the frequency of cerebellar hemorrhage is low, establishing the diagnosis is important because of the potentially serious outcome if not treated and the contrasting good prognosis after surgical treatment. Cerebellar hemorrhage usually originates in the region of the dentate nucleus, arising from distal branches of the posterior inferior cerebellar

Figure 13-16. Necropsy section of the pons and cerebellum shows a large cerebellar hemorrhage (*arrows*). The fourth ventricle is compressed and distorted from above. (Reprinted with permission from LR Caplan. Posterior Circulation Disease: Clinical Findings, Diagnosis, and Management. Boston: Blackwell, 1996.)

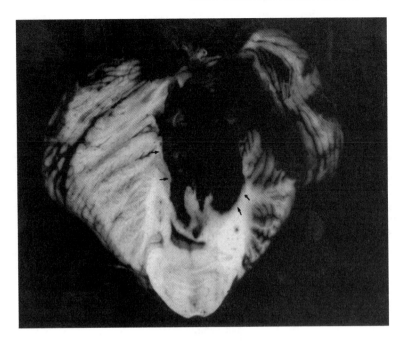

artery and the superior cerebellar artery. Hematomas collect around the dentate and spread into the cerebellar hemispheral white matter, frequently extending into the fourth ventricle. The adjacent brain stem is seldom directly involved, but is compressed from above by the lesion. Occasional cerebellar hemorrhages arise in the vermis in medial branches of the posterior inferior cerebellar artery or the superior cerebellar artery. Figure 13-16 shows a large cerebellar hemorrhage that is compressing the fourth ventricle.

The most consistent symptom is inability to walk.[157–160] Some patients even have difficulty remaining in a sitting or standing position, often leaning or tilting toward the side of the hematoma. Patients have been known to crawl, slide, or bump on their bottom to get to the bathroom or phone. Vomiting is also frequent, occurring in 68 (92%) of 72 patients from several series.[140] Headache is also common, usually affecting the occiput, neck, or frontal region. Dysarthria, hiccups, and tinnitus occur, but are less frequent. Loss of consciousness at onset is distinctly unusual, but by the time these patients reach the hospital, approximately one-third are obtunded.[157–160]

Neurologic signs include (1) an ipsilateral abducens or gaze palsy toward the side of the hematoma; (2) small pupils, with the ipsilateral pupil slightly smaller; (3) rebound overshoot of the rapidly elevated ipsilateral arm; and (4) gait ataxia. Hemiparesis probably does not occur in cerebellar hemorrhage, but cerebellar lesions do produce an apparent asthenia or slowness of the affected limbs.[157–160] Inferior extremity reflexes are usually symmetrically exaggerated, but plantar responses are flexor. Classic cerebellar-type incoordination of the arm on finger-to-nose or toe-to-object testing and frank intention tremor are uncommon. In my experience with patients with cerebellar infarction and hemorrhage, the single most useful cerebellar sign is elicited when the patient is asked to raise both arms together rapidly, then to brake the ascent quickly. Next, the patient is directed to drop the arms quickly, again braking the descent before the hands hit the bed or table. The arm on the side of the cerebellar lesion lags behind the other arm and overshoots the endpoint.

Patients with large cerebellar hematomas often have brain stem compression. The patients develop increasing stupor, lateral gaze palsy toward the side of the hematoma, and bilateral extensor plantar responses. Among those patients not comatose on admission in one series, only 20% had a smooth, uneventful recovery. Eighty percent deteriorated to coma, with 25% of these becoming comatose within 3 hours after onset.[157] In the series of Fisher et al.,[158] only 2 of 18 patients had a benign course. The other 16 patients developed coma, usually within a few hours. Because the hematoma usually affects the caudal cerebellum, the medulla is the portion of the brain stem compressed. Thus, vasomotor disturbances and respiratory arrest may develop. Untreated patients with cerebellar hemorrhage who become comatose invariably die of brain stem compression. CT and MRI not only document the size, locale, and position of the hematoma, but also give considerable information about posterior-fossa pressure. An expanding lesion obliterates the cerebellopontine angle and ambient cisterns, and displaces the fourth ventricle toward the opposite side. Usually, the fourth ventricle compression leads to hydrocephalus, with early dilatation of the temporal horns of the lateral ventricles.

Occasionally, patients with cerebellar hemorrhage have a more indolent course, presenting with symptoms and signs of hydrocephalus. Abulia, dementia, slow-stepped shuffling gait, and incontinence are the characteristic signs of hydrocephalus. The patient and family may fail to emphasize the preceding symptoms of dizziness, headache, and vomiting that had been interpreted as the flu. Other patients have laterally placed cerebellar hematomas that compress the cerebellopontine angle structures. These patients develop dysfunction of the fifth, sixth, seventh, and eighth cranial nerves, in addition to ataxia. Hemorrhage into the vermis, with headache, vomiting, and sudden coma, is more rare.[160]

Because the course of cerebellar hematomas is unpredictable and large lesions frequently cause coma and death, it is probably wise to drain lesions that are 3 cm or larger, especially if a decrease in level of alertness develops.[160,161] Some patients have been successfully treated by medical decompression (steroids and osmotic diuretic agents) or ventricular drainage.[160,162] Ventricular shunts do not treat brain stem compression and have been followed by delayed deterioration.[163]

Diagnosis, Prognosis, and Treatment

Diagnosis

Accurate bedside diagnosis of ICH rests on the presence of an appropriate ecologic background, such as hypertension or bleeding diathesis; the nonfluctuat-ing, usually gradually progressive course over minutes or hours; accompanying symptoms, such as headache and vomiting; and neurologic signs compatible with a deep lesion. CT has proven to be an excellent instrument for the diagnosis of ICH. Blood provides dense contrast, even acutely. One reported patient with ICH had an abrupt worsening of symptoms while in the CT scanner. The initial films had shown a small, round hyperdensity in the lentiform nucleus. A second film of the same area showed a much larger, hyperdense, irregular zone extending laterally from the putamen to the insula.[164] Other investigators have also described enlargement of hematomas on sequential CT scans.[14–17]

Findings on CT and MRI scans can help determine the age of the hematoma. Hematomas are at first regular and smooth. During the first 48 hours, large hematomas may show fluid-blood levels, indicating that the hematoma is partially liquid and has not solidified.[165] During the first 72 hours or longer, edema produces a hypodense area around the lesion and considerable mass effect is noted.[166,167] From 3 to 20 days after bleeding, the dense area becomes smaller, beginning at the periphery. The border develops an irregular contour, which is enhanced with the use of contrast.[166–168] Reduction of edema and mass effect also occurs during this period. Intraventricular blood has usually disappeared by 5 weeks.[169] The absorption coefficient of the hematoma decreases gradually, and the lesion develops a lucent appearance, with absorption characteristics resembling edema fluid or CSF. By 9 weeks, mass effect and enhancement are usually gone, and a local circumscribed region of slight hypodensity remains.[169] On MRI scans, the zone of altered attenuation or abnormal metabolism is usually much larger than the hypodensity seen on CT.

MRI is also effective in imaging acute hematomas[170,171] and is more useful than CT in recognizing hemorrhage in chronic lesions. In Chapter 4, I discuss MRI findings in hematomas in some detail. Table 4-1 tabulates the findings depending on various MR imaging techniques. Acute hematomas are isointense or hypointense on T1-weighted scans, sometimes with a darker hypointense rim, and they are bright and hyperintense on T2-weighted images.[167] Figure 13-12 shows a large acute hematoma in the thalamus, imaged by T2-weighted MRI. Later, the center of the hematoma appears dark on T2 and is surrounded by a bright rim. Chronic hematomas are bright on T2-weighted images.

Angiography is generally unnecessary unless the lesion is in an unusual locus or the patient has no risk factors for hemorrhage, such as hypertension or bleeding diathesis. Angiography is used to opacify AVMs or aneurysms that might have caused ICH.

Prognosis

Size and locale of the lesion on brain imaging scans renders useful prognostic information.[25] In putaminal hemorrhages, lesions larger than 140 mm² in one slice had a poorer outcome.[30] In thalamic hemorrhage, lesions larger than 3.3 cm in maximal diameter had a poor prognosis,[31] as did cerebellar lesions larger than 3 cm.[172] In six other studies, large-volume hematomas were associated with a poor outcome.[23,24,128,173-175] Pulse pressure, admission blood pressure, and level of consciousness, as measured by the Glasgow Coma Scale, are also important prognostic variables.[23,25,174,176] The presence of hydrocephalus in patients with supratentorial hemorrhages is also an adverse prognostic sign.[175]

During the acute phase of ICH, the mass effect of the developing hematoma presents a much greater risk of death than does a comparable-sized cerebral infarct. In the case of ICH, something extra (blood) has been added to the intracranial contents. In cerebral infarction, the already existing contents—brain tissue—are ischemic, but an acute mass has not been added. Later, infarcts and hematomas become edematous, increasing ICP. In the chronic phase, if the patient with ICH has survived, the prognosis for recovery is actually much better than cerebral infarcts of similar size and location. Hematomas have dissected and separated the cerebral cortex and other brain parts, but usually the surrounding cortex is preserved. In contrast, infarcts leave dead, nonfunctioning cortex when they heal. Unlike SAH, recurrence of ICH during the acute illness is rare. These simple facts dictate the approach to ICH treatment—that is, aggressively try to limit the expanding hematoma to prevent death and late morbidity. In patients with ICH, the concern is control of acute mass effect, whereas in SAH, the goal is to prevent rebleeding and arterial vasoconstriction.

Treatment

Careful medical management of patients with ICH may be lifesaving and is important, even in those patients who later have surgical drainage of their hematomas. Increased ICP causes decreased responsiveness and hypoventilation; in turn, hypoventilation causes a low arterial oxygen tension and high carbon dioxide tension, which lead to vasodilatation and further increase in ICP. Maintenance of a good airway and mechanical hyperventilation can reverse this process and quickly lower ICP. Control of systemic blood pressure helps stop intracranial bleeding, but must be done cautiously. In some patients with ICH, systemic blood pressure is further increased to ensure adequate perfusion of the brain. Increased ICP causes increased venous pressure, so elevated arterial pressure is needed to overcome the increased venous pressure to perfuse the tissues. Overzealous lowering of blood pressure can lead to underperfusion and clinical deterioration. Blood pressure should be lowered quickly, but not to hypotensive levels. Patients must be watched carefully during the treatment. Guidelines from the Stroke Council of the American Heart Association recommend maintaining the mean arterial pressure below 130 mm Hg.[177]

So-called medical decompression with corticosteroids, mannitol, or glycerol is widely used in patients with ICH. Few data exist, however, about their effectiveness. Concern exists that hypertonic agents could diffuse into the ICH and cause a secondary increase in volume of the hematoma because of ingress of fluid. Langfitt noted that mannitol and forced hyperventilation were effective in reducing ICP in a group of patients with ICH.[178] Poungvarin et al. studied the usefulness of dexamethasone treatment in patients with supratentorial ICH in a double-blind randomized trial. He found that it did not improve mortality, and infections and diabetic complications were more often found in the corticosteroid-treated group.[179]

When considering surgery and other therapies, hematomas, in practice, can be divided into the following three main groups:

1. Massive, rapidly developing lesions that effectively kill or devastate patients before they reach the hospital. For these lesions, little can or should be done.

2. Small hematomas, from which the patient will make an excellent spontaneous recovery. Treatment consists of controlling the etiologic factors, such as hypertension, to prevent recurrences.

3. Medium-sized hematomas—hematoma volumes between the two extremes—with developing mass effect after the patient reaches the hospital. Within this third group, medical measures and surgery are most helpful.

Because hematomas represent the development of so-called benign masses, the logical treatment for life-threatening lesions is surgical drainage. The factors outlined in the following sections should be considered in deciding on surgical therapy.

Size

Hematomas larger than 3 cm in their widest diameter have a higher mortality and a more delayed recovery rate than smaller lesions. Thus, the larger the lesion on CT, the more logical its drainage would be.

Location

Some hematomas are more accessible surgically, such as those in the cerebellum or cerebral lobes. Although putaminal hemorrhages can be drained through the sylvian fissures and insular cortex, large left basal-ganglionic hemorrhages usually leave patients aphasic and dependent. Thus, treatment should be less aggressive than for right-sided lesions. Cerebellar ICH can cause respiratory arrest without preceding gradual deterioration of neurologic function or alertness, and surgical removal of a portion of the cerebellum often leaves no important residual handicap. For these reasons, the threshold for recommending surgery for cerebellar hematomas is lower than other lesions of comparable size. Cerebellar, lobar, and right putaminal hemorrhages are most accessible to surgical drainage.

Mass Effect and Drainage Patterns

Size of the hematoma does not, by itself, solely determine mass effect. Older patients may have sufficient pre-existing atrophy to be able to accommodate a sizable hematoma without a critical rise in ICP or shift in intracranial compartments. Some lesions have a great deal of surrounding edema, whereas others have relatively little. Hydrocephalus can add to the increased mass effect. Does the hematoma compress the third or lateral ventricle? Has a shift of the midline occurred? Is uncal herniation present? In posterior fossa ICH, has displacement of the fourth ventricle been found? Are the ambient, cerebellopontine, and other cisterns effaced? Does the lesion drain into the ventricles or superficially into the subarachnoid space? Entry into the CSF may spontaneously decompress the lesion. Surgical drainage would be indicated more strongly for lesions with greater mass effect and no spontaneous decompression.

Etiology

Even after surgical drainage, hematomas caused by amyloid angiopathy may tend to bleed because of the fragility of the blood vessels.[180] Similarly, hemorrhages in patients with anticoagulant-related or other bleeding disorders also continue to bleed unless the coagulopathy is reversed before surgery. Ideally, surgeons like to remove the malformations when operating on hematomas caused by vascular malformations while also draining the hematoma. The threshold for surgical treatment should be most favorable for vascular malformations, moderately so for accessible lesions caused by hypertension, and least favorable for CAA or ICH caused by a bleeding diathesis.

Timing

During the first 24–36 hours, hematomas are still at least partly liquid and can be more easily drained. Later, hematomas solidify and become more difficult to drain. After 7–10 days, blood begins to be absorbed, and the lesion becomes softer again. Ideally, drainage should occur either early or after 7–10 days for technical reasons. In general, if the patient has survived the first week, improvement occurs as edema subsides. Thus, little argument for late drainage exists except for concurrent removal of a vascular malformation. Some have wondered whether late surgery (1–2 weeks) would speed recovery, but this argument is unsupported by data.

Clinical Course

Perhaps the most important factor to consider is whether the patient is improving, stable, or worsening. Patients who deteriorate and show a decrease in level of consciousness to severe lethargy or stupor have a poor outlook for recovery.[23,25] In patients with putaminal hemorrhage, other poor prognostic signs include the development of ipsilateral pupillary dilation, an ipsilateral extensor plantar response, or an ipsilateral conjugate gaze paresis. These signs are indicative of midline shift or early brain stem compression. In patients with cerebellar hemorrhage, development of bilateral extensor plantar responses is a poor prognostic sign.[158] In deteriorating patients with accessible lesions, surgery should not be delayed if medical decompression is not quickly beneficial. The effectiveness of surgical decompression of ICHs is controversial and has been extensively debated.[25,177,181–183]

Fleming and colleagues analyzed the Mayo Clinic experience regarding patients with lobar hematomas that deteriorated after hospital admission.[184] Because lobar and cerebellar hematomas are most often considered for surgery, this analysis is quite useful. Decreased consciousness (Glasgow Coma Scale score of <14) was the most important single predictor of deterioration.[184] Large hematoma volume (>60 ml), midline shift, effacement of the contralateral perimesencephalic and ambient cisterns, and dilatation of the contralateral temporal horn of the lateral ventricle are other predictive features.[184] Patients who deteriorate during the first 12 hours usually have enlargement of hematoma on follow-up CT scans. Those that deteriorate after the first day usually do so because of brain edema around the hematoma.

Advances in neuroimaging capabilities since the mid-1980s have made it possible to drain hematomas percutaneously using stereotaxic surgery.[177,185–188] A burr hole is made, and the drainage instrument is guided stereotactically, using CT or MRI, to the core of the hematoma, which is then evacuated. Fibrinolytic agents also can be instilled to soften and lyse the clot.[177,189–191] Thirty percent to 90% of the hematomas were removed using stereotactic procedures in various studies.[177] Stereotactic treatment using fibrinolytic agents is promising. Little experience exists, however, to allow comparison of open versus stereotactic drainage of hematomas.

A CT scan in JT showed a large, deep putaminal hemorrhage, with spread to the thalamus and lateral ventricles. At this time, he was comatose; had bilateral horizontal gaze palsies; dilated, unreactive pupils; and bilateral extensor plantar reflexes. I judged that nothing could or should be done to reverse his mortal bleed.

Much must be learned regarding therapy for patients with ICH. The technological revolution has made diagnosis easy. More well-designed studies of different modes of treatment in patients with lesions of various etiologies, sizes, locations, and varying levels of consciousness are needed.

References

1. Morgagni GB. De sedibus, et causis morborum per anatomen indagatis libri quinque.Vienna: Typographica Remondiana, 1761.
2. Cheyne J. Cases of apoplexy and lethargy with observations on comatose patients. London: Thomas Underwood, 1812.
3. Gowers W. A Manual of Diseases of the Nervous System, Vol 2. (2nd ed). London: J & A Churchill, 1892;384–421.
4. Osler W. The Principles and Practices of Medicine (5th ed). New York: Appleton, 1903;997–1008.
5. Aring C, Merritt H. Differential diagnosis between cerebral hemorrhage and cerebral thrombosis: clinical and pathological study of 245 cases. Arch Intern Med 1935; 56:435–456.
6. Kunitz S, Gross C, Heyman A, et al. The Pilot Stroke Data Bank: definition, design, and data. Stroke 1984;15:740–746.
7. Caplan LR, Hier DB, D'Cruz I. Cerebral embolism in the Michael Reese Stroke Registry. Stroke 1983;14:530–540.
8. Mohr JP, Caplan LR, Melski J, et al. The Harvard Cooperative Stroke Registry: a prospective registry. Neurology 1978;28:754–762.
9. Whisnant J, Fitzgibbons J, Kurland L, et al. Natural history of stroke in Rochester, Minnesota, 1945–1954. Stroke 1971;2:11–22.
10. Matsumoto N, Whisnant J, Kurland L, et al. Natural history of stroke in Rochester, Minnesota, 1955–1969. Stroke 1973;4:20–29.
11. Caplan LR, Mohr JP. Intracerebral hemorrhage: an update. Geriatrics 1978;33:42–52.
12. Fisher CM. Pathological observations in hypertensive cerebral hemorrhages. J Neuropathol Exp Neurol 1971; 30:536–550.
13. Herbstein D, Schaumburg H. Hypertensive intracerebral hematoma: an investigation of the initial hemorrhage and rebleeding using chromium Cr51 labelled erythrocytes. Arch Neurol 1974;30:412–414.
14. Kelly R, Bryer JR, Scheinberg P, Stokes IV. Active bleeding in hypertensive intracerebral hemorrhage: computed tomography. Neurology 1982;32:852–856.

15. Broderick JP, Brott TG, Tomsick T, et al. Ultra-early evaluation of intracerebral hemorrhage. J Neurosurg 1990;72: 195–199.

16. Fujii Y, Tanaka R, Takeuchi S, et al. Hematoma enlargement in spontaneous intracerebral hemorrhage. J Neurosurg 1994;80:51–57.

17. Kazui S, Naritomi H, Yamamoto H, et al. Enlargement of spontaneous intracerebral hemorrhage: incidence and time course. Stroke 1996;27:1783–1787.

18. Kase C, Robinson K, Stein R, et al. Anticoagulant-related intracerebral hemorrhage. Neurology 1985;35:943–948.

19. Kase CS. Bleeding Disorders. In CS Kase, LR Caplan (eds), Intracerebral Hemorrhage. Boston: Butterworth–Heinemann, 1994;117–151.

20. Kornyey S. Rapidly fatal pontile hemorrhage: clinical and anatomic report. Arch Neurol Psychiatry 1939;41:793–799.

21. Caplan LR. General Symptoms and Signs. In CS Kase, LR Caplan (eds), Intracerebral Hemorrhage. Boston: Butterworth–Heinemann, 1994;31–43.

22. Mello TP, Pinto AN, Ferro JM. Headache in intracerebral hematomas. Neurology 1996;47:494–500.

23. Tuhrim S, Dambrosia JM, Price TR, et al. Prediction of intracerebral hemorrhage survival. Ann Neurol 1988;24: 258–263.

24. Broderick JP, Brott TG, Duldner JE, et al. Volume of intracerebral hemorrhage. Stroke 1993;24:987–993.

25. Kase CS, Crowell RM. Prognosis and Treatment of Patients with Intracerebral Hemorrhage. In CS Kase, LR Caplan (eds), Intracerebral Hemorrhage. Boston: Butterworth–Heinemann, 1994;467–489.

26. Borison H, Wang S. Physiology and pharmacology of vomiting. Pharmacol Rev 1953;5:193–230.

27. Faught E, Peties D, Bartolucci A, et al. Seizures after primary intracerebral hemorrhage. Neurology 1989;39: 1089–1093.

28. Kilpatrick CJ, Davis SM, Tress BM, et al. Epileptic seizures in acute strokes. Arch Neurol 1990;47:157–160.

29. Berger AR, Lipton RB, Lesser ML, et al. Early seizures following intracerebral hemorrhage. Neurology 1988;38: 1363–1365.

30. Hier DB, Davis K, Richardson EP, et al. Hypertensive putaminal hemorrhage. Arch Neurol 1977;1:152–159.

31. Walshe T, Davis K, Fisher CM. Thalamic hemorrhage, a computed tomographic-clinical correlation. Neurology 1977;29:217–222.

32. Hier DB, Babcock DJ, Foulkes MA, et al. Influence of site on course of intracerebral hemorrhage. J Stroke Cerebrovasc Dis 1993;3:65–74.

33. Fisher CM. Some neuro-ophthalmological observations. J Neurol Neurosurg Psychiatry 1967;30:383–392.

34. Caplan LR. Intracerebral hemorrhage revisited. Neurology 1988;38:624–627.

35. Caplan LR. Hypertensive Intracerebral Hemorrhage. In CS Kase, LR Caplan (eds), Intracerebral Hemorrhage. Boston: Butterworth–Heinemann, 1994;99–116.

36. Cole F, Yates P. Intracerebral microaneurysms and small cerebrovascular lesions. Brain 1967;90:759–768.

37. Rosenblum WI. Miliary aneurysms and "fibrinoid" degeneration of cerebral blood vessels. Hum Pathol 1977; 8:133–139.

38. Santos-Buch CA, Goodhue W, Ewald B. Concurrence of iris aneurysms and cerebral hemorrhage in hypertensive rabbits. Arch Neurol 1976;33:96–103.

39. Takebayashi S, Kaneko M. Electron microscopic studies of ruptured arteries in hypertensive intracerebral hemorrhage. Stroke 1983;14:28–36.

40. Takebayashi S, Sakata N, Kawamura K. Re-evaluation of miliary aneurysms in hypertensive brain: recanalization of small hemorrhage. Stroke 1990;21(Suppl 1):59–60.

41. Bahemuka M. Primary intracerebral hemorrhage and heart weight: a clinicopathologic case-control review of 218 patients. Stroke 1987;18:531–536.

42. Brott T, Thalinger K, Hertzberg V. Hypertension as a risk factor for spontaneous intracerebral hemorrhage. Stroke 1986;17:1078–1083.

43. Caplan LR, Neely S, Gorelick PB. Cold-related intracerebral hemorrhage. Arch Neurol 1984;41:227.

44. Hines F, Brown G. A standard test for measuring the variability of blood pressure: its significance as an index of the prehypertensive state. Ann Intern Med 1933;7:209–217.

45. Barbas N, Caplan LR, Baquis G, et al. Dental chair intracerebral hemorrhage. Neurology 1987;37:511–512.

46. Cawley CM, Rigamonti D, Trommer B. Dental chair apoplexy. South Med J 1991;84:907–909.

47. Haines S, Maroon J, Janetta P. Supratentorial intracerebral hemorrhage following posterior fossa surgery. J Neurosurgery 1978;49:881–886.

48. Waga S, Shimosaka S, Sakakura M. Intracerebral hemorrhage remote from the site of the initial neurosurgical procedure. Neurosurgery 1983;13:662–665.

49. Sweet WH, Poletti CE. Complications of standard treatment for trigeminal neuralgia: need for mechanism for prompt reporting of complications (abstract). Poster presentation #82 in program of the annual meeting of the American Association of Neurological Surgeons. Denver, Colorado, 1986;243.

50. Sweet WH, Poletti CE, Roberts JT. Dangerous rises in blood pressure upon heating of trigeminal rootlets: increased bleeding times in patients with trigeminal neuralgia. Neurosurgery 1985;17:843-844.

51. Kehler CH, Brodsky JB, Samuels SI, et al. Blood pressure response during percutaneous rhizotomy for trigeminal neuralgia. Neurosurgery 1982;10:200–202.

52. Norregaard TV, Moskowitz MA. Substance P and sensory innervation of intracranial and extracranial feline cephalic arteries. Brain 1985;108:517–533.

53. Moskowitz MA. The neurobiology of vascular head pain. Ann Neurol 1984;16:157–168.

54. Caplan LR, Skillman J, Ojemann R, Fields W. Intracerebral hemorrhage following carotid endarterectomy: a hypertensive complication. Stroke 1978;9:457–460.

55. Bruetman MF, Fields WS, Crawford ES, DeBakey ME. Cerebral hemorrhage in carotid artery surgery. Arch Neurol 1963;9:458–467.

56. Wylie EJ, Hein MF, Adams JE. Intracerebral hemorrhage following surgical revascularization for treatment of acute strokes. J Neurosurg 1964;21:212–215.

57. Humphreys RP, Hoffman JH, Mustard WT, et al. Cerebral hemorrhage following heart surgery. J Neurosurg 1975;43:671–675.

58. Sila CA. Spectrum of neurologic events following cardiac transplantation. Stroke 1989;20:1586–1589.

59. Cole A, Aube M. Migraine with vasospasm and delayed intracerebral hemorrhage. Arch Neurol 1990;47:53–56.

60. Fisher CM, Adams RD. Observations on Brain Embolism with Special Reference to Hemorrhagic Infarction. In A Furlan (ed), The Heart and Stroke. London: Springer, 1987;17–36.

61. Wilson SAK, Bruce AN. Neurology (2nd ed). London: Butterworth, 1955;1367–1383.

62. Askey JM. Hemorrhage during long-term anticoagulant drug therapy: intracranial hemorrhage. Calif Med 1966; 104:6–10.

63. Babikian V, Kase CS, Pessin MS, et al. Intracerebral hemorrhage in stroke patients anticoagulated with heparin. Stroke 1989;20:1500–1503.

64. Kase CS, Pessin MS, Zivin JA, et al. Intracranial hemorrhage after coronary thrombolysis with tissue plasminogen activator. Am J Med 1992;92:384–390.

65. Caplan LR. Drugs. In CS Kase, LR Caplan, Intracerebral Hemorrhage. Boston: Butterworth–Heinemann, 1994; 201–220.

66. Caplan LR, Hier DB, Banks G. Stroke and drug abuse. Curr Concepts Cerebrovasc Dis (Stroke) 1982;17:9–14.

67. Harrington H, Heller HA, Dawson D, et al. Intracerebral hemorrhage and oral amphetamine. Arch Neurol 1983;40:503–507.

68. Citron B, Halpern M, McCarron M, et al. Necrotizing angiitis associated with drug abuse. N Engl J Med 1970;283:1003–1011.

69. Rumbaugh C, Bergeron R, Fang H, et al. Cerebral angiographic changes in the drug abuse patient. Radiology 1971;101:335–344.

70. Rumbaugh C, Bergeron R, Scanlon R, et al. Cerebral vascular changes secondary to amphetamine abuse in the experimental animal. Radiology 1971;101:345–351.

71. Lukes SA. Intracerebral hemorrhage from an arteriovenous malformation after amphetamine injection. Arch Neurol 1983;40:60–61.

72. Cahill D, Knipp HJ, Mosser J. Intracranial hemorrhage with amphetamine usage. Neurology 1981;31:1058–1059.

73. Yu YJ, Cooper DR, Wellenstein DE, Block B. Cerebral and intracerebral hemorrhage associated with methamphetamine abuse: case report. J Neurosurg 1983;58:109–111.

74. Levine SR, Welch KMA. Cocaine and stroke. Stroke 1988;19:779–783.

75. Levine SR, Brust JCM, Futrell N, et al. Cerebrovascular complications of alkaloid cocaine. N Engl J Med 1990; 323:699–704.

76. Eastman J, Cohen S. Hypertensive crisis and death associated with phencyclidine poisoning. JAMA 1975;231:1270–1271.

77. Bessen H. Intracranial hemorrhage associated with phencyclidine abuse. JAMA 1982;248:585–586.

78. Stratton M, Witherspoon J, Kirtley T. Hypertensive crisis and phencyclidine abuse. Va Med 1978;105:569–572.

79. Lasagna L. Phenylpropanolamine: a review. New York: Wiley, 1988.

80. Kikta DG, Devereux MW, Chandar K. Intracranial hemorrhage due to phenylpropanolamine. Stroke 1985;16:510–512.

81. Kase CS, Foster TE, Reed JE, et al. Intracerebral hemorrhage and phenylpropanolamine use. Neurology 1987;37: 399–404.

82. McDowell JR, Leblanc H. Phenylpropanolamine and cerebral hemorrhage. West J Med 1985;142:688–691.

83. Glick R, Hoying J, Cerullo L, Perlman S. Phenylpropanolamine: an over-the-counter drug causing cerebral nervous system vasculitis and intracerebral hemorrhage. Neurosurgery 1987;20:969–974.

84. Mueller S, Muller J, Asdell S. Cerebral hemorrhage associated with phenylpropanolamine in combination with caffeine. Stroke 1984;15:119–123.

85. Mueller S. Neurologic complications of phenylpropanolamine use. Neurology 1983;33:650–652.

86. Caplan LR, Thomas C, Banks G. Central nervous system complications of addiction to T's and blues. Neurology 1982;32:623–628.

87. Zenkevich GS. Role of congophilic angiopathy in the genesis of subarachnoid-parenchymatous hemorrhages in middle-aged and elderly persons. Zh Nevropatol Psikhiatr 1978;78:52–57.

88. Jellinger K. Cerebral hemorrhage in amyloid angiopathy. Ann Neurol 1977;1:604.

89. Jellinger K. Cerebrovascular amyloidosis with cerebral hemorrhage. J Neurol 1977;214:195–206.

90. Vinters H, Gilbert J. Cerebral amyloid angiopathy: incidence and complications in the aging brain: II. The distribution of amyloid vascular changes. Stroke 1983;14:923–928.

91. Lee S, Stemmerman G. Congophilic angiopathy and cerebral hemorrhage. Arch Pathol Lab Med 1978;102:317–321.

92. Gilbert J, Vinters H. Cerebral amyloid angiopathy: incidence and complications in the aging brain: I. Cerebral hemorrhage. Stroke 1983;14:915–923.

93. Kase CS. Cerebral Amyloid Angiopathy. In CS Kase, LR Caplan (eds), Intracerebral Hemorrhage. Boston: Butterworth–Heinemann, 1994;179–200.

94. Gilles C, Brucher J, Khoubesserian P, et al. Cerebral amyloid angiopathy as a cause of multiple intracerebral hemorrhages. Neurology 1984;34:730–735.

95. Finelli P, Kessimian N, Bernstein P. Cerebral amyloid angiopathy manifesting as recurrent intracerebral hemorrhage. Arch Neurol 1984;41:330–333.

96. Caplan LR. Head Trauma and Related Intracerebral Hemorrhage. In CS Kase, LR Caplan (eds), Intracerebral Hemorrhage. Boston: Butterworth–Heinemann, 1994; 221–241.

97. Alvarez-Sabin J, Turon A, Lozano-Sanchez M, et al. Delayed posttraumatic hemorrrhage, "spat-apoplexie." Stroke 1995;26:1531–1535.

98. Kase CS. Intracranial Tumors. In CS Kase, LR Caplan (eds), Intracerebral Hemorrhage. Boston: Butterworth–Heinemann 1994;243–261.

99. Kase CS. Vasculitis and Other Angiopathies. In CS Kase, LR Caplan (eds), Intracerebral Hemorrhage. Boston: Butterworth–Heinemann 1994;263–303.

100. Caplan LR, Kase CS. Mechanisms of Intracerebral Hemorrhage. In CS Kase, LR Caplan (eds), Intracerebral Hemorrhage. Boston: Butterworth–Heinemann, 1994;95–98.

101. Russell DS. The pathology of spontaneous intracranial hemorrhages. Proc R Soc Med 1954;47:689–693.

102. Mutlu N, Berry RG, Alpers BJ. Massive cerebral hemorrhage: clinical and pathological correlations. Arch Neurol 1963;8:74–91.

103. McCormick WF, Rosenfield DB. Massive brain hemorrhage: a review of 144 cases and an examination of their causes. Stroke 1973;4:946–954.

104. Schutz H. Spontane intrazerebrale hamatome: pathophysologie, klinik, und therapie. Heidelberg: Springer, 1988.

105. Jellinger K. Zur atiologie und pathogenese der spontanen intrazerebralen blutung. Therapiewoche 1972;22:1440–1450.

106. Weisberg LA. Computerized tomography in intrcranial hemorrhage. Arch Neurol 1979;36:422–26.

107. Quereshi AI, Suri MAK, Safdar K, et al. Intracerebral hemorrhage in blacks. Risk factors, subtypes, and outcome. Stroke 1997;28:961–964.

108. Ruiz-Sandoval JL, Cantu C, Barinagarrementeria F. Intracerebral hemorrhage in young people: analysis of risk factors, locations, causes, and prognosis. Stroke 1999;30:537–541.

109. Fisher CM. Clinical Syndromes in Cerebral Hemorrhage in Pathogenesis and Treatment of Cerebrovascular Disease. In W Fields (ed), Proceedings of the Annual Meeting of the Houston Neurological Society. Springfield, IL: Thomas, 1961;318–342.

110. Caplan LR. Putaminal Hemorrhage. In CS Kase, LR Caplan (eds), Intracerebral Hemorrhage. Boston: Butterworth–Heinemann, 1994;309–327.

111. Koba T, Yokoyama T, Kaneko M. Correlation between the location of hematoma and its clinical symptoms in the lateral type of hypertensive intracerebral hemorrhage. Stroke 1977;8:676–680.

112. Mizukami M, Nishijuma M, Kin H. Computed tomographic findings of good prognosis for hemiplegia in hypertensive putaminal hemorrhage. Stroke 1981;12:648–652.

113. Stein R, Caplan LR, Hier DB. Intracerebral hemorrhage: role of blood pressure, location, and size of lesions. Ann Neurol 1983;14:132–133.

114. Mizukami M, Kin H, Araki G, et al. Surgical treatment of primary intracerebral hemorrhage: I. New angiographical classification. Stroke 1976;7:30–36.

115. Metter EJ, Jackson C, Kempler D, et al. Left hemisphere intracerebral hemorrhages studied by (F-18)-fluorodeoxyglucose PET. Neurology 1986;36:1155–1162.

116. Stein R, Kase C, Hier DB, et al. Caudate hemorrhage. Neurology 1984;34:1549–1554.

117. Weisberg L. Caudate hemorrhage. Arch Neurol 1984;41: 971–974.

118. Caplan LR. Caudate Hemorrhage. In CS Kase, LR Caplan (eds), Intracerebral Hemorrhage. Boston: Butterworth–Heinemann, 1994;329–340.

119. Pedrazzi P, Bogousslavsky J, Regli F. Hematomes limites a la tete du Noyau Caude. Rev Neurol 1990;146:12:726–738.

120. Caplan LR. Thalamic Hemorrhage. In CS Kase, LR Caplan (eds), Intracerebral Hemorrhage. Boston: Butterworth–Heinemann, 1994;341–362.

121. Chung, CS, Caplan LR, Han W, et al. Thalamic haemorrhage. Brain 1996;119:1873–1886.

122. Barraquer-Bordas L, Illa I, Escartin A, et al. Thalamic hemorrhage: a study of 23 patients with diagnosis by computed tomography. Stroke 1981;12:524–527.

123. Caplan LR. "Top of the basilar" syndrome: selected clinical aspects. Neurology 1980;30:72–79.

124. Mohr JP, Walters W, Duncan G. Thalamic hemorrhage and aphasia. Brain Lang 1975;2:3–17.

125. Ciemins V. Localized thalamic hemorrhage: a cause of aphasia. Neurology 1970;20:776–782.

126. Samarel A, Wright T, Sergay S, et al. Thalamic hemorrhage with speech disorder. Trans Am Neurol Assoc 1975;101:283–285.

127. Watson R, Heilman K. Thalamic neglect. Neurology 1979;29:690–694.

128. Young WB, Lee KP, Pessin MS, et al. Prognostic significance of ventricular blood in supratentorial hemorrhage: a volumetric study. Neurology 1990;40:616–619.

129. Kawahara N, Sato K, Muraki M, et al. CT classification of small thalamic hemorrhages and their clinical implications. Neurology 1986;35:165–172.

130. Ikeda K, Yamashima T, Uno E, et al. Clinical manifestations of small thalamic hemorrhages. Brain Nerve 1985;37:171–179.

131. Gilner L, Avin B. A reversible ocular manifestation of thalamic hemorrhage: a case report. Arch Neurol 1977;34:715–716.

132. Waga S, Okada M, Yamamoto Y. Reversibility of Parinaud syndrome in thalamic hemorrhage. Neurology 1979;29: 407–409.

133. Kase C, Williams J, Wyatt D, et al. Lobar intracerebral hematomas: clinical and CT analysis of 22 cases. Neurology 1982;32:1146–1150.

134. Ropper A, Davis K. Lobar cerebral hemorrhages: acute clinical syndromes in 26 cases. Ann Neurol 1980;8:141–147.

135. Kase CS. Lobar Hemorrhage. In CS Kase, LR Caplan (eds), Intracerebral Hemorrhage. Boston: Butterworth–Heinemann, 1994;363–382.

136. Zhu XL, Chan MSY, Poon WS. Spontaneous intracranial hemorrhage: which patients need diagnostic cerebral angiography. A prospective study of 296 cases and review of the literature. Stroke 1997;28:1406–1409.

137. Caplan LR. Primary Intraventricular Hemorrhage. In CS Kase, LR Caplan (eds), Intracerebral Hemorrhage. Boston: Butterworth–Heinemann, 1994;383–401.

138. Butler A, Partain R, Netsky M. Primary intraventricular hemorrhage in adults. Surg Neurol 1977;8:143–149.

139. Little JR, Blomquist G, Ethier R. Intraventricular hemorrhage in adults. Surg Neurol 1977;8:143–149.

140. Kase C, Caplan LR. Parenchymatous Posterior Fossa Hemorrhage. In HJM Barnett, JP Mohr, B Stein, F Yatsu (eds), Stroke: Pathophysiology, Diagnosis and Management. New York: Churchill Livingstone, 1985; 621–641.

141. Caplan LR. Pontine Hemorrhage. In CS Kase, LR Caplan (eds), Intracerebral Hemorrhage. Boston: Butterworth–Heinemann, 1994;403–423.

142. Caplan LR, Zervas N. Survival with permanent midbrain dysfunction after surgical treatment of traumatic subdural hematoma: the clinical picture of a Düret hemorrhage. Ann Neurol 1977;1:587–589.

143. Steegman T. Primary pontile hemorrhage. J Nerv Ment Dis 1951;114:35–65.

144. Silverstein A. Primary Pontine Hemorrhage. In P Vinken, G Bruyn (eds), Handbook of Clinical Neurology, Vol 12,

Part 2. Vascular Diseases of the Nervous System. Amsterdam: North Holland, 1972;37–53.

145. Caplan LR, Goodwin J. Lateral tegmental brainstem hemorrhage. Neurology 1982;32:252–260.

146. Kase C, Maulsby G, Mohr JP. Partial pontine hematomas. Neurology 1980;30:652–655.

147. Graveleau P, DeCroix JP, Samson Y, et al. Deficit sensitive isole d'un hemicorps par hematome du pont. Rev Neurol (Paris) 1986;142:788–790.

148. Araga S, Fukada M, Kagimoto H, et al. Pure sensory stroke due to pontine hemorrhage. J Neurol 1987;235: 116–117.

149. Holtzman RNN, Zablozki V, Yang WC, et al. Lateral pontine tegmental hemorrhage presenting as isolated trigeminal sensory neuropathy. Neurology 1987;37:704–706.

150. Veerapen R. Spontaneous lateral pontine hemorrhage with associated trigeminal nerve root hematoma. Neurosurgery 1989;25:451–454.

151. Gobernado J, de Molina A, Gineno A. Pure motor hemiplegia due to hemorrhage in the lower pons. Arch Neurol 1980;37:393.

152. Kameyama S, Tanaka R, Tsuchida T. Pure motor hemiplegia due to pontine hemorrhage. Stroke 1989;20:1288.

153. Schnapper R. Pontine hemorrhage presenting as ataxic hemiparesis. Stroke 1982;13:518–519.

154. Kobatake K, Shinohara Y. Ataxic hemiparesis in patients with primary pontine hemorrhage. Stroke 1983;14:762–764.

155. Tuhrim S, Yang WC, Rubinowitz H, et al. Primary pontine hemorrhage and the dysarthria-clumsy hand syndrome. Neurology 1982;32:1027–1028.

156. Nakajima K. Clinicopathological study of pontine hemorrhage. Stroke 1983;14:485–493.

157. Brennan R, Berglund R. Acute cerebellar hemorrhage: analysis of clinical findings and outcome in 12 cases. Neurology 1977;27:527–532.

158. Fisher CM, Picard E, Polak A, et al. Acute hypertensive cerebellar hemorrhage: diagnosis and surgical treatment. J Nerv Ment Dis 1965;140:38–57.

159. Ott K, Kase C, Ojemann R, et al. Cerebellar hemorrhage: diagnosis and treatment. Arch Neurol 1974;31:160–167.

160. Kase CS. Cerebellar Hemorrhage. In CS Kase, LR Caplan (eds), Intracerebral Hemorrhage. Boston: Butterworth–Heinemann, 1994;425–443.

161. Ojemann R, Heros R. Spontaneous brain hemorrhage. Stroke 1983;14:468–474.

162. Shenkin H, Zavala M. Cerebellar strokes: mortality, surgical indications and results of ventricular damage. Lancet 1982;2:429–432.

163. Richardson AE. Spontaneous Cerebellar Hemorrhage. In P Vinken, G Bruyn (eds), Handbook of Clinical Neurology. Amsterdam: North Holland, 1972;54–67.

164. Longo M, Fiumara F, Pandolfo I, et al. CT observation of an ongoing intracerebral hemorrhage. J Comput Assist Tomogr 1983;7:362–363.

165. Zilkha A. Intraparenchymal fluid-blood level: a CT sign of recent intracerebral hemorrhage. J Comput Assist Tomogr 1983;7:301–305.

166. Pineda A. Computed tomography in intracerebral hemorrhage. Surg Neurol 1977;8:55–58.

167. Dul K, Drayer B. CT and MR Imaging of Intracerebral Hemorrhage. In CS Kase, LR Caplan (eds), Intracerebral Hemorrhage. Boston: Butterworth–Heinemann, 1994; 73–93.

168. Scott W, New P, Davis K, et al. Computerized axial tomography of intracerebral and intraventricular hemorrhage. Radiology 1974;112:73–80.

169. Herald S, Kummer R, Jaeger C. Follow-up of spontaneous intracerebral hemorrhage by computed tomography. J Neurology 1982;228:267–276.

170. Schellinger PD, Jansen O, Fiebach JB, et al. A standardized MRI protocol. Comparison with CT in hyperacute intracerebral hemorrhage. Stroke 1999;30:765–768.

171. Linfante I, Llinas RH, Caplan LR, Warach S. MRI features of intracerebral hemorrhage within 2 hours from symptom onset. Stroke 1999;30:2263–2267.

172. Little J, Blomquist G, Ethier R. Cerebellar hemorrhage in adults: diagnosis by computerized tomography. J Neurosurg 1978;48:575–579.

173. Radberg JA, Olsson JE, Radberg CT. Prognostic parameters in spontaneous intracer ebral hematomas with special reference to anticoagulant treatment. Stroke 1991; 22:571–576.

174. Terayama Y, Tanahashi N, Fukuuchi Y, Gotoh F. Prognostic value of admission blood pressure in patients with intracerebral hemorrhage. Keio Cooperative Stroke Study. Stroke 1997;28:1185–1188.

175. Diringer MN, Edwards DF, Zazulia A. Hydrocephalus: a previously unrecognized predictor of poor outcome from supratentorial intracerebral hemorrhage. Stroke 1998;29: 1352–1357.

176. Dandapani B, Suzuki S, Kelley RE, et al. Relation between blood pressure and outcome in intracerebral hemorrhage. Stroke 1995;26:21–24.

177. Broderick JP, Adams HP, Barsan W, et al. Guidelines for the management of spontaneous intracerebral hemorrhage: a statement for healthcare professionals from a special writing group of the Stroke Council, American Heart Association. Stroke 1999;30:905–915.

178. Langfitt T. Conservative Care of Intracranial Hemorrhage. In R Thompson, J Green (eds), Advances in Neurology, Vol 11. Stroke. New York: Raven, 1977;169–180.

179. Poungvarin N, Bhoopat W, Viriyavejakul A, et al. Effects of dexamethasone in primary supratentorial intracerebral hemorrhage. N Engl J Med 1987;316:1229–1233.

180. Tyler K, Poletti C, Heros R. Cerebral amyloid angiopathy with multiple intracerebral hemorrhages. Neurosurgery 1982;577:286–289.

181. Batjer HH, Reisch JS, Allen BC, et al. Failure of surgery to improve outcome in hypertensive putaminal hemorrhage. A prospective randomized trial. Arch Neurol 1990;47:1103–1106.

182. Morganstern LB, Frankowski RF, Shedden P, et al. Surgical treatment for intracerebral hemorrhage (STICH). A single-center randomized clinical trial. Neurology 1998; 51:1359–1363.

183. Hankey GJ. Surgery for primary intracerebral hemorrhage: is it safe and effective? A systematic review of case series and randomized trials. Stroke 1997;28: 2126–2132.

184. Fleming KD, Wijdicks EFM, St Louis EK, Li H. Predicting deterioration on patients with lobar haemorrhages. J Neurol Neurosurg Psychiatry 1999;66:600–605.

185. Matsumoto K, Honda H. CT guided stereotaxic evacuation of hypertensive intracerebral hematoma. J Neurosurg 1984;61:440–448.

186. Kandel EL, Peresadov VV. Stereotactic evacuation of spontaneous intracerebral hematomas. J Neurosurg 1985; 62:206–213.

187. Nizuma H, Suzuki J. Stereotactic aspiration of putaminal hemorrhage using a double track aspiration technique. Neurosurgery 1988;22:432–436.

188. Nguyen JP, Decq P, Brugieres P, et al. A technique for stereotactic aspiration of deep intracerebral hematomas under computed tomographic control using a new device. Neurosurgery 1992;31:330–335.

189. Mohadjer M, Eggert R, May J, Mayfrank L. CT-guided stereotactic fibrinolysis of spontaneous and hypertensive cerebellar hemorrhage: long-term results. J Neurosurg 1990;73:217–222.

190. Schaller C, Rhode V, Meyer B, Hassler W. Stereotactic puncture and lysis of spontaneous intracerebral hemorrhage using recombinant tissue-plasminogen activator (rtPA) after stereotactic aspiration: initial results. Neurosurgery 1995;36:328–335.

191. Findlay JM, Grace MG, Weir BK. Treatment of intraventricular hemorrhage with tissue plasminogen activator. Neurosurgery 1993;32:941–947.

Chapter 14
Stroke in Children and Young Adults

Strokes are not especially common in the young, but when they occur, clinical features and evaluation strategies are rather different from adult patients in the customary stroke age group (50–85 years). In this chapter, I briefly outline some of the key differences, and review the differential diagnoses of strokes in the young. I do not repeat descriptions of stroke syndromes and vascular disorders covered in more depth elsewhere in this book. Chapter 11 includes discussions of many of the conditions that cause stroke in the young.

General Features and Differences from Geriatric Age Strokes

Heterogeneity

Causes of stroke in the young are more heterogeneous than in the older population. The differential diagnosis list includes many genetic, congenital, metabolic, and systemic disorders that are rarely encountered in mature adult populations. Also, more often than in adults, the cause of childhood stroke remains obscure, even after evaluation.

Etiologic Variations Associated with Age

Causes of stroke differ considerably with age. For example, the differential diagnosis of stroke in a young baby is quite different from that in a 40-year-old adult, yet both are often referred to as *stroke in the young*. Three convenient groups can be distinguished—perinatal and neonatal, children (ages 1–15 years), and adolescents and young adults (ages 15–40 years). Each of these groups has different frequencies of various stroke etiologies. Causes also

vary considerably, depending on geographic, socioeconomic, and environmental factors. For instance, tuberculous meningitis is an important cause of stroke in India,[1] and neurocysticercosis is an important cause of stroke in Mexico and parts of central and South America.[2] These causes of stroke, however, are unusual in the United States.

Prevalence of Hemorrhagic Stroke

Hemorrhagic strokes, including subarachnoid hemorrhage (SAH) and intracerebral hemorrhage (ICH) are relatively more common in the young. In the geriatric years, the ischemic to hemorrhagic stroke ratio is approximately 4 to 1 (80% of strokes are ischemic), whereas in the young, the ratio is close to 0.6 to 1.0 (60% are hemorrhagic).[3,4] Accurate comparative statistics are hard to gather because hemorrhagic strokes are often cared for on neurosurgical units, and ischemic strokes are usually admitted to pediatric and adult neurology units.

Prevalence of Particular Etiologies of Stroke

In my experience, migraine, trauma (including dissection), and cardiac disease are especially important etiologies in children and young adults. Drugs and systemic, genetic, and hematologic causes are also important. Occlusion of dural venous sinuses is a more important cause of stroke in the young than in mature adults.

Locations of Lesions

Brain and vascular location of lesions are somewhat different in the young. Cerebral infarcts tend to be more often limited to deep regions of the hemispheres, especially the striatocapsular region. Vascular-occlusive lesions are more often intracranial, affecting especially the supraclinoid internal carotid artery (ICA), proximal middle cerebral artery (MCA), and basilar artery. Extracranial occlusive disease is much less common. When the occlusive process affects the MCA before the lenticulostriate branches, the striatum and internal capsule are involved. Because of the absence of extensive vascular disease, collateral circulation over the convexity is usually good, accounting for sparing of the cortical territory of the MCA.[5,6] Similarly, proximal posterior cerebral artery occlusion before the thalamogeniculate branches usually leads to thalamic infarcts, with sparing of the temporal and occipital lobes.[7,8] Vascular malformations are more often periventricular or intraventricular than in adults.

Clinical Presentations and Features

In youths, the clinical presentations and features of stroke are also different. In youths, apoplectic sudden onset is the rule. Transient ischemic attacks are unusual. Seizures are common and are often the presenting feature. Brain edema and increased intracranial pressure are also common. Less reserve space in the cranium exists because of the absence of brain atrophy than in geriatric patients. Aphasias in childhood are most often nonfluent, regardless of brain lesion location.[9] In children, agitation and general confusion are often described, but specific disorders of higher cognitive function are harder to recognize and are less well characterized than in adults. Abnormalities of posture and movement, such as dystonias, chorea, and athetosis, are more frequent features and sequelae of stroke than in adults.[10] These extrapyramidal disorders probably reflect the predominance of striatocapsular ischemia. In young children with ischemic damage to the basal ganglia and thalamus, these basal gray-matter tissues become hypermyelinated, giving them a marbled appearance, referred to as *status marmoratus*.[11]

Prognosis

In youths, the outlook for recovery is better than in adults with comparable lesions. The absence of generalized vascular disease and presence of good collateral circulation often minimizes the eventual brain damage, making the ultimate infarct smaller than in adults. Also, the developing brain shows more plasticity. Undamaged areas can frequently assume the functions of damaged regions. As a result, focal disorders of cognition and aphasia often improve, leaving no major speech deficit, although general intellectual function may be less than that expected before the stroke. Although the prognosis is better than in the geriatric age group, strokes in the young are far from benign. A 1994 study of the prognosis of strokes in patients 15–45 years showed that most stroke survivors had emotional, social, or physical impairments that adversely affected employment and reduced their quality of life.[12]

Strokes in Neonates

Hypoxic-ischemic injury is relatively common in neonates. Hypoxia and ischemia are most often caused by (1) intrauterine asphyxia; (2) birth-related problems, such as umbilical cord prolapse; (3) uterine and placental abruption; (4) respiratory insufficiency after birth, caused by aspirated meconium; (5) recurrent apnea; (6) hyaline-membrane disease in premature infants; and (7) severe congenital heart disease, with left-to-right shunts in premature and full-term neonates.[13–15] Cerebral blood flow is lower in preterm than term newborns (20 ml/100 g/min vs. 50–60 ml/100 g/min).[16] The neonatal brain has little autoregulatory capability, so it is much more vulnerable to falls or elevations in blood pressure. Neonatal ischemia is often caused by cardiac disease, sepsis with vascular collapse, and hypertension. The most vulnerable areas for hypoxic-ischemic injury are the cerebral cortex, especially the hippocampus; Purkinje cells of the cerebellar cortex; and the pontine nuclei in the brain stem.[13–16] Perinatal asphyxia also often causes severe damage to the putamen and thalamus on both sides. In addition, more severe hypoxic-ischemic insults damage the caudate nuclei and sensorimotor cortex around the central fissure.[14,17,18]

Three particularly common distributions of hypoxic-ischemic lesions exist in neonates—the parasagittal regions, deep periventricular white matter, and basal ganglia-thalami.[13–21] The parasagittal cortex between the anterior cerebral artery and

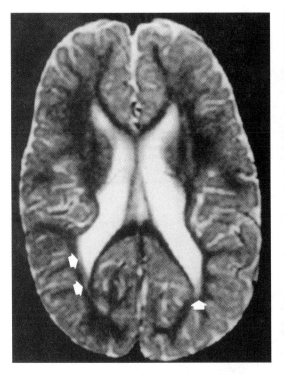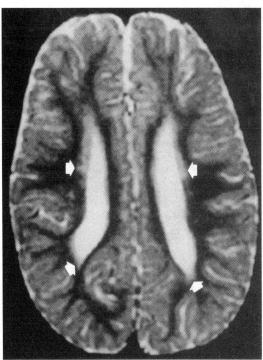

Figure 14-1. T2-weighted magnetic resonance imaging scans of a patient with spastic diplegia caused by periventricular leukomalacia. The scans were taken at 15 months and show irregularity of the ventricular walls, loss of white matter, and T2 prolongation in the periventricular white matter. Arrows point to periventricular abnormalities. (Reprinted with permission from N Aida, NA Nishimura, Y Hachiya, et al. Magnetic resonance imaging of perinatal brain damage: comparison of clinical outcome with initial and follow-up magnetic resonance findings. AJNR Am J Neuroradiol 1998;19:1909–1921.)

MCA, and between the MCA and posterior cerebral artery territories are watershed zones, frequently selectively damaged by hypotension in the full-term newborn infant.[13,19] The most frequent resulting clinical picture is weakness of the proximal limbs, especially the arms. Spastic quadriparesis, which is worse in the arms, is the most characteristic clinical picture.[13,19,20] Computed tomography (CT), magnetic resonance imaging (MRI), radionuclide studies, and positron emission tomography scanning can show the parasagittal distribution of ischemic damage.[13,19,22]

In premature infants, hypoxic-ischemic injury is often reflected in damage to the white matter around the ventricles, a process usually termed *periventricular leukomalacia.*[16,21,23–26] Sometimes, small isolated foci of necrosis exist at the angles of the ventricles. Often, the lesions are extensive and spread out from the ventricles toward the cortex. The periventricular lesions can be hemorrhagic and

are often associated with enlargement of the ventricular system. The predominant clinical sequela is spastic weakness of the legs (diplegia), with lesser involvement of the upper limbs. The white matter lesions near the anterior horns intercept the fibers coming from the parasagittal motor cortex, subserving control of the thighs, legs, and feet. CT, MRI, and ultrasound allow diagnosis during the neonatal period and sequential evaluation of the lesions. Figure 14-1 is an MRI that shows periventricular leukomalacia lesions.

Severe acute hypoxic-ischemic insults during the perinatal period can cause severe damage to the basal ganglia and thalami.[14,17,21] Figure 14-2 is an MRI that illustrates these lesions. The clinical findings during the neonatal period include tongue fasciculations and feeding problems, with impaired swallowing, irritability, and tonic posturing of the arms and legs.[14] Many individuals with these lesions die during the neonatal period. Survivors

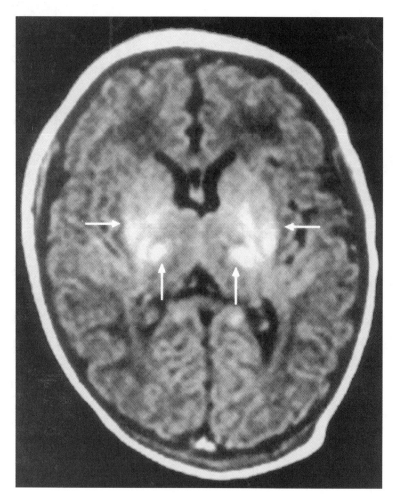

Figure 14-2. T1-weighted magnetic resonance imaging scan at 10 days shows abnormal signal intensities (*arrows*) in the lenticular nuclei and thalamus in a patient who had spastic quadriparesis, seizures, athetoid movements, and developmental delay. (Reprinted with permission from N Aida, NA Nishimura, Y Hachiya, et al. Magnetic resonance imaging of perinatal brain damage: comparison of clinical outcome with initial and follow-up magnetic resonance findings. AJNR Am J Neuroradiol 1998;19:1909–1921.)

often have spastic quadriparesis, chorea-athetosis, and feeding problems with recurrent aspiration and pulmonary infections.[14]

Focal arterial and venous infarcts are also often found in neonates, with seizures or hemiparesis.[13,21,27–29] Most of these lesions are in the territories of the major cerebral arterial distribution, most often affecting the MCA. The lesions may be large and cystic and on occasion communicate with the ventricular system, forming porencephalic cysts. For reasons that are unclear, focal asymmetric infarcts are sometimes found in asphyxiated infants with generalized hypoxia and ischemia. Focal infarcts are clearly more common than are presently diagnosed. In an autopsy study of 592 neonates, 32 (5.4%) had focal infarcts in a recognized arterial distribution.[27] Full-term neonates more often had focal infarcts than premature infants. Arterial embolization with sepsis and disseminated intravascular coagulation were common causes. Focal arterial territory infarcts in infants can also result from drugs, especially cocaine use, by the mother.[30] Traumatic occlusions of the cervical, carotid, and vertebral arteries and intracranial vessels during delivery are another important cause of stroke in neonates.[31,32]

Brain hemorrhages are an even more frequent and important cause of stroke in the perinatal period. Premature infants are especially susceptible to developing hemorrhages in the periventricular region, spreading into the ventricles.[13,16,33–35] These hemorrhages originate in the subependymal germinal matrix, a structure located over the head and body of the caudate nuclei at the level of the intraventricular foramina. The matrix contains fragile capillaries and loose supporting tissue. By full term, the germinal matrix is no longer visible. In the absence of effective autoregulation, increase in blood pressure or blood volume can lead to breakage of these fragile vessels and ICH. Also, an increase in venous pressure, as might be found in asphyxia or hyaline-membrane disease, might facilitate hematoma formation. Hemorrhages usually extend into the adjacent ventricle. Regions of necrosis often surround the hematomas. In full-term infants, periventricular and intraventricular hemorrhages arise from residual matrix tissue or directly from the choroid plexus vasculature.

Most germinal matrix hemorrhages occur during the first 3 postnatal days, especially during the first postpartum hours, but some develop in utero.[35] Clinically, infants with germinal-matrix hemorrhages may appear desperately ill with coma, respiratory abnormalities, and poor muscle tone, or they may appear to be faring normally. At times, a gradual deterioration of function occurs. Ultrasound and CT are effective ways to diagnose and follow children with hemorrhages. Intraventricular hemorrhages can cause temporary hydrocephalus, which resolves itself, or progressive hydrocephalus, requiring ventricular drainage or shunting. Lumbar puncture, with removal of cerebrospinal fluid, is another effective treatment. Ventricular size should be carefully followed by ultrasound or CT.

Since the mid-1970s, cerebellar hemorrhage has been recognized more often during the early neonatal period, especially in premature infants.[16,32,36,37] Cerebellar hemorrhage occurs in an estimated 15–25% of preterm infants.[32,38] In the late stages of gestation, a cerebellar germinal matrix is present. This probably accounts for the high risk of bleeding in preterm babies. Asphyxia and hyaline-membrane disease are contributing factors. Trauma is the principal cause of parenchymatous cerebellar bleeding in full-term babies. Often, cerebellar hemorrhage causes catastrophic loss of function. Seizures; falling hematocrit; signs of brain stem compression, such as ocular bobbing or skew deviation; and acute hydrocephalus may result. Ultrasound and CT allow diagnosis. Surgical decompression is often required and can be lifesaving.[32]

Subarachnoid bleeding is extremely common, and some red blood cells are found in the cerebrospinal fluid of nearly every baby delivered vaginally. Bleeding is most often trivial. More severe birth trauma or coagulation abnormalities can lead to more severe subarachnoid bleeding and diminished alertness in the neonate.[16] Trauma can also cause significant subdural collections of blood.

Strokes in Children (1–15 Years of Age)

Infantile hemiplegia and childhood stroke have been recognized for centuries. Gowers commented in his 1888 textbook of neurology, "Hemiplegia of sudden onset is not uncommon in children, especially in young children."[39] Despite considerable interest, information about etiology did not come about until the work of Ford and Schaffer.[40] A study in Rochester, Minnesota, estimated the rate as 2.52 cases per 100,000 children per year,[41] but the rates are undoubtedly higher in Japan and India. In the Rochester study, 31 childhood strokes were hemorrhagic, whereas 38 were ischemic.[41]

Hemorrhagic Stroke in Children

In preadolescent children, vascular malformations are the most frequent cause of intracranial bleeding.[32,42,43] If all individuals younger than 20 years are included, however, aneurysms are a more common cause of bleeding than vascular malformations. Among 124 young patients with SAH in one series, 50 patients had aneurysms and 33 had arteriovenous malformations (AVMs).[44] Among three series, 36% of young patients had aneurysmal bleeding, whereas 27% bled from AVMs.[44]

Aneurysms generally become symptomatic before the age of 2 years or after the age of 10 years.[32,45] Aneurysms are more common in individuals with coarctation of the aorta, polycystic renal disease, and Ehlers-Danlos syndrome.[32] In childhood, bacterial endocarditis with embolism to the vasorum of intracranial arteries, and mycotic aneurysm formation are especially important causes of SAH. Aneurysms that rupture in childhood have a somewhat different distribution than those found in adults. Shucart and Wolpert analyzed the site of rupture of 100 congenital intracranial aneurysms in children younger than 15 years.[46] Compared with adult series, the intracranial ICA was more often the site of anterior-circu-

Table 14-1. Differential Diagnosis of Pediatric Brain Ischemia (Age 1–15 Years)

Migraine

Trauma: dissection and other vascular injuries; abuse, including whiplash-shake injuries; oral foreign-body trauma to the internal carotid artery

Cardiac: congenital heart disease with right-to-left shunts, tetralogy of Fallot, transposition of great vessels, tricuspid atresia, atrial and ventricular septal defects, cardiomyopathies, endocarditis, pulmonary arteriovenous fistula

Drugs, especially cocaine and heroin

Infections: bacterial meningitis, especially *Haemophilus influenzae*, pneumonococci, and streptococci; facial, otitic, and sinus infections; acquired immunodeficiency syndrome; dural sinus occlusion and infection; tuberculous meningitis

Genetic and metabolic: neurofibromatosis, hereditary disorders of connective tissue (Marfan's and Ehlers-Danlos syndromes), pseudoxanthoma elasticum, homocystinuria, Menkes' kinky hair syndrome, hypoalphalipoproteinemia, familial hyperlipidemias, methylmalonic aciduria, MELAS syndrome (*Mito*chondrial, *E*ncephalopathy, *L*actic *A*cidosis, and *S*troke-like episodes)

Hematologic and neoplastic: sickle cell anemia, purpuras, leukemia, L-arginase and aminocaproic acid (Amicar) treatment, radiation vasculopathy, hypercoagulable states (e.g., caused by decrease in natural inhibitors, such as antithrombin III)

Systemic disease: rheumatic, gastrointestinal, renal, hepatic, pulmonary, moyamoya syndrome

Others: arteritis, collagen vascular disease, local infections, Takayasu's syndrome, Behçet's syndrome, venous sinus thrombosis, head and neck infections, dehydration, coagulopathy, paroxysmal nocturnal hemoglobinuria, puerperal or pregnancy-related

lation bleeding in children, whereas the posterior and anterior communicating arteries were less often implicated in children.[46] Posterior-circulation aneurysms were relatively more common in children (23% of the total) than in adults. They especially involved the intracranial vertebral artery and basilar artery apex.[46] Evaluation and treatment of aneurysms are similar in children and adults.

Intracranial vascular malformations are undoubtedly present at birth, but do not become symptomatic in most patients until adulthood. Although AVMs are the most frequent cause of intracranial bleeding in preadolescents, less than 10% of malformations are diagnosed before the age of 10 years.[32]

Mackenzie noted in 1953 that 29 of his 50 patients (58%) with brain angiomas developed initial symptoms before age 20 years.[47] In adolescents and older children, the most frequent symptoms relate to hemorrhage. Most often, bleeding is into the brain (ICH), but superficial lesions and those abutting on ependymal surfaces can cause SAH or primary intraventricular bleeding. Approximately 20% of arteriovenous malformations in children are infratentorial, approximately equally divided between the cerebellum and brain stem.[48] Supratentorial arteriovenous malformations are typically superficial and cone-shaped, with the base located on the cortical surface and the apex closer to the ventricle.[49] Approximately 10% are deep, involving the basal ganglia and thalamus.[49] Focal neurologic signs often develop gradually and can be associated with signs of increased intracranial pressure. Epilepsy and headache are other less frequent presentations of vascular malformations.

Neonates and young children often harbor a type of malformation that is rarely, if ever, first discovered in adulthood—vein of Galen malformations. In this condition, the vein of Galen is greatly enlarged, forming a large varix, and the straight sinus is also large and tortuous. The malformation is usually fed by posterior choroidal arteries. The typical CT appearance is that of a round hyperdense mass behind the third ventricle, connected to a prominent torcula by the dilatated midline straight sinus. Hydrocephalus is also occasionally associated in approximately one-third of cases. The most common presenting syndrome during the neonatal period and infancy is high-output congestive heart failure, caused by the large volume of shunted blood.[32] A loud cranial bruit is usually audible. Older infants and young children may present with SAH or intraventricular hemorrhage, seizures, or signs of hydrocephalus. If left untreated, these malformations usually prove fatal early in life. I also discuss this malformation in Chapter 13.

Ischemic Strokes in Children

Differential diagnosis of brain infarcts in children is quite wide (Table 14-1), and many patients escape etiologic diagnosis, even after full evaluation. Deep basal ganglia, internal capsule, and thalamic infarcts are relatively more common in children than older age groups. Brower and colleagues described the clinical findings, imaging features, and causes among 36 children (newborn to 13 years old) with striatocapsular and thalamic infarcts at their medical center during a 6-year period.[50] Most children presented with an acute hemiplegia that usually resolved within 1 week, leaving minor motor residua. Sensory and cognitive abnormalities were unusual unless infarction was bilateral.[50] A wide variety of vasculopathies were responsible. The deep pattern is probably best explained by involvement of the proximal portions of the ICAs or MCAs, or both, and the posterior cerebral artery in the presence of good collateral circulation, which continues to supply adequate blood flow to the cerebral cortex.

In my experience and that of others, four risk factors are unusually common in children with ischemic stroke: cardiac disease, infection, trauma, and migraine. In addition, sickle cell anemia may cause brain infarction, particularly among African-American youths. Various coagulopathies are also found in some young stroke patients.

Brain infarcts in patients with cardiac disease are most often caused by embolism, but infection (bacterial endocarditis) and in situ arterial and venous occlusion secondary to polycythemia also occur. Congenital heart disease, especially with shunting of blood (atrial and ventricular septal defects and patent ductus arteriosis), and complex congenital defects are frequent.[51] Children with stroke and congenital heart disease are often cyanotic and have chronic hypoxia and polycythemia. Brain abscess is also common in this situation and must be distinguished from infarction. Rheumatic heart disease, endocarditis, cardiomyopathies, and myocarditis are important acquired heart diseases associated with brain embolism.[52] Diagnostic techniques, especially transesophageal echocardiography and transcranial Doppler sonography after intravenous injection of air bubbles, have led to the detection of small atrial shunts (intra-atrial septal defects and patent foramen ovale) in children and young adults with otherwise unexplained brain infarcts.

Infection was cited as an important predisposing cause of hemiplegia in children in the 1927 report of Ford and Schaffer[40] and in other early writings.[32] Most often, the infections were respiratory or systemic, and the mechanism of stroke was uncertain.

In a 1991 study of childhood stroke in the Tohoku district of Japan, 10 of 54 patients (18.5%) had upper respiratory tract infections or fevers of unknown origin.[53] Tonsillitis can occasionally lead to occlusive changes in the adjacent pharyngeal portion of the ICA. Influenza and *Mycoplasma pneumoniae* have been occasionally implicated as causes of brain infarction.[32,54,55] The mechanism is thought to be a cerebral vasculitis. In herpes zoster in adults, the virus can be detected in the vascular endothelium, often without an inflammatory response. Endothelial viral infection could cause thrombosis by activating platelets and triggering the coagulation cascade. Systemic infection can lead to changes in circulating globulins, with activation of serine protein coagulation factors, such as factor VIII.

Head and neck traumas, even trivial ones, are frequently mentioned as a predisposing factor by the parents of children with ischemic strokes. Ten of the 54 patients (18.5%) in the previously cited Japanese series of children with ischemic strokes had head trauma in the home within the 2 days before the strokes.[53] Oral trauma by penetrating objects can cause ICA occlusions.[56,57] Young children may fall while keeping pencils and tooth brushes in their mouths. The pharynx is lacerated or contused, and the ICA is injured during its course behind the faucial pillars. Extracranial carotid and vertebral artery dissection can develop after head or neck injuries, especially involving sudden twisting movements and blunt trauma to the neck. Neck, jaw, or throat pain or headache may be the earliest symptoms. Brain infarction occurs when the blood within the arterial wall dissects into the arterial lumen and embolizes intracranially. At times, the intramural clot occludes the lumen sufficiently that a luminal thrombus forms in situ because of the sluggish flow and activation of clotting factors.

I have seen several patients in whom seemingly trivial head trauma led to severe intracranial arterial dissections. A young girl developed a fatal intracranial ICA and MCA dissection after her head hit the top of a car when it hit a bump.[58] A young boy fell and hit his head while trick-or-treating on Halloween. Although he appeared uninjured to his mother, he developed a hemiplegia and bilateral motor signs the next day, later shown to be caused by an angiographically documented basilar artery dissection.

Table 14-2. Differential Diagnosis of Ischemia in Young Adults (Age 15–40 Years)

Migraine

Arterial dissection

Drugs, especially cocaine and heroin

Premature atherosclerosis, hyperlipidemias, hypertension, diabetes, smoking, homocystinuria

Female hormone–related (oral contraceptives, pregnancy, puerperium): eclampsia, dural sinus occlusion, arterial and venous infarcts, peripartum cardiomyopathy

Hematologic: deficiency of antithrombin III, protein C, protein S, factor V Leiden, prothrombin gene mutations, fibrinolytic system disorders, deficiency of plasminogen activator, antiphospholipid antibody syndrome, increased factor VIII, cancer, thrombocytosis, polycythemia, thrombotic thrombocytopenic purpura, disseminated intravascular coagulation

Rheumatic and inflammatory: systemic lupus erythematosus, rheumatoid arthritis, sarcoidosis, Sjögren's syndrome, scleroderma, polyarteritis nodosa, cryoglobulinemia, Crohn's disease, ulcerative colitis

Cardiac: intra-atrial septal defect, patent foramen ovale, mitral valve prolapse, mitral annulus calcification, myocardiopathies, arrhythmias, endocarditis

Penetrating artery disease (lacunes): hypertension, diabetes

Others: moyamoya syndrome, Behçet's syndrome, neurosyphilis, Takayasu's syndrome, Sneddon's syndrome, fibromuscular dysplasia, Fabry's disease, Cogan's disease

Migraine is also common in children with brain infarcts. The frequency of its recognition depends on how vigorously physicians have explored the past personal and family history of headache. In 1990, I reported a 6-year-old boy who had severe headache preceding a basilar artery occlusion[59]; he also had a strong family history of migraine. In another young boy, a striatocapsular infarct associated with narrowing of the MCA was followed by the development of typical unilateral throbbing migraine headaches, with photophobia, nausea, and vomiting. Migraine probably causes brain infarcts caused by prolonged vasoconstriction or the formation of local thrombi related to vascular narrowing and activation of the clotting system.[59,60]

Sickle cell anemia is an important cause of brain infarction, especially in African-American children and young adults. In the study of Wood, three-fourths of patients with cerebrovascular complications of sickle cell disease were younger than 15 years.[61] Patients with stroke often have a more severe form of the disease, with frequent sickle crises and lower hematocrits than other patients with the disease. Strokes often occur during a clinical sickle crisis.[32,62] Strokes in sickle cell disease involve large and penetrating small arteries.[63] Sickle cell disease is discussed in Chapter 11. Hemoglobin sickle cell disease is also occasionally complicated by ischemic strokes. Thrombocytosis, congenital deficiency of antithrombin III, proteins C and S, and the C_2 component of complement are also implicated among the causes of strokes in childhood.[32] Advances in genetics have led to detection of resistance to the anticoagulant function of activated protein C, most often caused by factor V Leiden, and prothrombin gene mutations, in some children and young adults with venous thromboses and strokes.

The true incidence of coagulopathies in childhood and the frequency with which they cause ischemic stroke are unknown because coagulation factors and functions have seldom been systematically investigated in large series of children, with or without strokes. Activation of clotting factors could underlie many brain infarcts in children with systemic diseases, infections, and injuries.

In some children and young adults, mitochondrial and other metabolic disorders produce stroke-like episodes. These patients develop confusion; visual abnormalities, including hemianopia and visual neglect; and sometimes seizures and headache. Brain imaging often shows white matter abnormalities predominantly, but not exclusively, in the posterior portions of the cerebral hemispheres in the occipital-temporal and parietal regions. Vascular imaging is usually normal. The pathogenesis is related to energy depletion. MELAS syndrome (*M*itochondrial, *E*ncephalopathy, *L*actic *A*cidosis, and *S*troke-like episodes) is the best-known disorder that causes stroke-like episodes. This and other mitochondrial disorders are discussed in Chapter 11.

Strokes in Young Adults (15–40 Years of Age)

Causes of brain hemorrhage and infarction change as individuals progress from childhood to adulthood. The differential diagnosis of ischemic stroke in this age group is listed in Table 14-2. The topic of stroke in young adults has received increasing attention, and many series report the relative frequencies of various conditions.[1,4,12,64–84] The series, however, are not comparable because of the wide variation in socioeconomic-environmental factors, including age, sex, and race of patients; the time of accrual of the series data, with widely varying available technologies for investigation; and the investigations performed to arrive at the stroke etiology. Drug use, tuberculosis, and oral contraceptive use, for example, vary widely among the United States, India, and Japan, accounting for the variability of these specific etiologies. Cardiac disease was assiduously sought by some authors using modern echocardiography,[72,73,77,79,82] but in other series, this technology was not available or was not systematically used. In some series, few patients had angiography, whereas in one series of 148 patients, all patients had angiography.[76] In another series, 234 out of 300 patients (78%) had angiography with abnormalities detected in 130 (56%).[84]

In some diagnoses, the key data come from the history (e.g., history of the use of illicit drugs and oral contraceptive agents, historical features suggestive of migraine, and the presence of preceding head trauma). The frequency of detection of these causes varies, depending on the preliminary hypotheses and biases of the investigators and on whether the series was prospective, allowing the authors to collect the history, or retrospective, gleaned from the charts. Medical records are notoriously poor in historical detail, especially in terms of negative factors. The history in the medical record may not note that the patient did not have migraine, head, or neck trauma; a recent infection; and so forth. In some series, various etiologies were not considered. In other series, factors, such as oral contraceptive use, migraine, and trauma, were only noted when they were considered etiologically related to the stroke, whereas others simply noted the percentage of subjects in which the factors were present. Table 14-3 summarizes the data from those series that quantitated their data sufficiently to allow tabulation.

In some series, premature atherosclerosis becomes an important cause of stroke in individuals older than 20 years. Louis and McDowell analyzed risk factors in their patients younger than 50 years with stroke caused by atherosclerosis.[64] Among 50 patients, 21 were diabetic. Seventeen patients out of 30 with available lipid measurement had hypercholesterolemia. Thirty-one patients (54%) had hypertension.[64] In the series of Adams et al. among 144 patients aged 15–45 years with ischemic strokes, 38 (27%) were attributed to atherosclerosis.[70] Hypertension, smoking, and diabetes were the principal risk factors, whereas only three patients had hyperlipidemia.[70] In two large series of young Mexican stroke patients, only 10% of men and 5% of women were hypertensive, and 10% of men and 2% of women had hyperlipidemia.[79,84] In one series of patients younger than 30 years who were predominately female, only 5% of ischemic strokes were attributed to premature atherosclerosis.[72] Although premature strokes and coronary artery disease are prevalent in series of patients with severe familial hyperlipidemia, hyperlipidemia was not an important risk factor among the series of young stroke patients reviewed.

Because angiography was not consistently performed in most series, the diagnosis of premature atherosclerosis was often based on the presence of risk factors. Among 148 patients studied by angiography in one series, atherosclerotic lesions were found in 22% of patients, and 19% had thrombotic occlusions (three-fourths involving the carotid circulation and one fourth-being vertebrobasilar).[76]

Cardiac-origin embolism is an important cause of stroke in young adults. The cardiac disorders responsible are, however, somewhat different than those found in childhood series. Rheumatic heart disease, prosthetic valves, and various cardiomyopathies are frequently mentioned cardiac sources of emboli. Intra-atrial septal defects and patent foramen ovale are also commonly detected in some series, depending on the technology available. Table 14-4 shows the cardiac conditions identified in four series of young stroke patients.

Lechat and his French colleagues found that 40% of young patients with ischemic stroke had patent foramen ovale, compared with 10% of controls the same age without stroke.[85,86] Intracardiac shunts can be detected readily by using bubbles introduced intravenously while studying patients with transesophageal echocardiography or transcranial Doppler ultrasound. Few of the series cited routinely used these techniques. Mitral valve prolapse was common in the series of Bogousslavsky and Regli[72] (12 out of 41, 29%) but was infrequent in other series (i.e., 3 out of 144,[70] 3 out of 100,[66] 8 out of 133,[73] and 13 out of

Table 14-3. Series of Strokes in Young Adults

Reference (Year:Site)	Number	Age/Sex	Hemorrhage	Premature Atherosclerosis (%)	Cardiac Emboli (%)	Trauma (%)	Dissection (%)	Oral Contraceptive Use Peripartum (%)	Migraine (%)	Other[a] Unknown[b] (%)
Hart, Miller[66] 1983:USA	100 Ischemia	<40 yrs/NM	—	18	31	2	2	9/5	12	15
Snyder et al.[65] 1980:USA	61 Ischemia	16–49/62% M	—	47	11	NM	NM	11/1	NM	8
Bougousslavaski, Regli[72] 1987:Switzerland	41 Ischemia	<30/27% M	—	5	29/MVP	NM	21	65 NM	15	20
Gautier et al.[73] 1989:France	133 All strokes	9–45/51% M	9	15	12	13	21	34?NM	14	14
Adams et al.[70] 1986:USA	144 Ischemia	15–45/51% M	—	27	24	NM	6	4/5	14	42
Hilton-Jones, Warlow[68] 1985:UK	75 All strokes	<45/66% M	20	9	7	17	NM	9/NM	13	7
Berlit[74] 1990:Germany	168 Ischemia	<40/46% M	—	32	9	4	2	12/4	10	18
Lisovoski, Rousseau[76] 1991	148 Ischemia	5–40/51% M	—	22	13	NM	10	11	17	—
Baringarrementaria et al.[84] 1996:Mexico	300 Ischemia	11–40/46% M	—	4	24	NM	15	NM	3	22
Baringarrementaria et al.[71] 1998:Mexico	130 Ischemia	11–40/all F	—	0	36	NM	11	12/2	7	22
Giovannoni, Fritz[81] 1993:South Africa	75 Ischemia	<45/44% M	—	37	38	NM	0	5/NM	9	24

Study										
Williams et al.[77] 1997:USA	75 TIA	18–45/52% M	—	16	14	NM	15	NM	NM	32
Kristensen et al.[83] 1997:North Sweden	116 Ischemia	11–44/59% M	—	12	33	NM	NM	3/NM	1	30
Carolei et al.[82] 1993:Italy	107 Ischemia	15–44/52% M	—	34	24	NM	0.3	4/NM	1	8
Kapelle et al.[12] 1994:USA	333 Ischemia	15–45/53%	—	22	21	NM	NM	5 of 10 patients/NM	NM	42

F = females; M = males; MVP = mitral valve prolapse; NM = not mentioned; TIA = transient ischemic attack.
The percentages in every study do not add to 100. Some authors cite oral contraceptive use, migraine, and trauma, only when thought to cause stroke. Others list all patients with these factors. Some patients have more than one condition (e.g., migraine and oral contraceptives, trauma and dissection).
[a]Other includes known or probable cause other than those specified in this chart (e.g., moyamoya syndrome, inflammatory diseases, coagulopathy).
[b]Unknown, usually meant the cause was not determined.

Table 14-4. Cardiac Disease Identified in Various Series of Young Adult Stroke Patients

Disease	Barrinagarrementaria[84] n = 300 Echo = 67	Barrinagarrementaria[79] n = 130 Females, Echo = 85	Williams[77] n = 116	Carolei[82] n = 333 Echo = 323
Rheumatic heart disease	38	29	—	7
Prosthetic valve	6	9	—	7
Aortic valve disease	1	—	—	4
Mitral valve prolapse	13	—	—	28
Myxoma	2	1	—	—
Ventricular septal defect	1	—	—	—
Patent foramen ovale/atrial septal defect	1	8	5	—
Myocarditis/endocarditis	—	—	3	3
Congenital heart disease	—	—	—	2
Acute myocardial infarction	—	—	—	3
Chronic cardiac ischemia	2	—	—	13
Cardiomyopathy	2	—	—	2
Atrial fibrillation	—	—	—	2
Other	—	—	6	—

300[84]). In the series studied by Gautier et al., five of the eight patients with mitral valve prolapse also had a patent foramen ovale.[73]

Trauma is a common risk factor for ischemia in young adults. In the series studied by Hilton-Jones and Warlow, 13 of 75 patients had head or neck trauma at varying intervals before stroke.[68] Few of these patients had other stroke risk factors. Trauma is infrequently mentioned in other series. Arterial dissections were common in some series; the frequency of its detection varied with the extent of angiography. Gautier et al. identified 23 cases of dissection among their 112 (20%) arterial infarcts. One-third of patients with dissection gave a history of recent trauma.[73] In their angiography series, Lisovoski and Rousseaux found that 15 of 148 patients (10.1%) had arterial dissections.[76] Arterial dissections were found in 17 out of 116 patients (14.5%),[77] and 45 out of 300 (15%)[84] in other series. In an Italian series, only 1 out of 333 patients had dissections, despite the fact that 72% of patients had angiography.[82] The authors of this series posited that the low frequency of dissection might be explained by the admission of all patients with head and neck trauma to surgical services.[83] I believe that cervical and intracranial dissections are much more common than are appreciated. This entity is greatly underdiagnosed. Dissections are discussed in detail in Chapter 11.

Many strokes in young women were related to pregnancy, the puerperium, or use of oral contraceptive agents. In India especially, puerperal stroke, usually caused by dural venous sinus occlusion, was very important.[1,67] Srinivasan reviewed the experience in Madurai, India,[67] where puerperal stroke accounted for 15–20% of strokes in the young. One hundred and forty-five cases had been seen during a decade. Usually, symptoms began during the first 3 weeks after normal childbirth in multiparous women. Seizures (80%); reduced alertness (50%); transient focal signs, such as unilateral weakness (60%); and raised increased cranial pressure (18%) were common early findings.[67] The vast majority of patients had dural-sinus occlusion. Fibrinogen levels were considerably raised in 104 out of 120 measured (86%). Mortality was high. Pulmonary embolism and puerperal cardiomyopathy were also problems in these patients.[67] Series of young women who develop dural and venous sinus thrombosis always include a large number of patients who develop the occlusions during pregnancy or the puerperium. Oral contraceptive use was common among young women with strokes, although the relationship to etiology was usually uncertain. Although 34% of young women in the series of Gautier et al. used oral contraceptives, this was not significantly different from the estimated rate of use in the population of the same age (32%).[73] Lower-dose oral contraceptive agents have less risk of stroke. Published series antedate the widespread use of lower-dose contraceptives or do not report the strength of estrogen and progesterone used.

In some series, oral contraceptive use and migraine were combined risk factors. Migraine was mentioned prominently in some series,[68,70,72,73,75,79,82,84] but the mechanism by which it related to stroke was most often not identified. Some series tabulated all patients that gave a history of migraine, whereas other series listed only patients in whom the authors considered that migraine was the etiology of the brain infarct.

Infections seem to be less important as an etiology of stroke in young adults than in children. Neurosyphilis is an important cause of stroke in young adults in India, as is tuberculous meningitis.[67] Neurocysticercosis was an important cause of stroke in Mexican young adults, accounting for 14 of the 80 cases of nonatherosclerotic vasculopathies found among 300 patients.[84]

An important factor that may have been unrecognized is the use of drugs. Illicit drugs, especially cocaine, have become an important and frequent cause of ischemia and hemorrhage in young adults.[4] A history of drug use was seldom mentioned in the series reviewed and was seldom pursued vigorously as a possible etiology. In a case-control study of individuals aged 15–44 years, the estimated overall relative risk for stroke was 6.5 and was 11.2 for patients younger than 35 years.[87] The Baltimore-Washington Young Stroke Study investigators specifically sought data regarding stroke among 422 patients with first ischemic strokes (age range, 17–44 years).[88] Any drug use was acknowledged in 94 patients (22%), and 51 individuals (12%) used drugs within the 48 hours before stroke onset.[88] In 20 of these 51 patients (39%) with recent drug use, no other cause of stroke was identified. Strokes were attributed directly to the drug use.[88] Cocaine was the most commonly used drug in this and other series. I discuss drug-related stroke in more detail in Chapter 11.

Few reports analyze the causes of hemorrhagic stroke in young adults. Because hemorrhagic stroke patients are often cared for on neurosurgical services and ischemia is usually treated on neurologic

units, the relative frequencies of the two types of stroke are difficult to determine. Hemorrhagic strokes probably make up a smaller proportion of strokes in the ages 15–45 years than before age 15 years. The ratio of hemorrhage to ischemia varies considerably with the race, sex, and location of stroke patients. In Osaka, Japan, for example, among 252 young stroke patients aged 16–40 years, 175 had hemorrhagic strokes (70%),[75] whereas in a British series of patients younger than 45 years, only 20% had hemorrhages.[68] In a French series, only 9% of 133 patients had intracranial hemorrhages.[73]

In general, the etiology of ICH in patients younger than 45 years is similar to those older than 45 years, except for an overrepresentation of AVMs, drug abuse, and early life bleeding disorders such as hemophilia. Amyloid angiopathy is not encountered in young adults, and warfarin-related hemorrhages are less frequent than in older patients. Hypertension remains a frequent cause of intraparenchymatous bleeding in both age groups. Toffol and colleagues reviewed the Iowa experience with nontraumatic ICH in patients 15–45 years of age.[71] The most common location was lobar (41 out of 72, 57%); 11 were putaminal (15%), and four were intraventricular. Etiologies included AVMs (21 out of 55, 39%), hypertension (11 out of 72, 15%), aneurysm (7 out of 72, 10%), and drug use with amphetamines or phenylpropanolamine, or both (5 out of 72, 7%).[71] Among the 15 cases of ICH included in the British series, six were caused by AVMs and two by hypertension.[68] In a Japanese neurologic series among 25 young patients with ICH, seven had AVMs. In 16 patients, hemorrhages were attributed to hypertension.[75] Aneurysms (51%) accounted for more ICHs than AVMs (19%) among Japanese patients treated on a neurosurgical service.[75] In a Mexican study of 200 patients younger than 40 years with ICHs, AVMs and cavernous angiomas were the most common causes.[78] In this series, only 22 (11%) hemorrhages were attributed to hypertension. The majority of hemorrhages (55%) were lobar.[78] Table 13-2 records the etiologies of hemorrhage in this series and the locations of the hemorrhages in relation to etiology.

Aneurysms in young adults have the same locations and clinical findings as in older patients. SAHs before and after age 40 years are diagnosed and managed in the same fashion.

Differences in Evaluation

In young adults and children, clinicians face a dilemma regarding the extensiveness of the evaluation. A patient's youth, with nearly a lifetime remaining of potential risks of future stroke and other vascular diseases and the vast number of diagnostic possibilities are factors that argue for extensive evaluation. On the other hand, the tendency for young patients to improve dramatically irrespective of treatment, the knowledge that a high proportion of cases go undiagnosed despite intensive testing, and the high cost of technology and testing argue for conservatism when ordering tests.

In my opinion, clinicians should spend more time with the clinical encounter. The history should include questions about smoking, headache, trauma, cardiac symptoms, past bleeding, miscarriages, thrombophlebitis, and prior strokes or ischemic attacks. The use of medicines and drugs of any kind (especially cocaine, amphetamines, and other illicit drugs) and oral contraceptive agents is particularly important. The history should include a thorough review of systems, searching for symptoms that might indicate systemic disease. Family history is important. Information about premature atherosclerosis, hypertension, hyperlipidemia, migraine, and metabolic and hereditary diseases in family members should be sought.

The general physical examination should include careful inspection of the skin for rashes and other lesions. Palpation of pulses and cardiac, neck, and cranial auscultation are especially important. Blood tests, including coagulation studies; neuroimaging; and cardiac evaluation are probably needed in every young person with stroke. Ultrasound and angiography may be indicated, depending on the findings from the clinical encounter and early investigations. The yield of angiography is high. In one series, two-thirds of angiograms were abnormal, often allowing an etiologic diagnosis.[76] Magnetic resonance and CT angiography and extracranial and intracranial ultrasound may allow clinicians to noninvasively acquire more data about the vasculature without risk to the patients. Physicians should order contrast angiography only when preliminary screening vascular imaging suggests a vascular lesion, but does not define it sufficiently to select and monitor treatment.

References

1. Chopra JS, Prabhakar S. Clinical features and risk factors in stroke in young. Acta Neurol Scand 1979;60:289–300.
2. Caplan LR. How to manage patients with neurocysticercosis. Eur Neurol 1997;37:124–131.
3. Nencini P, Inzitari D, Baruffi MC, et al. Incidence of stroke in young adults in Florence, Italy. Stroke 1988;19:977–981.
4. Stern B, Kittmer S, Sloan M, et al. Stroke in the young. Maryland Med J 1991;40:453–462, 565–571.
5. Walsh LE, Garg B. Isolated acute subcortical infarctions in children: clinical description and radiographic correlation. Ann Neurol 1990;28:458–459.
6. Caplan LR, Babikian V, Helgason C, et al. Occlusive disease of the middle cerebral artery. Neurology 1985;35:975–982.
7. Caplan LR, DeWitt LD, Pessin MS, et al. Lateral thalamic infarcts. Arch Neurol 1988;45:959–964.
8. Caplan LR. Posterior Cerebral Artery Disease. In LR Caplan (ed). Posterior Circulation Disease. Boston: Blackwell, 1996;444–491.
9. Ferro JM, Crespo M. Young adult stroke: neuropsychological dysfunction and recovery. Stroke 1988;19:982–986.
10. Dooling EC, Adams RD. The pathological anatomy of posthemiplegic athetosis. Brain 1975;98:29–48.
11. Malamud N. Status marmoratus: a form of cerebral palsy following either birth injury or inflammation of the central nervous system. J Pediatr 1950;37:610–619.
12. Kappelle LJ, Adams HP, Heffner ML, et al. Prognosis of young adults with ischemic stroke. A long-term follow-up study assessing recurrent vascular events and functional outcome in the Iowa Registry of Stroke in Young Adults. Stroke 1994;25:1360–1365.
13. Hill A, Volpe JJ. Stroke and Hemorrhage in the Premature and Term Neonate. In MB Edwards, HJ Hoffman (eds), Cerebral Vascular Diseases in Children and Adolescents. Baltimore: Williams & Wilkins, 1989;179–194.
14. Roland E, Poskitt K, Rodriguez E, et al. Perinatal hypoxic-ischemic thalamic injury: clinical features and neuroimaging. Ann Neurol 1998;44:161–166.
15. Leech RW, Alvord EC Jr. Anoxic-ischemic encephalopathy in the human neonatal period: the significance of brain stem involvement. Arch Neurol 1977;34:109–113.
16. Rorke LB, Zimmerman RA. Prematurity, postmaturity, and destructive lesions in utero. AJNR Am J Neuroradiol 1992;13:517–536.
17. Johnston MV. Selective vulnerability in the neonatal brain. Ann Neurol 1998;44:155–156.
18. Martin LJ, Brambrink A, Koehler RC, Traystman RJ. Primary sensory and forebrain motor systems in the newborn brain are preferentially damaged by hypoxia-ischemia. J Comp Neurol 1997;377:262–285.
19. Volpe JJ. Value of MR in definition of the neuropathology of cerebral palsy in vivo. AJNR Am J Neuroradiol 1992;13:79–83.
20. Volpe JJ, Pasternak JF. Parasagittal cerebral injury in neonatal hypoxic-ischemic encephalopathy: clinical and neuroradiologic features. J Pediatr 1977;91:472–476.

21. Aida N, Nishimura NA, Hachiya Y, et al. MR imaging of perinatal brain damage: comparison of clinical outcome with initial and follow-up MR findings. AJNR Am J Neuroradiol 1998;19:1909–1921.

22. Volpe JJ, Herscovitch P, Perlman JM, et al. Positron emission tomography in the asphyxiated term newborn: parasagittal impairment of cerebral blood flow. Ann Neurol 1985;17:287–296.

23. Banker BQ, Larroch JC. Periventricular leukomalacia of infancy: a form of neonatal anoxic encephalopathy. Arch Neurol 1962;7:386–410.

24. DeReuck J, Chattha AS, Richardson EP Jr. Pathogenesis and evolution of periventricular leukomalacia in infancy. Arch Neurol 1972;27:229–236.

25. Truwit CL, Barkovich AJ, Koch TK, Ferriero DM. Cerebral palsy: MR findings in 40 patients. AJNR Am J Neuroradiol 1992;13:67–78.

26. Kuban KC, Leviton A. Cerebral palsy. N Engl J Med 1994;330:188–195.

27. Barmada MA, Moossy J, Shuman RM. Cerebral infarcts with arterial occlusion in neonates. Ann Neurol 1979;6:495–502.

28. Mantovani JF, Gerber GJ. "Idiopathic" neonatal cerebral infarction. Am J Dis Child 1984;138:359–362.

29. Rollins NK, Morris MC, Evans D, et al. The role of early MR in the evaluation of the term infant with seizures. AJNR Am J Neuroradiol 1994;15:239–248.

30. Chasnoff IJ, Bussey ME, Savich R, et al. Perinatal cerebral infarction and maternal cocaine use. J Pediatr 1986;108:456–459.

31. Roessmann CC, Miller RT. Thrombus of the middle cerebral artery associated with birth trauma. Neurology 1980;30:889–892.

32. Roach ES, Riela AR. Pediatric Cerebrovascular Disorders. Mount Kisco, NY: Futura, 1988.

33. Ahmann PA, Lazzara A, Dykes FD, et al. Intraventricular hemorrhage in the high-risk preterm infant: incidence and outcome. Ann Neurol 1980;7:118–124.

34. Papile LA, Burstein J, Burstein R, et al. Incidence and evolution of subependymal and intraventricular hemorrhage: a study of infants with birth weights of less than 1500 gm. Pediatrics 1978;92:529–534.

35. Garcia JH, Pantoni L. Strokes in childhood. Semin Pediatr Neurol 1995;2:180–191.

36. Grunnet ML, Shields WD. Cerebellar hemorrhage in the premature infants. J Pediatr 1976;88:605–608.

37. Martin R, Roessmann U, Fanaroff A. Massive intracerebellar hemorrhage in low birth-weight infants. J Pediatr 1976;89:290–293.

38. Volpe JJ. Neonatal periventricular hemorrhage: past, present and future. J Pediatr 1978;92:693–696.

39. Gowers WR. A manual of diseases of the nervous system. Philadelphia: P Blakiston, 1888:839.

40. Ford FR, Schaffer AJ. The etiology of infantile acquired hemiplegia. AMA Arch Neurol Psychiatry 1927;18:323–347.

41. Schoenberg BS, Mellinger JF, Schoenberg DG. Cerebrovascular disease in infants and children: a study of incidence, clinical features, and survival. Neurology 1978;28:763–768.

42. So SC. Cerebral arteriovenous malformations in children. Childs Brain 1978;4:242–250.

43. Ventureyra EC, Herder S. Arteriovenous malformations in children. Childs Nerv Syst 1987;3:12–18.

44. Sedzimir CB, Robinson J. Intracranial hemorrhages in children and adolescents. J Neurosurg 1973;38:269–281.

45. Orozco M, Trigueros F, Quintana F, et al. Intracranial aneurysms in early childhood. Surg Neurol 1978;9:247–252.

46. Shucart WA, Wolpert SM. Intracranial arterial aneurysms in childhood. Am J Dis Child 1974;127:288–293.

47. Mackenzie I. The clinical presentation of the cerebral angioma. Brain 1953;76:184–213.

48. Humphreys RP. Infratentorial Arteriovenous Malformations. In MS Edwards, HJ Hoffman (eds), Cerebral Vascular Disease in Children and Adolescents. Baltimore: Williams & Wilkins, 1989;309–320.

49. Martin NA, Edwards MS. Supratentorial Arteriovenous Malformations. In MS Edwards, HJ Hoffman (eds), Cerebral Vascular Diseases in Children and Adolescents. Baltimore: Williams & Wilkins, 1989;283–308.

50. Brower MC, Rollins N, Roach ES. Basal ganglia and thalamic infarction in children. Cause and clinical features. Arch Neurol 1996;53:1252–1256.

51. Terplan AK. Patterns of brain damage in infants and children with congenital heart disease. Am J Dis Child 1973;125:176–185.

52. Caplan LR. Brain Embolism. In LR Caplan. JW Hurst, M Chimowitz (eds), Clinical Neurocardiology. New York: Marcel Dekker, 1999;35–185.

53. Satoh S, Shirane R, Yoshimoto T. Clinical survey of ischemic cerebrovascular disease in children in a district of Japan. Stroke 1991;22:586–589.

54. Zilkha A, Mendelsohn F, Borofsky LG. Acute hemiplegia in children complicating upper respiratory infections. Clin Pediatr 1976;15:1137–1142.

55. Parker P, Puck J, Fernandez F. Cerebral infarction associated with *Mycoplasma pneumoniae*. Pediatrics 1981;67:373–375.

56. Pitner SE. Carotid thrombosis due to intraoral trauma—an unusual complication of a common childhood accident. N Engl J Med 1966;274:764–767.

57. Pearl PL. Childhood stroke following intraoral trauma. J Pediatr 1987;110:574–575.

58. Duncan A, Rumbaugh C, Caplan LR. Cerebral embolic disease: a complication of carotid aneurysms. Radiology 1979;133:379–384.

59. Caplan LR. Migraine and vertebrobasilar ischemia. Neurology 1990;41:55–61.

60. Caplan LR. Migraine. In LR Caplan (ed), Posterior Circulation Disease, Boston: Blackwell, 1996;544–548.

61. Wood DH. Cerebrovascular complications of sickle-cell anemia. Stroke 1978;9:73–75.

62. Grotta JC, Manner C, Pettigrew LC, et al. Red blood cell disorders and stroke. Stroke 1986;17:811–816.

63. Adams RJ, Nichols FT, McKie V, et al. Cerebral infarction in sickle cell anemia: mechanism based on CT and MRI. Neurology 1988;38:1012–1017.

64. Louis S, McDowell F. Stroke in young adults. Ann Intern Med 1967;66:932–938.

65. Snyder BD, Ramirez-Lassepas M. Cerebral infarction in young adults: long term prognosis. Stroke 1980;11:149–153.

66. Hart RG, Miller VT. Cerebral infarction in young adults: a practical approach. Stroke 1983;14:110–114.

67. Srinivasan K. Ischemic cerebrovascular disease in the young: two common causes in India. Stroke 1984;15:733–735.

68. Hilton-Jones D, Warlow CP. The causes of stroke in the young. J Neurol 1985;232:137–143.

69. Radhakrishnan K, Ashek PP, Sridharan R, Mousa ME. Stroke in the young: incidence and pattern in Benghazi, Libya. Acta Neurol Scand 1986;73:434–438.

70. Adams HP, Butler MJ, Biller J, Toffol GJ. Nonhemorrhagic cerebral infarction in young adults. Arch Neurol 1986;43:793–796.

71. Toffol GJ, Biller J, Adams HP. Nontraumatic intracerebral hemorrhage in young adults. Arch Neurol 1987;44:483–485.

72. Bogousslavsky J, Regli F. Ischemic stroke in adults younger than 30 years of age. Arch Neurol 1987;44:479–482.

73. Gautier JC, Pradat-Diehl P, Loron PL, et al. Accidents vasculaires cérébraux des sujets jeunes. Une etude de 133 patients ages de 9 à 45 ans. Rev Neurol 1989;145:437–442.

74. Berlit P. Cerebral ischemia in young adults. Ann Neurol 1990;28:258.

75. Yamaguchi T, Yoshinaga M, Yonekawa Y. Stroke in the young—Japanese perspective. Abstracts International Conference on Stroke. Geneva, Switzerland: May 30–June 1, 1991.

76. Lisovoski F, Rousseaux P. Cerebral infarction in young people: a study of 148 patients with early angiography. J Neurol Neurosurg Psychiatry 1991;54:576–579.

77. Williams LS, Garg BP, Cohen M, et al. Subtypes of ischemic stroke in children and young adults. Neurology 1997;49:1541–1545.

78. Ruiz-Sandoval JL, Cantu C, Baringarrementaria F. Intracerebral hemorrhage in young people. Analysis of risk factors, locations, causes, and prognosis. Stroke 1999;30:537–541.

79. Baringarrementaria F, Gonzalez-Duarte A, Miranda L, Cantu C. Cerebral infarction in young women: analysis of 130 cases. Eur Neurol 1998;40:228–233.

80. Kittner SJ, Stern BJ, Wozniak M, et al. Cerebral infarction in young adults. The Baltimore-Washington Cooperative Young Stroke Study. Neurology 1998;50:890–894.

81. Giovannoni G, Fritz VU. Transient ischemic attacks in younger and older patients. A comparative study of 798 patients in South Africa. Stroke 1993;24:947–953.

82. Carolei A, Marini C, Ferranti E, et al. A prospective study of cerebral ischemia in the young. Analysis of pathogenic determinants. Stroke 1993;24:362–367.

83. Kristensen B, Malm J, Carlberg B, et al. Epidemiology and etiology of ischemic stroke in young adults aged 18 to 44 years in Northern Sweden. Stroke 1997;28:1702–1709.

84. Baringarrementaria F, Figueroa T, Huebe J, Cantu C. Cerebral infarction in people under 40 years. Etiologic analysis of 300 cases prospectively evaluated. Cerebrovasc Dis 1996;6:75–79.

85. Lechat P, Mas JL, Lescault G, et al. Prevalence of patent foramen ovale in patients with strokes. N Engl J Med 1988;318:1148–1152.

86. Lechat P, Lascault G, Thomas D, et al. Patent foramen ovale and cerebral embolism. Circulation 1985;72(Suppl 3):134.

87. Kaku DA, Lowenstein DH. Emergence of recreational drug abuse as a major risk factor for stroke in young adults. Ann Intern Med 1990;113:821–827.

88. Sloan MA, Kittner SJ, Feeser BR, et al. Illicit drug-associated ischemic stroke in the Baltimore-Washington Young Stroke Study. Neurology 1998;49:1688–1693.

Chapter 15
Spinal Cord Strokes

Strokes affect the human spinal cord, but spinal cord strokes represent a minute fraction of all patients with central nervous system vascular disease. The rarity of spinal cord strokes and lack of accessibility to study the spinal cord vascular system during life have prevented complete understanding of spinal cord vascular disease. To compound ignorance, the spinal cord and its vascular system are seldom examined in detail at necropsy. Nonetheless, when sought, spinal ischemic lesions are found. In London, Ontario, Canada, a systematic search for examples of hypoxic myelopathy uncovered 52 cases among 1,200 consecutive necropsies (4%).[1,2]

Unique Anatomy of the Spinal Cord

The unique anatomy of the spinal cord makes the clinician's approach to spinal lesions quite different from brain lesions. Anatomic definition requires placing the lesion in two planes, longitudinally (rostrocaudally) and in depth. Imaging the lesion with magnetic resonance imaging (MRI) or standard angiography requires localization to the craniospinal junction region, cervical cord, thoracic cord, lumbar cord, or cauda equina. Lesions at different rostrocaudal levels have different likely etiologies.

Three depths of lesions with clinical importance are: (1) within the epidural space; (2) inside the dura, but outside the spinal cord (intradural extramedullary); and (3) intramedullary. Most epidural lesions reflect disease of the bony fortress and its connective tissue elements that surround the spinal cord. Lesions inside the dura are most often benign tumors, hematomas, or abscesses. Intramedullary

lesions have a wide differential diagnosis that includes infarcts and hematomas.

Rostrocaudal localization depends on the level of findings affecting the long motor (pyramidal) and sensory (spinothalamic and posterior column proprioceptive) tracts, and the presence of local segmental signs.[3] Root or dermatomal distribution of sensory, reflex, or lower motor neuron loss accurately identifies the rostrocaudal level of the process. Local bone tenderness and pain are also usually reliable in pointing to the segment involved.

Depth localization is more difficult. Epidural processes usually involve the vertebral column, and bone and root pain usually precede symptoms related to dysfunction of the spinal cord. Intradural lesions cause root pain, but bony findings are absent clinically and by x-ray. Intramedullary lesions are most often, but not always, painless. Asymmetric signs, sparing of distal sensory fibers, and dissociated sensory loss are other clues to an intramedullary localization. This subject is discussed in more depth elsewhere.[3]

Spinal Cord Vascular System

I did not include diagnosis or discussion of the spinal vascular system in the general discussion of anatomy in Chapter 2. I find it easiest to understand and visualize the system by first focusing on a spinal cord segment in axial section (Figure 15-1). A large single anterior spinal artery runs in the ventral midline rostrally from the spinomedullary junction at the foramen magnum caudally to the tip of the spinal cord, the filum terminale. In contrast, paired smaller posterior spinal arteries exist on the dorsal

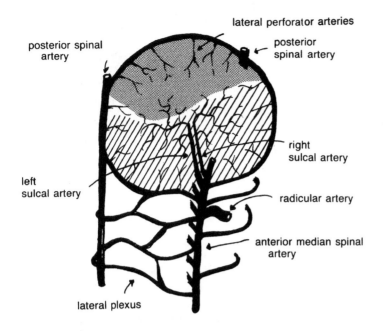

lateral perforator arteries

posterior spinal artery

posterior spinal artery

right sulcal artery

left sulcal artery

radicular artery

anterior median spinal artery

lateral plexus

Figure 15-1. Cross section of spinal cord shows arterial patterns of supply. The anterior spinal artery is a single midline artery that courses in the anterior fissure. This artery divides into left and right sulcal arteries, which supply the anterior horns and white matter. Two posterior spinal arteries exist, one on each side, which form an anastomotic rete from which branches emerge to supply the posterior gray horns and posterior columns.

surface, which often form a plexus of small vessels. The anterior spinal artery gives off deep branches, which course along the ventral sulcus and then branch as they reach the central gray matter to supply left and right branches to the anterior horn regions on each side.[4,5] Lateral circumferential arteries and their penetrators course laterally from the midline anterior spinal artery to supply the ventral white matter, tips of the anterior horns, and pyramidal tracts.[4,5] This pattern is similar to that found in the brain stem, in which paramedian penetrators and short and long circumferential arteries branch from the vertebral and basilar arteries (see Figure 2-14). The posterior spinal artery plexus also gives off penetrating branches to the posterior columns and posterior gray horns.[1,4,5] The regions of supply of the anterior and posterior spinal arteries are shaded diagrammatically on Figure 15-1. The area between the two zones of supply in the central portion of the cord has often been called the *border zone* or *watershed region of supply*.[6]

The anterior spinal supply comes from five to 10 usually single, unpaired radicular arteries, which feed into the anterior spinal artery at various levels (Figure 15-2). The most rostral supply comes from the intracranial vertebral artery. Each intracranial vertebral artery in its distal segment gives off a ramus, which joins with that of the con-

tralateral vertebral artery to form a midline anterior spinal artery. The midline anterior spinal artery feeds the medulla and descends in the midline through the foramen magnum to supply the cervical spinal cord. Branches from the thyrocervical and costocervical branches of the subclavian arteries and branches of the nuchal vertebral artery feed into the spinal cord at the cervical enlargement. The thoracic portion of the anterior spinal artery is fed by radicular branches of the deep cervical and intercostal arteries and by branches of the aorta. Blood supply is most marginal in the upper thoracic region (T2–T4). This has been referred to as a *longitudinal spinal cord watershed region*. The largest artery usually arises in the lower thoracic or upper lumbar segments, most often between T9 and T12, but can arise as low as L2. This artery is usually referred to as the *artery of Adamkiewicz*; it usually comes from the left and supplies the lumbar enlargement of the cord. The sacral cord and cauda equina are nourished anteriorly from the hypogastric or obturator arteries.

In contrast, many more posterior radicular arteries exist, which enter along nerve roots from each side at nearly every spinal level to supply the plexus of vessels that lie on the posterior cord surface.[4] Some additional segmental arteries arise from the vertebral, aorta, and iliac arteries to supply the paraspinous structures and then end on the anterior and posterior nerve roots without supplying the spinal cord or penetrating the dura. These vessels are often the origin of spinal arteriovenous malformations (AVMs).[7]

The venous spinal cord anatomy has also been well worked out and studied.[8] Similar to the arterial supply, anterior and posterior venous drainage systems exist. Radicular veins are plentiful and drain into the paravertebral and intravertebral plexus into the pelvic veins. The posterior portions of the cord drain into a large midline posterior vein. The anterior and posterior venous system forms an extensive network, virtually encircling the spinal cord. Venous spinal cord infarction is probably more common than venous brain infarcts. This kind of infarction is most often caused by mechanical compression, infection, and inflammation, which obliterate the veins, and to vascular malformations, which cause increased venous pressure. Venous hypertension is an important contributor to spinal cord infarction in patients with spinal dural fistulas.

Spinal Cord Ischemia and Infarction

In many ways, the history of the development of ideas about spinal cord infarction parallels the evolution of knowledge about the mechanism of brain infarcts. Most of the details of the vascular anatomy of the spinal cord were worked out by Düret, Adamkiewicz, and others in the late-nineteenth century.[1,6] Early in the twentieth century, clinicians recognized that most spinal cord infarcts involved the anterior portion of the spinal cord. Clinicians attributed spinal cord infarcts to anterior spinal artery occlusion. The putative cause was intrinsic disease of this artery, especially due to syphilis, diabetes, or atherosclerosis. Recall that during this same era, intracranial anterior circulation infarcts were invariably diagnosed as middle cerebral artery occlusions. Later, it was shown that intracranial arteries were less often the seat of disease than extracranial arteries. Embolism was a more frequent explanation for intracranial arterial occlusion than in situ atherothrombosis. Similarly, it has become clear that infarction in the distribution of the anterior spinal artery is most often caused by disease of the parent artery (usually the aorta), and

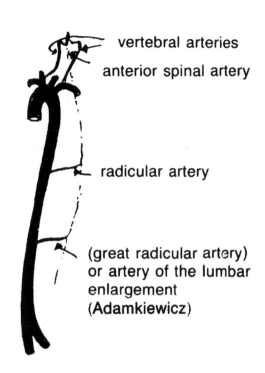

Figure 15-2. Aorta and its branches show important feeders at various levels. The cervical feeders come from the vertebral arteries. The others come from the aorta.

less often by embolism. Intrinsic disease of intraspinal arteries is much less common.

Disease of the aorta is undoubtedly the most commonly recognized cause of spinal cord infarction. Most often, paraplegia is recognized after repair of thoracic and abdominal aortic aneurysms.[5,6,9–12] During repair, flow through radicular supply arteries to the anterior spinal artery is compromised. When the thoracic cord is involved, usually a flaccid paraplegia is noted directly after surgery, with incontinence and a thoracic sensory level. Later, the lower limbs become spastic. When the lumbar cord is involved, a conus medullaris infarct develops, with hypotonia; wasting and areflexia of the legs; loss of sphincter function; and variable loss of touch and pinprick sensation in the lower limbs, perineum, and lower abdomen.

Similar findings are noted in unruptured aneurysms, dissections of the aorta, traumatic rupture of the aorta, thromboembolic aortic occlusions, and ulcerative aortic plaque disease. Thrombi and plaques can obstruct the orifices of radicular spinal arteries. Dissections can tear or interrupt the orifices of spinal cord feeding arteries, sometimes over a long area. Cholesterol crystals and other plaque materials can embolize into spinal arteries and block branches. In some patients, spinal ischemia develops gradually and insidiously. Spinal ischemia can be misdiagnosed as motor neuron disease or diabetic amyotrophy because of selective ischemia in the anterior horns and, sometimes, the pyramidal tracts.[13] In contrast to brain ischemic strokes, transient ischemic attacks are quite unusual, but do occur.[11] Often, the posterior columns are spared, and vibration sense is retained. The regions of spinal cord softening can be imaged on newer-generation MRI scanners.[5,12] Transesophageal echocardiography may show aortic plaques in patients who present with acute paraplegia.[14] Imaging signs of vertebral bone infarction may accompany spinal cord infarction caused by aortic disease.

Embolism can and does cause spinal cord infarction. I have seen several patients with bacterial endocarditis with spinal and brain embolic infarcts, and such have been reported by others.[1,11] Atrial myxoma and nonbacterial thrombotic (marantic) endocarditis are other disorders in which small particles can embolize to the spinal cord.

Since the early 1980s, pathologists and clinicians have become aware that cartilaginous material from intervertebral disks can somehow invade the spinal arteries and veins and cause devastating spinal cord strokes.[3,15] Most reported cases are cervical and involve young women. Some patients have been pregnant, puerperal, or on oral contraceptives. Minor trauma, sudden neck motion, or lifting was commonly mentioned. The first symptoms are usually pain in the neck or upper back, or radicular pain. Then, a rapidly progressive, sometimes asymmetric, spinal cord syndrome with quadriparesis develops. Syringomyelia-like dissociated sensory loss, with loss of pain and temperature (but preserved touch sensation), may be found in the upper limbs or cape region. I have not seen or read of reversal of symptoms once paralysis developed. The same syndrome can affect the lumbar spinal cord and cause conus medullaris infarction.[3] Myelography and other studies usually fail to show herniated disks with compression of the cord or nerve roots. Infarction is usually bland, but can be hemorrhagic.[3] Undoubtedly, this syndrome occurs more often than is presently diagnosed.

Infarction and inflammation of the meningeal coverings of the spinal cord can spread to the spinal arteries, causing acute spinal strokes. The phenomenon is similar to Heubner's arteritis found in the brain in the presence of tuberculosis and syphilis. These two disorders, as well as fungal infections and Lyme borreliosis, probably account for the vast majority of infectious spinal arteritis. Almost invariably, the spinal fluid provides the clue to this problem.

Chronic adhesive arachnoiditis from any cause can also lead to scarring and obliteration of spinal penetrating arteries and ischemic necrosis of the central portion of the spinal cord.[16] The clinical findings are similar to syringomyelia, except that any level of the spinal cord can be involved. Arachnoidal scarring can be caused by trauma, hemorrhage, or infection. The signs and symptoms develop gradually, sometimes years after the spinal injury, bleed, or meningitis.[16]

Spinal cord ischemia may also develop during shock or cardiac arrest. Damage is most likely to affect the thoracic spinal cord between the T4 and T8 segments, the most vulnerable region of the spinal cord.[11] Nearly always, spinal cord signs and symptoms are overshadowed by brain hypoxic-ischemic injury. The deeply comatose patient remains hypotonic and areflexic because of accompanying spinal ischemia. A pure spinal syndrome rarely complicates systemic hypoperfusion.

Venous infarction is an important cause of cord ischemia. The infarcts may remain bland[17] or become frankly hemorrhagic.[3,18] Venous infarcts can be attributed to one of three different mechanisms—spinal dural AVMs,[3,7,18-22] coagulopathies with venous thrombosis, or mechanical compression of veins by epidural mass lesions.[17,23]

Spinal Vascular Malformations

Contrary to the situation within the cranium, spinal vascular malformations often present with ischemia rather than hemorrhage, and some malformations cause bleeding and ischemia. Because of their distinctive characteristics and the fact that many neurologists and stroke experts are inexperienced with the usual findings and diagnosis in such cases, I believe it best to consider spinal vascular malformations separately rather than in relation to the topics of ischemia or hemorrhage.

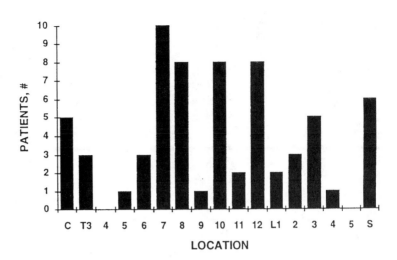

Figure 15-3. Location of spinal dural arteriovenous fistulas in 66 patients. (C = cranial; L = lumbar; S = sacral; T = thoracic.) (Reprinted with permission from JL Gilbertson, GM Miller, MS Goldman, WR Marsh. Spinal dural arteriovenous fistulas: magnetic resonance and myelographic findings. AJNR Am J Neuroradiol 1995;16:2049–2057.)

Spinal malformations should be divided into two large groups, which have differing blood supplies, presentations, and clinical findings—the dural and intradural groups.[7,24,25] So-called type I malformations, often referred to as *dural*, derive their blood supply from arteries located in the dural sleeves of spinal roots.[7,20] The small nidus of arteriovenous communication is fed by dural branches of a radicular artery. The arteriovenous fistulas drain intradurally by one or more arterialized, enlarged, usually tortuous veins, which course on the dorsal surface of the spinal cord, usually above, but occasionally below, the feeders. The dural feeding arteries do not participate in the blood supply of the spinal cord. These lesions occur predominantly in men (4 to 1 ratio) between 40 and 70 years of age, and involve mostly the lower thoracic and lumbosacral segments. In one series, 26 of 27 type I malformations were fed by arteries in the thoracic or lumbar regions, and the remaining one malformation was sacral.[25] In another series of 13 dural fistulas, eight were located between T8 and T12, two were at S1, and one each was at L1 and L5.[20] Figure 15-3[26] shows the distribution of 66 arteriovenous fistulas in one large series. Most often, one feeder exists, but, at times, two or three arterial feeders have been found.[7] Among a series of 27 such lesions, 24 had one feeder and three had two feeders.[25] Usually, this type of AVM is referred to as *low-flow* because angiography results only in slow, low-volume filling of the lesions. These lesions are not associated with arterial or venous aneurysms.[7,25] Cutaneous angiomas are not seen, and bruits are not audible.

The most frequent presentation of dural malformations is that of progressive neurologic worsening, often with acute deteriorations.[20] They usually do not cause subarachnoid bleeding, except when the lesions are cervical.[22,27] The cervical fistulas that cause subarachnoid hemorrhage (SAH) are fed by the vertebral artery and are often located near the cervico-medullary junction. Thoracic, lumbar, and sacral fistulas rarely, if ever, present with SAH, but epidural hemorrhage occasionally develops. Pain is present in approximately 40% of patients. Pain can be radicular, sometimes mimicking sciatic pain. Symptoms often worsen after exercise. One of my patients had two episodes of leg paralysis and numbness that occurred while she was driving a car.[28] Her husband had to grab the wheel and foot controls to avert a crash. Soon, strength and feeling returned. Another patient had a Brown-Séquard distribution attack while in hospital that lasted several hours.[28] Activity worsened symptoms in 19 of 27 patients (27%) in the National Institutes of Health series.[25] Signs usually progress if the lesion is untreated, and most patients become unable to walk within 5 years of the onset of weakness. These lesions probably cause symptoms because of venous hypertension and occasional thrombosis of the venous drainage system.[19–21]

Type I dural lesions are often not well seen by MRI, but increased T2 signal in the cord and spinal

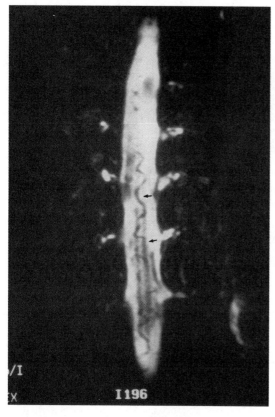

Figure 15-4. Coronal heavily T2-weighted magnetic resonance imaging scan of the thoracolumbar spine shows serpiginous vessels (*arrows*) along the dorsal surface of the spinal cord. (Reprinted with permission from J Kleefield. Magnetic Resonance and Radiologic Imaging in the Evaluation of Back Pain. In GM Aranoff [ed], Evaluation and Treatment of Chronic Pain. Baltimore: Williams & Wilkins, 1998;477–504.)

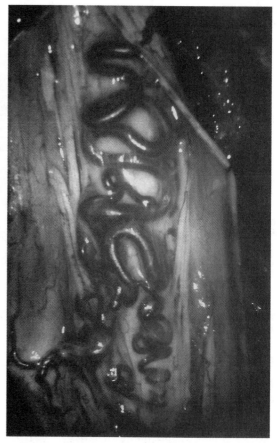

Figure 15-5. Intraoperative view of the surface of the spinal cord after the dura has been opened. Tortuous, dilatated veins can be seen along the surface of the cord. (Courtesy of Roberto Heros, M.D., University of Miami School of Medicine.)

cord edema are common.[26,29] Myelography is the key diagnostic test because coiled, enlarged serpiginous veins are usually visible along the dorsal cord surface.[24,26,29] Films should be taken with the patients lying supine on their backs to show the abnormal veins. Selective spinal angiography in expert, experienced hands often shows the feeding arteries, but sometimes the feeding arteries cannot be opacified.[26] MRI can occasionally show these serpiginous dilatated veins (Figure 15-4). Magnetic resonance angiography usually shows these abnormal veins,[30,31] and phase display after contrast injection can show the direction of flow within the epidural veins to indicate the likely location of

arterial feeders.[31] Figure 15-5 shows the appearance of these dilatated, enlarged tortuous veins at surgery. I urge surgical exploration when the clinical findings are typical and abnormal veins are clearly present on myelography or magnetic resonance angiography examinations. Ligation of arterial feeders usually prevents worsening, so the venous structures need not be removed.[7]

Some dural fistulas are located in the spine or paravertebral region, but drain into epidural veins and often into the intradural venous system.[32] The enlarged epidural veins can cause a compressive myelopathy. The venous hypertension that results from these paravertebral fistulas can cause venous hypertension and a congestive myelopathy in the same way as dural AVMs.[32] MRI may show hyperintensity on T2-weighted sequences, spinal cord edema, and prominent perimedullary vessels. Dilatated tortuous epidural veins are often visible on magnetic resonance sequences and angiography.[32]

The remainder of spinal AVMs are intradural. Type II malformations are usually intramedullary, but can be partially intramedullary, and partially between the dura and the cord. Intradural malformations are divided into various types: (1) glomus, referring to a tightly packed localized nidus of abnormal vessels within the cord; (2) juvenile, in which abnormal vessels occupy the entire spinal cord and are fed by numerous arterial feeding vessels at different levels; (3) direct arteriovenous fistulas, involving branches of arteries feeding the spinal cord; and (4) cavernous angiomas, which have no major feeding arteries and resemble cavernous angiomas of the brain. Increased availability of MRI leads frequently to identification of spinal cavernous malformations.

Usually, patients with intradural lesions are younger than those with dural lesions, but again, a strong male predominance is present. In one series, 65% of patients were younger than 25 years at first presentation.[25] These lesions have high flow, and hemorrhage is relatively common.[7,25] Intradural lesions are more widely distributed along the spinal axis and are often cervical. Spinal aneurysms, extraspinal aneurysms, other AVMs, and arterial bruits are common in patients with intradural AVMs. Most lesions are intramedullary (80% in the National Institutes of Health series)[25] and symptoms and signs are progressive.

Intradural AVMs are usually well-imaged and diagnosed by MRI. Glomus and juvenile lesions and cavernous angiomas have a nidus in the cord parenchyma. The spinal cord is usually enlarged, and multiple serpiginous signal voids are seen.[29] Increased signal on T1-weighted images may represent methemoglobin from a prior hemorrhage. Low, dark signals on T1- and T2-weighted images can represent hemosiderin.[29] Spinal angiography usually readily shows intradural AVMs. Surgical treatment is not as successful for intradural AVMs as for dural ones, but glomus lesions and cavernous angiomas can be removed.

Cavernous angiomas are shown well by MRI.[33–36] Spinal cavernous angiomas usually present during the second to sixth decades and are slightly more common in women.[35] Symptoms can begin abruptly or progress gradually.[35,36] Symptoms may worsen with pregnancy, in the puerperium, and after trauma. As in the cranium, these lesions are angiographically occult. Appearance on MRI is similar to that of brain angiomas—heterogeneous, well-circumscribed, discrete lesions. Cavernous angiomas are well circumscribed and can be removed surgically.[36] When removed surgically, cavernomas appear as well-circumscribed, dark blue-brown, intramedullary, mulberry-shaped lesions that are surrounded by gliosis and hemosiderin staining.[34]

Intradural AVMs can cause chronic arachnoiditis due to bleeding, with subsequent scarring of small cord-feeding arteries and cord ischemia. Veins can thrombose. The so-called Foix-Alajouanine syndrome,[37] a subacute necrotizing ascending myelopathy, probably was, in retrospect, caused by such thrombosed vascular malformations of the dural or intradural variety.[38]

Spinal Hemorrhages

Hematomyelia describes bleeding into the substance of the spinal cord parenchyma. The most common cause is trauma. Onset can be immediate or delayed. Usually, the area around the central canal and gray matter are involved, most often in the cervical region. Neck pain; weakness; and areflexia in the arms, associated with a cape-like distribution of pain and temperature loss, are the usual signs. Other causes include AVMs, anticoagulation, hemophilia and other bleeding disorders, and hemorrhage into spinal cord tumors, as well as (rarely) syrinxes. The spinal fluid is bloody, and MRI and myelography reveal a swollen blood-filled cord.

Spinal SAH is unusual. Unlike intracranial SAH, the most common causative lesions are AVMs. Aneurysms on spinal arteries rarely rupture.[39] Local back pain is often followed by a stiff neck and pain that radiates along a root distribution or down the back or legs. Often, headache ensues, caused by spillage of blood intracranially. Bleeding diatheses and anticoagulants may cause spinal SAH.

Spinal epidural and subdural hematomas are rarer than intracranial hemorrhages in these compartments. Epidural hematomas are approximately four times more common than subdural hematomas. Each most often occurs in patients who are on anticoagulants.[40,41] Some patients have had liver disease and portal hypertension.[40] Lumbar punctures have been known to precipitate these bleeds in patients on anticoagulants. At times, these hemorrhages begin after exertion or straining, and, in some patients, no cause is found, even after full evaluation.[40] Degenerative disk disease could be an etiologic factor.[42] The earliest symptom is pain in the back, usually in the neck. This is followed by radicular pain, usually in one or both arms. The earliest symptoms closely mimic disk herniation syndromes. Within hours, or rarely, days, sensory and motor signs develop in the legs, bowel, and bladder, and sexual dysfunction ensues. Usually, weakness and sensory loss are symmetric, but a Brown-Séquard distribution may be found.[40,43]

Diagnosis of spinal epidural or subdural hematoma has usually been made by myelography. A block is most often found. Computed tomography and MRI show the blood. MRI is superior in defining the location and extent of hematomas. Signs are almost invariably progressive, unless the lesions are decompressed. Anticoagulation should be reversed, using vitamin K or fresh frozen plasma. Decompression is urgent and should be pursued as soon as the prothrombin time reaches approximately 40–50% of the control values.[40] Outcome depends on the severity of the deficit before surgery, the duration of spinal cord compression, and the rapidity of onset of the paraplegia. Chronic spinal subdural hematomas or hygromas are rare and are usually related to prior trauma or small bleeds.[44]

References

1. Buchan AM, Barnett HJM. Infarction of the Spinal Cord. In HJM Barnett, JP Mohr, B Stern, F Yatsu (eds), Stroke: Pathophysiology, Diagnosis and Management. New York: Churchill Livingstone, 1986;707–719.
2. Vinters HV, Gilbert JJ. Hypoxic myelopathy. Can J Neurol Sci 1979;6:380.
3. Caplan LR. Case records of the Massachusetts General Hospital: Case 5–1991. N Engl J Med 1991;324:322–332.
4. Gillilan L. The arterial blood supply of the human spinal cord. J Comp Neurol 1958;110:75–103.
5. Mawad ME, Rivera V, Crawford S, et al. Spinal cord ischemia after resection of thoracoabdominal aortic aneurysms: MR findings in 24 patients. AJNR Am J Neuroradiol 1990;11:987–991.
6. Hogan EL, Romanul FCA. Spinal cord infarction occurring during insertion of aortic graft. Neurology 1966;16:67–74.
7. Heros R. Arteriovenous Malformations of the Spinal Cord. In RG Ojemann, RC Heros, RM Crowell (eds), Surgical Management of Cerebrovascular Disease (2nd ed). Baltimore: Williams & Wilkins, 1988;451–466.
8. Gillilan L. Veins of the spinal cord: anatomic details—suggested clinical applications. Neurology 1970;20:860–868.
9. Dodson WE, Landau W. Motor neuron loss due to aortic clamping in repair of coarctation. Neurology 1973;23:539–542.
10. Ross RT. Spinal cord infarction in diseases and surgery of the aorta. Can J Neurol Sci 1985;12:289–295.
11. Cheshire WP, Santos CC, Massey EW, Howard JF Jr. Spinal cord infarction: etiology and outcome. Neurology 1996;47:321–330.
12. Mawad ME, Rivera V, Crawford S, et al. Spinal cord ischemia after resection of thoracoabdominal aortic aneurysms: MR findings in 24 patients. AJNR Am J Neuroradiol 1990;11:987–991.
13. Herrick MK, Mills PE. Infarction of spinal cord: two cases of selective grey matter involvement secondary to asymptomatic aortic disease. Arch Neurol 1971;24:228–241.
14. Walsh DV, Uppal JA, Karalis DG, Chandrasekaran K. The role of transesophageal echocardiography in the acute onset of paraplegia. Stroke 1992;23:1660–1661.
15. Srigley JR, Lambert CD, Bilbao JM, Pritzker KP. Spinal cord infarction secondary to intervertebral disc embolism. Ann Neurol 1981;9:296–301.
16. Caplan LR, Noronha A, Amico L. Syringomyelia and arachnoiditis. J Neurol Neurosurg Psychiatry 1990;53:106–113.
17. Kim RC, Smith HR, Henbest ML, Choi BH. Nonhemorrhagic venous infarction of the spinal cord. Ann Neurol 1984;15:379–385.
18. Hughes JT. Venous infarction of the spinal cord. Neurology 1971;21:794–800.
19. Larsson EM, Desai P, Hardin CW, et al. Venous infarction of the spinal cord resulting from dural arteriovenous fistula: MR imaging findings. AJNR Am J Neuroradiol 1991;12:739–743.
20. Bradac GB, Daniele D, Riva A, et al. Spinal dural arteriovenous fistulas: an underestimated cause of myelopathy. Eur Neurol 1993;34:87–94.
21. Hurst RW, Kenyon LC, Lavi E, Raps EC, Marcotte P. Spinal dural arteriovenous fistula: the pathology of venous hypertensive myelopathy. Neurology 1995;45:1309–1313.
22. Hemphill JC III, Smith WS, Halbach VV. Neurologic manifestations of spinal epidural arteriovenous malformations. Neurology 1998;50:817–819.
23. Roa KR, Donnenfeld H, Chusid JG, Valdez S. Acute myelopathy secondary to spinal venous thrombosis. J Neurol Sci 1982;56:107–113.
24. DeChiro G, Doppman JL, Ommaya AK. Radiology of spinal cord arteriovenous malformations. Prog Neurol Surg 1971;4:329–354.

25. Rosenblum B, Oldfield EH, Doppman JL, DiChiro G. Spinal arteriovenous malformations: a comparison of dural arteriovenous fistulas and intradural AVMs in 81 patients. J Neurosurg 1987;67:795–802.

26. Gilbertson JR, Miller GM, Goldman MS, Marsh WR. Spinal dural arteriovenous fistulas: MR and myelographic findings. AJNR Am J Neuroradiol 1995; 16:2049–2057.

27. Do HM, Jensen ME, Cloft HJ, et al. Dural arteriovenous fistula of the cervical spine presenting with subarachnoid hemorrhage. AJNR Am J Neuroradiol 1999;20:348–350.

28. Teal PA, Wityk RJ, Rosengart A, Caplan LR. Spinal TIAs—a clue to the presence of spinal dural AVMs. Neurology 1992;42(Suppl 3):341.

29. Greenberg J. Neuroimaging of the spinal cord. Neurol Clin 1991;9:696–698.

30. Bowen BC, Fraser K, Kochan JP, et al. Spinal dural arteriovenous fistulas: evaluation with MR angiography. AJNR Am J Neuroradiol 1995;16:2029–2043.

31. Mascalchi M, Quillici N, Ferrito G, et al. Identification of the feeding arteries of spinal vascular lesions via phase-contrast MR angiography with three-dimensional acquisition and phase display. AJNR Am J Neuroradiol 1997;18: 351–358.

32. Goyal M, Willinsky R, Montanera W, terBrugge K. Paravertebral arteriovenous malformations with epidural drainage: clinical spectrum, imaging features, and results of treatment. AJNR Am J Neuroradiol 1999;20:749–755.

33. Lopate G, Black JT, Grubb RL. Cavernous hemangioma of the spinal cord: report of two unusual cases. Neurology 1990;40:1791–1793.

34. Cosgrove GR, Bertrand G, Fontaine S, et al. Cavernous angiomas of the spinal cord. J Neurosurg 1988;68:31–36.

35. McCormick PC, Michelson WJ, Post KD, et al. Cavernous malformations of the spinal cord. Neurosurgery 1988; 23:459–463.

36. Ogilvy CS, Louis DN, Ojemann RG. Intramedullary cavernous angiomas of the spinal cord: clinical presentation, pathological features, and surgical management. Neurosurgery 1992;31:219–230.

37. Foix C, Alajouanime T. La myelite necrotique subaique. Rev Neurol 1926;2:1–42.

38. Criscuolo GR, Oldfield EH, Doppman JL. Reversible acute and subacute myelopathy in patients with dural arteriovenous fistulas. J Neurosurg 1989;70:354–359.

39. Garcia C, Dulcey S, Dulcey J. Ruptured aneurysm of the spinal artery of Adamkiewicz during pregnancy. Neurology 1979;29:394–398.

40. Mattle H, Sieb JP, Rohner M, Mumenthaler M. Nontraumatic spinal epidural and subdural hematomas. Neurology 1987;37:1351–1356.

41. Post MJD, Becerra JL, Madsen PW, et al. Acute spinal subdural hematoma: MR and CT findings with pathological correlates. AJNR Am J Neuroradiol 1994;15:1895-1905.

42. Gundry CR, Heithoff KB. Epidural hematoma of the lumbar spine: 18 surgically confirmed cases. Radiology 1993; 187:427–431.

43. Russman BS, Kazi K. Spinal epidural hematoma and the Brown-Séquard syndrome. Neurology 1971;21:1066–1068.

44. Black P, Zervas N, Caplan LR, Ramirez L. Subdural hygroma of the spinal meninges: a case report. Neurosurgery 1978;2:52–54.

Chapter 16
Strokes, Cerebrovascular Disease, and Surgery

Surgery is being performed in patients who are increasingly older and sicker than patients in the past. Surgical considerations play an increasingly frequent role in the thoughts and activities of neurologists and other clinicians who care for individuals with cerebrovascular disease. Often, neurologists and other physicians consider surgery on their own patients or in a patient seen in consultation. Clinicians are also often asked to see patients in whom a stroke or other neurologic complication has developed after surgery. Surgeons and physicians must become fully knowledgeable about the indications, nature, and complications of surgical procedures. In this chapter, I selectively review the most common surgical situations that confront clinicians—coronary artery and other cardiac surgery, and carotid endarterectomy (CEN) and other extracranial vascular surgery. I also briefly discuss some causes of stroke after general surgery.

Carotid Endarterectomy

Carotid artery surgery is one of the most commonly performed procedures in the United States. The frequency of CEN varies dramatically in countries throughout the world. The United States has the highest per capita rate of CENs in the world. The difference in the rates between the United States and elsewhere has fueled controversy about the explanation. Are the rates of carotid artery surgery in the United States too high? Are the rates elsewhere too low? Or are both of these postulates true—that is, are too many surgeries performed by some and too few by others? Chapters 5 and 6 include discussions

of CEN and carotid artery angioplasty. I do not review in any detail the results of the CEN trials, but instead discuss only selected aspects.

Indications

Reports of the North American[1,2] and European[3,4] CEN trials showed that patients with symptoms, such as transient ischemic attacks (TIAs) or small strokes related to severe carotid artery stenosis (>70% luminal narrowing), clearly benefit from CEN when surgery is performed by selected surgeons with excellent low rates of complications. For the benefit to risk ratio to favor CEN, the operative morbidity and mortality should not exceed 2% mortality and 5–6% morbidity.[1–8] The benefit for surgery in patients with 50–70% stenosis (as measured by the North American Symptomatic Carotid Endarectomy Trial method) is modest and depends more on the surgical morbidity and mortality record of the surgeon and hospital where the surgery will be performed.[2] When brain infarcts are large and cause a severe neurologic deficit, not much further at-risk ischemic tissue exists and little can be gained by reperfusion. Also, complication rates are high. The European Carotid Surgery Trial showed that patients with minor degrees of carotid stenosis (<30% luminal narrowing) do not benefit from CEN.[3,4]

Reports of four carotid surgery trials for asymptomatic carotid artery stenosis have been published,[9–12] and fifth and sixth trials are nearing completion in Europe.[13,14] The results of the completed trials have been widely reviewed. The merits of surgery on asymptomatic patients have been extensively discussed and hotly debated.[5,7,15–17] The largest trial, the Asymptomatic Carotid Atherosclerosis Study, enrolled 1,602 patients.[9] This study showed that the addition of carotid surgery to medical management (325 mg of aspirin each day and risk factor reduction) was better than medical treatment alone in preventing stroke among patients with asymptomatic carotid artery stenosis of 60% or more.[9,15] The follow-up period in the Asymptomatic Carotid Atherosclerosis Study was projected at 5 years, but an independent monitoring board stopped the study prematurely after a median follow-up of 2.7 years when the results became statistically significant. The surgical combined mortality and morbidity rate (2.3%) was low; approximately one-half of the complications were attributable to angiography. The 5-year calculated stroke rate was 11% for the medically treated group versus 5.1% for the surgical group.[9] The benefit for women was less than that for men. The benefit was modest in comparison with the results of the symptomatic carotid surgery studies. In the Asymptomatic Carotid Atherosclerosis Study, patients with serious coronary artery disease were excluded. Many patients with severe carotid artery disease, however, also have significant coronary artery disease and myocardial ischemia.

The randomized trials of symptomatic and asymptomatic individuals considered and stratified patients by severity of carotid artery stenosis. Some have also advocated surgery on patients with ulcerated lesions, even when stenosis is minor. In fact, most ulcers are found in severely stenotic arteries, so ulceration and stenosis usually coexist. Ulcers do occur in nonstenotic arteries, but not often. I am not convinced that ulcers found on angiography should be an important factor favoring surgery. Recognition of ulcers is difficult, and the accuracy of the radiologic diagnosis is low. As plaques grow and encroach further on the lumen, plaque complications, including ulceration and mural thrombi, become more frequent. Examination of CEN specimens from tightly stenotic arteries shows a high incidence of these atherosclerotic plaque complications.[18] The natural history of ulcers in nonstenosing plaques is unknown; they may heal well. Agents that alter platelet function, such as aspirin, might be effective in preventing white platelet-fibrin clots from embolizing from these plaques. I use patient's symptoms and the severity of luminal

narrowing as the major factors when deciding on CEN. A residual lumen smaller than 2 mm favors surgery in symptomatic patients. I would only suggest CEN for ulceration in a nonstenotic artery if all medical therapy had failed, a circumstance I have not personally encountered.

At times, large thrombi are found within the internal carotid artery (ICA).[19,20] These may be attached to plaques or found without plaques and may be the result of a hypercoagulable state. Anticoagulants and surgery have been used to treat these thrombi, but I favor anticoagulants after evaluation of coagulation functions. Thrombi within a stenotic artery increase the risk of stroke during carotid surgery.

Decisions on Surgery

The patient's preferences should be given considerable weight when deciding on surgery.[21] Each individual lives in a unique socioeconomic-psychological environment. Given the same information, different patients make different decisions. Some patients find the diagnosis of a severe carotid artery lesion difficult to live with. Told that they have an imminent, permanent risk of a disabling stroke, these patients perceive the sword continually hovering over them. This leads to great stress and altered behavior. Some individuals gamble risk for removal of the sword. They choose the knife (CEN) over the sword (stroke related to the stenotic artery). Others do not find the news untenable. These patients are aware of the risks associated with this illness. They do not let the knowledge of their carotid artery disease interfere with their lives. These patients are content to pursue medical therapy and clinical monitoring. These individuals would not gamble the risk of a surgical stroke complication if the risk is avoidable. Furthermore, if these patients had a stroke during surgery, it would immediately affect them, whereas the risk of stroke without surgery is spaced over the years ahead. I believe that patients should be provided with information regarding the pros and cons of each alternative, including angioplasty. Doctors should convey their own advice and opinion, but ultimately, the patient has the right and responsibility to choose.

When considering the decision regarding CEN, I weigh the benefit of surgery (potential prevention of stroke) versus the risk of surgery in the individual patient. The benefit depends on the risk of stroke without surgery, which relies on the presence or absence of symptoms and the severity of stenosis. In deciding on the risks of surgery, I follow the schema proposed by Sundt, with some modifications[21,22] (Table 16-1). Risks for CEN include neurologic, vascular-specific, and cardiac factors and other comorbidity. The degree of neurologic stroke deficit and the presence of neurologic deficits, such as dementia, are clearly important considerations. Vascular risk factors include the length of the stenotic lesion, presence of tandem intracranial disease in the ICA siphon and middle cerebral artery (MCA), involvement of the common carotid artery and the external carotid artery, and location of the carotid artery bifurcation (a high bifurcation increases the technical difficulty of the vascular surgery). Myocardial infarction (MI) is the most important and severe nonneurologic complication of CEN; the presence of coronary artery disease is also of great importance and is discussed in more depth subsequently. Other diseases, such as pulmonary disease and cancer, clearly affect surgical risk and other treatment decisions.

Indications and contraindications for alternative, nonsurgical treatment of carotid artery disease should be considered. Intolerance to aspirin and other antiplatelet aggregants, bleeding disorders, and active peptic ulcers make aspirin and warfarin unattractive therapeutic alternatives. Angioplasty is also an alternative treatment. Trials of angioplasty versus surgery in comparable patients have begun.

The surgeon, hospital, and surgical team are also important. Studies in Springfield, Illinois,[23] Cincinnati, Ohio,[24] and New York State[25] show dramatic variability in complication rates among hospitals, even among surgeons in the same hospital. In New York, the in-hospital mortality rates for CENs performed by surgeons who conduct less than five carotid surgeries a year, and for hospitals in which less than 100 CENs are performed annually, are significantly higher than those for surgeons and hospitals that have higher surgical volumes.[25] To establish the benefit to risk ratio of CEN for a given individual, the morbidity and mortality results of the surgeon who performs the CEN, and the hospital where the surgery is planned are critical information. When these morbidity and

Table 16-1. Risks of Carotid Endarterectomies

Neurologic risks
    Progressive course
    Recent stroke
Vascular anatomy risks
    High bifurcation
    Long lesion (>3 cm distally in internal carotid artery or 5 cm into common carotid artery)
    Clot
    Contralateral internal carotid artery stenosis or occlusion
    Intracranial stenosis or occlusion
Medical risks
    Hypertension
    Coronary artery disease
    Diabetes
    Obesity
    Smoking
    Chronic obstructive pulmonary disease
    Congestive heart failure

Source: Modified from TM Sundt, BA Sandok, JP Whisnant. Carotid endarterectomy complications and preoperative assessment of risk. Mayo Clin Proc 1975;50:301–306.

mortality rates are high and surgery is clearly indicated, the patient should be referred to a surgeon and hospital with better CEN results. The patient deserves the best surgical care, even if that care is at another hospital or locale and even if the insurance carrier opposes the referral.

Complications

Major complications of CEN are death, ischemic stroke, MI, brain edema, and intracerebral hemorrhage. The most frequently fatal complications are medical, especially perioperative MI. Callow reviewed CEN complications at the New England Medical Center during 1958–1967 and 1968–1979.[26] During the first decade, the operative morbidity (3.4%) was nearly all accounted for by stroke, but during the second decade, all mortality was caused by MI.[26] Patient selection and improved technique explain the difference. Postoperative MI is especially common when an MI has occurred within the preceding 3 months and when the operative procedure is performed under general anesthesia. One series showed a 27% rate of perioperative MI, all fatal, in such patients.[27] Cardiac evaluation is mandatory in any patient who undergoes CEN and has cardiac symptoms. Recent MI, unstable angina, gallop rhythm, and heart failure are high-risk factors.[28] Serious noncardiac medical complications of CENs are unusual, except for pulmonary embolism. Most relate to pre-existing disorders, such as obstructive uropathy, chronic lung disease, and so forth.

Perioperative and postoperative strokes are a major cause of morbidity and a great worry for all concerned. Many episodes of ischemia are transient and may occur after the immediate postoperative period. Among a total of 358 CENs performed in a number of centers in Toronto, Canada, 18 patients had postoperative TIAs, 14 had brain infarcts, and two fatal brain hemorrhages occurred.[29] Nine of the ischemic strokes and both hemorrhages occurred after the immediate postoperative period. Steed and colleagues timed the onset of neurologic deficits in patients they operated on under local anesthesia.[30] Among 345 CENs, three TIAs occurred during ICA dissection, one stroke during carotid clamping, and two strokes on release of the clamp; five patients had TIAs immediately after surgery, and 10 patients had delayed onset of ischemia.[30] The mechanisms of perioperative ischemia include reocclusion of the ICA; embolization of plaque, clot, or fibrin during or after the surgery; and hemodynamic decrease in flow during surgery or perioperative hypotension. Most ischemic events are caused by artery-to-artery emboli. The frequency of reocclusion immediately after surgery and shortly thereafter varies, but is probably between 5% and 10%.[6,31]

Suddenly opening up the ICA into a chronically underperfused region can cause a so-called hyperperfusion syndrome,[32,33] characterized by headache and severe, migraine-like neurologic accompaniments,[33,34] seizures, and brain edema. Brain edema and brain hemorrhage are the most serious components of the hyperperfusion syndrome after CEN. Careful monitoring of blood pressure after CEN shows that many patients become hypertensive, probably because of surgical injury to the baroreceptors in the carotid sinus.[33,35,36] This risk is higher in patients who have been hypertensive in the past. Severe hypertension can lead to brain hemorrhage, either into an area of infarction or at sites common for hypertensive intracerebral hemorrhage. If the patient has neurologic signs and computed tomography (CT) or magnetic resonance imaging (MRI) shows infarction, it is probably wise to delay CEN for 4–6 weeks. All patients must have careful monitoring of blood pressure in the days after CEN. I have seen an intracerebral hemorrhage develop as long as 3 days after CEN.[37] Brain edema is another serious complication and may develop 4–7 days after surgery, usually preceded by increased blood pressure, headache, focal neurologic signs, and seizures.[33] Hypertension and diminished autoregulatory function after a prolonged period of hypoperfusion explain the hyperperfusion syndrome. Because the syndrome can develop between 4 and 7 days after surgery, and most often after hospital discharge, blood pressure should be carefully monitored at home during the week after CEN. Transcranial Doppler (TCD) measurements of MCA flow-velocities can be helpful after CEN when predicting the occurrence of the hyperperfusion syndrome.[33]

Other complications are usually less serious and are reversible. They include wound hematomas, continued wound bleeding, and wound infection. Retraction on cranial and cervical nerves and their branches, and the cutting of cranial nerves and cutaneous branches can lead to focal regions of numbness or weakness. Complications are listed in Table 16-2.

Overall, morbidity and mortality figures are so variable that a standard average rate is hard to choose. As I have noted, the results of the surgeon who will perform the procedure are most important to the patient undergoing CEN. The two largest and most representative series are those of the Toronto Cerebrovascular Surgeons[29] study previously cited, and a retrospective review audit undertaken by a neurosurgical society[38] (Table 16-3).

Combined Carotid and Coronary Artery Disease

Atherosclerosis is a systemic disease that hits hardest at the aorta, coronary arteries, extracranial brain arteries, and large arteries to the limbs. Severe coronary artery and cerebrovascular disease frequently coexist. Asymptomatic neck bruits are found in approximately 10% of preoperative coronary bypass patients. Approximately one-half of the patients with bruits have significant carotid artery stenosis by ultrasound testing.[39] An arteriographic study of 100 coronary artery bypass graft

Table 16-2. Types of Carotid Endarterectomy Complications

Serious
- Death, usually cardiac
- Myocardial infarction
- Perioperative ischemic stroke
- Postoperative intracerebral hemorrhage
- Postoperative brain edema
- Pulmonary embolism

Usually Minor
- Hypertension
- Wound hematoma
- Wound infection
- Numbness in local region of jaw or neck ipsilaterally
- Facial (VII), hypoglossal (XII), and superior laryngeal branch of vagus (X) nerve palsies

Source: Reprinted with permission from European Carotid Surgery Trialists' Collaborative Group. Randomized trial of endarterectomy for recently symptomatic carotid stenosis: final results of the MRC European Carotid Surgery Trial (ECST). Lancet 1998;351:1379–1387.

Table 16-3. Cardiac and Cerebrovascular Complications of Carotid Endarterectomy—Two Large Series

Complication	Fode et al.[22, a]	Toronto[14, b]
Cerebrovascular		
Transient ischemic attacks	82 (12.5%)	18 (5.4%)
Strokes	140 (4.2%)	16 (4.8%)
Minor	44 (1.3%)	—
Major	96 (2.8%)	—
Stroke deaths	40 (1.2%)	3 (0.8%)
Cardiac: myocardial infarctions	—	8 (seven myocardial infarctions and one cardiac arrest)
Deaths		
Total	66 (2%)	5 (1.5%)
Myocardial infarction deaths	26 (0.8%)	1 (0.3%)
Stroke deaths	40 (1.2%)	3 (0.9%)

[a]Total of 3,328 patients at 44 institutions.
[b]Total of 333 patients.

(CABG) patients with neck bruits, of whom one-third had some cerebrovascular symptoms, showed that one-half had carotid stenosis.[40,41] Evaluation of patients with carotid artery disease shows a high incidence of concurrent symptomatic and asymptomatic coronary artery disease. Rokey and colleagues found significant coronary artery disease in 29 of 50 patients (58%) who presented with TIAs or stroke.[42,43] In a coronary angiography study, Hertzer et al. found that 35% of all patients with symptomatic carotid artery disease or asymptomatic bruits had severe coronary artery disease.[44]

I find that the data persuasively show that patients undergoing CEN should be evaluated for coexistent coronary artery disease. As has been discussed in relation to complications of CEN, both MI and cardiac death are frequent and important sequelae of CEN. Riles et al. studied the MI rate in 683 consecutive CEN procedures, among whom 203 patients had pre-existing coronary artery disease.[45] Among patients with coronary artery disease, 14 had MIs, five of which were fatal, whereas among the 288 patients without coronary artery disease, only two had MIs, and no deaths occurred.[45] Similar results were found by Hertzer and Lees, who reported on 335 CEN patients treated at the Cleveland Clinic.[46] Five of 217 patients with coronary artery disease had an MI within 30 days of CEN, all of which were fatal, compared with only one fatal MI among those without historical or electrocardiogram evidence of coronary artery disease.[46]

Noninvasive testing for the presence of coronary artery disease is effective. A careful history, looking especially for past MI and angina, is mandatory. Electrocardiogram, echocardiography, myocardial perfusion imaging, and exercise electrocardiogram are useful in predicting the presence and severity of coronary artery disease.[43,47] Particularly helpful is thallium-201-dipyridamole radionuclide scanning, which has a high sensitivity and specificity for the diagnosis of coronary artery disease.[47–49] Some patients with angina and positive findings from noninvasive testing need coronary angiography to define the location and severity of the coronary artery disease. The presence of active coronary artery disease or unstable angina clearly presents a prohibitive risk if untreated. Patients with unstable angina who do not respond to medical therapy or have evidence of silent ischemia have a reduced 1-year survival rate. Coronary artery disease needs medical or surgical management before, during, or after treatment of the carotid artery lesion.[50]

Physicians have long deliberated on the best way to manage patients with combined severe coronary artery and cerebrovascular disease. They worry that if CEN is performed first, the risk of MI and death from coronary disease will be high. If, on the other hand, CABG is performed first, physicians worry about the risk of stroke. I have already indicated that the risk of MI and death has been shown unequivocally to be high in patients with active coronary artery disease.[43,51,52] Studies show that the risk of stroke during CABG is high in those patients who have had past strokes and symptomatic carotid artery disease, but is rather low in patients with asymptomatic carotid artery disease.[41,43] Angioplasty of the carotid or coronary arteries, or both, is an alternative that could be performed before coronary or carotid surgery.

Ropper and colleagues showed that bruits did not predict stroke complication risk after a variety of elective surgical operations.[53] Neck bruits were found in 104 of 735 patients (14%) preoperatively. One patient with a history of transient monocular blindness had a stroke within 3 days of CABG. Among 631 patients without bruits, four had strokes during the perioperative period. No difference in the incidence of stroke in patients with and without bruits existed.[53] Breslau et al. used duplex scanning in 102 patients undergoing CABG.[54] Eighteen had more than 50% carotid artery stenosis. None of these patients had perioperative strokes, whereas 2 of 84 patients (2.4%) without stenosis had strokes.[43,54] Turnipseed and colleagues studied 330 CABG patients.[55] Severe carotid artery stenosis or occlusion was found in 103 patients by TCD using spectral analysis of flow. The stroke rate after CABG in patients with severe carotid artery disease and those without was an identical 5%.

Some studies show that the stroke rate after CABG is related to the severity of carotid artery stenosis as determined by angiography.[56] In a retrospective study in which angiography had been performed before CABG, Furlan et al. identified 155 stenotic carotid arteries (>50% stenosis) among 144 patients. Stroke ipsilateral to a stenotic carotid artery developed in 1 of 90 patients (1%) with 50–90% stenosis, 1 of 16 (6%) with 90–99% stenosis, and in 1 of 49 (2%) with

carotid artery occlusion.[57] Schwartz and colleagues found that none of the 52 patients with unilateral 50–79% carotid artery stenosis had a stroke after CABG, but 4 of 75 patients (5.3%) with unilateral 80–99% stenosis, bilateral 50–99% stenosis, or unilateral occlusion with contralateral greater than 50% stenosis had strokes.[58] In a prospective study of 1,631 consecutive CABG patients, the risk of stroke was 0% in patients without carotid stenosis, 3.2% in patients with greater than 70% stenosis, and 27% in patients with carotid artery occlusion.[59]

The initial strategy in dealing with patients with combined coronary and carotid artery disease was to perform the two procedures, CEN and CABG, together under the same anesthetic. The perioperative stroke, MI, and mortality figures proved high, much higher than with either procedure alone. Pettigrew tabulated 22 reports that described the results of staged or simultaneous cardiac and carotid surgery procedures among a total of 1,076 patients.[43] Perioperative complications included 34 MIs (3.2%), 57 TIAs or strokes (5.3%), and 47 deaths (4.4%).[43]

Considering the foregoing data, I advise a treatment paradigm similar to that of Hertzer and his Cleveland Clinic colleagues.[60] Their recommendations are summarized in Table 16-4.

What if the Patient Has Severe Coronary Artery Disease and Asymptomatic Carotid Artery Stenosis?

If the patient has severe coronary artery disease and asymptomatic carotid artery stenosis, CABG or coronary angioplasty, if indicated, is warranted. The patient could then be subsequently evaluated for possible CEN. Fisher said, "If the patient[s] can stand up, they can lie down." By this, Fisher meant that if patients can perform daily living activities in an upright posture, they can safely lie down for surgery. The data bear this out.[41,43,56]

What if the Patient Has Severe Symptomatic Carotid Artery Disease and the Coronary Disease Is Stable or Inactive?

I favor CEN when patients have severe symptomatic carotid artery disease, without concurrent CABG. The choice of medical therapy, coronary angioplasty, or a later CABG would be left to a cardiologist.

What if the Patient Has Both Active Symptomatic Coronary and Carotid Artery Disease?

Patients with both active symptomatic coronary and carotid artery disease have unstable angina or silent myocardial ischemia, and TIAs or recent strokes in the territory of the narrowed carotid artery. In this circumstance, I advise combined CABG and CEN under the same anesthetic; the risk of either procedure alone or of the staged procedures is high. Angioplasty on the coronary or carotid arteries seems to be a reasonable alternative before carotid or coronary artery surgery in this situation.

Vertebral Artery Surgery

The number of posterior circulation surgical reconstructions is minimal when compared with the number of anterior circulation procedures. Yet, surgery for posterior circulation occlusive disease has been performed by selected surgeons with good results and low complication rates.[61–70] The most common procedures involve the vertebral artery (VA) origin region, including the parent subclavian artery.[61–65] Bypass intracranial procedures, [66–68] and even endarterectomy of the intracranial vertebral artery (ICVA)[69,70] have been performed. In sharp contrast to the situation in the anterior circulation, in which both CEN[1–5] and extracranial/intracranial bypass[71] have been studied in formal trials, no trials or controlled data apply to the posterior circulation, and as far as I know, none is on the drawing board or planned.

Subclavian Artery Surgery for Subclavian Steal

Studies have shown that subclavian steal is generally a benign syndrome, with a low frequency of stroke.[72,73] A high incidence of concurrent carotid artery disease is present. Surgery on the subclavian artery is complex and often requires a thoracotomy for repair. The morbidity is higher than neck surgery. Subclavian artery angioplasty has been performed, but the benefit to risk ratio of angioplasty and VA surgery have not been studied in comparable patients. In my opinion, only two circumstances warrant consideration for subclavian surgery: (1) when disabling arm ischemia is

Table 16-4. Recommendations for Combined Carotid and Coronary Disease

Carotid Disease	Coronary Disease	Recommendation
Active,[a] severe	Inactive	Carotid endarterectomy
Inactive	Active,[b] severe	Coronary artery bypass graft
Active, severe	Active, severe	Coronary artery bypass graft and carotid endarterectomy combined

[a]Active carotid disease: ipsilateral hemispheral or retinal transient ischemic attacks or recent stroke and severe internal carotid artery stenosis (<2 mm residual lumen or 75% stenosis).
[b]Active coronary disease: unstable angina, silent ischemia, or a recent myocardial infarction with severe surgically operable disease by coronary angiography.

present (e.g., athletes, especially baseball pitchers and golfers, are susceptible to the development of subclavian artery disease, and arm ischemia may limit their performance),[73–75] and (2) when the occlusive disease involves the right side—the innominate or right subclavian artery. Subclavian clots may extend proximally and embolize into the right carotid artery territory, causing right-hemisphere strokes.[73,75,76] As in the carotid artery, surgery should be considered in those circumstances only if the stenosis is severe.

Vertebral Artery Origin Disease

Although surgery on the extracranial vertebral artery (ECVA) origin region can be done safely, the indications are unclear. Most surgeons do not do an endarterectomy, but perform some type of shunting procedure into the carotid system. At times, the local VA bypass is accompanied by a CEN on the same side. After the stenotic ICA is repaired, the VA is divided, the proximal end is tied, and the distal end is anastomosed to the ICA.[61–65] Atherostenosis of the ECVA origin seldom causes persistent hemodynamic symptoms because even in the event of occlusion, excellent collateral circulation develops from the thyrocervical trunk and external carotid artery branches.

Even bilateral ECVA-origin disease is usually well tolerated.[73,77] When one VA is stenosed or occluded intracranially, however, stenosis of the opposite ECVA can be problematic, especially if some ipsilateral tandem intracranial disease is present. The ECVA can also serve as the nidus for embolism into the posterior circulation.[73,78] Possible indications for ECVA-origin surgery are embolism from the ECVA origin; persistent hemodynamic insufficiency, especially when contralateral intracranial VA disease is present; and at the time of CEN, when the ICA and ECVA on the same side are tightly stenotic. VA angioplasty is an alternative consideration, although the morbidity and complication rate of this procedure have not been thoroughly studied.

Intracranial Posterior Circulation Bypass Surgery

Shunts within the posterior circulation most often involve anastomoses between the occipital artery branch of the external carotid artery and the posterior inferior cerebellar artery, or one of its branches.[66–68] Less often, the occipital artery is grafted to the anterior inferior cerebellar artery. The superficial temporal artery can also be used as a donor, with the superior cerebellar artery or posterior cerebellar artery as recipients. Nearly always, the indication for surgery has been persistent ischemic attacks, despite medical therapy. The advent of angioplasty on the ICVAs makes it possible in patients with severe ICVA stenosis on one side and severe ICVA stenosis or occlusion on the contralateral side to augment flow to the lower brain stem by angioplasty of one of the stenotic ICVAs. Basilar artery angioplasty has also been performed, but carries a higher risk of compromise of penetrating artery branches to the pons. When the basilar artery is occluded, usually collaterals from the ICA–posterior communicating arteries provide natural collaterals to the distal basilar artery. The perforating arteries at the level of occlusion are not fed, but a bypass does not help this situation either. The remaining single indication for posterior circulation bypass is bilateral ICVA occlusions with persistent major symptoms, despite optimal medical therapy.

Cardiac Surgery

I have discussed the indications for CABG in patients with cerebrovascular disease earlier in this chapter. All too often, neurologists are called on to see patients after open heart surgery, so they must be familiar with the common complications.

The reported incidence of neurologic abnormalities during the postoperative period varies from 7% to 61% for transient, and from 1.6% to 23% for permanent complications.[79–81] The complication rate is much higher in prospective series, in which patients are routinely examined postoperatively, rather than in retrospective reviews of charts. In one study among 312 patients, transient complications were noted in fully 61% of patients.[81] At the Cleveland Clinic among a series of 421 CABG patients, 16.8% had prolonged encephalopathy or stroke.[82] Complications can be readily divided into four groups: (1) encephalopathy, (2) stroke, (3) cognitive dysfunction, and (4) peripheral nervous system complications.

Encephalopathy

A wide spectrum of neuropsychiatric findings, including delirium, confusion, disorientation, drowsiness, and altered behavior without focal neurologic abnormalities, are often bundled together under the broad term encephalopathy. Imaging tests do not show new large focal brain infarcts. In the Cleveland Clinic series of CABG operations, 11.6% of patients were considered encephalopathic on the fourth postoperative day.[82] In another large series, 57 of 1,669 CABG patients (3.4%) had severe postoperative mental changes, including delirium and encephalopathy.[83] Undoubtedly, the causes are multiple. Encephalopathy is especially common among older patients and those with a history of alcohol abuse and renal disease. Some patients have a hypoxic-ischemic encephalopathy caused by prolonged time on the pump, during which their brain was poorly perfused. An important number of cases are explained by medications. Sedatives; analgesics, especially narcotics; and, most important, haloperidol are common offenders. Haloperidol often produces depressed alertness, stiffness, inertia, and drowsiness, and the drug stays in the body a long time. Haloperidol has been shown to retard recovery in animals with brain lesions.[84,85] In my opinion, this drug should not be used in older surgical and medical patients, especially those with abnormal brains.

The initial recognition that the neurobehavioral changes were not psychiatric in origin was made by Gilman in 1965, when he prospectively followed a series of open heart surgery patients.[86] Early research drew the conclusion that embolization of particulate matter related to the pump and its filters leads to encephalopathy.[56,87] The introduction of membrane, rather than bubble, oxygenators and in-line filtration led to a decrease in the risk of macroembolic particles larger than 25 μm, reaching the systemic circulation.[87] A 1990 report of the necropsy findings in five patients and six dogs who had cardiac surgery has aroused new interest in this subject.[88] Focal small capillary and arteriolar dilatations were widely scattered in 10 of these 11 brains. Approximately one-half of the focal small capillary and arteriolar dilatations contained birefringent crystalline material within the dilatated capillary regions.[88] The vascular lesions affected medium-sized arterioles, terminal arterioles, and capillaries; they were often distributed in multiples in the same vessels or in clusters near each other. Two other patients had a small number of focal small capillary and arteriolar dilatations. The authors thought that the findings were most consistent with iatrogenically induced release into the system of small particles of air or fat.[88] Microemboli are likely to be an important cause of encephalopathy and persistent cognitive abnormalities after cardiopulmonary bypass surgery.

Pugsley and colleagues studied 100 patients who had cardiopulmonary bypass, 50 with an arterial line filter and 50 without a filter.[89] TCD was used to monitor microemboli. All patients were given neuropsychological tests before and after surgery. Neuropsychological deficits at 8 days and 8 weeks postoperatively were more common in patients who had cardiopulmonary bypass without the arterial filter, and neuropsychological abnormalities correlated with the number of microemboli.[89]

Strokes

Focal neurologic deficits are the most feared complication of cardiac surgery because they are often persistent and can be disabling. The frequency of focal deficits that qualify as strokes ranges from 4.7% to 5.2% in various series.[81,82,90] Intracardiac operations, such as valve replacements, carry a higher risk of postoperative strokes, ranging from 4.2% to 13%.[90] Among 2,264 patients having CABG with and without intracardiac procedures, the frequency of neurologic deficits was approximately doubled in those who had intracardiac procedures in addition to CABG.[90,91] Among the Cleveland Clinic series were 22 of 421 patients (5.2%) who had postoperative strokes, but the deficits were severe in only 2% of the total series.[82] Twelve infarcts involved a cerebral hemisphere (seven right, five left), five involved the brain stem, five involved the retina, and two involved an optic nerve.[82] Using neuroimaging data, infarcts are multiple in 65% of patients. Infarcts are typically small and numerous and involve preferentially the cerebellum, occipital lobes, borderzone territories between the MCAs and posterior cerebral arteries, and territories supplied by MCA branches.[90] Many strokes are first noted after the patient awakens from anesthesia, but strokes also often develop during the first few postoperative days.

In my opinion, the vast majority of brain infarcts after cardiac surgery are caused by embolism from the heart and aorta. A major worry of cardiac surgeons, cardiologists, and neurologists has been that hemodynamic circulatory stress during heart surgery might lead to underperfusion of tenuous zones of pre-existing extracranial vascular stenosis. This concern was the driving force behind early use of preoperative auscultation for bruits and later use of noninvasive and angiographic demonstration of the extracranial vascular system before cardiac surgery. If carotid artery disease was found, CEN was performed before or during the same anesthetic as cardiac surgery. The morbidity and mortality of this approach proved high.[60]

It is known that true hemodynamic insufficiency in regions of prior vascular compromise is quite rare. Patients with carotid bruits have a low rate of stroke after elective surgery.[53] I have already cited studies of patients with carotid stenosis documented by ultrasound who had a low rate of ipsilateral ischemic infarcts in the perioperative periods.[43,54,55] In a retrospective study of CABG patients with known carotid artery disease, 144 patients had severe atherostenosis (>50% luminal narrowing) affecting 155 arteries, as shown by preoperative angiography.[57] Strokes ipsilateral to the stenosis occurred in only 1.1% of arteries with 50–90% stenosis, in 6.2% of arteries with greater than 90% stenosis, and in only 2% of arteries with carotid occlusion.[57] Von Reutern and colleagues monitored the MCA of patients using TCD during cardiac surgery. Even patients with severe carotid stenosis usually showed no important changes during surgery.[92]

Brain infarcts often develop in the period after cardiac surgery. Because hemodynamic stress is maximal intraoperatively, underperfusion should cause damage noted on awakening after surgery. In one study, 5 of 30 postoperative strokes (17%) were noted immediately after cardiac surgery,[93] 14 others developed deficits within 24 hours, and seven did so during the subsequent 24- to 48-hour period. In two patients, strokes occurred 5 and 11 days, respectively, after surgery. The distribution and multiplicity of the postoperative infarcts on CT scans were most consistent with embolism.[93] The authors concluded, "Our findings support the contention that in patients who suffer cerebral infarction associated with coronary artery bypass grafting, the main mechanism of injury is cerebral embolization, rather than cerebral hypoperfusion."[93]

Some emboli originate from cardiac lesions known to exist before heart surgery, such as valve lesions, ventricular aneurysms, and myocardial akinetic zones. Atrial fibrillation and other arrhythmias may have been present before surgery or may first appear during the postoperative period. Atrial fibrillation often develops after surgery and may be transient. Some patients had taken warfarin or aspirin before surgery, but this was discontinued before and during the operation and was not restarted until after the embolic stroke had occurred.

Mounting evidence also links postoperative embolism to ulcerative atherosclerotic lesions of the ascending aorta.[56,90,94–100] Aortotomy or cross-clamping of the aorta to anastomose the vein graft may liberate cholesterol crystals and calcific plaque debris. Yellow aortic plaques are often visible and can be palpated by the surgeon. When the aorta is clamped, an audible crunch is often heard. Figure 16-1 is a photograph of the descending aorta at necropsy that contains many ulcerative lesions in a patient who did not awaken after CABG surgery. The transesophageal echocardiography of this patient showed severe aortic disease with multiple mobile plaques.

The most important risk factor for stroke after cardiopulmonary bypass surgery is aortic atheromatosis. The frequency of aortic atheromas increases dramatically with age, from 20% in the fifth decade at necropsy, to 80% in patients older than 75 years.[90,101] The stroke rate after CABG also increases sharply with age, from 1% in patients age 51 to 60 years, to 9% in patients older than 80 years.[90] The correlation between aortic atheromas and stroke after CABG was first shown at necropsy in a study that involved 221 patients.[101] Atheroemboli were found in 37% of patients who had severe atherosclerosis of the ascending aorta, but in only 2% of patients who did not have significant ascending aortic atheromas.[101] In another study, cardiac surgeons retrospectively reviewed the records of 3,279 consecutive patients with CABG at Johns Hopkins, seeking risk factors for postoperative stroke.[100] Severe atherosclerosis of the ascending aorta was one of the most definitive risk factors found.[100]

Embolization can be detected and quantified before, during, and after surgery using ultrasound. TCD recording over the MCAs can detect the arrival of microemboli in the cranial arteries. Figures 16-2 and 16-3 represent TCD recordings taken during cardiac surgery at various times during the procedure. Intraoperative transesophageal echocardiography can be used to detect the passage of emboli into and through the aorta. Figure 16-4 is a transesophageal echocardiography recorded during cardiac surgery that shows a shower of emboli entering the aortic lumen. More emboli are detected during intracardiac surgery because these patients often have valve calcifications, valve vegetations, and intracardiac thrombi. By using TCD monitoring during closed cardiac operations, the number of microemboli vary from 0 to 1,200 within one MCA (average, 130).[90] The numbers of emboli detected in the aorta by transesophageal echocardiography is in the thousands, reflecting the fact that only a fraction of the microembolic particles reach the brain.[90,102]

Embolization is not evenly distributed during the various stages of surgery. Maneuvers that involve manipulation of the aorta, such as clamping and unclamping, account for more than 60% of the total number of emboli.[90,102] Flurries of emboli are detected during aortic cannulation and at the start and termination of cardiopulmonary bypass. During open cardiac procedures, the number of emboli detected by TCD is especially high during cardiac ejection, after the release of aortic cross-

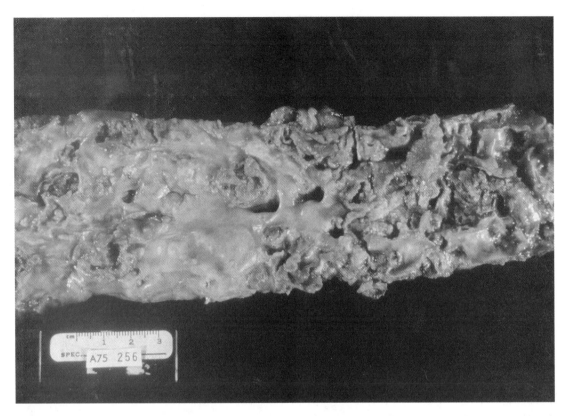

Figure 16-1. Descending aorta at necropsy from a patient whose transesophageal echocardiography before surgery showed severe disease of the ascending aorta and aortic arch with mobile protruding plaques. This patient died after coronary artery bypass graft surgery having never awakened after the procedure. (Courtesy of Denise Barbut, M.D., Cornell University Medical College and the New York Hospital.)

clamps, and immediately after bypass.[90] Figure 16-2 is a TCD recording during cardiac surgery that shows a "white-out" created by a massive shower of emboli that occurred immediately after release of aortic clamps. Many of the microemboli are gaseous particles. Aortic clamping and clamp release are followed by a snowstorm-like appearance of intensely echogenic, well-defined particles within the aorta and a corresponding flurry of particles within the brain arteries.[90] The mean diameter of these particles is 0.85 mm. These microembolic particles are most likely atheromatous debris from the aorta. They are small enough to enter the brain circulation, although only a small fraction do so.

Transesophageal echocardiography can detect and quantitate ulcerative aortic plaques before surgery. Figure 16-4 shows such a mobile protruding plaque. Some cardiac surgeons use transesophageal echocardiography during surgery (before clamping) to detect aortic atheromas and so indicate the regions of the aorta to avoid during clamping. Mar-shall and colleagues used an intraoperative B-mode ultrasound probe placed on the aorta to search for protruding plaques.[103] Ultrasonic imaging was more effective in showing plaques than visual inspection and palpation. Furthermore, the amount and location of plaque often altered the procedure performed.[103] Cardiac surgeons have begun to introduce filter devices into the aorta when the aortic clamps are removed to catch debris and cholesterol crystals. Figure 16-5 shows cholesterol crystals and other particulate debris caught in one of these filters.

Occasionally, intracerebral hemorrhages develop after cardiac surgery. Most often, this occurs after repair of congenital heart disease and cardiac transplantation.[104–107] The most common congenital heart lesions whose repair is followed by brain hemorrhage are transposition of the great vessels and ventricular septal defects.[104] In these patients and those who have received cardiac transplants, cardiac output has been abruptly increased by cardiac surgery. The brain hemorrhages are most likely

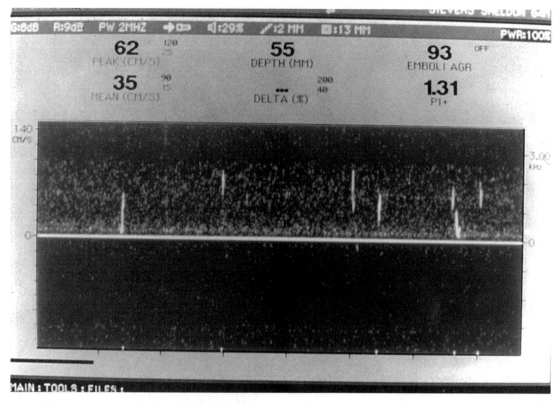

Figure 16-2. Transcranial Doppler recording from the middle cerebral artery during steady state cardiac bypass surgery at a time when the aorta was being manipulated. The white streaks represent microemboli. (Courtesy of Denise Barbut, M.D., Cornell University Medical College and the New York Hospital.)

attributable to the sudden change in brain blood flow, with relative cerebral hyperperfusion, in patients who had chronic reduced brain perfusion and likely altered cerebral autoregulation.[108]

Cognitive Dysfunction

Cognitive dysfunction without accompanying focal motor, sensory, or visual dysfunction is the most common complication of CABG surgery. Some patients have obvious loss of intellect, whereas others have subtle problems detectable only by formal neuropsychological evaluation. Estimates of the frequency of cognitive dysfunction after CABG range from 30%[109] to 88%,[110] depending on the timing and extent of neuropsychological testing. The most frequent cognitive abnormalities are defective memory, concentration, attention, and rapidity of response to stimuli.[110] Although many patients improve considerably within a few months, studies show that a substantial number of patients have persistent loss of intellectual functions. Cognitive dysfunction was present in 35% of patients 1 year postoperatively,[111] and in 20%[112] of patients at 3 years in two different studies. In a well-designed prospective study, 127 patients who had CABG surgery were tested in eight cognitive domains before surgery and at 1 month and 1 year after surgery. Only 12% of patients had no loss of function after surgery.[110] Among the 88% of patients who showed cognitive loss in at least one domain, 10% had persistent decline in the domains of verbal memory, visual memory, attention, and visual-related construction after 1 year.[110] Depression was also common after CABG.

Advanced age and length of bypass are important risk factors for cognitive dysfunction after

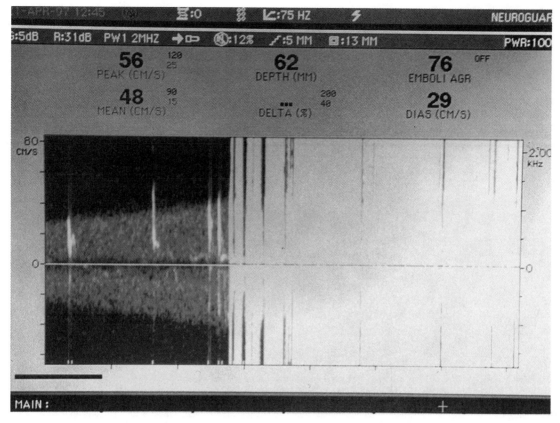

Figure 16-3. Transcranial Doppler recording from the middle cerebral artery during cardiac bypass surgery. A few distinct emboli (*left white streaks*) are followed by a massive shower of emboli ("white-out") at the time of the release of aortic clamps. (Courtesy of Denise Barbut, M.D., Cornell University Medical College and the New York Hospital.)

cardiopulmonary bypass.[113] Prospective studies provide evidence that microembolism is the most important cause of cognitive deficits after cardiac surgery using cardiopulmonary bypass.[56,89,90,114,115] Patients with cognitive deficits have more microemboli during surgery, compared with patients who have no cognitive decline. Pugsley and colleagues found that 43% of patients with intraoperative embolic counts greater than 1,000 had cognitive abnormalities at 8 weeks after cardiac surgery, compared with only 8% of patients with less than 200 emboli.[89] Barbut et al. found that the average number of microemboli at the time of removal of aortic clamps was 166 in six patients with cognitive abnormalities, compared with 73 microemboli in 11 patients who showed no loss of cognitive function.[114]

Prevention of Post–Coronary Artery Bypass Graft Strokes, Encephalopathy, and Cognitive Dysfunction

In my opinion, all patients who are going to have cardiac surgery should have preoperative transesophageal echocardiography. This should allow detection of potential cardiac and aortic sources of embolization. When the chest is opened, epiaortic ultrasound is also helpful. The presence of potential cardiac sources helps guide the use of heparin during and after surgery. Knowledge of aortic disease guides clamping sites and technique. Some patients can be operated on without aortic clamping—hypothermic fibrillatory arrest without aortic cross-clamping, graft replacement of the ascending aorta, and CABG without cardiopulmonary

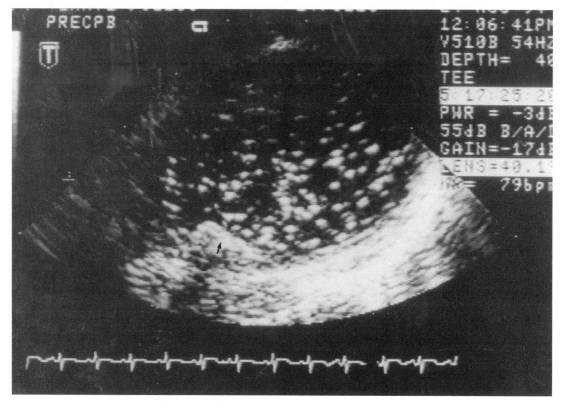

Figure 16-4. Transesophageal echocardiography recording during cardiac surgery from the aorta at the level of the origin of the left subclavian artery. A mobile plaque is seen protruding into the aortic lumen (*arrow*). This recording was taken after the release of aortic clamps and shows a "shower" of emboli within the aortic lumen beyond where the aorta was previously clamped. (Courtesy of Denise Barbut, M.D., Cornell University Medical College and the New York Hospital.)

bypass.[56] Placement of a filtering device in the aorta during and after release of aortic clamps is another useful maneuver to prevent microemboli from reaching the brain and other organs.

Peripheral Nervous System Complications

Brachial plexus and peripheral nerve lesions often develop after heart surgery, and the symptoms can be confused with a stroke. In one large series among 421 patients, 63 new peripheral nervous system deficits occurred among 55 patients (13%).[116] The most common syndrome is characterized by shoulder pain and numbness and weakness of the hand. This results from a brachial plexus intraoperative injury related to positioning of the arm, with traction on the brachial plexus.

Ulnar, peroneal, and saphenous nerve injuries are also common and relate to positioning. Diaphragmatic and vocal cord paralysis relate to local injury to the phrenic and recurrent laryngeal nerves during surgery.[116]

General Surgery

General anesthesia can augment brain edema, so general anesthesia should ordinarily not be given to patients recovering from a sizable brain infarct or hematoma. Stroke risk factors rarely, if ever, should postpone or delay general surgery, unless the patient is having active brain ischemia (TIAs within 2 weeks or stroke within a month). Cardiac risk factors are more important because MI and cardiac death are greater surgical risks than stroke.

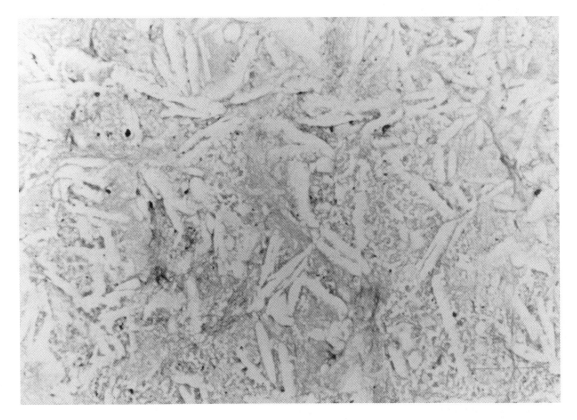

Figure 16-5. Cholesterol crystals and other particulate debris caught in a filter placed in the aorta at the time that aortic clamps are removed. (Courtesy of Denise Barbut, M.D., Cornell University Medical College and the New York Hospital.)

Goldman et al. have outlined the relative risk factors for cardiac morbidity and mortality in relation to general surgery.[28]

Strokes do occur after general surgery. Some relate to known medical disorders antedating surgery, such as polycythemia, thrombocytosis, arrhythmia, bleeding diathesis, and so forth. Puncture of the carotid artery[82] or ECVA[117] during attempted jugular vein cannulation can lead to thrombosis of these arteries, with subsequent stroke.

As my colleagues and I reported in 1993, we studied a group of patients who developed brain stem and cerebellar infarcts after general, noncardiac, and nonvascular surgery.[118] The surgical procedures were often minor (i.e., bunion removal, fracture repair, appendectomy). Most were orthopedic or gynecologic. During the immediate postoperative period or the first 36 hours, the patients developed vestibulocerebellar symptoms and signs of stupor with reduced levels of consciousness. CT showed cerebellar and rostral basilar artery territory infarcts. None of these patients had known atherosclerosis or a cardiac-source embolism. I believe that the most likely mechanism of stroke was abnormal positioning in relation to surgery, which was performed using general anesthesia and intubation in all patients. Thrombus probably formed in one ECVA in the neck during positioning in one neck posture. After the surgery was over and patients could move freely, clot was then discharged intracranially to block the ICVA (causing a cerebellar infarct) or the top of the basilar artery (causing thalamic, superior cerebellar, or posterior cerebral-hemisphere infarcts). These are the same areas affected by intra-arterial emboli in patients who have not had surgery.[78]

Vertebral artery dissection can also complicate surgery, and it is possible that carotid artery dissection might be precipitated by unusual head and neck positioning. The incidence of stroke during general surgery is not known, but stroke occurrence is probably more common than is presently recognized. Careful preoperative screening for cardiac and hematologic diseases and meticulous patient positioning during and after surgery, especially in the recovery room, are key factors in stroke prevention.

References

1. North American Symptomatic Carotid Endarterectomy Trial (NASCET) Collaborators. Beneficial effects of carotid endarterectomy in symptomatic patients with high-grade carotid stenosis. N Engl J Med 1991;325: 445–453.
2. Barnett HJM, Taylor DW, Eliasziw M, et al. Benefit of carotid endarterectomy in patients with symptomatic moderate or severe stenosis. The North American Symptomatic Carotid Endarterectomy Trial Collaborators. N Engl J Med 1998;339:1415–1425.
3. European Carotid Surgery Trialists' Collaborative Group. MRC European Carotid Surgery trial: interim results of symptomatic patients with severe (70–99%) or with mild (0–29%) carotid stenosis. Lancet 1991;1:1235–1243.
4. European Carotid Surgery Trialists' Collaborative Group. Randomized trial of endarterectomy for recently symptomatic carotid stenosis: final results of the MRC European Carotid Surgery Trial (ECST). Lancet 1998;351:1379–1387.
5. Moore WS, Barnett HJM, Beebe HG, et al. Guidelines for carotid endarterectomy. A multidisciplinary consensus statement from the Ad Hoc Committee, American Heart Association. Circulation 1995;91:566–579.
6. Caplan LR, Pessin MS. Symptomatic carotid artery disease and carotid endarterectomy. Ann Rev Med 1988;39:273–299.
7. Chassin MR. Appropriate use of carotid endarterectomy. N Engl J Med 1998;339:1468–1471.
8. Goldstein LB, Hasselblad V, Matchar DB, McCrory DC. Comparison and meta-analysis of randomized trials of endarterectomy for symptomatic carotid artery stenosis. Neurology 1995;45:1965–1970.
9. Asymptomatic Carotid Atherosclerosis Study Group. Carotid endarterectomy for patients with asymptomatic carotid artery stenosis. JAMA 1995;273:1421–1428.
10. The CASANOVA Study Group. Carotid surgery versus medical therapy in asymptomatic carotid stenosis. Stroke 1991;22:1229–1235.
11. Mayo Asymptomatic Carotid Endarterectomy Study group. Results of a randomized controlled trial of carotid endarterectomy of asymptomatic carotid stenosis. Mayo Clin Proc 1992;67:513–518.
12. Hobson RW, Weiss DG, Fields WS, et al. Efficacy of carotid endarterectomy for asymptomatic carotid stenosis. N Engl J Med 1993;328:221–227.
13. Halliday AW, Thomas D, Mansfield A. The Asymptomatic Carotid Surgery trial (ACST). Rationale and design. Steering Committee. Eur J Vasc Surg 1994;8:703–710.
14. Lagneau P. Stenoses carotidiennes asymptomatiques J Mal Vasc 1993;18:209–212.
15. Brott T, Toole JF. Medical compared with surgical treatment of asymptomatic carotid artery stenosis. Ann Intern Med 1995;123:720–722.
16. Barnett HJM, Meldrum HE, Eliasziw M. The dilemna of surgical treatment for patients with asymptomatic carotid disease. Ann Intern Med 1995;123:723–725.
17. Warlow C. Surgical treatment of asymptomatic carotid stenosis. Cerebrovasc Dis 1996;6(suppl 1):7–14.
18. Fisher CM, Ojemann R. A clinico-pathological study of carotid endarterectomy plaques. Rev Neurol 1986;142: 573–589.
19. Caplan LR, Stein R, Patel D, et al. Intraluminal clot of the carotid artery detected radiographically. Neurology 1984;34:1175–1181.
20. Pessin MS, Abbott BE, Prager R, et al. Clinical and angiographic features of carotid rculation thrombus. Neurology 1986;36:518–523.
21. Caplan LR, Clinical crossroads. A 79 year old musician with asymptomatic carotid artery disease. JAMA 1995; 274:1383–1389.
22. Sundt TM, Sandok BA, Whisnant JP. Carotid endarterectomy complications and pre-operative assessment of risk. Mayo Clin Proc 1975;50:301–306.
23. Easton JD, Sherman DO. Stroke and mortality rate in carotid endarterectomy: 228 consecutive operations. Stroke 1977;8:565–568.
24. Brott TG, Thalinger K. The practice of carotid endarterectomy in a large metropolitan area. Stroke 1984;15:950–955.
25. Hannan EL, Popp AJ, Tranner B, et al. Relationship between provider volume and mortality for carotid endarterectomies in New York State. Stroke 1998;29:2292–2297.
26. Callow AD. An overview of the stroke problem in the carotid territory: the David M. Hume Memorial Lecture. Am T Surg 1980;140:181–191.
27. Tarhan S. Moffitt FR, Taylor W, Guiliani E. Myocardial infarction after general anesthesia. JAMA 1972;220:1451–1454.
28. Goldman L, Caldera DL, Nussbaum SR, et al. Multifactorial index of cardiac risk in non-cardiac surgical procedures. N Engl J Med 1977;297:845–850.
29. Toronto Cerebrovascular Study Group. Risks of carotid endarterectomy. Stroke 1986;17:848–852.
30. Steed DL, Pertzman AB, Grandy B. Webster M. Causes of stroke in carotid endarterectomy. Surgery 1982;92:634–641.
31. Diaz FG, Patel S, Bordas R, et al. Early angiographic changes after carotid endarterectomy. Neurosurg 1982;10: 151–161.
32. Sundt TM. The ischemic tolerance of nerve tissue and the need for monitoring and selective shunting during carotid endarterectomy. Stroke 1983;14:93–98.
33. Breen JC, Caplan LR, DeWitt LD, et al. Brain edema after carotid surgery. Neurology 1996;46:175–181.
34. Leviton A, Caplan LR, Salzman EW. Severe headache following carotid endarterectomy. Headache 1975;13:201–210.
35. Lehv MS, Salzman EW, Silen W. Hypertension complicating carotid endarterectomy. Stroke 1970;1:307–313.
36. Caplan LR, Skillman J. Ojemann R, Fields WS. Intracerebral hemorrhage following carotid endarterectomy: a hypertensive complication. Stroke 1978;9:157–160.
37. Pessin MS, Kwan ES, Scott RM, Hedges TR. Occipital infarction with hemianopia from carotid occlusive disease. Stroke 1989;20:409–411.
38. Fode NC, Sundt T, Robertson J, et al. Multicenter retrospective review of results and complications of carotid endarterectomy. Stroke 1986;17:370–376.

39. Hart RG, Easton JJ. Management of cervical bruits and carotid stenosis in preoperative patients. Stroke 1983;14:290–297.

40. Mehigan JT, Birch WS, Pipkin RD, Fogarty TJ. A planned approach to coexistent cerebrovascular disease in coronary artery bypass candidates. Arch Surg 1977;112:1403–1409.

41. Easton JD, Hart RG. Asymptomatic Carotid Artery Disease in Patients Undergoing Open Heart Surgery: A Neurologic Viewpoint. In AJ Furlan (ed), The Heart and Stroke. London: Springer, 1987;319–327.

42. Rokey R, Rolak LA, Harati Y, et al. Coronary artery disease in patients with cerebral vascular disease: a prospective study. Ann Neurol 1984;16:50–53.

43. Pettigrew LC. Surgical Considerations. In LA Rolak, R Rokey (eds), Coronary and Cerebral Vascular Disease. Mount Kisco, NY: Futura, 1990;349–377.

44. Hertzer NR, Young JR, Beven KG, et al. Coronary angiography in 506 patients with extracranial cerebral vascular disease. Arch Intern Med 1985;145:849–852.

45. Riles TS, Kopelman I, Imparato AM. Myocardial infarction following carotid endarterectomy: a review of 683 operations. Surgery 1979;85:249–252.

46. Hertzer NR, Lees CD. Fatal myocardial infarction following carotid endarterectomy. Ann Surg 1981;194:212–218.

47. Verani M, Rokey R. Coronary Artery Disease: Diagnosis and Clinical Features. In LA Rolak, R Rokey (eds), Coronary and Cerebral Vascular Disease. Mount Kisco, NY: Futura, 1990;19–49.

48. Boucher CA, Brewster DC, Darling RC, et al. Determination of cardiac risk by dipyridamole-thallium imaging before peripheral vascular surgery. N Engl J Med 1985;312:389–394.

49. Gould KL, Sorenson SG, Albro P, et al. Thallium-201 myocardial imaging during coronary vasodilatation induced by oral dipyridamole. J Nucl Med 1986;27:31–36.

50. Chimowitz M. Asymptomatic Coronary Artery Disease in Patients with Carotid Stenosis: Incidence, Prognosis, and Treatment. In LR Caplan, JW Hurst, M Chimowitz (eds), Clinical Neurocardiology, New York, Marcel Dekker, 1999;287–297.

51. Gottlieb SO, Weisfeldt ML, Ouyang P, et al. Silent ischemia as a marker for early unfavorable outcome in patients with unstable angina. N Engl J Med 1986;314:1214–1219.

52. Gazes PC, Mobley EM Jr, Faris HM Jr, et al. Preinfarctional (unstable) angina—a prospective study: ten year follow-up. Circulation 1973;48:331–337.

53. Ropper AH, Wechsler LR, Wilson LS. Carotid bruit and the risk of stroke in elective surgery. N Engl J Med 1982;307:1388–1390.

54. Breslau PJ, Fell G, Ivey TD, et al. Carotid arterial disease in patients undergoing coronary artery bypass operations. J Thorac Cardiovasc Surg 1981;82:765–767.

55. Turnipseed WD, Berkhoff HA, Belzer FO. Postoperative stroke in cardiac and peripheral vascular disease. Ann Surg 1980;192:365–368.

56. Chimowitz M. Neurological Complications of Cardiac Surgery. In LR Caplan, JW Hurst, M Chimowitz (eds), Clinical Neurocardiology. New York: Marcel Dekker, 1999;226–257.

57. Furlan A, Craciun A. Risk of stroke during coronary artery bypass graft surgery in patients with internal carotid artery disease documented by angiography. Stroke 1985;16:797–799.

58. Schwartz L, Bridgman A, Kieffer R, et al. Asymptomatic carotid artery stenosis and stroke in patients undergoing cardiopulmonary bypass. J Vasc Surg 1995;21:146–153.

59. Mickleborough L, Walker P, Takagi Y, et al. Risk factors for stroke in patients undergoing coronary artery bypass grafting. J Thorac Cardiovasc Surg 1996;112:1250–1258.

60. Hertzer NR, Loop FD, Beven KG. Management of Coexistent Carotid and Coronary Artery Disease: A Surgical Viewpoint. In AJ Furlan (ed), The Heart and Stroke. London: Springer, 1987;305–318.

61. Lee RE. Reconstruction of the Proximal Vertebral Artery. In R Berguer, LR Caplan (eds), Vertebrobasilar Arterial Disease. St. Louis: Quality Medical, 1991;211–223.

62. Berguer R, Kiefer E. Surgery of the Arteries to the Head. New York: Springer, 1992.

63. Kieffer E, Koskas F, Bahnini A, et al. Long-term Results After Reconstruction of the Cervical Vertebral Artery. In LR Caplan, EG Shifrin, AN Nicolaides, WS Moore (eds), Cerebrovascular Ischaemia—Investigation & Management. London: Med-Orion, 1996;617–625.

64. Pauliukas PA, Barkauskas EM, Shifrin EG, Portnoi IM. Experience with reconstruction of vertebral arteries. In LR Caplan, EG Shifrin, AN Nicolaides, WS Moore (eds), Cerebrovascular Ischaemia—Investigation & Management. London: Med-Orion, 1996;577–601.

65. Spetzler RF, Hadley MN, Martin NA, et al. Vertebrobasilar insufficiency: I. Microsurgical treatment of extracranial vertebrobasilar disease. J Neurosurg 1987;66:648–661.

66. Hopkins LN, Martin NA, Hadley MN, et al. Vertebrobasilar insufficiency: II. Microsurgical treatment of intracranial vertebrobasilar disease. J Neurosurg 1987; 66:662–674.

67. Sundt T, Whisnant J, Piepgras D, et al. Intracranial bypass grafts for vertebro-basilar ischemia. Mayo Clin Proc 1978; 53:12–18.

68. Roski R, Spetzler R, Hopkins L. Occipital artery to posterior inferior cerebellar artery bypass for vertebrobasilar ischemia. Neurosurgery 1982;10:44–49.

69. Allen G, Cohen R, Preziosi T. Microsurgical endarterectomy of the intracranial vertebral artery for vertebrobasilar transient ischemic attacks. Neurosurgery 1981;81:56–59.

70. Ausman JI, Diaz FG, Pearce JE, et al. Endarterectomy of the vertebral artery from C_2 to posterior inferior cerebellar artery intracranially. Surg Neurol 1982;18:400–404.

71. The EC/IC Bypass Study Group. Failure of the extracranial-intracranial arterial bypass to reduce the risk of ischemic stroke. N Engl J Med 1985;313:1191–1200.

72. Hennerici M, Klemm C, Rautenberg W. The subclavian steal phenomenon: a common vascular disorder with rare neurologic deficits. Neurology 1988;38:669–673.

73. Caplan LR. Proximal Extracranial Occlusive Disease: Subclavian, Innominate, and Proximal Vertebral Arteries. In LR Caplan. Posterior Circulation Disease: Clinical Findings, Diagnosis, and Management. Boston: Blackwell, 1996;198–230.

74. Fields WS. Neurovascular syndromes of the neck and shoulders. Semin Neurol 1981;1:301–309.

75. Fields WS, Lemak NA, Ben-Menachem Y. Thoracic outlet syndrome: review and reference to a stroke in a major league pitcher. AJNR Am J Neuroradiol 1986;7:73–78.

76. Symonds C. Two cases of thrombosis of subclavian artery with contralateral hemiplegia of sudden onset, probably embolic. Brain 1927;50:259–260.

77. Fisher CM. Occlusion of the vertebral arteries. Arch Neurol 1970;22:13–19.
78. Caplan LR. The 1991 Graeme Robertson Lecture: vertebrobasilar embolism. Clin Exp Neurol 1991;28:1–23.
79. Slogoff S, Girgis KZ, Keats AS. Etiologic factors in neuropsychiatric complications associated with cardiopulmonary bypass. Anesth Analg 1982;61:903–911.
80. Gilman S. Neurological complications of open heart surgery. Ann Neurol 1990;28:475–476.
81. Shaw PJ, Bates D, Cartledge NEF. Early neurological complications of coronary artery bypass surgery. BMJ 1985;391:1384–1387.
82. Breuer AC, Furlan AJ, Hanson MR, et al. Central nervous system complications of coronary artery bypass graft surgery: prospective analysis of 421 patients. Stroke 1983;14:682–687.
83. Coffey CE, Massey EW, Roberts KB, et al. Natural history of cerebral complication of coronary artery bypass graft surgery. Neurology 1983;33:1416–1421.
84. Feeney DM, Gonzalez A, Law WA. Amphetamine, haloperidol and experience interact to affect the rate of recovery after motor cortex injury. Science 1982;217:855–857.
85. Houda DA, Feeney DM. Haloperidol blocks amphetamine induced recovery of binocular depth perception of the bilateral visual cortex abilities in the cat. Proc West Pharmacol Soc 1985;28:209–211.
86. Gilman S. Cerebral disorders after open heart operations. N Engl J Med 1965;272:489–498.
87. Sila C. Neuroimaging of cerebral infarction associated with coronary revascularization. AJNR Am J Neuroradiol 1991;12:817–818.
88. Moody DM, Bell MA, Challa VR, et al. Brain microemboli during cardiac surgery or aortography. Ann Neurol 1990;28:477–486.
89. Pugsley W, Klinger L, Paschalis C, et al. The impact of microemboli during cardiopulmonary bypass on neuropsychological functioning. Stroke 1994;25:1393–1399.
90. Barbut D, Caplan LR. Brain complications of cardiac surgery. Curr Probl Cardiol 1997;22:447–476.
91. Wolman RL, Kanchuger MS, Newman MF, et al. Adverse neurological outcome following cardiac surgery. Anesth Analg 1994;78(Suppl):S484.
92. Von Reutern G, Hetzel A, Birnbaum D, et al. Transcranial Doppler ultrasound during cardiopulmonary bypass in patients with internal carotid artery disease documented by angiography. Stroke 1988;19:674–680.
93. Hise JH, Nipper MN, Schnitker JC. Stroke associated with coronary artery bypass surgery. AJNR Am J Neuroradiol 1991;12:811–814.
94. Barbut D, Gold JP. Aortic atheromatosis and risks of cerebral embolization. J Cardiothorac Vasc Anesth 1996;10:24–30.
95. Blauth CI, Cosgrove DM, Webb BW, et al. Atheroembolism from the ascending aorta. An emerging problem in cardiac surgery. J Thorac Cardiovasc Surg 1992;103:1104–1112.
96. Masuda J, Yutani C, Ogata J, et al. Atheromatous embolism to the brain: a clinicopathologic analysis of 15 autopsy cases. Neurology 1994;44:1231–1237.
97. Katz ES, Tunick PA, Rusinek H, et al. Protruding aortic atheromas predict stroke in elderly patients undergoing cardiopulmonary bypass: experience with intraoperative transesophageal echocardiography. J Am Coll Cardiol 1992;20:70–77.
98. Mills NL, Everson CT. Atherosclerosis of the ascending aorta and coronary artery bypass. Pathology, clinical correlates and operative management. J Thorac Cardiovasc Surg 1991;102:546–553.
99. Yao FSF, Barbut D, Hager DN, et al. Detection of aortic emboli by transesopageal echocardiography during coronary artery bypass surgery. J Cardiothorac Vasc Anesth 1996;10:314–317.
100. Gardner TJ, Horneffer PJ, Manolio TA, et al. Stroke following coronary artery bypass grafting: a ten-year study. Ann Thorac Surg 1985;40:574–581.
101. Warehag TH, Davila-Roman VG, Barzilai B, et al. Management of the severely atherosclerotic aorta during cardiac operations. J Thorac Cardiovasc Surg 1992;103:453–462.
102. Barbut D, Yao FS, Hager DN, et al. Comparison of transcranial Doppler ultrasonography and transesophageal echocardiography during coronary artery bypass surgery. Stroke 1996;27:87–90.
103. Marshall WG, Barzilai B, Kouchoukos NT, et al. Intraoperative ultrasonic imaging of the ascending aorta. Ann Thorac Surg 1989;48:339–344.
104. Humphreys RP, Hoffman HJ, Mustard WT, et al. Cerebral hemorrhage following cardiac surgery. J Neurosurg 1975;43:671–675.
105. Sila CA. Spectrum of neurologic events following cardiac transplantation. Stroke 1989;20:1586–1589.
106. Andrews BT, Hershon JJ, Calanchini P, et al. Neurologic complications of cardiac transplantations. West J Med 1990;153:146–148.
107. Ferro JM, Mendes M, Guimaraes, et al. Intracerebral hemorrhage following cardiac transplant. Cerebrovasc Dis 1993;3:375–376.
108. Caplan LR. Intracerebral hemorrhage revisited. Neurology 1988;38:624–627.
109. Sotaniemi K, Mononen H, Hokkanen T. Long-term cerebral outcome after open-heart surgery. Stroke 1986;17:410–416.
110. McKann G, Goldsborough M, Borowicz L, et al. Cognitive outcome after coronary artery bypass: a one-year prospective study. Ann Thorac Surg 1997;63:510–515.
111. Venn G, Klinger L, Smith P. Neuropsychological sequelae of bypass twelve months after coronary artery surgery. Br Heart J 1987;57:565.
112. Martzke J, Murkin J, Baird D, et al. Perioperative predictors of neuropsychological outcome 3 years after coronary artery bypass surgery. Anesth Analg 1996;82:SCA 37.
113. Borowicz I, Goldsborough M, Selnes O, McKann G. Neuropsychologic change after cardiac surgery. A critical review. J Cardiothorac Vasc Anesth 1996;10:105–111.
114. Barbut D, Hinton R, Szatrowski, et al. Cerebral emboli detected during bypass surgery are associated with clamp removal. Stroke 1994;25:2398–2402.
115. Hammon J, Stump D, Kon N, et al. Risk factors and solutions for the development of neurobehavioral changes after coronary aartery bypass grafting. Ann Thorac Surg 1997;63:1613–1618.
116. Lederman RJ, Breuer AC, Hanson MR, et al. Peripheral nervous system complications of coronary artery bypass graft surgery. Ann Neurol 1982;12:297–301.
117. Sloan MA, Mueller JD, Adelman LS, Caplan LR. Fatal brainstem stroke following internal jugular vein catheterization. Neurology 1991;41:1092–1095.
118. Tettenborn B, Caplan LR, Sloan MA, et al. Postoperative brainstem and cerebellar infarcts. Neurology 1993;43:471–477.

Chapter 17
Cerebral Venous Thrombosis

Most brain ischemia is caused by thromboembolism and occlusive arterial disease. Brain infarcts and brain edema rarely result from thrombosis of dural sinuses and cerebral and cerebellar veins. Relatively little has been written about this problem when compared with the voluminous literature on arterial diseases because of the rarity of venous occlusive disease. Until the advent of magnetic resonance imaging (MRI), magnetic resonance angiography (MRA), and venography, the diagnosis of venous occlusion could only be made by cerebral angiography. I discuss the anatomy of the venous system in Chapter 2.

Development of Ideas

Venous occlusions were first reported in the 1820s. In 1825, Ribes described the first case of dural sinus thrombosis.[1–3] Ribes' patient was a 45-year-old man who developed epilepsy, severe headaches, and delirium. The delirium improved within a month, but headaches persisted and seizures increased in frequency. He died 6 months later. At necropsy, the superior sagittal and left lateral sinuses were thrombosed. Carcinomatous metastases were present in the brain. Three years later, John Abercrombie described the first case of puerperal sinus thrombosis.[4] A 24-year-old woman developed a severe headache after the delivery of her second child. Later, a sense of uneasiness in her head and numb feelings in her occiput and neck were followed by sudden weakness and numbness of her right hand, loss of speech, and twisting of her mouth. Frequent seizures were followed by coma and death. At necropsy, the sagittal sinus was occluded and the draining veins were distended and turgid. The brain showed softening and hemorrhage.[4]

Tonnelle[5] published a review of thrombosis of the dural sinuses in 1829 and Cruveilher[6] included a chapter on inflammation of the dural sinuses in his popular pathologic anatomy atlas. These authors noted that dural sinus thrombosis was common in children, especially those with fever and infections. In addition, Tonnelle and Cruveilher noted that dural sinus thrombosis occurred during the puerperium and in older, ill individuals, so-called senile cases. At the end of the nineteenth century, Quinke, the clinician usually given credit for originating lumbar puncture, described patients who had headache, visual symptoms, papilledema, and evidence of raised intracranial pressure who often recovered and did not have brain tumors.[7,8] At necropsy, one of Quinke's patients had occlusion of both transverse sinuses and the vein of Galen. Sir Charles Symonds deserves credit for bringing the phenomenology of benign intracranial hypertension and its relation to dural sinus occlusion and cerebral venous thrombophlebitis to the attention of clinicians. Symonds, in a series of key papers that spanned a quarter of a century, described the phenomenology of so-called otitic hydrocephalus and its relation to lateral sinus thrombosis and disease of the ears and mastoid air cells.[9–12]

In 1967, Kalbag, a neurosurgeon, and Woolf, a neuropathologist, wrote a monograph on the topic of cerebral venous thrombosis.[1] These physicians reviewed the history of recognition of this disorder, ideas about pathogenesis, and past contributions. The increased ability to recognize dural sinus and venous occlusions using magnetic resonance technology has led to a dramatic increase in knowledge about venous occlusive disease during the 1990s. This increased knowledge has led investigators and clinicians to publish comprehensive reviews and monographs on the topic of venous and dural sinus occlusions.[13–16]

Etiologies

Infections

In the pre-antibiotic era and perhaps until the 1970s, infections were the most common cause of dural sinus occlusions. Otitic and mastoid infections were a particularly common cause of lateral sinus thrombosis, and facial and paranasal sinus infections could lead to septic cavernous sinus infection. Past authors divided the etiologies of venous occlusive disease into infective and noninfective causes. In the pre-antibiotic era, occlusion of the lateral and sigmoid sinuses was almost exclusively caused by spread of infection from the mastoid air cells through emissary veins or directly into the adjacent lateral sinuses. The infectious process sometimes spread from the lateral sinus to the inferior petrosal sinus and then to the cavernous sinus. Lateral sinus occlusion was found predominantly in young patients with acute and chronic otitis media and those with inflammatory cholesteatomas. Most infections were pyogenic, but tuberculosis also involved the ear structures and mastoid cells and often spread to the meninges and dural sinuses. Facial infections were the most common cause of septic cavernous sinus thrombosis before the introduction of antibiotics; ethmoid and sphenoid sinusitis are the most important infectious causes.[17] During infections of the structures of the middle third of the face, including the nose, paranasal sinuses, orbits, tonsils, and palate, bacteria can enter the facial veins and pterygoid venous plexus to drain into the cavernous sinus via the superior and inferior ophthalmic veins.[17,18]

Dural sinus infection may follow open, direct, septic, traumatic injuries and brain and epidural abscesses. Meningitis is also occasionally complicated by dural sinus occlusion. High fever and dehydration, especially in children and the elderly, can also precipitate dural sinus thrombosis. Infections are known to increase the concentrations of acute phase reactants, including serine proteins that are involved in the coagulation process. The increased coagulability that results probably also promotes venous and dural sinus occlusion.

Hormonal Factors

Since Abercrombie, physicians have recognized that hormonal factors in women are important in patients with dural sinus and venous occlusions. The most common such circumstance is the puerperium, but dural sinus occlusions also probably occur more often than expected during pregnancy and in women who take oral contraceptive pills.[19–25] The United States National Hospital Discharge Survey showed that 5,723 cases of intracranial venous thrombosis reported between 1979–1991 among 50,264,631 deliveries occurred, yielding a frequency of 11.4 per 100,000 deliveries.[25] Dural sinus occlusion during pregnancy and the puerperium is especially common, or at least frequently reported, in India[22–24] and Mexico.[20,21] Venous occlusions are more common in the postpartum period than pregnancy. Among a series of 113 patients with nonseptic cranial venous thromboses studied in Mexico, 67 women were diagnosed during the puerperium, five during pregnancy, and one after an abortion.[20] In another series of 20 Mexican women with intracranial sinus thrombosis, 13 women were puerperal.[21] Six women took oral contraceptive pills. The great majority of postpartum cases occurred during the first 3 weeks after delivery, but venous thromboses can occur at any time during pregnancy. Postpartum cerebral venous thrombosis is more common in patients who have had venous thromboses outside the nervous system during previous pregnancies (pelvic or lower extremity phlebothrombosis and pulmonary embolism), multiparous women, women from lower socioeconomic strata who have had less prenatal care, and after deliveries at home. Among 135 patients with cerebral venous thrombosis collected by Bousser during a 20-year period in Paris, four occurred in women during pregnancy and 17 occurred during the puerperium.[16]

Hormonal changes might also be important in males. A healthy 31-year-old man was reported to develop extensive dural sinus occlusions after taking intramuscular injections of androgens for body building.[26] Among 27 patients with anemia treated with androgen therapy in one series, three patients developed sagittal sinus thrombosis.[27]

Cancer

Cancer, with its increase in acute phase reactants and enhanced coagulability, is another common cause of thrombosis. Adenocarcinomas, especially from the pancreas and gastrointestinal tract, are especially likely to be accompanied by thrombotic complications. Hickey et al. reported three patients with cancer (two with breast cancer and one with lung adenocarcinoma) who had intracranial venous sinus thrombosis.[28] They also reviewed 13 prior case reports. All patients had breast cancer, lung cancer, or hematologic malignancies, including lymphoma and leukemia. The clinical syndromes related to the intracranial venous thrombosis were indistinguishable from noncancer patients, but coexisting limb venous thromboses and pulmonary emboli were often present. In some cancer patients, the sinovenous occlusive disease was extensive. One patient with lung cancer at necropsy had occlusion of both renal arteries and veins, both internal carotid arteries, the splenic and portal veins, the pulmonary artery, the superior sagittal sinus (SSS), vein of Galen, and numerous cortical veins. In two patients, dural sinus thrombosis was the presenting problem occurring before the diagnosis of cancer. Migratory thrombophlebitis, Trousseau's sign, was first described in patients with pancreatic cancer. Trousseau's sign is common, especially in patients with mucinous adenocarcinomas.[29–31]

Cranial neoplasms can invade the dura mater and cause occlusions of the adjacent dural sinuses. This probably occurs most often in patients with meningiomas. Metastatic tumors that invade the skull, such as breast cancer and myeloma, may spread to the subjacent dura and dural sinuses and cause thrombosis. Six of the 135 patients (4.5%) in the series of Bousser had cancer, including two with carcinomatous meningitis.[16] Neck tumors and abscesses, which involve the pharynx that blocks the jugular veins, can also cause propagation of clot into the lateral sinuses.[32]

Abnormalities of the Blood and Coagulation System

Acquired and congenital abnormalities of the blood and coagulation system are also important causes of dural sinus and cerebral venous thrombosis. Thrombocytosis,[33] polycythemia vera,[34–36] parox-ysmal nocturnal hemoglobinuria,[37] and antiphospholipid antibody syndrome[38,39] have all been reported to cause dural sinus and cerebral venous occlusions. Some reported patients with dural sinus thrombosis have had severe anemia as the only predisposing cause.[16] Patients with systemic lupus erythematosus and lupus anticoagulant have also been reported to develop dural sinus occlusions, presumably because of hypercoagulability.[40,41] Sickle cell disease, protein C and protein S deficiencies, antithrombin III deficiency, plasminogen deficiency,[42] disseminated intravascular coagulation, and thrombosis associated with heparin-induced thrombocytopenia have all been reported to cause dural sinus occlusions. Resistance to activated protein C caused most often by the presence of factor V Leiden is an important cause of cerebral venous thrombosis, especially if patients with this genetic mutation take oral contraceptives or become pregnant.[43–45] Among 40 patients with cerebral venous thrombosis studied for coagulation abnormalities, three had increased antiphospholipid antibodies, six had thrombophilia, one had protein C deficiency, one had protein S deficiency, and four had factor V Leiden.[46] Other congenital disorders that produce a prothrombotic state, such as prothrombin gene mutations, can also cause cerebral venous thrombosis.

Some systemic illnesses predispose to venous and dural sinus occlusions. Patients with nephrotic syndrome may have renal vein and dural sinus occlusions probably related to deficiencies in coagulation proteins caused by the heavy proteinuria.[47,48] Dehydrated patients probably develop thrombosis because of a relatively high hematocrit and increase in viscosity and coagulability. In ill, cachectic elderly patients, a combination of dehydration and activation of coagulation factors probably cause so-called senile marantic venous sinus thrombosis. Congestive heart failure is also an important cause of cerebral venous thrombosis, presumably because of elevated venous pressure.

Systemic inflammatory diseases, especially ulcerative colitis,[16,49–51] Crohn's disease,[16,52,53] and Behçet's disease,[16,54–58] are known causes of dural sinus and cerebral venous occlusions. Among a series of 76 patients with cerebral venous thrombosis studied in Paris, 11 patients had Behçet's disease. Behçet's disease may cause a pseudotumor syndrome with papilledema[54] and has been

Table 17-1. Etiologies of Cerebral Venous Thromboses in Various Series

Etiologies	Bousser et al.[59] Number (%)	Cantu and Barinagarrementeria[20] Number (%)	Daif et al.[58] Number (%)	Bousser et al.[16] Number (%)
Idiopathic	17 (22)	25 (22)	10 (25)	29 (21)
Female hormonal	12 (16)	74 (65.5)	2 (5)	31 (23)
Pregnancy	1	5	—	4
Puerperal	4	62	1	13
Oral contraceptive*	7	7	1	14
Infections	8 (10.5)	0	3 (7)	8 (6)
Behçet's disease	11 (15)	0	10 (25)	18 (13)
Head injury	6 (8)	0	—	7 (5)
Cancer	6 (8)	1	3 (7)	6 (4.5)
Coagulopathy	5 (6.5)	11 (10)	9 (25)	10 (7.5)
Vascular malformation	1 (1)	2	0	3 (2)
Systemic lupus	1 (2.5)	0	3 (7)	2 (1.5)
Nephrotic syndrome	1 (2.5)	0	—	2 (1.5)
Others	8 (10.5)	0	—	19 (14)
Total	**38**	**113**	**40**	**135**

*Among the 29 patients who took oral contraceptives, 15 also had other predisposing causes.

reported as an important cause of intracranial venous occlusive disease. Among 250 patients with Behçet's disease followed in Paris, 25 patients (10%) had angiographically confirmed cerebral venous thromboses.[57] The outcome in the Paris series of patients with Behçet's disease and venous occlusions was quite good when the patients were treated with heparin and corticosteroids. In a series of patients with dural sinus thrombosis studied in Saudi Arabia, Behçet's disease accounted for one-fourth of the cases.[58]

Other Causes

Patients with dural arteriovenous fistulas may have accompanying thrombosis of dural venous sinuses and draining veins. The venous thrombosis can predispose to the development of a fistula, and fistulas can be the cause of subsequent venous thrombosis. This topic is discussed in Chapter 12. Head trauma can also lead to dural sinus thrombosis.[16]

The cause of intracranial venous thrombosis is undetermined in many patients despite extensive investigations. In the initial series of 76 patients reported by Bousser,[59] 17 patients (22%) were idiopathic. In the later Bousser series, 29 of 135 patients (21%) had no recognized etiology.[16] Twenty-five of 113 (22%) cases studied by Cantu and Barinagarrementeria could not be assigned an etiology.[20] In the series of cases from Saudi Arabia, 10 of 40 patients (25%) were idiopathic even after thorough evaluation.[58] Table 17-1 tabulates the etiologies of cerebral venous thromboses in several series of patients.[16,20,58,59]

Demography

Intracranial venous occlusive disease predominantly affects women and relatively young individuals. Among five series of patients,[20,58,60–62] 363 individuals were studied, including 241 girls or women (66%) and 122 boys or men (34%). Two-thirds of the patients were girls or women. Ages spanned 6 days to 77 years, with an average age of 33 years. The average age in all of the series was quite young: age 26 years in puerperal women with venous sinus thrombosis[20]; age 36 years in non-puerperal men and women[20]; and 38.7 years, 34.3 years,[60] 27.8 years,[58] and 33.3 years of age[62] in series that included both sexes. All reviewed series showed female predominance except that of Bousser et al., which included 21 men (55%) and 17 women,[13] and Daif et al.,[58] which included 20 men and 20 women. The sex and age predominance of patients with cerebral venous thrombosis contrasts dramatically with that found in patients with thromboembolic arterial disease, which has a male predominance and an average age at least three decades older.

Clinical Findings

Some clinical findings relate to occlusion of intracranial venous structures in general, whereas others are relatively specific for the location of thrombosis. General symptoms are reviewed first. Focal symptoms are discussed when various locations of venous thrombosis are analyzed.

> CD, a 57-year-old man, worked in the anatomy department of a medical school as a repairman. One day, a neuroanatomist working in the laboratory saw him suddenly stop speaking in the midst of a conversation. He repeated "I can't, I can't" and his right arm briefly shook. He was brought to the emergency room where he was noted to have difficulty speaking. While being examined, he had a grand mal seizure heralded by turning of his head to the right. Blood pressure was 160/100 mm Hg, but gradually returned to normal (125/80 mm Hg). Postictal agitation and aphasia were present. The aphasia was fluent and consisted of paraphasic errors and difficulty naming. He had a right superior quadrantanopia. Comprehension and repetition of speech were relatively spared. When he was able to discuss his symptoms, he reported that he had awakened that morning with a headache. He felt well the day before his attack. During the preceding weeks, he had intense headaches. He was being treated with nifedipine for hypertension. A year ago, he had an episode of thrombophlebitis and was treated with warfarin for 4 months. He was not taking coumadin or aspirin at the time of his attack.

Onset and Course

The presentation of patients with dural sinus thrombosis may be acute, as in CD, but, in general, venous occlusions seem to develop and propagate much more slowly than arterial occlusions. In most series, a gradual or stepwise development of symptoms and signs is more common than sudden abrupt onset.[2] Progression of symptoms after onset is also common and observed more often than in patients with arterial infarcts.

In the series of Cantu and Barinagarrementeria, acute onset was found more often in women who had puerperal venous thromboses when compared with nonpuerperal patients (82% vs. 54%).[20] Subsequent progression was also more common in puerperal thromboses (72% vs 52%).[20] Acute onset is more common during and after pregnancy and when the cause is infectious. Gradual increase in symptoms and a fluctuating course are the rule in patients with other causes of venous thromboses.[2,16] Ameri and Bousser found that the onset of symptoms was acute (<48 hours) in 31 (28%) patients, subacute (2 days–1 month) in 46 (42%) patients, and chronic (>1 month) in 33 (30%) patients.[60] Insidious onset, usually without focal neurologic signs, has often led to delays in admission to the hospital and presentation to doctors. In some patients, symptoms are present for longer than 6 months when the diagnosis is made. Among 102 patients with angiographically proven intracranial venous thromboses in one series, the mean day of admission after symptom onset was the fifth day, whereas the average was the fourteenth day.[63] Eleven patients in this series came to the hospital more than 1 month after symptom onset.[63] Gutschera-Wang analyzed 102 reports and found that nine (10%) patients had a history of headache for longer than 6 months before the diagnosis of venous thrombosis was made.[64]

Necropsy studies sometimes document venous thrombi at different stages of formation and organization.[63,65] Radiologically confirmed extension of thrombosis within the dural sinuses and veins has been noted after anticoagulants are stopped. The slow and gradual onset of symptoms and signs can be explained by the slow evolution and propagation of thrombosis and the potentially broad collateralization potential of the cranial venous and sinus drainage patterns. Collateralization of venous drainage patterns is more likely when thrombosis is gradual rather than when the occlusion is abrupt.

Headache

Head discomfort or pain is an extremely common symptom in patients with intracranial venous occlusive disease. CD had headaches before and at the onset of his neurologic symptoms. Headache is the only symptom in some patients, but is a major symptom in most patients. Headache is much more common in patients with venous thrombosis than in patients with arterial thromboembolic disease. Table 17-2 lists the symptoms that occurred during the course of illness among various reported series of patients with cerebral venous thromboses.[16,20,58,60–62,66]

In the series of Cantu and Barinagarrementeria, headache was the most common presenting symptom in the puerperal group. Headache was also the most common symptom in the group of patients who did not have venous thrombosis in relation to pregnancy or the postpartum period.[20] Headache was the most frequent symptom present in at least 340 of the total 439 patients (77%) in these various series. This frequency of headache is most likely a minimal figure because some obtunded and con-fused or aphasic patients might not have been able to report the presence of headache.

The presence of headache is best explained by two major factors: (1) the local process within the veins and dural sinuses and (2) the development of increased intracranial pressure. Unlike the brain itself, the dura and overlying skull and venous sinuses are invested with pain-sensitive fibers. Distention of the sinuses, especially when caused by inflammation, activates these pain-sensitive fibers. Thrombosis causes obstruction (at least temporarily) to venous drainage from intracranial structures. The resulting increased venous pressure causes increased intracranial pressure, brain edema, brain hemorrhage and infarction, and decreased absorption of cerebrospinal fluid. These findings cause increased intracranial pressure, often with papilledema. Papilledema was noted in 196 of 439 (45%) patients in which this sign was sought (see Table 17-2). In the series of 76 patients reported by Bousser and Barnett,[66] 38% had a pseudotumor syndrome characterized by headache, papilledema, and sixth nerve palsy. The pseudotumor syndrome, also often called *benign intracranial hypertension*, is characterized by headache, transient visual obscuration, papilledema, and raised intracranial pressure (as measured by lumbar puncture) without important

Table 17-2. Frequency of Various Clinical Findings in Patients with Intracranial Venous Thromboses in Various Reported Series

Clinical Finding	Cantu and Barinagarrementeria[20] (Puerperal) n = 67 (%)	Cantu and Barinagarrementeria[20] (Nonpuerperal) n = 46 (%)	Ameri and Bousser[60] n = 110 (%)	Einhaupl et al.[61] n = 71 (%)	Tsai et al.[62] n = 29 (%)	Bousser and Barnett[66] n = 76 (%)	Daif et al.[58] n = 40
Headache	59 (88)	32 (70)	83 (75)	63/69 (91)	9 (31)	61 (80)	33 (82)
Seizures	40 (60)	29 (63)	41 (37)	34 (48)	3 (10)	22 (29)	4 (10)
Focal findings	53 (79)	35 (76)	57 (52)	47 (66)	9 (31)	34 (48)	11 (27)
Altered consciousness	42 (63)	27 (59)	33 (30)	40 (56)	27 (93)	18 (27)	4 (10)
Papilledema	27 (40)	24 (52)	54 (49)	19 (27)	2 (7)	38 (50)	32 (80)

Source: Modified from M-G Bousser, R Ross Russell. Cerebral Venous Thrombosis. London: WB Saunders, 1997.

neurologic signs. Sixth nerve palsies and vision loss can result from the increased intracranial pressure. A pseudotumor syndrome was the most common clinical syndrome in the series of Bousser and Barnett[66] and is the usual presentation in patients with lateral sinus thrombosis caused by otologic infection.

Focal Neurologic Signs and Symptoms

Venous occlusive disease leads to focal parenchymal abnormalities, including edema, hemorrhage, ischemia, and infarction, which cause focal neurologic signs and symptoms. A focal neurologic sign, aphasia, was the presenting symptom in patient CD. Edema is probably the most common brain abnormality. Edema may be localized to the region drained by the occluded venous channel or be more generalized. Bilateral symmetric brain edema can produce a picture of small, slit-like ventricles on neuroimaging scans. When draining venous sinuses are occluded, the intravascular pressure in the feeding arteries must increase to a level above venous pressure to achieve an arterial-venous gradient sufficient for brain perfusion. Increased pressure at a capillary level leads to capillary leakage and edema in the interstitial spaces. Edema can also form around infarcts and hemorrhages.

A relatively abrupt increase in intravascular pressure in smaller arteries and arterioles often causes brain hemorrhages. Petechiae, hemorrhagic infarction, and frank hematoma formation are common in patients with cerebral venous and dural sinus occlusions. Hemorrhages may be bilateral when the SSS or bilateral sinuses are occluded. Some hemorrhages are subcortical and multifocal; in other patients, multiple petechiae are present amidst regions of ischemia. In the series of Tsai et al., 26 of 29 patients (90%) had some degree of mass effect, nine patients had hemorrhages, and five patients had infarcts.[62] Among 102 patients studied by Villringer et al., 43 patients (42%) had some degree of intracranial hemorrhage.[63] In the series of Bousser et al. among 38 patients, three had hemorrhages, seven had infarcts, seven had significant edema, two localized, and five had diffuse brain edema.[13] Infarction is most often precipitated and related to propagation and spread of thrombi to draining superficial and deep draining veins.

Focal neurologic symptoms and signs are present in approximately one-half of patients with dural sinus occlusions. The signs vary considerably, depending on which dural sinuses are involved and whether the deep venous system is also occluded. Most large series of patients do not divide signs according to the sinus involved. Hemiparesis is probably the most common sign. Hemianopia, ataxia, neglect, and aphasia are particularly common when the posterior dural sinuses are occluded. Aphasia was the first sign in patient CD. The aphasia and agitation were caused by focal dysfunction of the left temporal lobe.

Seizures

A grand mal seizure developed in CD shortly after onset of aphasia. In contrast to thromboembolic arterial disease in which seizures are rare during the acute period, seizures are quite common in patients with venous occlusive disease. Seizures are the presenting symptom in approximately 12–15% of cases. Seizures were present in 173 of 439 patients (39.5%) with intracranial venous thrombosis at some time during the course of illness (see Table 17-2). Seizures are approximately equally divided between focal and generalized. Often, the onset of focal seizures or generalized seizures with focal onset is followed by the appearance of residual focal neurologic signs. Edematous or partially ischemic nerve cells may have more potential for discharge than cells rendered nonfunctional by ischemia. Reversibly injured neurons must be quite common judged by the high frequency of reversible neurologic signs and reversible brain-imaging abnormalities.[63]

Decreased Level of Consciousness

Although diminished consciousness is not a common presenting symptom, 191 of 439 reported patients with cerebral venous occlusive disease (43.5%) had an alteration in their level of alertness at some time during the course of their illness.[16] In one series of patients with intracranial venous thromboses diagnosed by neuroimaging techniques, 27 of 29 patients (93%) had some reduction in mentation or level of alertness.[62] This frequency of altered consciousness is much higher than any series of patients with arterial disease except cases of extensive basilar artery thrombosis and pseudotumoral cerebellar infarcts. In patients with intracranial venous occlusive disease, the alteration in level of consciousness is usually reversible (as contrasted to the other two situations). Brain edema and raised intracranial pressure probably account for the decreased level of consciousness found in patients who have dural sinus occlusive disease. In patients with deep venous occlusions, bilateral involvement of the medial thalami also contributes to the occurrence of drowsiness, stupor, and coma.

Distribution of Venous Structure Involvement and Findings Related to Specific Locations

Figure 17-1 shows important intracranial dural sinuses.[17] These structures are also shown in Figure 2-17. Figure 17-2 shows the major venous structures as they appear in the venous phase of a normal angiogram. In this chapter, I use the term *lateral sinus* to include the transverse and sigmoid sinuses. Some authors use the terms *lateral sinus* and *transverse sinus* interchangeably. I list in Table 17-3 the distribution of involvement of the various venous structures among reported series of patients.[17,20,58,60,62,66] The determination of the sinuses involved should be viewed as approximate estimates because many of the studies are based on incomplete neuroradiologic studies. Cerebral and cortical vein involvement was sometimes not sought specifically and probably was often missed by the brain and vascular imaging performed in these series.

The SSS was the most commonly involved venous structure in all of the studies cited except that of Southwick et al., which was limited to only septic cases.[17] The SSS was involved alone in 87 of 260 cases (34%) in which this determination was commented on. The lateral sinus was the next most commonly involved venous structure, involved almost as often as the SSS in most studies. The frequency of isolated lateral sinus thrombosis was, however, less than that found in isolated SSS thrombosis. Only 28 of 213 patients (13%) had unilateral lateral sinus thromboses. Occlusions of the deep venous system were much less common than dural sinus occlusions. Cerebral cortical veins were commonly involved, but almost never in iso-

lation. Cerebellar cortical veins are rarely involved. The incidence of multiple venous channel involvement was high. Approximately two-thirds of patients had thrombosis of more than one venous channel (237 of 368 patients, 64.5%) among the series that tabulated multiple channel involvement.[20,58,60,62,66]

The studies cited in Table 17-3 include patients who have had many different etiologies. In puerperal patients, the SSS seems to be involved much more often than in patients with thrombosis unrelated to female hormonal changes. Septic thrombosis involves preferentially the lateral and cavernous sinuses because of the drainage of the ear and paranasal sinus structures into these dural sinuses.

Cavernous Sinus Thrombosis

Thrombosis of the cavernous sinus is most commonly caused by sepsis and is a serious disease with high mortality. The veins draining the medial portions of the face, orbit, nose, and nasal sinuses lead into the cavernous sinus. The cavernous sinus, in turn, drains via the petrosal sinuses into the lateral sinus and ultimately into the jugular vein.

The most common organism implicated in septic cavernous sinus thromboses is *Staphylococcus aureus*.[17,67] *Pneumococci*, streptococcal species, gram-negative bacteria, and fungi, especially *Aspergillus* species, account for the remainder of cases.[16] The earliest symptoms of septic cavernous sinus thrombosis are headache, facial pain, and fever. The eyelid and eye become red. The eye becomes proptotic. The face may become edematous and red. Orbital and retinal congestion develop, and ophthalmoplegia is found on examination. The oculomotor and trochlear nerves and the ophthalmic and maxillary branches of V course along the lateral wall of the cavernous sinus. The abducens nerve and internal carotid artery with its surrounding sympathetic nerve fibers run more in the center of the sinus. Any and all of these structures may be involved. Ophthalmoplegia may be complete or partial and is often accompanied by sensory abnormalities in the distribution of V1 and V2.

Head trauma, surgery on facial structures, prothrombotic states, and thrombosis of dural arteriovenous fistulas can cause nonseptic cavernous sinus thrombosis.[16] The onset of symptoms and

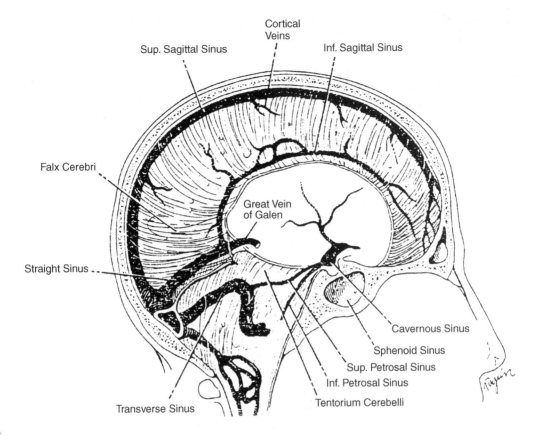

A

Figure 17-1. Dural sinus anatomy. **(A)** Lateral and **(B)** horizontal cross sections show the locations of major dural venous sinuses and their relation to the paranasal sinuses and mastoid air cells. (INF = inferior; L = left; R = right; SUP = superior; V = vein.) (Reprinted with permission from FS Southwick, EP Richardson, MN Swartz. Septic thrombosis of the dural venous sinuses. Medicine [Baltimore] 1986;65: 82–106.)

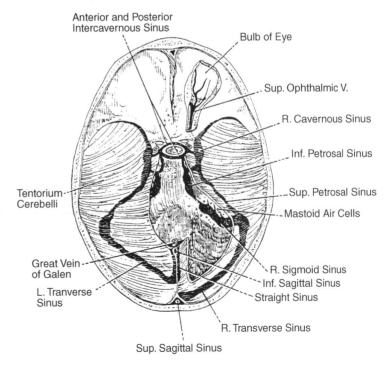

B

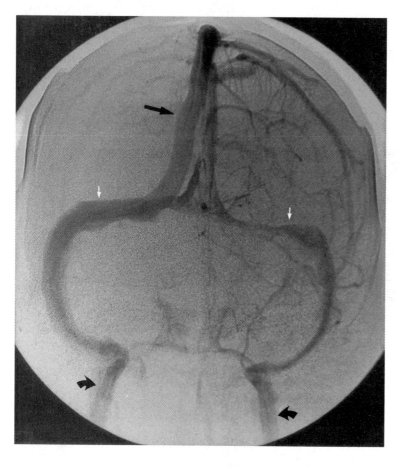

Figure 17-2. Venous phase of an angiogram shows the normal venous structures. The sagittal sinus (*straight black arrow*), transverse sinuses (*white arrows*), and jugular veins (*curved black arrows*) are shown clearly. The left transverse sinus is smaller than the right transverse sinus. (Courtesy of Rafael Llinas, M.D., Beth Israel Deaconess Hospital.)

signs in nonseptic cases may be gradual and indolent. Proptosis and redness of the eye may be only moderate in severity.

Sagittal Sinus Thrombosis

The SSS is the most common location of dural venous sinus thrombosis. The sagittal sinus is the favorite location for occlusion during the puerperium. Parasagittal meningiomas, neoplastic disease of the meninges, head trauma, Behçet's disease, and prothrombotic states are other frequent causes. Symptoms and signs depend greatly on the involvement of cerebral veins that drain into the sinus and on involvement of the lateral and other dural sinuses.

When thrombosis is limited to the sagittal sinus, the presentation may be that of pseudotumor cerebri with isolated increased intracranial pressure as the only clinical manifestation.[16] Extension of thrombus into rolandic and parietal veins is common and is often associated with the development of focal motor or sensory signs, or both, and focal or generalized seizures.[16] Sometimes, the neurologic signs are transient and closely resemble transient ischemic attacks of arterial origin. Often, the neurologic signs are bilateral, an occurrence that should always bring to mind the possibility of sagittal sinus thrombosis. Edema and hemorrhages are often found on brain imaging in the medial and dorsal portions of the cerebral hemispheres. Reduced consciousness and coma are common when the brain becomes severely edematous and bilateral hemorrhages and hemorrhagic infarcts are present. Papilledema is common.

Lateral Sinus Thrombosis

Lateral sinuses are the second most commonly involved dural sinus. Within the posterior circula-

Table 17-3. Distribution of Venous Structures Involved in Various Studies

Vein	Cantu and Baringar-rementeria[20] (Puerperal) n = 67 (%)	Cantu and Baringar-rementeria[20] (Nonpuerperal) n = 46 (%)	Ameri and Bousser[60] n = 110 (%)	Southwick et al.[17] (Septic) n = 179 (%)	Tsai et al.[62] n = 29 (%)	Bousser and Barnett[66] n = 76 (%)	Daif et al.[58] n = 40 (%)
SSS	60 (22)	45 (11)	79 (14)	23 (7)*	19 (11)	53	34 (22)
LS	23 (1)	20 (1)	78 (10)	64 (4)*	15 (8)	55	13 (4)
SS	0	0	3 (1)	—	3	10	3
CS	0	0	3	92 (8)*	0	2	0
DV	17 (4)	10	9 (1)	—	1	3	4 (1)
CCV	13	14	30 (2)	—	0	29	0
>1	39	34	85	—	9	56	14

CCV = cortical or cerebellar superficial vein; CS = cavernous sinus; DV = deep venous system; LS = lateral sinus; SS = straight sinus; SSS = superior sagittal sinus; >1 = more than one venous structure involved.
Numbers in parentheses represent cases in which only that structure alone was involved.
*Numbers in parentheses represent personally studied cases. The rest are from literature review.
Source: Reprinted with permission from M-G Bousser, R Ross Russell. Cerebral Venous Thrombosis. London: WB Saunders, 1997.

tion, the lateral sinus is by far the most commonly occluded dural sinus. Lateral sinus thrombosis is caused by coagulopathies and other systemic conditions; however, a much higher proportion of patients with lateral sinus thrombosis than sagittal sinus occlusions have an infectious etiology almost entirely caused by spread of infection from acute or chronic ear and mastoid infections. The infective process within the otologic structures often leads to a local thrombophlebitis. Infections spread through emissary veins or directly through a thin sinus plate into the lateral sinus. The sigmoid portion of the lateral sinus lies adjacent to the mastoid air cells from its origin to the jugular bulb. Infection can spread from the lateral sinus into the jugular vein.

Lateral sinus thrombosis caused by otologic infections and mastoiditis has undoubtedly become less common because of the widespread use of antibiotics. In the past, otitis media was also often complicated by other septic intracranial complications. The clinical findings in patients with lateral sinus thrombosis caused by otitic infections are quite characteristic.[17,68–71] Boys and men are more often affected than girls and women. Nearly all patients have had chronically draining ears and show acute infection or perforations of the eardrum. Fever, headache, neck pain, and neck tenderness are important and frequent signs.[69,71] Pain and tenderness are usually centered along the anterior border of the

sternocleidomastoid muscle on one side. The mastoid region is often sensitive and uncomfortable to finger percussion. Pain is usually also felt behind the ear. Headache is common and usually described as severe, persistent, and rather diffuse, located mostly in the frontotemporal and occipital areas of one or both sides.[17] If meningitis develops, bilateral neck stiffness and rigidity develop.

Vertigo, nausea, and vomiting are also often present. Diplopia caused by sixth nerve palsy and signs of fifth nerve irritation in the form of temporal and retro-orbital pain are often present. The combination of fifth and sixth nerve involvement, called the *Gradenigo's syndrome*, indicates involvement of these nerves at the petrous apex in or near Dorello's canal. Decreased alertness may be present and is explained by the elevated intracranial pressure. Elevated intracranial pressure and papilledema are more common after right-sided lateral sinus thrombosis. Structures on either side of the tentorium may be involved because both the inferior portions of the temporal lobe and cerebellum drain into the lateral sinuses. Combined temporal lobe and cerebellar involvement on one side suggests lateral sinus thrombosis. Aphasia, agitation, and a right hemianopia or superior quadrantanopia are the most common signs. These signs were all present in patient CD, who was found to have left temporal lobe dysfunction related to a left lateral sinus occlusion. Right temporal lobe involvement usually causes an agitated state with a left visual field defect. Nystagmus and gait ataxia are the most common signs of cerebellar involvement. Spread of thrombus into the jugular vein can be accompanied by pulmonary embolism, a serious, but not common, complication.

Plain x-rays of the mastoid regions usually show abnormalities, including increased density with loss of the mastoid air cell trabeculae, bony sclerosis, or lytic lesions of the temporal and parietal bones.[17] Cholesteatomas are common and have sometimes eroded through the temporal bone.[17,71] Spread of the occlusive process to other adjacent dural sinuses and jugular vein is common.

Deep Venous System Occlusions

Occlusion of the deep venous system, including the internal cerebral veins and vein of Galen, is much less common than dural sinus thrombosis. The straight sinus may also be occluded in patients with deep venous occlusions. The straight sinus and vein of Galen receive venous inflow from both thalami, the basal ganglia, midbrain, geniculate bodies, and the cerebellum. In the past, thrombosis of the deep venous system was thought to be almost exclusively a disorder of babies and young children and uniformly fatal. Since the 1980s, the condition has become recognized in adults, and the course is often much more benign than previously thought.[72–75] Necropsy studies of patients dying of deep vein thrombosis usually show bilateral thalamic and, often, basal ganglionic hemorrhagic infarcts.[72,73] Figure 17-3 is an MRI that shows bilateral basal ganglia and thalamic lesions in a patient with extensive thrombosis of deep veins. The causes of deep vein thrombosis are similar to dural sinus occlusion. Sepsis; dehydration, especially in babies; sickle cell disease; ulcerative colitis[75]; and oral contraceptives[73] have been reported as etiologic factors. In some cases, the cause is not discovered.

Patients with internal cerebral vein and vein of Galen thrombosis usually have reduced consciousness and are often stuporous or comatose. Headache may precede other symptoms and may be severe. Stiffness of the limbs with decerebrate postures, coma, and vertical gaze palsy are the most common clinical findings in patients with extensive basal ganglionic and thalamic hemorrhagic infarcts and edema.[2,16] Some patients present with apathy and are found on examination to be abulic. Poor memory is a predominant sign. When patients who present with stupor or coma recover, they often show residual signs of lack of initiative and spontaneity (abulia) and may also have poor memory.

Cortical Cerebral and Cerebellar Vein Thrombosis

Isolated thrombosis of cortical veins without associated dural sinus occlusion has long been recognized as an entity, but before MRI, this diagnosis was seldom made except at surgery or necropsy. Modern neuroimaging allows diagnosis and suspicion of this diagnosis.[76–79] Most reported patients have had seizures as a presenting or major symptom. The seizures have most often been focal or have had focal onsets with secondary generalization. Focal neurologic signs, such as hemiparesis and aphasia, are common. Headache is also a common sign. Reduced consciousness and increased intracranial pressure are less common than in dural sinus occlusions. Brain imaging shows a focal region of brain edema often with hemorrhage located along the pial surface of one cerebral hemisphere. In reported cases, occlusion has often involved the vein of Labbe.[78,79]

Cerebellar venous occlusions with cerebellar infarction have only rarely been described.[13,80,81] One reported patient had a sudden, severe headache mimicking subarachnoid hemorrhage, and another patient had multiple cranial nerve palsies, cerebellar type incoordination, and papilledema, a syndrome that mimicked a posterior fossa tumor.[13] Another patient has been described who also had a pseudotumoral syndrome.[80] One reported diabetic patient presented with seizures and coma during a severe hyperosmolar state.[81] He was found to have occlusion of the straight sinus and presumed occlusion of draining cerebellar veins. He also had bilateral large cerebellar hemorrhagic infarcts and hematomas. He died of brain stem compression caused by cerebellar lesions.[81] The clinical findings in patients with arterial and venous cerebellar infarcts are probably quite similar.

Figure 17-3. Diffusion-weighted magnetic resonance imaging shows bilateral basal ganglionic and thalamic abnormalities. The two arrows on the left point to the lesion in the putamen and the arrow on the right points to the lesion in the right thalamus. (Courtesy of Rafael Llinas, M.D., Beth Israel Deaconess Hospital.)

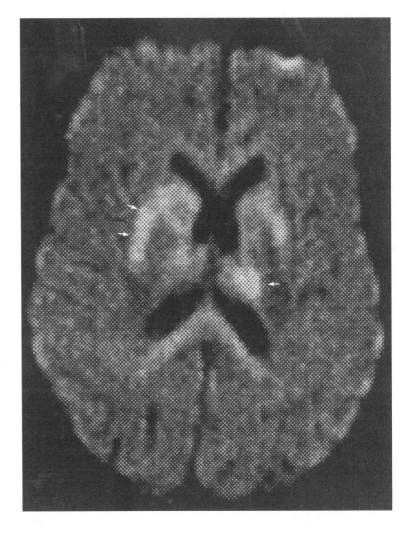

Diagnosis

Recognition of the presence of occlusion of the dural sinuses or intracranial venous system depends on a combination of clinical and neuro-radiologic findings. The demographics and risk factors for intracranial venous occlusive disease are quite different from those found in patients with arterial occlusions. Patients with venous occlusions are younger, usually female, and have low frequencies of hypertension, coronary artery disease, diabetes, and smoking when compared with patients with arterial occlusive disease. The conditions and circumstances that should alert clinicians to the possibility of venous occlusive disease are as follows:

1. Infants and babies with dehydration and sepsis
2. Puerperal and pregnant women and those taking oral contraceptives
3. Patients with known cancers, especially adenocarcinomas, leukemias, and lymphomas
4. Meningitis and other intracranial infections
5. Acute and chronic otitis media and mastoid infections
6. Acute sinusitis
7. The presence of inflammatory diseases, such as Behçet's disease, ulcerative colitis, and Crohn's disease
8. Nephrotic syndrome
9. Sepsis
10. Cachexia, malnutrition, and dehydration, especially in the young and old

11. Known hematologic disorders, which predispose to hypercoagulability
12. The presence of past recurrent leg vein thrombosis with pulmonary embolism
13. Intracranial tumors, such as meningiomas, that involve or abut on venous sinuses
14. The presence of dural vascular malformations
15. Penetrating cranial traumatic injuries

Clinical findings are also helpful in diagnosis. Headache is usually the earliest clinical symptom and often antedates any neurologic symptoms or signs. Seizures and decreased alertness are much more common in sinovenous occlusive disease than in patients with arterial occlusion-related infarcts. Increased intracranial pressure, especially in the absence of severe neurologic deficits, is also helpful in suggesting the possibility of venous occlusive disease. Usually, the evolution of the clinical course in patients with venous occlusive disease is slower and more indolent than in patients with arterial occlusions. The absence of cardiac and vascular abnormalities on echocardiography, MRA and computed tomography (CT) angiography, and extracranial and transcranial ultrasound in patients with clinical and imaging-documented brain infarcts should also raise the possibility of venous thrombosis. The clinical findings in patients with dural and cerebral venous occlusions are often indistinguishable from patients with intracranial infections, such as encephalitis, brain abscess, subdural empyema, and brain tumors, all of which are important differential diagnostic considerations.

Imaging and neuroradiologic investigations have dramatically improved the ability of clinicians to confirm the diagnosis of intracranial venous thrombosis. Although plain x-rays of the skull, paranasal sinuses, and mastoid air cells can show important abnormalities, CT allows for better definition of bony abnormalities and sinus disease. CT is probably the most common initial brain imaging test ordered. CT can show abnormalities within the bony structures of the skull, such as evidence of paranasal sinus infection, erosion of the middle ear structures, and changes in the mastoid regions. Infection-related erosion and thinning of the sinus plate are also sometimes evident. CT also effectively shows the parenchymatous brain lesion and may even show abnormalities within the veins and dural sinuses.

In patient CD, the CT scan showed a hemorrhage in the inferior portion of the left temporal lobe, which extended from the pial surface nearly to the sylvian fissure (Figure 17-4A). The hematoma was surrounded by a rim of lucent brain. A focal region of hyperdensity in the left transverse sinus region was also present. A later CT scan (Figure 17-4B) showed that a large hemorrhagic infarct had developed above the hemorrhage that was previously seen. MRI was unsatisfactory because of motion, but confirmed the temporal lobe hemorrhage, edema, and infarction. Angiography showed early filling of the left basal vein of Rosenthal, nonfilling of the left vein of Labbe, and no opacification of the left transverse and sigmoid portions of the left lateral sinus (Figure 17-5). The left jugular vein was not filled.

In patient CD, the vein of Labbe was occluded in addition to thrombosis of the lateral sinus and may have been most responsible for his temporal lobe hemorrhagic infarction. Most patients with lateral sinus thrombosis without cortical vein involvement have only a pseudotumor syndrome.

Evidence for venous and dural sinus occlusion on CT can derive from direct evidence of a sinus or vein abnormality or by parenchymatous abnormalities.[2,16,82–87] The dural sinuses or deep veins can appear as hyperdense, round, or triangular ("dense triangle" sign) structures on noncontrast axial CT scan sections, indicating the presence of a thrombus within a venous channel. This sign is rarely found. The so-called "cord sign," in which a cerebral cortical vein is imaged as a high-density, linear, thin, cylindric structure that contains thrombus, is rare. When present, however, the cord sign is specific for venous occlusive disease. These direct evidences of venous occlusion are not common on plain CT scans. Parenchymatous changes include regions of hypodensity, representing infarction and edema; hemorrhages; and brain edema with small, compressed ventricles. Often, the distribution of the parenchymal abnormalities, including diffuse edema, bilaterality of infarcts and hemorrhages, predominance of hemorrhagic changes, and the presence of a lesion, which does not conform to a typical arterial distribution, suggests venous occlusive disease.

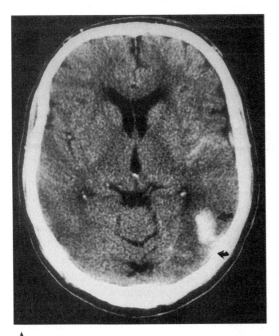

A

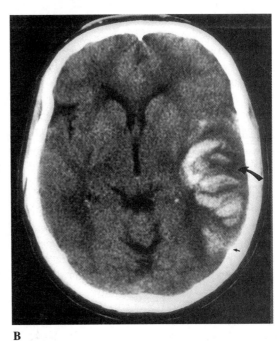

B

Figure 17-4. Computed tomography scans of patient CD. **(A)** Left temporal lobe hemorrhage (*large arrow*). Near the surface the thrombosed lateral sinus images as a hyperdensity (*curved arrow*). **(B)** Computed tomography scan taken days later shows a large hemorrhagic zone of infarction (*curved large arrow*) that has developed above the area of hemorrhage, which is still seen below (*small arrow*).

Figure 17-5. Angiogram, venous phase, in patient CD. The right lateral sinus is well opacified and drains into the right jugular vein (*black arrow*). The left lateral sinus (*open arrow*) does not fill, and no opacification of the left jugular vein exists. The left vein of Labbe also did not fill. (Reprinted with permission from LR Caplan. Venous and Dural Sinus Thrombosis in Posterior Circulation Disease. Clinical Findings, Diagnosis, and Management. Boston: Blackwell, 1996;569–592.)

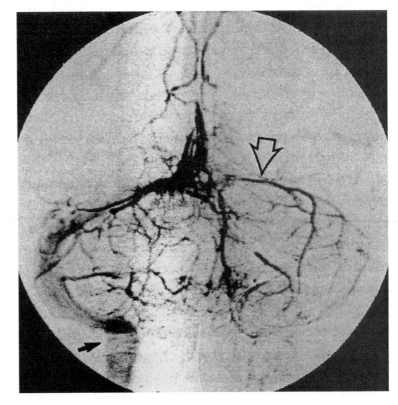

More information is usually obtained from contrast-enhanced CT scans than from plain scans.[83] Perhaps most important is the so-called empty delta sign,[82–87] a finding that has only been described in patients with sagittal sinus thrombosis. Contrast enhances the smaller collateral veins and walls of the sinus, but the middle region representing the thrombosed lumen does not enhance. In other patients after contrast, a filling defect is present within opacified sinuses. Cortical and medullary veins may appear dilatated on contrast-enhanced scans because of dilatation of collateral draining channels.[83] Contrast enhancement in a gyral pattern may also occur as it does in arterial disease–related infarcts. The tentorium or other dural structures may enhance in the region of a thrombosed dural sinus. Evidence of brain infarction and edema is more often found on CT scans than direct evidence of venous occlusion. In patients with cerebellar venous infarction, hydrocephalus and compression of the fourth ventricle may be found. CT venography is a reliable means of opacifying the normal venous structures and often can show evidence of venous occlusive disease.[88]

CT scans are helpful in the diagnosis of occlusion of the deep venous system. The characteristic finding is bilateral hypodensity, involving the thalami and basal ganglia. Hyperdensities in these same regions representing hemorrhages or hemorrhagic infarction also suggest the diagnosis of deep vein occlusions.[73] Severe edema with compression of the third ventricle may occur. The occluded sinuses and deep veins may appear as hyperdense structures on unenhanced CT scans. After contrast, nonopacification of the vein of Galen, straight sinus, and retention of contrast for a prolonged period in the usual draining veins, such as the thalamostriate veins and basal vein of Rosenthal, suggest occlusion of the deep venous system.[73]

Magnetic resonance scans are more likely than CT to provide definitive evidence of intracranial sinus or venous thrombosis.[2,16,87,89–95] MRI shows a variety of parenchymatous changes, including early infarction, hemorrhage, hemorrhagic infarction, focal edema, and diffuse edema. Gyral enhancement may be shown after gadolinium enhancement. In some patients, mass effect is found without any abnormalities of signal within the edematous regions.[93] Susceptibility-weighted images may show small areas of hemorrhage containing hemosiderin in late stages of evolution.

Direct evidence of abnormal flow in the dural venous sinuses is more often found on MRI scans than on CT. The findings, however, depend heavily on the MRI sequences used and the stage of the thrombosis. Dormont and colleagues studied 53 patients with cerebral venous thromboses imaged at various clinical stages.[89] Table 17-4, derived

Table 17-4. Nature of Dural Sinus Magnetic Resonance Imaging Signals and Their Intensity in Patients with Dural Sinus Thromboses

Stage	Normal	Early (First Week)	Intermediate (Weeks 2–4)	1–2 Months	Late (>6 Months)
Signal intensity[89]					
T1-weighted	—	—	—	—	—
T2-weighted	Variable	Iso-signal	High signal	Iso-signal	Isointense
Flow sensitive	No signal	Low signal	High signal	High signal	Hyperintense
	High signal	Iso-signal	High signal	Iso-signal	Iso-signal
Signal nature[90]	Normal	Sometimes expanded, homogeneous signal	Target sign	Often not homogeneous signal	Heterogeneous

Source: Adapted from LR Caplan. Venous and Dural Sinus Thrombosis in Posterior Circulation Disease. Clinical Findings, Diagnosis, and Management. Boston: Blackwell, 1996;569–592; D Dormont, R Axionnat, S Evrard, et al. IRM des thromboses veineuses cerebrales. J Neuroradiol 1994;21:81–99; and CH Isensee, J Reul, A Thron. Magnetic resonance imaging of thrombosed dural sinuses. Stroke 1994;25:29–34.

Figure 17-6. Magnetic resonance imaging scan of patient with multiple thromboses of dural sinuses. The superior sagittal sinus thrombosis is shown as a hyperintense signal (*two small arrows*). The straight sinus is also occluded and shows a hyperintense signal (*large arrow*). The sagittal sinus proximal to the hyperintensity (*small black arrow*) is patent.

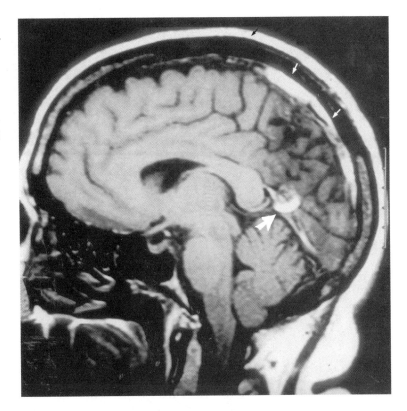

from two different studies,[90] notes the types of signals obtained on T1- and T2-weighted images and on flow-sensitive gradient echo sequence images at various stages of the clinical course. During the first week after thrombosis, the occluded sinuses appear as iso-signals on T1-weighted scans and a low-intensity signal on T2-weighted images. Flow-sensitive gradient echo images at this time show an iso-signal within the sinus instead of the normal high signal appearance, indicating a lack of flow in the sinus. In patients with cortical vein thrombosis, the lumens of the thrombosed veins may appear hyperintense on T1-weighted images.[77] During the next few weeks when most images are obtained, the dural sinus thrombi appear as high-signal intensity structures on all images. During the chronic stages longer than a month after onset, the sinuses most often appear as iso-signals on T1-weighted and flow-sensitive images and have an increased signal on T2-weighted images.[89,90,94]

Isensee et al. studied 23 patients with dural sinus thrombosis using multiplanar spin-echo and flow-sensitive sequences.[90] They described similar signal intensities on various magnetic resonance sequences, but also noted that during the first 5 days after thrombosis, the thrombus signal was always homogeneous and the sinus itself appeared expanded by the thrombus.[90] During days 6–15, the signal from the thrombus was always hyperintense, irrespective of the magnetic resonance sequence used. Figure 17-6 is an MRI that shows increased signal in the sagittal sinus on a T2-weighted scan. Sometimes, a "target sign," consisting of a central isointensity surrounded by peripheral circumferential hyperintensity, was shown. The absence of cardiac and vascular abnormalities on echocardiography, MRA and computed tomography angiography, and extracranial and transcranial ultrasound in patients with clinical and imaging-documented brain infarcts should also raise the possibility of venous thrombosis. Depending on recanalization, the thrombus signal decreased on all sequences. The signal became inhomogeneous in the late stages. When the sinus completely recanalizes, the signals becomes normal. Mas and colleagues showed that some patients with dural sinus thrombosis continued to have hyperintensity on T2-weighted images when studied 6 months after symptom onset.[95] The

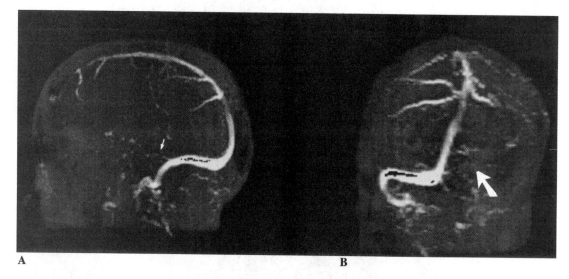

Figure 17-7. Magnetic resonance venogram in the patient whose magnetic resonance imaging scan is shown in Figure 17-2. **(A)** Sagittal view. The vein of Galen and straight sinus are not seen. The small arrow points to their usual location. **(B)** Axial view. The deep veins, straight sinus, and lateral sinus on the right of the figure are not seen. The arrow points to the location of the lateral sinus. (Courtesy of Rafael Llinas, M.D., Beth Israel Deaconess Hospital.)

signal changes within the dural sinuses depend on the presence or absence of flow; presence of deoxy-hemoglobin, which produces hypointensity on T2-weighted images; and extracellular methemoglobin. The signal changes related to chemical transformation of hemoglobin within the thrombus proceed from the periphery to the center of the thrombus, explaining the occurrence of a target sign.[90]

The lateral sinuses are often of unequal size; the larger sinus is the one with a more direct connection to the SSS. The right lateral sinus usually drains the SSS. The straight sinus usually drains into the left lateral sinus. The left lateral sinus is sometimes hypoplastic and in one study did not opacify in 14% of normal angiograms.[91] Mas et al. used MRI to study patients in whom angiography had shown nonvisualization or poor visualization of one or both lateral sinuses at angiography to determine if magnetic resonance studies could distinguish between hypoplastic and thrombosed lateral sinuses.[91] Hypoplastic sinuses were smaller, asymmetric structures on parasagittal MRI images without abnormal signal intensities along the course of the sinus. In contrast, occluded sinuses had increased intraluminal signals on all pulse sequences.[91]

In the chronic phase of dural sinus thrombosis, enhancement of chronic thromboses often occurs after the injection of gadolinium dimeglumine.[92,93] This enhancement is explained by organization of the thrombus, which is changed to vascularized connective tissue. On three-dimensional time-of-flight MRA images taken after enhancement, the thrombosed sinuses may be indistinguishable from normal sinuses because of this organized thrombus enhancement and may give a false-negative result on MRA. Hyperemia of dural structures that lie adjacent to thrombosed sinuses may appear on gadolinium-enhanced images as thickened and enhanced meninges, including the tentorium.[87]

MRA techniques, especially magnetic resonance venography, are particularly useful in defining dural sinus and cerebral and cerebellar venous occlusions by abnormalities in the normal flow signals, non-opacification of sinuses, and by showing collateral venous channels. Figure 17-7 illustrates the absence of the deep veinous structures on magnetic resonance venography, confirming the diagnosis of deep vein occlusion. With the advent of CT angiography and venography[88] and newer magnetic resonance techniques, which allow dural sinus and venous imaging, catheter angiography, once considered the "gold standard," is used much less often than in the past.

Conventional catheterization angiography, when necessary, can be performed using conventional filming or by digitalized intra-arterial filming techniques. Anteroposterior and lateral films are required with opacification of the entire venous system. Sometimes, oblique films are also useful, but are most helpful in patients with suspected sagittal sinus thrombosis. The partial or complete lack of opacification of venous channels is the primary angiographic evidence of venous occlusion. In patient CD, nonfilling of the left lateral sinus confirmed the clinical diagnosis (see Figure 17-5). For comparison, Figure 17-2 is an angiogram of the venous phase, which shows normal lateral sinuses and jugular veins. Delayed emptying and dilatation of collateral venous channels are other signs that are often present.[13,87,96] Because of wide variability in the development of the lateral sinuses, the entire lateral sinus, especially the sigmoid portion, should fail to opacify to be certain of occlusion. Neck films help to show whether the jugular bulb and vein are thrombosed. Delayed venous filling and emptying are common and are found in one-half of the patients with dural sinus occlusions.[13] Dilatated and tortuous cortical veins are more often seen at angiography than transcerebral collaterals.

Images of the dural sinuses can also be obtained by introducing catheters into the venous system and introducing contrast. Retrograde jugular catheterization with installation of contrast and dural sinus venography are usually done only when the angiographer intends to instill local fibrinolytic agents into the thrombosed venous sinuses.

Transcranial Doppler (TCD) ultrasonography has been used to diagnose and follow patients with dural sinus thrombosis.[97–100] In normal individuals and in patients, venous signals can be detected and displayed from the region of the basal vein of Galen, which lies adjacent to the P2 portion of the posterior cerebral artery, and from the straight sinus and superior and inferior portions of the sagittal sinus. In patients with dural sinus occlusions, the veins of Labbe and Rosenthal often serve as collateral channels. Increased blood flow in these veins increases the blood-flow velocities measured by TCD. Intravenous instillation of echo-contrast material helps to image the sinuses, using transcranial color-coded real-time sonography.[97,100] In patients studied, the mean blood-flow velocities in the region of the basal vein of Rosenthal have been elevated acutely and later returned to normal after treatment and presumed recanalization of the origi-

nal dural sinus occlusion.[98,99] TCD may be most useful in monitoring changes in venous flow and documenting the effect of treatment. Data about the use of TCD is preliminary. Too few patients have been studied to know the effect of the location of the dural sinus occlusion on the frequency and reliability of the TCD results.

Treatment

Antibiotics and surgical drainage of paranasal sinus infections and middle ear and mastoid infections remain the most important treatments in patients with septic dural sinus thrombosis. Anticonvulsants for seizure control are important in patients who have seizures. Raised intracranial pressure can be managed with osmotic diuretics, such as mannitol, corticosteroids, acetazolamide, and lumbar punctures.[101] In patients with pseudotumor syndromes, the intracranial pressure can usually be managed using lumbar punctures and acetazolamide. Temporary ventricular drains and shunts are seldom necessary. Among 110 patients in the series of Ameri and Bousser, only two required shunting procedures.[60] Mannitol and steroids may be useful in patients who have severe brain edema with small, slit-like ventricles as long as sepsis, when present, is appropriately treated with antibiotics.

> CD was treated with anticonvulsants. Heparin was begun on the sixth hospital day despite the large temporal lobe hematoma. Lupus anticoagulant studies were positive. The platelet count was slightly reduced and the prothrombin time was slightly accelerated. A new phlebothrombosis in the leg was identified and an inferior vena cava filter was placed. CD gradually improved, but remained aphasic.

The use of anticoagulants was once controversial in patients with dural sinus thrombosis, especially in patients with hemorrhagic infarcts and frank hematomas. Anticoagulants were first used to treat patients with puerperal intracranial venous thrombosis by Stansfield[102] and by Martin and Sheenan[103] in the early 1940s. In their monograph on cerebral venous thrombosis published in 1967, Kalbag and Woolf favored early anticoagulation before thrombosis spread to cortical veins.[1] In the same year, Krayenbuhl noted that patients treated with anticoagulants and antibiotics had a 7% mortality compared with 37% mortality in those treated only with antibiotics and compared with 70% mortality in those not given antibiotics or anticoagulants.[104] Krayenbuhl wrote that he never had a patient who developed intracranial hemorrhage during well-controlled anticoagulant treatment of intracranial venous thrombosis.[104] Despite the opinions of these authorities, most clinicians considered anticoagulants to be too dangerous because of the risk of further brain hemorrhage. The known tendency for intracranial venous thrombosis to be associated with hemorrhage persuaded many that anticoagulants were risky. An important reason to use anticoagulants was to prevent pulmonary embolism from the venous clots, which often extended into the jugular vein. Like any other peripheral venous occlusion, venous clots can extend to the heart. Diaz and colleagues reported a patient with SSS thrombosis who died of a fatal pulmonary embolus.[105] They reviewed the available literature on patients with dural sinus occlusion studied between 1942 and 1990. Diaz and colleagues found that in 23 of 203 patients (11%), dural sinus thrombosis was complicated by pulmonary embolism. All but 1 of these 23 patients died.[105]

Case reports and retrospective reviews showed that patients did not seem to worsen or have new hemorrhagic changes after institution of heparin or other anticoagulants.[106,107] Ameri and Bousser noted that among 82 patients treated with heparin, no deaths occurred, and 77% of patients had a complete recovery.[60] Austrian clinicians published the results of 42 patients with cerebral dural sinus thrombosis treated with heparin followed by oral anticoagulants.[108] Partial or complete recanalization of the thrombosed sinus was achieved in 36 of 40 (90%) patients; 40 patients improved clinically, among whom 26 recovered completely. Only one patient had a hemorrhagic transformation, but this patient did not worsen clinically.[108] Table 17-5 reviews retrospective, nonrandomized results from other case reports and series of patients with intracranial venous thromboses treated or not treated with anticoagulants. Among 79 patients given anticoagulants, 94% improved and survived, whereas only approximately one-half of the 157 patients not given anticoagulants survived.[107] Although these studies cannot prove effectiveness, they show that anticoagulants are probably seldom harmful.

A small, randomized, double-blind, prospective trial of heparin use in patients with intracranial venous thrombosis was reported by Einhaupl and colleagues.[109] During 1982–1984, they studied 28 patients with angiographically proven dural sinus thrombosis. Ten of the 20 patients that met inclusion criteria were given heparin by intravenous bolus of 3,000 IU and then 25,000–65,000 IU each day by continuous intravenous infusion. The dose was adjusted to double the initial prothrombin time, but not to exceed 120 seconds (target, 80–100 seconds). The other 10 patients were given placebo. At

Table 17-5. Retrospective Nonrandomized Studies of the Effects of Anticoagulation in Patients with Intracranial Venous Thrombosis

	Anticoagulated		Not Anticoagulated	
	Survived/ Improved	Died n (%)	Survived/ Improved	Died n (%)
Krayenbuhl[104]	16	1	32	24
Bousser et al.[13]	23	0	11	4
Case reports, 1942–1987	25	3 bled	25	44
Walker (*unpublished*)	6	0	7	1
Jacewicz and Plum[107]	4	1 (veg)	4	5
Total	**74 (94)**	**5 (6)**	**79 (50)**	**78 (50)**

Source: Reprinted with permission from M Jacewicz, F Plum. Aseptic Cerebral Venous Thrombosis. In KM Einhaupl, O Kempski, A Baethman (eds), Cerebral Sinus Thrombosis: Experimental and Clinical Aspects. New York: Plenum Press, 1990;157–170.

the start of treatment, three patients in the heparin-treated group and two patients in the placebo group had hemorrhages on CT scans.[109] A specially designed severity score (1–9, with 9 = death) and the development of intracerebral hemorrhage (ICH) on treatment were the outcome measures studied. To evaluate the occurrence of brain hemorrhage, at least two CT scans were performed on each patient. A CT scan was also performed at any suspicion of hemorrhage. The investigators planned to admit 60 patients with an interim analysis after the first 20 patients. The interim analysis was considered so positive for anticoagulation that the study was terminated after the first 20 patients were entered. Complications in the group treated with heparin included hematuria, a groin hematoma, and a stillbirth. One patient in the placebo group died after pulmonary embolism. No patient in the heparin-treated group had a new brain hematoma. In the placebo group, three patients with new brain hemorrhages were present, two of whom did not have a hemorrhage at onset. In the three patients with brain hemorrhages present before heparin treatment, two had a complete recovery.[109]

Einhaupl et al. also retrospectively analyzed their data from 102 patients with angiographically proven intracranial dural sinus and venous occlusions studied between 1977 and 1991.[109,110] Among the 102 patients, 43 had an ICH. Two patients had their first ICH after heparin treatment. One patient who had an ICH before treatment had another while receiving heparin. Altogether, six patients had ICH after heparin. Thirty-three patients not treated with heparin had new hemorrhages. They also analyzed data from 40 patients who had known ICH before heparin treatment (27 patients) and before no heparin treatment (13 patients). The patients not treated with heparin fared worse and had a higher mortality.[109,110]

Another randomized trial studied the use of low-molecular-weight heparin in patients with dural sinus thrombosis.[111] No difference existed in outcome between the 30 patients treated with low-molecular-weight heparin and those given placebo. No patient had a new symptomatic hemorrhage. One patient treated with low-molecular-weight heparin had a major gastrointestinal hemorrhage, and one patient in the placebo-treated group died of pulmonary embolism.[111] I find the data quite convincing that heparin and low-molecular-weight

heparin are not associated with clinical worsening and do not predispose to ICH. Heparin should be given to patients with intracranial dural and venous thrombosis unless a strong contraindication is present. Heparin is customarily administered during acute hospitalization and is followed by coumadin, which is usually given for a period of months. Longer-term coumadin is used in patients with severe prothrombotic conditions.

Thrombolytic agents have been used to treat patients with dural sinus thrombosis. The results, however, are still preliminary.[62,112–119] These reports include 66 patients. The dural sinus involvement in these cases was lateral sinus (24 patients), SSS (12 patients), SSS and lateral sinus (20 patients), or SSS and straight sinus (1 patient). In nine patients, multiple dural sinuses and deep veins were thrombosed, usually including the SSS, one or both lateral sinuses and, often, the straight sinus (six also had occlusion of the vein of Galen and other deep veins). Dural sinus venography was performed before infusion of thrombolytic agents. Infusion of the thrombolytic drug was then given locally through catheters introduced into the regions of the occluded sinuses. In some patients, a single infusion was given for approximately 60–75 minutes.[113,116] In one study, thrombolytic infusion was given for 82–244 hours (average, 163 hours).[113] In another study, urokinase was infused for 12–84 hours, with total doses ranging from 1,500,000 to 7,000,000 IU.[117] When follow-up imaging was performed and reported, the treated sinuses were usually recanalized. Complications were usually not reported but in one study, two patients treated with prolonged infusions had venous stenoses, which were treated with percutaneous angioplasty.[115] In another study, 2 of 12 patients had hemorrhages, one of which was evacuated surgically.[119] Heparin was given with and after thrombolytic treatment. These studies were all uncontrolled. They show that dural sinus venography is feasible. Thrombi can be lysed, but the dose of thrombolytic drugs used and the infusion times are much higher than those used to treat patients with arterial thromboses. It is difficult to make any conclusions from the preliminary data on thrombolytic therapy. The role of thrombolysis in patients with dural sinus thromboses is unclear.[120]

Direct surgery on the dural sinuses has been occasionally performed.[121] In the late 1960s and early 1970s, Yasargil[122] and Donaghy,[123] pioneers in the field of microneurosurgery for intracranial vascular disease, performed a number of reparative surgeries on the dural sinuses mostly for repair of traumatic injuries. Since then, a handful of surgeons have performed various procedures, including venous bypass and disobliteration of an occluded sinus in patients with dural sinus thrombosis. Surgery has most often been performed in patients with dural arteriovenous fistulas and sinus thrombosis.[124,125] Jugular vein ligation was at one time a popular surgical procedure in patients with lateral sinus thrombosis. Tying of the jugular vein was thought to effectively isolate the septic source in the lateral sinus from the general circulation and prevent pulmonary embolism. This procedure was often followed by septic complications and could promote retrograde thrombosis and interrupt drainage of venous blood from the head. Internal jugular vein ligation is seldom performed today. Most neurologists and neurosurgeons agree that the treatment of dural sinus thrombosis is medical except for patients with dural sinus thrombosis related to dural fistulas. Occasionally, patients with pseudotumoral cerebellar infarcts may need decompressive surgery. Hydrocephalus may require a ventricular shunt procedure in some patients.

Outcome

Unlike the situation in patients with brain infarction caused by arterial disease, patients with venous occlusive disease usually have complete recovery or die. Among various series that I tabulated, complete recovery without residual signs occurred in 250 of 383 (65%) patients, a much higher figure than found in any series of arterial infarcts.[2] Forty-eight of the 383 patients died (12.5%). Slight residual deficits were found in 14%. Severe residual deficits were found in only 8% of patients.[2] The nature of the residual deficits varied widely. In the study of Bousser et al. among 38 patients, seven patients had residual deficits; three patients had hemiparesis; two had optic atrophy; one was aphasic; and one had a sixth nerve palsy, slight incoordination and nystagmus.[13] In the series of Tsai et al., only one of 29 patients had a residual deficit (bilateral blindness); all other patients recovered or died.[62] The treatment of patients in these various series differed greatly. For

example, none of the patients in the series of Cantu and Barinagarrementeria[20] received anticoagulants, whereas 82 of 110 (75%) patients in the series of Ameri and Bousser[60] were treated with anticoagulants,[62] and thrombolytic therapy was used in 18 of 29 (62%) patients by Tsai and colleagues, but was not used in any of the other series that I tabulated. Treatment for brain edema also probably varied greatly among the series cited.

Outcome depends on the following criteria:

1. Extent of thrombosis within the dural venous sinuses
2. Spread to cortical and deep veins
3. Nature of the underlying causative disease
4. Presence and extent of parenchymal infarcts and hemorrhages
5. Use of anticoagulants and thrombolytic agents
6. Treatment of raised intracranial pressure

References

1. Kalbag RM, Woolf AL. Cerebral venous thrombosis. London: Oxford University Press, 1967.
2. Caplan LR. Venous and Dural Sinus Thrombosis in Posterior Circulation Disease. Clinical Findings, Diagnosis, and Management. Boston: Blackwell,1996; 569–592.
3. Ribes MF. Des recherches faites sur la phlebite. Revue Medicale Francaise et etrangere et Jornal de clinique de l'Hotal-Dieu et de la Charite de Paris 1825;3:5–41.
4. Abercrombie J. Pathological and practical researches on diseases of the brain and spinal cord. Edinburgh: Waugh & Innes, 1828;83–85.
5. Tonnelle M-L. Memoire sur les maladies des sinus veineux de la dure-mere. J Hebd Med 1829;5:337–403.
6. Cruveilhier J. Anatomie pathologique du corps humain: descriptions avec figures lithographiées et caloriées des diverses alterations morbides dont le corps humain est susceptible. Paris: J.B. Bailliere, 1842;1835–1842.
7. Quinke H. Ueber meningitis serosa. Inn Med Nr 1891;23: 655–694.
8. Quinke H. Ueber meningitis serosa und verwandte Zustande. Dtsch Z Nervenheilk 1896;9:149–168.
9. Symonds CP. Otitic hydrocephalus. Brain 1931;54:55–71.
10. Symonds CP. Hydrocephalus and focal cerebral symptoms in relation to thrombophlebitis of dural sinuses and cerebral veins. Brain 1937;60:531–550.
11. Symonds CP. Cerebral thrombophlebitis. BMJ 1940;2: 348–352.
12. Symonds CP. Otitic hydrocephalus. Neurology 1956;6: 681–685.
13. Bousser M-G, Chiras J, Bories J, Castaigne P. Cerebral venous thrombosis—a review of 38 cases. Stroke 1985; 16:199–213.

14. Einhaupl KM, Kempski O, Baethman A. Cerebral Sinus Thrombosis: Experimental and Clinical Aspects. New York: Plenum, 1990.

15. Einhaupl KM, Masuhr F. Cerebral venous and sinus thrombosis. An update. Eur J Neurol 1994;1:109–126.

16. Bousser M-G, Ross Russell R. Cerebral venous thrombosis. London: Saunders, 1997.

17. Southwick FS, Richardson EP, Swartz MN. Septic thrombosis of the dural venous inuses. Medicine (Baltimore) 1986;65:82–106.

18. Tveteras K, Kristensen S, Dommerby H. Septic cavernous and lateral sinus thrombosis. J Laryngol Otol 1988;102:877–882.

19. Donaldson JO. Neurology of pregnancy. Philadelphia: Saunders, 1978.

20. Cantu C, Barinagarrementeria F. Cerebral venous thrombosis associated with pregnancy and puerperium. Review of 67 cases. Stroke 1993;24:1880–1884.

21. Estanol B, Rodriguez A, Conte G, et al. Intracranial venous thrombosis in young women. Stroke 1979;10:680–684.

22. Srinivasan K. Cerebral venous and arterial thrombosis in pregnancy and puerperium, a study of 135 patients. Angiology 1983;34:733–746.

23. Chopra JS, Banerjee AK. Primary Intracranial Sinovenous Occlusions in Youth and Pregnancy. In PJ Vinken, GW Bruyn, HL Klawans (eds), Handbook of Clinical Neurology, Vol 10. Amsterdam: Elsevier, 1989;425–452.

24. Srinivasan K. Puerperial cerebral venous and arterial thrombosis. Semin Neurol 1988;8:222–225.

25. Lanska DJ, Kryscio R. Stroke and intracranial venous thrombosis during pregnancy and puerperium. Neurology 1998;51:1622–1628.

26. Jaillard AS, Hommel M, Mallaret M. Venous sinus thrombosis associated with androgens in a healthy young man. Stroke 1994;25:212–213.

27. Shiozawa Z, Yamada H, Mabuchi C, et al. Superior sagittal sinus thrombosis associated with androgen therapy for hypoplastic anemia. Ann Neurol 1982;12:578–580.

28. Hickey WF, Carnick MB, Henderson IC, Dawson DM. Primary cerebral venous thrombosis in patients with cancer—a rarely diagnosed paraneoplastic syndrome. Report of three cases and review of the literature. Am J Med 1982;73:740–750.

29. Sproul EE. Carcinoma and venous thrombosis: the frequency of association of carcinoma in the body or tail of the pancreas with multiple venous thrombosis. Am J Cancer 1938;34:566–585.

30. Miller SP, Sanchez-Avalos J, Stefanski T, Zuckerman L. Coagulation disorders in cancer: I. Clinical and laboratory studies. Cancer 1967;20:1452–1465.

31. Amico L, Caplan LR, Thomas C. Cerebrovascular complications of mucinous cancers. Neurology 1989;39:523–526.

32. Poe LB, Manzione JV, Wasenko JJ, Kellman RM. Acute internal jugular vein thrombosis associated with pseudoabscess of the retropharyngeal space. AJNR Am J Neuroradiol 1995;16:892–896.

33. Mitchell D, Fisher J, Irving D, et al. Lateral sinus thrombosis and intracranial hypertension in essential thrombocythaemia. J Neurol Neurosurg Psychiatry 1986;49:218–219.

34. Haan J, Caebeke, JFV, van der Meer FJM, Wintzen AR. Cerebral venous thrombosis as a presenting sign of myelo-proliferative disorders. J Neurol Neurosurg Psychiatry 1988;51:1219–1220.

35. Pouillot B, Pecker J, Guegan Y, et al. Benign intracranial hypertension in polycythemia which had caused a lateral sinus thrombosis. Neurochirurgie 1984;30:131–134.

36. Lauvin R, Lore P, Pinel JF, et al. Intracranial hypertension caused by lateral sinus thrombosis in Vaquez's disease. Rev Med Interne 1985;6:158–161.

37. Johnson RV, Kaplan SR, Blailock Z. Cerebral venous thrombosis in paroxysmal nocturnal hemoglobinuria. Neurology 1970;20:681–686.

38. Mokri B, Jack CR Jr, Petty GW. Pseudotumor syndrome associated with venous sinus occlusion and antiphospholipid antibodies. Stroke 1993;24:469–472.

39. Agah R, Rice L, Winikates J. Fatal cerebral venous thrombosis as the initial manifestation of the antiphospholipid syndrome. J Neurol Neurosurg Psychiatry 1996;98:189–191.

40. Vidailhet M, Piette J-C, Wechsler B, et al. Cerebral venous thrombosis in systemic lupus erythematosis. Stroke 1990; 21:1226–1231.

41. Levine SR, Kieran S, Puzio K, et al. Cerebral venous thrombosis with lupus anticoagulants: report of two cases. Stroke 1987;18:801–804.

42. Schutta HS, Williams EC, Baranski BG, Sutula TP. Cerebral venous thrombosis with plasminogen deficiency. Stroke 1991;22:401–405.

43. Zuber M, Toulon P, Marnet L, et al. Leiden mutation in cerebral venous thrombosis. Stroke 1996;27:1721–1723.

44. Dulli D, Luzzio CC, Williams EC, Schutta HS. Cerebral venous thrombosis and activated protein C resistance. Stroke 1996;27:1731–1733.

45. Brey RL, Coull BM. Cerebral venous thrombosis. Role of activated protein C resistance and Factor V gene mutation. Stroke 1996;27:1719–1720.

46. Deschiens M-A, Conard J, Horellou MH, et al. Coagulation studies, factor V leiden, and anticardiolipin antibodies in 40 cases of cerebral venous thrombosis. Stroke 1996;27:1724–1730.

47. Barthelemy M, Bousser M-G, Jacobs C. Thrombose veineuse cerebrale au cours d'un syndrome nephrotique. Nouv Presse Med 1980;9:367–369.

48. Lau SU, Bock GH, Edson JR, Michael AF. Sagittal sinus thrombosis in the nephrotic syndrome. J Pediatr 1980; 97:948–950.

49. Harrison MJG, Truelove SC. Cerebral venous thrombosis as a complication of ulcerative colitis. Am J Digest Dis 1967;12:1025–1028.

50. Das R, Vasishta RK, Banerjee AK. Aseptic cerebral venous thrombosis associated with idiopathic ulcerative colitis: a report of two cases. Clin Neurol Neurosurg 1996;98:179–182.

51. Silburn PA, Sandstrom PA, Staples C, et al. Deep cerebral venous thrombosis presenting as an encephalitic illness. Postgrad Med J 1996;72:355–357.

52. Sigsbee B, Rotenberg DA. Sagittal sinus thrombosis as a complication of regional enteritis. Ann Neurol 1978;3:450–452.

53. Motte S, Flamme F, Depianeux M, et al. Venous thromboangiitis associated with regional enteritis. Internal Angiology 1992;11:237–240.

54. Pamir MN, Kansu T, Erbengi A, Zileli T. Papilledema in Behcet's syndrome. Arch Neurol 1981;38:643–645.

55. Bousser M-G, Bletry O, Launay M, et al. Thrombose veineuse cerebrale au cours de la maladie de Behcet. A propos deux cas. Rev Neurol 1980;136:753–762.

56. Rougemont D, Bousser M-G, Wechsler B, et al. Manifestations neurologiques de la maladie de Behcet: 24 observations. Rev Neurol (Paris) 1982;138:493–505.

57. Wechsler B, Vidailhet M, Piette JC, et al. Cerebral venous thrombosis in Behçet's disease: clinical study and long-term follow-up of 25 cases. Neurology 1992;42:614–618.

58. Daif A, Awada A, Al-Rajeh S, et al. Cerebral venous thrombosis in adults. A study of 40 cases from Saudi Arabia. Stroke 1995;26:1193–1195.

59. Bousser M-G. Thromboses veineuses cerebrales. A propos de 76 cas. J Mal Vasc 1991;16:249–255.

60. Ameri A, Bousser M-G. Cerebral venous thrombosis. Neurol Clin 1992;10:87–111.

61. Einhaupl K, Villringer A, Haberl RL, et al. Clinical Spectrum of Sinus Venous Thrombosis. In K Einhaupl, O Kemski, A Baethmann (eds), Cerebral Sinus Thrombosis, Experimental and Clinical Aspects. New York: Plenum, 1990;149–155.

62. Tsai F, Wang A-M, Matovich VB, et al. MR staging of acute dural sinus thrombosis: correlation with venous pressure measurements and implications for treatment and prognosis. AJNR Am J Neuroradiol 1995;16:1021–1029.

63. Villringer A, Mehraein S, Einhaupl KM. Pathophysiological aspects of cerebral sinus venous thrombosis (SVT). J Neuroradiol 1994;21:72–80.

64. Gutschera-Wang L. Zur klinik von letalen hirnvenen-und sinus thrombosen anhand von 102 fallen. Erwachsener in der literatur. Inaug. dissertation. Munich, 1982

65. Cervos-Navarro J, Kannuki S. Neuropathological Findings in the Thromboses of Cerebral Veins and Sinuses:Vascular Aspects. In K Einhaupl, O Kempski, A Baethmann (eds), Cerebral Sinus Thrombosis, Experimental and Clinical Aspects. New York: Plenum, 1990;15–25.

66. Bousser M-G, Barnett HJM. Cerebral Venous Thrombosis. In HJM Barnett, JP Mohr, BM Stein, F Yatsu (eds), Stroke Pathophysiology, Diagnosis, and Management (2nd ed). New York: Churchill Livingstone, 1992;517–537.

67. DiNubile MJ. Septic thrombosis of the cavernous sinus. Arch Neurol 1988;45:567–572.

68. Samuel J, Fernandes CM. Lateral sinus thrombosis. a review of 45 cases. J Laryngol Otol 1987;101:1227–1229.

69. Mathews TJ. Lateral sinus pathology. 22 cases managed at Groote Schuur hospital. J Laryngol Otol 1988;102:118–120.

70. Tveteras K, Kristensen S, Dommerby H. Septic cavernous and lateral sinus thrombosis; modern diagnostic and therapeutic principles. J Laryngol Otol 1988;102:877–882.

71. Singh B. The management of lateral sinus thrombosis. J Laryngol Otol 1993;107:803–808.

72. Bots GAM. Thrombosis of the Galenic system veins in the adult. Acta Neuropathol 1971;17:227–233.

73. Haley EC, Brashear R, Barth JT, et al. Deep cerebral venous thrombosis. clinical, neuroradiological, and neuropsychological correlates. Arch Neurol 1989;46:337–340.

74. Johnsen S, Greenwood R, Fishman MA. Internal cerebral vein thrombosis. Arch Neurol 1973;28:205–207.

75. Averback P. Primary cerebral venous thrombosis in young adults: the diverse manifestations of an underrecognized disease. Ann Neurol 1978;3:81–86.

76. Jacobs K, Moulin T, Bogousslavsky J, et al. The stroke syndrome of cortical vein thrombosis. Neurology 1996;47:376–382.

77. Leach JL, Bulas RV, Ernst RJ, Cornelius RS. MR imaging of isolated cortical vein thrombosis: the hyperintense vein sign. J Neurovasc Dis 1996;1:32–38.

78. Dorndorf D, Wessel K, Kessler C, Kompf D. Thrombosis of the right vein of Labbe: radiological and clinical findings. Neuroradiology 1993;35:202–204.

79. Cambria S. Infarctus cerebral hemorrhagique par thrombose de la veine de Labbe. Rev Neurol (Paris) 1980;136:321–326.

80. Rousseaux P, Lesoin F, Barbaste P, Jomin M. Infarctus cerebelleux pseudotumoral d'origine veineuse. Rev Neurol (Paris) 1987;144:209–211.

81. Eng LJ, Longstreth WT, Shaw CM, et al. Cerebellar venous infarction: case report with clinicopathologic correlation. Neurology 1990;40:837–838.

82. Buonanno FS, Moody DM, Ball MR, et al. Computed cranial tomographic findings in cerebral sinovenous occlusion. J Comput Assist Tomogr 1978;2:281–290.

83. Rao CV, Knipp HC, Wagner EJ. Computed tomographic findings in cerebral sinus and venous thrombosis. Radiology 1981;140:391–398.

84. Tovi F, Hirsch M. Computed tomographic diagnosis of septic lateral sinus thrombosis. Ann Otol Rhinol Laryngol 1991;100:79–81.

85. De Slegte RGM, Kaiser MC, van der Baan S, Smit L. Computed tomographic diagnosis of septic sinus thromboses and their complications. Neuroradiology 1988;30:160–165.

86. Irving RM, Jones NS, Hall-Craggs MA, Kendall B. CT and MR imaging in lateral sinus thrombosis. J Laryngol Otol 1991;105:693–695.

87. Bousser M-G, Goujon C, Ribeiro V, Chiras J. Diagnostic Strategies in Cerebral Sinus Vein Thrombosis. In K Einhaupl, O Kempski, A Baethmann (eds), Cerebral Sinus Thrombosis, Experimental and Clinical Aspects. New York: Plenum, 1990;187–197.

88. Wetzel SG, Kirsch E, Stock KW, et al. Cerebral veins: comparative study of CT venography with intraarterial digital subtraction angiography. AJNR Am J Neuroradiol 1999;20:249–255.

89. Dormont D, Axionnat R, Evrard S, et al. IRM des thromboses veineuses cerebrales. J Neuroradiol 1994;21:81–99.

90. Isensee Ch, Reul J, Thron A. Magnetic resonance imaging of thrombosed dural sinuses. Stroke 1994;25:29–34.

91. Mas J-L, Meder J-F, Meary E, Bousser M-G. Magnetic resonance imaging in lateral sinus hypoplasia and thrombosis. Stroke 1990;21:1350–1356.

92. Dormont D, Sag K, Biondi A, et al. Gadolinium-enhanced MR of chronic dural sinus thrombosis. AJNR Am J Neuroradiol 1995;16:1347–1352.

93. Yuh WTC, Simonson TM, Wang A-M, et al. Venous sinus occlusive disease: MR findings. AJNR Am J Neuroradiol 1994;15:309–316.

94. Bianchi D, Maeder P, Bogousslavsky J, Schnyder P, Meuli RA. Diagnosis of cerebral venous thrombosis with routine magnetic resonance: an update. Eur Neurol 1998;40:179–190.

95. Mas J-L, Meder JF, Meary E. Dural sinus thrombosis: long-term follow-up by magnetic resonance imaging. Cerebrovasc Dis 1992;2:137–144.

96. Krayenbuhl H. Cerebral venous thrombosis. The diagnostic value of cerebral angiography. Schweiz Arch Neurol Neurochir Psychiat 1954;74:261–287.

97. Becker G, Bogdahn U, Gehlberg C, et al. Transcranial color-coded real-time sonography of intracranial veins. J Neuroimaging 1994;5:87–94.

98. Wardlaw JM, Vaughan GT, Steers AJW, Sellar RJ. Transcranial Doppler ultrasound findings in venous sinus thrombosis. J Neurosurg 1994;80:332–335.

99. Valdueza JM, Schultz M, Harms L, Einhaupl KM. Venous transcranial Doppler ultrasound monitoring in acute dural sinus thrombosis. Report of two cases. Stroke 1995;26:1196–1199.

100. Ries S, Steinke W, Neff KW, Hennerici M. Echocontrast-enhanced transcranial color-coded sonography for the diagnosis of transverse sinus venous thrombosis. Stroke 1997;28:696–700.

101. Hanley DF, Feldman E, Borel CO, et al. Treatment of sagittal sinus thrombosis associated with cerebral hemorrhage and intracranial hypertension. Stroke 1988;19:903–909.

102. Stansfield FR. Puerperial cerebral thrombophlebitis treated by heparin. BMJ 1942;1:436–438.

103. Martin JP, Sheenan HL. Primary thrombosis of cerebral veins (following childbirth) BMJ 1941;1:349.

104. Krayenbuhl H. Cerebral venous and sinus thrombosis. Clin Neurosurg 1967;14:1–24.

105. Diaz JM, Schiffman JS, Urban ES. Superior sagittal sinus thrombosis and pulmonary embolism: a syndrome rediscovered. Acta Neurol Scand 1992;86:390–396.

106. Levine SR, Twyman RE, Gilman S. The role of anticoagulation in cavernous sinus thrombosis. Neurology 1988;38:517–522.

107. Jacewicz M, Plum F. Aseptic Cerebral Venous Thrombosis. In K Einhaupl, O Kempski, A Baethmann (eds), Cerebral Sinus Thrombosis, Experimental and Clinical Aspects. New York: Plenum, 1990;157–170.

108. Brucker AB, Vollert-Rogenhofer H, Wagner M, et al. Heparin treatment in acute cerebral sinus venous thrombosis: a retrospective clinical and MR analysis of 42 cases. Cerebrovasc Dis 1998;8:331–337.

109. Einhaupl KM, Villringer A, Meister W, et al. Heparin treatment in sinus venous thrombosis. Lancet 1991;338:597–600.

110. Meister W, Einhaupl K, Villringer A, et al. Treatment of Patients with Cerebral Sinus and Vein Thrombosis with Heparin. In K Einhaupl, O Kempski, A Baethmann, (eds), Cerebral Sinus Thrombosis, Experimental and Clinical Aspects. New York: Plenum, 1990;225–230.

111. de Bruijn SF, Stam J. Randomized, placebo-controlled trial of anticoagulant treatment with low-molecular-weight heparin for cerebral sinus thrombosis. Stroke 1999;30:484–488.

112. Scott JA, Pascuzzi RM, Hall PV, Becker GJ. Treatment of dural sinus thrombosis with local urokinase infusion. J Neurosurg 1988;68:284–287.

113. Higashida RT, Helmer E, Halbach VV, Heishima G. Direct thrombolytic therapy for superior sagittal sinus thrombosis. AJNR Am J Neuroradiol 1989;10:S4–S6.

114. Tsai F, Higashida R, Matovich V, Alfieri K. Acute thrombosis of the intracranial dural sinus: direct thrombolytic treatment. AJNR Am J Neuroradiol 1992;13:1137–1141.

115. Smith TP, Higashida R, Barnwell S, et al. Treatment of dural sinus thrombosis by urokinase infusion. AJNR Am J Neuroradiol 1994;15:801–807.

116. Griesmer DA, Theodorou A, Berg RA, Spera TD. Local fibrinolysis in cerebral venous thrombosis. Pediatr Neurol 1994;10:78–80.

117. Horowitz M, Purdy P, Unwin H, et al. Treatment of dural sinus thrombosis using selective catheterization and urokinase. Ann Neurol 1995;38:58–67.

118. Kim SY, Suh JH. Direct endovascular thrombolytic therapy for dural sinus thrombosis: infusion of alteplase. AJNR Am J Neuroradiol 1997;18:639–645.

119. Frey JL, Muro GJ, McDougall CG, et al. Cerebral venous thrombosis. Combined intrathrombus rtPA and intravenous heparin. Stroke 1999;30:489–494.

120. Bousser M-G. Cerebral venous thrombosis. Nothing, heparin, or local thrombolysis? Stroke 1999;30:481–483.

121. Gratzl O. Neurosurgery of the Cerebral Venous and Sinus System. In K Einhaupl, O Kempski, A Baethmann (eds), Cerebral Sinus Thrombosis. Experimental and Clinical Aspects. New York: Plenum, 1990;219–224.

122. Yasargil MG. Microsurgery. Stuttgart: Thieme, 1969.

123. Donaghy P, Wallman LJ, Flanagan MJ, Numoto M. Sagittal sinus repair. J Neurosurg 1973;38:244–248.

124. Sundt T, Piepgras DG. The surgical approach to arteriovenous malformations of the lateral and sigmoid dural sinuses. J Neurosurg 1983;59:32–39.

125. Awad IA, Barrow DL (eds). Dural Arteriovenous Malformations. Park Ridge, IL: American Association Neurological Surgeons, 1993.

Part III
Prevention, Complications, and Rehabilitation

Chapter 18
Stroke Prevention and Risk Factors

> When meditating over a disease, I never think of finding a remedy for it, but instead a means of preventing it.
>
> —Louis Pasteur[1]

Prevention of stroke is much more likely to have a major impact on the health and welfare of the population than even the most effective treatment after stroke has occurred. For this cogent reason, much effort is aimed at identifying and modifying, whenever possible, risk factors for cerebrovascular disease.

Despite these efforts, much of the population is still woefully ignorant about stroke. The medical profession and media have been relatively successful in educating the public about heart attacks, cancer, and acquired immunodeficiency syndrome. Stroke, although the third leading cause of death in the United States, has received much less public attention and remains poorly understood by most Americans. Publicity about thrombolysis has increased public awareness about stroke and may increase general knowledge. The San Francisco Chapter of the American Heart Association sponsored a survey of 500 representative local residents to compare knowledge about stroke and heart disease.[2] Nearly one-half of those surveyed were unable to name any early warning signs of stroke; those who did answer often gave incorrect responses. Nine of 10 respondents could identify, however, at least one major sign of heart attacks. Most could name two or more signs. Nearly two-thirds of those surveyed reported having changed a habit, activity, or way of life to reduce their perceived risk for heart attacks.

The American Heart Association's Stroke Subcommittee sponsored a national survey using a sample of 1,253 respondents to study knowledge about stroke in regards to other common diseases.[3] The survey results include the following:

1. Most were aware that stroke is among the three major causes of death in the United States.
2. When asked the question, "A stroke occurs when the blood supply is cut off to what part of the body," 29% did not select "brain" from the choices of "heart," "brain," "don't know," and "other."
3. Approximately 7% of individuals thought arthritis was a major cause of stroke.
4. Only 44% of individuals identified weakness or loss of feeling in one arm or leg as a symptom of stroke as opposed to heart attack.
5. The respondents overestimated the proportion of stroke patients who are permanently disabled or require institutionalization after stroke.

These surveys were performed in the mid-1980s. Kothari and colleagues in 1997 interviewed patients admitted to the emergency room with possible strokes at the University of Cincinnati Medical Center.[4] Their interviews consisted of open-ended questions and were conducted during the first 48 hours after hospital admission. Among 163 patients, 63 (39%) did not know a single symptom or sign of stroke. Unilateral weakness (26%) and numbness (22%) were the most often mentioned symptoms.[4] Persons older than 65 years were less knowledgeable than younger patients.

Despite the lack of public knowledge about stroke, an important decline in stroke incidence and mortality has occurred during the second half of the twentieth century.[5–7] This fact is probably explained by a number of factors. The public is definitely more health conscious. Good eating habits; regular exercise; and avoidance of cigarettes, alcohol, and dietary excesses have been an educational and media theme. Reduction in risk factors perceived in the public mind as related to heart attacks has reduced cerebrovascular disease as well. An emphasis on check-ups and screenings for high blood pressure, diabetes, and high cholesterol have also had an impact. Physicians' aggressive treatment of hypertension and better technology for assessing vascular disease have also played a role. More public and physician education, however, is needed for further gains in stroke prevention.

Risk Factors

Extensive information has been accumulated and analyzed regarding risk factors for the general category of stroke[8–16] and brain ischemia.[14–23] With regard to some stroke mechanisms, such as subarachnoid hemorrhage (SAH),[24–26] intracerebral hemorrhage (ICH),[27] and brain embolism of cardiac origin,[28] ample data exist. I discuss causes of hemorrhage in detail in Chapters 12 and 13. The major risk factors for cardiac-origin embolism are those that predispose to the various cardiac conditions. These are described in Chapter 10. Relatively less information is available about other specific stroke mechanisms, especially within the broad group of patients with brain ischemia. Most analyses of risk factors do not differentiate among patients with stenotic lesions of the extracranial arteries; those with stenosis of the large intracranial vessels, such as the middle cerebral arteries, and those with disease of penetrating arteries, such as the lenticulostriate arteries. Evidence exists that various risk factors, such as race and sex, have a differential effect on various pathologic lesions and on lesions at various loci within the vasculature.[22,27,29–32] Further data, especially in patients with specific stroke subtypes studied prospectively, are needed.

Despite these limitations, the currently identified risk factors are of great significance. These risk factors help identify individuals at risk for stroke in whom modification of lifestyle might reduce the chance of stroke and other cardiovascular diseases. In this section, I briefly discuss only some of these

risk factors because larger, more detailed reviews of the subject are available.[8,10,13–16] When risk factors are identified, the evidence is usually an epidemiologic relationship between the factor and the occurrence of stroke; correlation does not mean causation. For example, being female is strikingly associated with becoming pregnant, but clearly this does not cause the condition.

Nonmodifiable Demographic Risk Factors

Parents cannot be selected, nor can race and sex. Time cannot be turned back to reverse the aging process. Age, race, sex, and family history of cardiovascular risk factors and disease are among the most important risk factors for stroke.

Age is probably the risk factor best correlated with stroke. The Framingham Study showed that as a person ages, his or her risk of stroke increases, with incidence rates per 10,000 increasing from 22% to 32% to 83% in the age groups 45–55, 55–64, and 65–74 years, respectively.[33] With increasing age, an exponential increase occurs in the frequency of stroke. The great majority of ischemic strokes occur in individuals older than 65 years.[22] The incidence of SAH also rises steadily with age.[25] Data on age in patients with ICH also show a high frequency in the elderly. Despite the best efforts, aging is inevitable. Stroke also occurs in younger patients. Ischemic stroke in patients younger than 45 years is correlated with more frequent cardiac-origin embolism and less common occlusive lesions, whereas in stroke patients older than 65 years, intrinsic large and small artery diseases are most common, closely followed by cardiac-origin embolism.

Race and sex also influence the occurrence and subtypes of stroke.[29–32] African Americans and Asians have a higher risk of ICH than whites.[27,34] African Americans, persons of Asian descent, and women have more intracranial occlusive disease and less extracranial occlusive disease than white men.[29–32] Men have a greater frequency of stroke than women, but because life expectancy is higher in women, women often outnumber men in many stroke studies.[22] During the premenopausal years, women have fewer strokes than men, but the incidence levels off after age 60 years.

A history of stroke or other important cardiovascular disease among first-degree relatives, including coronary artery disease, peripheral vascular disease, and hypertension, is an important risk factor for stroke even after adjustment for other personal stroke risk factors.[35-38] I once heard an informal presentation by a seventh-grade school teacher from the South. During a discussion about health in her classroom, this teacher discovered that few of her students knew about illnesses within their own families. She then gave her students a homework assignment to inquire in detail about the medical conditions that affected close relatives. Doctors volunteered to test the students for various conditions. Children whose parents both had hypertension had a high frequency of elevated blood pressure themselves. Those with a strong family history of diabetes often had high blood sugars. Students whose family history was affected by elevated cholesterol levels frequently had high serum cholesterol levels when tested. In 1983, a routine examination showed that my cholesterol level was quite high. When I later tested my six children (ages 7–20 years at the time), five of them also had abnormally high cholesterol levels.

When neurologists and other physicians care for patients with risk factors, such as high cholesterol, severe hypertension, and diabetes, they should urge patients to test their children, especially if risk factors have been prevalent in their family histories. It is known that some risk factors are found at relatively early ages, even in children and young adults. Finding and modifying risk factors at an early age is far superior to modification only after an index cardiac or cerebrovascular event.

Hypertension

After age, hypertension is the risk factor that most significantly correlates with stroke. The degree of elevation of systolic and diastolic pressure is correlated with the risk of stroke. The risk curve is a continuum without any clear point separating the stroke-prone from the non–stroke-prone individual.[33,39-41] Hypertension plays a role in multiple mechanisms of stroke. Without a prior history of diabetes or hypertension, lacunar disease is rarely found at necropsy. Also, the association between hypertension and cardiac disease is well known, making cardioembolic brain infarction more likely. Hypertension plays a role in the atherodegenerative process in large blood vessels, resulting in occlusive and artery-to-artery embolic strokes. Hypertension also plays a role in the rupture of cerebral

aneurysms.[24-26] ICH in the basal ganglia, thalamus, pons, and cerebellum is more commonly found in the setting of acute and chronic hypertension.

For stroke in general and atherothrombotic brain infarction, no evidence exists that shows that women tolerate hypertension better than men, nor do studies exist that prove the effects of hypertension wane in the elderly.[33,41,42] Hypertension is more prevalent in women after age 65 years than men. Women incur as many, if not more, complications of hypertension than men.[43] The Framingham data strongly suggest that control of hypertension is as critical for stroke prevention in patients older than 80 years as it is in younger age groups.[33,39,41] Systolic blood pressure is at least as important as diastolic blood pressure.[23,33,39,41] In the Systolic Hypertension in the Elderly Program, studies show that treating isolated systolic hypertension in the geriatric years reduces the incidence of stroke and other cardiovascular events.[44-46] Patients with isolated systolic hypertension who were given antihypertensive drugs had fewer lacunar infarcts than those given placebo.[46] Antihypertensive treatment with low-dose chlorthalidone, lowering systolic pressure to 143 mm Hg in the treatment group versus 155 mm Hg in the placebo group, reduced the total stroke incidence by 36%—that is, by 30 strokes per 1,000 patients during 5 years.[44] Other clinical studies have also shown a reduction in stroke incidence and mortality when hypertension is treated.[47-51] In Japan, studies using ambulatory blood pressure monitoring have shown that patients with excessively high and abnormally low nocturnal blood pressures have a higher frequency of new strokes and hypertension-related white matter damage than patients who have normal nocturnal blood pressures.[52,53] In the United States between 1972 and 1977, age-adjusted death rates for hypertension-related cardiovascular diseases declined 20%, whereas unrelated cardiovascular disease declined only 9%.[8] It is generally agreed that aggressive and effective control of hypertension over many years has contributed to the decline in stroke incidence and mortality.

In patients with acute stroke, the effects of many years of hypertension on blood vessel walls cannot be reversed in 1 or 2 days by precipitously lowering blood pressure. In fact, radical decrease in blood pressure may reduce cerebral perfusion, which can lead to profound worsening of neurologic deficits. I aim for effective treatment of hypertension across many months. In some individuals with flow-dependent strokes, blood pressures that are usually excessive must be tolerated during the weeks it takes for collateral circulation to become firmly established.

Cardiac Disease

Cardiac disease is also highly correlated with stroke. Cardiac disease is a direct cause of stroke when the heart is a donor source of emboli to the brain. Heart disease, usually related to hypertension or coronary artery disease, coexists with hypertensive and atherosclerotic disease of the cervicocranial arteries in other patients. Cardioembolic stroke occurs in the setting of mitral or aortic valve disease, atrial fibrillation of any cause, prosthetic heart valves, endocarditis, myocardiopathies, akinetic myocardial segments, and ventricular aneurysms. Atrial fibrillation is the most common cardiac source of brain embolism. The frequency of atrial fibrillation increases with age.[54] The overall prevalence of atrial fibrillation is 0.89%. The median age of patients with atrial fibrillation is age 75 years.[54] Atrial fibrillation is present in 2.3% of individuals older than 40 years and in 5.9% of those older than 65 years.[54] Other indices of cardiac impairment, such as coronary artery disease, congestive heart failure, and left ventricular hypertrophy as measured by electrocardiography, chest x-ray, or echocardiography, are associated with increased stroke risk. Particularly important is that heart disease is the major cause of death in patients with strokes, transient ischemic attacks (TIAs), and carotid bruits.[55] Stroke is a major risk factor for heart disease even if no overt cardiac disease is observed. Patients with extracranial artery occlusive disease have an especially high frequency of coexistent coronary artery occlusive disease.[56,57] Physicians must diligently search for and treat heart disease in patients with stroke. The treatment of heart disease in association with stroke plays a major role in prolonging life and avoiding significant morbidity.

Diabetes Mellitus

Diabetes is associated with an increased risk of ischemic stroke and increased mortality in patients with stroke.[23,58–60] Hemorrhagic strokes are relatively less common in diabetic than in nondiabetic

individuals.[60] Hypertension is more common among patients with diabetes, so some of the effects attributed to diabetes may be related to accompanying hypertension.[58] The increased risk of stroke is present in insulin-dependent and non–insulin-dependent diabetic patients and does not diminish with advancing age in either sex. Among non–insulin-dependent diabetic patients, the presence of autonomic neuropathy[61] and an elevated serum uric acid[62] increases the relative risk of stroke. Diabetes is a risk factor for intracranial and extracranial large artery occlusive disease and penetrating artery disease. Intracranial branch artery atheromatous disease is particularly common among diabetic patients.[63,64] Atheromatous branch disease affects predominantly the paramedian pontine penetrating arteries, anterior choroidal arteries, and anterior inferior cerebellar arteries.[63,64] No clear data exist to support the notion that strict control of diabetes alters the risk of stroke.

Smoking

In the first edition of this book, the importance of cigarette smoking as a risk factor for stroke was still uncertain. Convincing epidemiologic data now strongly relate cigarettes to an increased risk of stroke and extracranial and intracranial atherosclerosis.[23,65–70] The increased stroke risk applies to middle-aged and older individuals and men and women, but is especially important in the young. The amount and duration of smoking are important factors. In the Framingham Study, smoking was a significant risk factor for atherothrombotic brain infarction only in men younger than 65 years.[71] In a series of young adults (ages 15–45 years) in Iowa, a smoker was 1.6 times more likely to have a brain infarct than a nonsmoker.[66] Paffenbarger and Williams found that smoking was one of the most important risk factors among college students who later had ischemic strokes.[72] In a series of patients with extracranial carotid artery disease studied at the Mayo Clinic, the total years of cigarette smoking was the single, most significant, independent predictor of the presence of severe occlusive disease.[67] Duration of cigarette smoking and hypertension were the most important predictors of intracranial internal carotid artery disease in another study.[68] Stopping smoking mitigates the risk of stroke[73] as it does with other conditions. In regard to SAH, cigarette smoking seems to be a risk factor only when combined with the use of high-dose estrogen and contraceptive pill use in women.[24,74]

Elevated Blood Lipids

Abnormalities of blood lipids, especially cholesterol, triglycerides, and high- and low-density lipoproteins, are less closely correlated with stroke than coronary heart disease. Studies do confirm, however, that elevated low-density lipoprotein cholesterol and low high-density lipoprotein cholesterol levels do increase the risk of stroke.[75] In the Framingham Study and others, the risk is primarily documented in patients younger than 55 years.[76] A relationship between low cholesterol and ICH has been shown in several reports.[77,78] The risk of ICH is especially high in patients with low cholesterol levels (<160–190 mg/dl).[79,80] The mechanism of how low cholesterol levels increase the risk for brain and SAH remain obscure.

In one large series of more than 350,000 men, a significant relationship existed between morbidity from ischemic stroke and high serum cholesterol levels.[78] In a study of ischemic stroke mortality among 8,586 Israeli men, low high-density lipoprotein cholesterol levels were related to an increased risk of death caused by stroke.[81] Elevated levels of low-density lipoproteins, a decrease in concentrations of high-density lipoproteins, and the presence of lipoprotein(a) correlate better with coronary and extracranial atherosclerosis than do total cholesterol levels.[82,83] Patients with ischemic cerebrovascular disease have an increased frequency of elevated levels of lipoprotein(a).[84] Low levels of high-density lipoprotein cholesterol do correlate with carotid atherosclerosis in men,[85] but serum lipids and lipoprotein levels are not as powerful predictors of extracranial internal carotid artery disease as are hypertension and cigarette smoking.[86] One of the strongest indicators that cholesterol may have an important role in extracranial and intracranial atherosclerosis and ischemic stroke is the effectiveness of β-hydroxyl-β-methyglutaryl-coenzyme A reductase inhibitors in decreasing the growth of atherosclerotic plaques in the carotid arteries and reducing the incidence of stroke.[87] Although these drugs may have effects on plaques and vascular endothelia in addition to their cholesterol lowering effects, reduction of low-density lipoprotein cholesterol is their predominant action.

Alcohol Use

The status of alcohol ingestion as a risk factor for ischemic stroke remains controversial.[88] A relationship between alcohol consumption and brain hemorrhage exists. Finnish studies, not well controlled, clearly linked heavy alcohol consumption and recent alcohol use to the occurrence of SAH.[89] ICH can be caused by the hypoprothrombinemia accompanying cirrhosis of the liver. In the Honolulu Heart Study, alcohol consumption was associated with intracranial hemorrhage, not with ischemic stroke.[77,90]

Most epidemiologists describe a J-shaped curve in relation to alcohol consumption and the risk of ischemic stroke. Light-to-moderate regular consumption of alcohol seems to be inversely related to carotid artery and systemic atherosclerosis, yet acute and chronic heavy use of alcohol positively correlate with the incidence of ischemic stroke.[91–93] The effect of alcohol as a stroke risk factor is at least partially explained by the frequent coexistence of hypertension and cigarette smoking.[94,95] The effect of the type of alcohol consumed has not been well studied. In a study performed in Copenhagen, regular wine consumption did confer a protective effect, whereas intake of beer and other spirits did not.[96] Some have attributed the salutary effects of wine to its nonalcoholic contents, especially to antioxidant flavonoids and tannins, which are posited to have a protective effect against atherosclerosis.[96–98] Grape juice might have the same effects as alcohol, although this hypothesis has not been systematically studied. Acute alcohol intoxication may precipitate ischemic strokes.[99]

Atherosclerosis of Extracranial and Peripheral Limb Arteries

Atherosclerosis is a systemic disease. Patients with carotid plaques and thickened carotid arterial walls have atherosclerosis and so have a higher risk of ischemic strokes and silent brain infarcts.[100–102] The risk increases proportionately to the severity of carotid artery stenosis and also correlates with the presence of ulcerated carotid artery plaques. Narrowing and plaques within the proximal portion of the vertebral artery also correlate with the presence of carotid artery and coronary artery disease.[103,104] The availability of duplex carotid and vertebral artery ultrasound scanning make it possible to objectively detect and measure the severity of atherosclerotic abnormalities within the extracranial arteries. The progression or regression of these abnormalities over time and after treatment gives clinicians a means of monitoring the atherosclerotic process in the arteries studied. The presence of a neck bruit should not be used as a risk factor because some bruits are not associated with carotid or vertebral artery disease. Ultrasound studies should be performed in patients who have bruits thought to indicate atherosclerotic narrowing to identify and quantify the disease.

Peripheral vascular arterial occlusive disease is a strong predictor of extracranial cerebrovascular and coronary artery disease. Patients with claudication and peripheral arterial disease have a high frequency of stroke and cardiovascular mortality.[105,106] I have already commented earlier in this chapter on the close association between coronary artery and extracranial arterial disease and stroke.

Transient Ischemic Attacks

When properly diagnosed, TIAs are an indication that occlusive cerebrovascular disease has already become established. In fact, some patients with clinical TIAs have computed tomography evidence of infarction in regions that correlate with the symptoms.[107–109] Nicolaides and Zukowski found that among 36 patients with clinical TIAs, 23 (64%) had computed tomography positive infarcts.[110] The frequency of infarcts in patients with clinical TIAs is even higher when magnetic resonance imaging is performed.[108] Patients with TIAs are also, of course, at risk for subsequent TIAs, stroke, and myocardial infarction.[56,57,111] Risk factors and prognosis are similar for patients with TIAs and those with minor strokes because the underlying vascular diseases are identical.[18] Recognition and appropriate treatment for patients with TIAs probably do not influence the total stroke incidence as much as control of the factors that prevent the establishment of atherosclerotic disease.

For the individual stroke patient, failure to recognize that a TIA has occurred and failure to diagnose and treat potentially remediable abnormalities can be a great personal and family tragedy. All too often, patients do not understand the importance of temporary focal nervous system and ocular symptoms. Patients often do not report these transient symptoms to their physicians. In my experience, doctors often reassure patients that the spells are not important. This is most often the case with transient monocular blindness. When the nature of the spells is correctly identified, treatment often involves overzealous carotid artery surgery or automatic prescription of the latest panacea for ischemic stroke (i.e., warfarin, vasodilators, and aspirin). Thoughtful and thorough evaluation of the cause in the individual patient followed by treatment of the specific abnormalities found are the exceptions, not the rule.

Oral Contraceptive Use

Perhaps the most controversial of all the putative stroke risk factors is the use of oral contraceptives. The American Heart Association Committee on Risk Factors in Stroke could not agree in 1984 on whether the use of oral contraceptives was an independent risk factor and, if it was, to what degree.[8] Retrospective case studies do suggest that oral contraceptive use conveys a four- to 13-fold increase in the risk of cerebral infarction.[8,74,112–114] Hypertension, migraine, diabetes, hyperlipidemia, cigarette smoking, age older than 35 years, and prolonged use of oral contraceptive pills compound the risk of ischemic stroke in oral contraceptive users.[8] Some evidence also indicates that oral contraceptives may also slightly increase the risk for SAH, especially in women who smoke cigarettes.[24,115,116]

Most of the data on the relationship between stroke and oral contraceptives are in patients who use pills with a relatively high estrogen content (50 μg of ethinyl estradiol or estranes). Lower-dose estrogen (20–40 μg of ethinyl estradiol) combined with newer progestational drugs are now usually prescribed as oral contraceptive agents. These low-dose estrogen pills have much less tendency to predispose to venous and arterial thromboses. Some studies show that young women who take these lower-dose pills do not have an important increased risk of stroke.[117–121] Among users of low-dose contraceptives, strokes most often occur in older women who have other stroke risk factors, such as age, hypertension, and cigarette smoking.[121] Genetics also probably plays a role, but this has been inadequately explored. Patients with prothrombin gene mutations have an increased risk of stroke when they take oral contraceptives.[122] The presence of factor V Leiden; prothrombin gene mutations; other causes of resistance to activated protein C; abnormalities of antithrombin III, protein C, and protein S; and other genetic-related disorders of coagulation proteins might make women who take oral contraceptives or smoke cigarettes especially susceptible to thrombosis.

The influence of female hormones on stroke frequency and subtypes has also been explored by studies on pregnancy and stroke. Women with six or more pregnancies are at a higher risk for stroke and cerebral infarction than women who have had fewer pregnancies.[123] One study showed that the risk of stroke was not increased during pregnancy, but the risk of brain infarction and brain hemorrhage were significantly increased during the 6 weeks after delivery.[124] The risk of cerebral venous thrombosis is especially high during the puerperium.

Obesity

Obesity probably has an important role in atherogenesis. Being considerably overweight increases the frequency of associated hypertension, hyperlipidemia, glucose intolerance, and hyperinsulinemia. In the Honolulu Heart Program, elevated body mass was associated with an increased risk of thromboembolic stroke in nonsmoking men aged 55–68 years who did not have other stroke risk factors.[125] Obesity increases the risk of coronary and other heart diseases[126,127] and increases the risk of cardiogenic brain embolism.

Lack of Exercise

During the 1990s, the effect of physical activity and exercise has been given attention in relation to cardiovascular disease. In a study of 7,735 British middle-aged men, regular, moderate-degree physical activity reduced the risk of stroke and heart attacks, but more vigorous physical activity did not confer any further protection.[128] Similarly, in the North Manhattan Stroke Study,[129] Copenhagen City Heart Study,[130] Reykjavik (Iceland) Study,[131] and patients in Seoul Korea,[132] participation in at least moderate-degree physical activity had a protective effect against stroke when compared with individuals who did not exercise regularly. This finding was true for men and women. Lee and Paffenbarger studied the relationship between physical activity (walking, climbing stairs, sports participation, and recreational physical activities) and stroke risk among 11,130 men who were Harvard University alumni.[133] They found that decreased stroke risk was found at energy expenditures of 1,000–1,999 kcal per week, with further decrements found at 2,000–2,999 kcal per week. Higher rates of exercise did not further decrease the risk of stroke.[133] In the Physicians Health Study among 21,823 male physicians, regular exercise that was vigorous enough to produce a sweat was associated with a decreased stroke risk.[134] The authors of this study posited that the effect of exercise was mediated through a salutary effect on weight, blood pressure, blood lipids, and glucose tolerance.[134] In two prospective studies, the risk for subsequent development of hypertension was much lower in individuals who performed vigorous exercise.[135,136] Less vigorous exercise (i.e., walking to work) decreased the risk for hypertension among 6,017 Japanese men studied in the Osaka Health Survey.[137]

Geographic Location

In the United States, physicians and epidemiologists have long been aware of a so-called "stroke belt." This region of high incidence of stroke and stroke mortality is located within the southeastern portion of the United States, with extreme mortality rates in Georgia and the Carolinas.[138–140] Clusters of regions with high stroke-mortality rates also exist along the Mississippi and Ohio river valleys.[138] Residence within these regions conveys to men and women of all races a strikingly higher rate of stroke than in other locations within the United States.[139] The reason for the presence of such a stroke belt remains mostly obscure, but many factors, such as the genetic makeup of the people; distribution of stroke risk factors, including hypertension and cigarette smoking; dietary habits; and even the constituents of the water have been posited.

Factors Determined by Blood and Urine Tests and Genetically Determined Conditions

Results of blood tests of certain factors also correlate with the probability of an individual developing a stroke. Pathologically elevated and high normal hematocrits have been associated with increased stroke and TIA risk even when hypertension and cigarette smoking are considered.[141,142] Higher hemoglobin levels are also correlated with the presence of brain infarction[143] and larger brain infarcts.[144] This correlation might be partly caused by the fact that chronic hypoxemia, pulmonary disease, and smoking may have caused high hematocrits. The adverse effect of high hematocrits could also relate to increased whole-blood viscosity.[144,145]

The plasma level of fibrinogen is also an important determinant of stroke risk. Studies have shown that individuals with high levels of fibrinogen have an increased risk of developing myocardial infarction and stroke.[146–148] Fibrinogen levels relate to age, sex, female hormone status, smoking, body weight, alcohol intake, and the presence of vascular and inflammatory diseases.[147] Fibrinogen is an important participant in the development of red and white thrombi. Along with the hematocrit, fibrinogen is an important determinant of whole blood viscosity.[149,150] Abnormalities in the fibrinolytic system (plasma levels of tissue plasminogen activator and plasma activator inhibitor), which produce acquired hypofibrinolysis, also increase the risk of developing ischemic stroke.[148] Because of increased or decreased blood clotting, abnormalities of the serine protein components of the coagulation cascade increase the risk of ischemic stroke and brain hemorrhage. Many of the disorders of the coagulation system are genetically determined. These genetic disorders may interact with behavioral factors, such as cigarette smoking and the use of oral contraceptives, to compound the risk of stroke.[122]

Convincing data show that elevated levels of plasma homocysteine substantially increase the risk of developing myocardial infarction and stroke.[151–153] High plasma homocysteine levels and low concentrations of folic acid and vitamin B_6 (probably because of their role in homocysteine metabolism) are associated with increased risk of carotid artery atherosclerosis in elderly individuals.[154]

Glycosuria and heavy proteinuria predispose to stroke. Even relatively small amounts of protein in the urine may be a risk factor for stroke. In a study of 186 older men and women (average age, 65 years), the presence of microalbuminuria (20–200 mg/liter) was three times more prevalent in patients with recent stroke when compared with normal, healthy individuals and individuals with risk factors for stroke who did not have a recent stroke.[155] One study showed that intensive, multifactorial, therapeutic interventions in patients with non–insulin-dependent diabetes and microalbuminuria did decrease the incidence of macrovascular events (myocardial infarcts and stroke).[156]

Some genetic disorders, such as Fabry's disease, homocystinuria, Ehlers-Danlos syndrome, and pseudoxanthoma elasticum, are recognized to confer increased stroke risk. Other specific disorders, such as CADASIL (*c*erebral *a*utosomal *d*ominant *a*rteriopathy with *s*ubcortical *i*nfarcts and *l*eukoencephalopathy) and MELAS syndrome (*m*itochondrial *m*yopathy, *e*ncephalopathy, *l*actic *a*cidosis, and *s*troke-like episodes), are genetically determined. I discuss these disorders in Chapter 11. Research on genetic determinants of atherosclerosis, hypertension, stroke, and other vascular disease is progressing at a rapid rate. This progression gives promise for unlocking some of the present mysteries and uncertainties about stroke development, especially among the young.[157]

Stroke Prevention

Prevention is usually separated into primary prevention (strategies to prevent stroke in patients who have never had a stroke) and secondary prevention (strategies to prevent a stroke recurrence).

Primary Prevention

For primary prevention, I favor public education. Improvement in general health practices in the population undoubtedly decreases modifiable stroke risk factors in many patients. Educating the public in general to implement good general health measures probably would have a large impact on the frequency of stroke and other cardiovascular disease. The public should be encouraged to stop smoking, avoid excessive alcohol intake, exercise regularly, make time for leisure activities, avoid becoming overweight, and decrease intake of foods high in fat and cholesterol. The risk of stroke, however, varies greatly among different individuals and depends heavily on individual factors present in each person. For example, some individuals can eat large quantities of eggs, milk, ice cream, and red meat and still have quite normal serum cholesterol and lipid values, whereas in others, simply smelling foods high in cholesterol seems to send their cholesterol levels skyrocketing. I have already emphasized the importance of hereditary diseases in the family. I believe that each individual should become aware of the cardiovascular disorders and stroke and heart disease risk factors prevalent in their families. Periodic check-ups with physicians who monitor blood pressure, weight, blood sugar and lipid levels, and who inquire about habits and health practices are important. This strategy is especially important for the children of patients who have had a myocardial infarct, stroke, or important stroke risk factors, such as hypertension, diabetes, and hypercholesterolemia.

When multiple risk factors are considered together, patients at particular risk for stroke can be identified. When systolic hypertension, elevated serum cholesterol, glucose intolerance, cigarette smoking, and electrocardiogram findings of left ventricular hypertrophy are combined, a population accounting for one-third of the strokes can be identified.[71] Wolf and his colleagues have created a stroke risk-factor score based on data obtained from the Framingham Study, which reflects an individual's 10-year probability of having a stroke.[158,159] This scoring system and the 10-year stroke probabilities for middle-aged men and women are shown in Tables 18-1 and 18-2.

Secondary Prevention

For secondary stroke prevention, identification of the mechanism of the initial stroke is most important. In patients who have lacunar infarcts caused by penetrating artery disease due to hypertension and in patients who have hypertensive ICHs, control of blood pressure is the most important strategy. In patients with severe carotid artery stenosis, surgery or angioplasty of the involved carotid artery may be the best strategy for secondary prevention. In patients with nonstenosing plaques, β-hydroxyl-β-methyglutaryl-coenzyme A reductase inhibitors and an agent that decreases platelet functions, such as aspirin, clopidogrel, or combined low-dose aspirin and modified release dipyridamole, are probably most effective. In patients who have had brain embolism caused by atrial fibrillation, anticoagulation with coumadin represents the best strategy for secondary stroke prevention unless contraindications to the use of coumadin are present. In the majority of patients, recurrent strokes are caused by the same mechanism as the initial stroke.[160] Sometimes, second and third strokes, however, have a different stroke mechanism than the initial stroke.[160–162] For example, some patients with atrial fibrillation also have hypertension and carotid artery disease. Their initial stroke may have been caused by their carotid artery disease, but atrial fibrillation poses a threat for brain embolism. The results of the North American Symptomatic Carotid Endarterectomy Trial, which included patients with various severities of carotid artery occlusive disease and excluded patients with cardiac lesions thought to carry high risk of cardioembolism, found that a significant number of strokes were caused by cardioembolism and penetrating artery disease.[162] Identification of all stroke risk factors by thorough cardiac, cerebrovascular, and blood evaluations at the time of the initial stroke allows factors and lesions present in the individual to be recognized and creates a database for the logical selection of strategies for secondary prevention of stroke and myocardial infarction.[161] Even when stroke has already occurred, treatment of identifiable stroke risk factors, such as hypertension, was shown in one study to decrease the expected mortality and stroke recurrence rate during the 5 years after the first stroke.[163]

The incidence of stroke is declining, but much more can be done. Advances will probably involve the following:

1. Improved general health measures initiated by individuals concerned about their bodies—A reduction in cardiopulmonary disease clearly lowers the incidence of stroke.
2. Education for patients regarding the symptoms and significance of hypertension and TIAs—Patients should become educated consumers who recognize and seek the most competent care.
3. Education for the public about the brain and symptoms that might indicate stroke and other brain diseases.

Table 18-1. Probability of Stroke within 10 Years for Men Ages 55–84 Years and Free of Prior Stroke

Risk Factors						Points					
	0	1	2	3	4	5	6	7	8	9	10
Age (yrs)	54–56	57–59	60–62	63–65	66–68	69–71	72–74	75–77	78–80	81–83	84–86
Syst BP	95–105	106–116	117–126	127–137	138–148	149–159	160–170	171–181	182–191	192–202	203–213
Hyp Rx	No	—	Yes	—	—	—	—	—	—	—	—
DM	No	—	Yes	—	—	—	—	—	—	—	—
Smoking	No	—	—	Yes	—	—	—	—	—	—	—
CVD	No	—	—	Yes	—	—	—	—	—	—	—
AF	No	—	—	—	Yes	—	—	—	—	—	—
LVH	No	—	—	—	—	—	Yes	—	—	—	—

Total Points	10-Yr Probability (%)	Total Points	10-Yr Probability (%)
1	2.6	16	22.4
2	3	17	25.5
3	3.5	18	29
4	4	19	32.9
5	4.7	20	37.1
6	5.4	21	41.7
7	6.3	22	46.6
8	7.3	23	51.8
9	8.4	24	57.3
10	9.7	25	62.8
11	11.2	26	68.4
12	12.9	27	73.8
13	14.8	28	79
14	17	29	83.7
15	19.5	30	87.9

AF = history of atrial fibrillation; CVD = history of claudication, congestive heart failure, myocardial infarct, angina pectoris, or coronary insufficiency; DM = diabetes mellitus; Hyp Rx = presently on antihypertensive therapy; LVH = left ventricular hypertrophy on electrocardiogram; Syst BP = systolic blood pressure.
Source: Reprinted with permission from PA Wolff, AJ Belanger, RB D'Agostino. Quantifying stroke risk factors and potentials for risk reduction. Cerebrovasc Dis 1993;(Suppl 1):7–14.

4. Education of general physicians—Physicians should know about the warning signs of stroke, stroke risk factors, and how to manage cerebrovascular disease.
5. Education of neurologists, vascular surgeons, neurosurgeons, and other stroke specialists— These specialists should know when and how to manage risk factors, as well as how to treat the presenting stroke problem.
6. Research—Advance the present capabilities for diagnosing and treating stroke patients and stroke-prone individuals.

References

1. Pasteur L. Address to the Fraternal Association of former students of the École Centrale des Arts et Manufactures, Paris, May 15, 1884.
2. American Heart Association, San Francisco Chapter. San Francisco Public Awareness Survey: Study 62202. San Francisco: Opinion Research Corporation, 1984.
3. American Heart Association. Stroke Awareness Study. Dallas: SRI Research Center, 1985.
4. Kothari R, Sauerbeck L, Jauch E, et al. Patients' awareness of stroke signs, symptoms, and risk factors. Stroke 1997;28:1871–1875.
5. Garraway WM, Whisnant JP, Furlan AJ, et al. The declining incidence of stroke. N Engl J Med 1979;300:449–452.

Table 18-2. Probability of Stroke within 10 Years for Women Ages 55–84 Years and Free of Prior Stroke

Risk Factors	Points										
	0	1	2	3	4	5	6	7	8	9	10
Age (yrs)	54–56	57–59	60–62	63–65	66–68	69–71	72–74	75–77	78–80	81–83	84–86
Syst BP	95–104	105–114	115–124	125–134	135–144	145–154	155–164	165–174	175–184	185–194	195–204
Hyp Rx	No	If yes, see below*									
DM	No	—	—	Yes	—	—	—	—	—	—	—
Smoking	No	—	—	Yes	—	—	—	—	—	—	—
CVD	No	—	Yes	—	—	—	—	—	—	—	—
AF	No	—	—	—	—	—	Yes	—	—	—	—
LVH	No	—	—	—	Yes	—	—	—	—	—	—

Total Points	10-Yr Probability (%)	Total Points	10-Yr Probability (%)
1	1.1	15	16
2	1.3	16	19.1
3	1.6	17	22.8
4	2	18	27
5	2.4	19	31.9
6	2.9	20	37.3
7	3.5	21	43.4
8	4.3	22	50
9	5.2	23	57
10	6.3	24	64.2
11	7.6	25	71.4
12	9.2	26	78.2
13	11.1	27	84.4
14	13.3		

AF = history of atrial fibrillation; CVD = history of claudication, congestive heart failure, myocardial infarct, angina pectoris, or coronary insufficiency; DM = diabetes mellitus; Hyp Rx = presently on antihypertensive therapy; LVH = left ventricular hypertrophy on electrocardiogram; Syst BP = systolic blood pressure.

*If under hypertensive therapy, add points depending on systolic blood pressure.

Source: Reprinted with permission from PA Wolff, AJ Belanger, RB D'Agostino. Quantifying stroke risk factors and potentials for risk reduction. Cerebrovasc Dis 1993;(Suppl 1):7–14.

6. Bonita R, Stewart A, Beaglehole R. International trends in stroke mortality: 1970–1985. Stroke 1990;21:989–992.
7. Sytkowski PA, Kannel WB, D'Agostino RB. Changes in risk factors and the decline in mortality from cardiovascular disease. N Engl J Med 1990;322:1635–1641.
8. Wolf P, Dyken M, Barnett HJM, et al. Risk factors in stroke. Stroke 1984;15:1105–1111.
9. Shaper AG, Phillips AN, Pocock SJ, et al. Risk factors for stroke in middle aged British men. BMJ 1991;302:1111–1115.
10. Matchar DB, McCrory DC, Barnett HJM, Feussner JR. Medical treatment for stroke prevention. Ann Intern Med 1994;121:41–53.
11. Bronner LL. Kanter DS, Manson JE. Primary prevention of stroke. N Engl J Med 1995;333:1392–1400.
12. Kalra L, Perez I, Melbourn A. Stroke risk management. Change in mainstream practice. Stroke 1998;29:53–57.
13. Gorelick PB, Sacco RL, Smith DB, et al. Prevention of a first stroke. A review of guidelines and a multidisciplinary consensus statement from the National Stroke Association. JAMA 1999;281:1112–1120.
14. Whisnant JP. Stroke populations, cohorts, and clinical trials. Boston: Butterworth–Heinemann, 1993.
15. Dorndorf W, Marx P. Stroke prevention. Basel: Karger, 1994.
16. Norris JW, Hachinski VC. Prevention of Stroke. New York: Springer, 1991.

17. Sobel E, Altu M, Davanipour Z, et al. Stroke in the Lehigh Valley: combined risk factors for recurrent ischemic stroke. Neurology 1989;39:669–672.

18. Dennis MS, Bamford JM, Sandercock PA, Warlow CD. A comparison of risk factors and prognosis for transient ischemic attacks and minor ischemic strokes. Stroke 1989; 20:1494–1499.

19. Davis PH, Dambrosia JM, Schoenberg BS, et al. Risk factors for ischemic stroke: a prospective study in Rochester, Minnesota. Ann Neurol 1987;22:319–327.

20. Simons LA, McCallum J, Friedlander Y, Simons J. Risk factors for ischemic stroke. Dubbo study of the elderly. Stroke 1998;29:1341–1346.

21. Whisnant JP, Wiebers DO, O'Fallon WM, et al. A population-based model of risk factors for ischemic stroke: Rochester, Minnesota. Neurology 1996;47:1420–1428.

22. Sacco RL. Risk factors, outcomes, and stroke subtypes for ischemic stroke. Neurology 1997;49(Suppl 4):S39–S44.

23. Sacco RL. Ischemic Stroke. In PB Gorelick, M Alter (eds), Handbook of Neuroepidemiology. New York: Marcel Dekker, 1994;77–121.

24. Longstreth WT, Koepsell T, Yerby M, et al. Risk factors for subarachnoid hemorrhage. Stroke 1985;16:377–385.

25. Teunissen LL, Rinkel GJE, Algra A, van Gijn J. Risk factors for subarachnoid hemorrhage. A systematic review. Stroke 1996;27:544–549.

26. Longstreth WT. Nontraumatic Subarachnoid Hemorrhage. In PB Gorelick, M Alter (eds), Handbook of Neuroepidemiology. New York: Marcel Dekker, 1994;123–140.

27. Broderick JP. Intracerebral Hemorrhage. In Gorelick PB, Alter M (eds), Handbook of Neuroepidemiology. New York: Marcel Dekker, 1994;141–167.

28. Caplan LR. Brain Embolism. In Caplan LR, Hurst JW, Chimowitz M (eds), Clinical Neurocardiology. New York: Marcel Dekker, 1999;35–185.

29. Gorelick PB, Caplan LR, Hier DB, et al. Racial differences in the distribution of anterior circulation occlusive cerebrovascular disease. Neurology 1984;34:54–59.

30. Gorelick PB, Caplan LR, Hier DB, et al. Racial differences in the distribution of posterior circulation occlusive disease. Stroke 1985;16:785–790.

31. Caplan LR. Race, sex, and occlusive cerebrovascular disease: a review. Stroke 1986;17:648–655.

32. Caplan LR. Cerebral Ischemia and Infarction in Blacks. Clinical, Autopsy, and Angiographic Studies. In RF Gillum, PB Gorelick, ES Cooper (eds), Stroke in Blacks. Basel: Karger, 1999;7–18.

33. Kannel WB. Current status of the epidemiology of brain infarction associated with occlusive vascular disease. Stroke 1971;2:295–318.

34. Gebel J, Broderick J. Primary Intracerebral Hemorrhage and Subarachnoid Hemorrhage in Black Patients: Risk Factors, Diagnosis, and Prognosis. In RF Gillum, PB Gorelick, ES Cooper (eds), Stroke in Blacks. Basel: Karger, 1999;29–35.

35. Kiely DK, Wolf PA, Cupples LA, et al. Family aggregation of stroke: the Framingham Study. Stroke 1993;24:1366–1371.

36. Liao D, Myers R, Hunt S, et al. Family history of stroke and stroke risk. The Family Heart Study. Stroke 1997;28: 1908–1912.

37. Wannamethee SG, Shaper AG, Ebrahim S. History of parental death from stroke or heart trouble and the risk of stroke in middle-aged men. Stroke 1996;27:1492–1498.

38. Jousilahri P, Rastenyte D, Tuomilehto J, et al. Parental history of cardiovascular disease and risk of stroke. A prospective follow-up of 14,371 middle-aged men and women in Finland. Stroke 1997;28:1361–1366.

39. Kannel WB, Wolf PA, Verter J, et al. Epidemiologic assessment of the role of blood pressure in stroke: the Framingham study. JAMA 1970;214:301–310.

40. Whisnant JP. Epidemiology of stroke: emphasis on transient cerebral ischemic attacks and hypertension. Stroke 1974;5:68–75.

41. Kannel WB. Blood pressure as a cardiovascular risk factor. Prevention and treatment. JAMA 1996;275:1571–1576.

42. Howard G, Manolio TA, Burke GL et al. Does the association of risk factors and atherosclerosis change with age? Stroke 1997;28:1693–1701.

43. Wenger NK. Hypertension and other cardiovascular risk factors in women. Am J Hypertens 1995;8:94S–99S.

44. SHEP Cooperative Research Group. Prevention of stroke by antihypertensive drug treatment in older persons with isolated systolic hypertension. JAMA 1991;265:3255–3264.

45. Sutton-Tyrrell K, Alcorn HG, Herzog H, et al. Morbidity, mortality, and antihypertensive treatment effects by extent of atherosclerosis in older adults with isolated systolic hypertension. Stroke 1995;26:1319–1324.

46. Davis BR, Vogt T, Frost PH, et al. Risk factors for stroke and type of stroke in persons with isolated systolic hypertension. The Systolic Hypertension in the Elderly Program (SHEP) Research Group. Stroke 1998;29:1333–1340.

47. Management Committee. The Australian therapeutic trial in mild hypertension. Lancet 1980;1:1261–1267.

48. Taguchi J, Faris E. Partial reduction of blood pressure and prevention of complications in hypertension. N Engl J Med 1974;29:329–331.

49. Veterans Administration Cooperative Study Group on Antihypertensive Agents. Effect of treatment on morbidity in hypertension: I. Results in patients with diastolic blood pressures averaging 115 through 129 mm Hg. JAMA 1969; 202:1028.

50. Veterans Administration Cooperative Study Group on Antihypertensive Agents. Effects of treatment on morbidity in hypertension: II. Results in patients with diastolic blood pressures averaging 90 through 114 mm Hg. JAMA 1970;213:1143–1152.

51. Spence JD. Antihypertensive drugs and prevention of atherosclerotic stroke. Stroke 1986;17:808–810.

52. Watanabe N, Imai Y, Nagai K, et al. Nocturnal blood pressure and silent cerebrovascular lesions in elderly Japanese. Stroke 1996;27:1319–1327.

53. Yamamoto Y, Akiguchi I, Oiwa K, et al. Adverse effect of nighttime blood pressure on the outcome of lacunar infarct patients. Stroke 1998;29:570–576.

54. Feinberg WM, Blackshear JL, Laupacis A, et al. Prevalence, age distribution, and gender of patients with atrial fibrillation. Arch Intern Med 1995;155:469–473.

55. Toole FJ, Janeway R, Choi K, et al. Transient ischemic attacks due to atherosclerosis: a prospective study of 160 patients. Arch Neurol 1975;32:5–12.

56. Chimowitz MI, Weiss DG, Cohen SL, et al. Veterans Affairs Cooperative Study Group 167. Cardiac prognosis of patients with carotid stenosis and no history of coronary artery disease. Stroke 1994;25:759–765.

57. Chimowitz MI. Asymptomatic Coronary Artery Disease in Patients with Carotid Artery Stenosis: Incidence, Prognosis, and Treatment. In LR Caplan, JW Hurst, M Chimowitz (eds), Clinical Neurocardiology. New York: Marcel Dekker, 1999;287–295.

58. Schoenberg BS, Schoenberg DG, Pritchard DA, et al. Differential risk factors for completed stroke and transient ischemic attack (TIA): study of vascular disease (hypertension, cardiac disease, peripheral vascular disease) and diabetes mellitus. Trans Am Neurol Assoc 1980;105:165–167.

59. Burchfiel CM, Curb D, Rodriguez B, et al. Glucose intolerance and 22-year stroke incidence. The Honolulu Heart Program. Stroke 1994;25:951–957.

60. Jorgenson H, Nakayama H, Raaschou HO, Olsen TS. Stroke in patients with diabetes. The Copenhagen Stroke Study. Stroke 1994;25:1977–1984.

61. Toyry JP, Niskanen LK, Lansimies EA, et al. Autonomic neuropathy predicts the development of stroke in patients with non-insulin dependent diabetes mellitus. Stroke 1996;27:1316–1318.

62. Lehto S, Niskanen L, Ronnemaa T, Laakso M. Serum uric acid is a strong predictor of stroke in patients with non-insulin-dependent diabetes mellitus. Stroke 1998;29:635–639.

63. Caplan LR. Intracranial branch atheromatous disease: a neglected, understudied, and underused concept. Neurology 1989;39:1246–1250.

64. Caplan LR. Diabetes and brain ischemia. Diabetes 1996;45(Suppl 3):595–597.

65. Higa M, Davanipour Z. Smoking and stroke. Neuroepidemiology 1991;10:211–222.

66. Love BB, Biller J, Jones MP, et al. Cigarette smoking: a risk factor for cerebral infarction in young adults. Arch Neurol 1990;47:693–698.

67. Whisnant JP, Homer D, Ingall TJ, et al. Duration of cigarette smoking is the strongest predictor of severe extracranial carotid artery atherosclerosis. Stroke 1990;21:707–714.

68. Ingall TJ, Homer D, Baker HL, et al. Predictors of intracranial carotid artery atherosclerosis: duration of cigarette smoking and hypertension are more powerful than serum lipid levels. Arch Neurol 1991;48:687–691.

69. Colditz GA, Bonita R, Stampfer MJ, et al. Cigarette smoking and risk of stroke in middle-aged women. N Engl J Med 1988;318:937–941.

70. Donnan GA, You R, Thrift A, McNeil JJ. Smoking as a risk factor for stroke. Cerebrovasc Dis 1993;3:129–138.

71. Wolf P, Kannel WB, Verter J. Current Status of Risk Factors for Stroke. In HJM Barnett (ed), Neurologic Clinics, Vol 1. Cerebrovascular Disease. Philadelphia: Saunders, 1983;317–343.

72. Paffenbarger R, Williams J. Chronic disease in former college students: V. Early precursors of fatal stroke. Am J Public Health 1967;57:1290–1299.

73. Kawachi I, Colditz GA. Smoking cessation and decreased risk of stroke in women. JAMA 1993;269:232–236.

74. Collaborative Group for the Study of Stroke in Young Women. Oral contraceptives and stroke in young women: associated risk factors. JAMA 1975;231:718–722.

75. Tell GS, Crouse JR, Furberg CD. Relation between blood lipids, lipoproteins, and cerebrovascular atherosclerosis. A review. Stroke 1988;19:423–430.

76. Kannel WB. Epidemiology of Cerebrovascular Disease. In RW Ross-Russel (ed), Cerebral Arterial Disease. New York: Churchill Livingstone, 1976;1–23.

77. Kagan A, Popper J, Rhoads G. Factors related to stroke incidence in Hawaiian Japanese men: the Honolulu heart study. Stroke 1980;11:14–21.

78. Stemmerman G, Hayashi T, Resch J, et al. Risk factors related to ischemic and hemorrhagic cerebrovascular disease at autopsy: the Honolulu heart study. Stroke 1984;15: 23–28.

79. Iso H, Jacobs DR, Wentworth D, et al. Serum cholesterol levels and six year mortality from stroke in 350,977 men screened for the multiple risk factor intervention trial. N Engl J Med 1989;320:904–910.

80. Yano K, Reed DM, Maclean CJ. Serum cholesterol and hemorrhagic stroke in the Honolulu Heart Program. Stroke 1989;20:1460–1465.

81. Tanne D, Yaari S, Goldbourt U. High-density lipoprotein cholesterol and risk of ischemic stroke mortality. A 21-year follow-up of 8586 men from Israeli Ischemic Heart Disease Study. Stroke 1997;28:83–87.

82. Steinberg D, Parthasarthy S, Carcio TE, et al. Beyond cholesterol: modification of low-density lipoprotein that increases its atherogenicity. N Engl J Med 1989;320:915.

83. Scanu A, Lawn RM, Berg K. Lipoprotein (a) and atherosclerosis. Ann Intern Med 1991;115:209–218.

84. Pedro-Botet J, Senti M, Nogues X, et al. Lipoprotein and apolipoprotein profile in men with ischemic stroke. Role of lipoprotein (a), triglyceride-rich lipoproteins, and apolipoprotein E polymorphism. Stroke 1992;23:1556–1562.

85. Wilt TJ, Rubins HB, Robins SJ, et al. Carotid atherosclerosis in men with low levels of HDL cholesterol. Stroke 1997;28:1919–1925.

86. Homer D, Ingall TJ, Baber HL, et al. Serum lipids and lipoproteins are less powerful predictors of extracranial carotid artery atherosclerosis than are cigarette smoking and hypertension. Mayo Clin Proc 1991;66:259–267.

87. Bucher HC, Griffith LE, Guyatt GH. Effect of HMGCoA reductase inhibitors on stroke. A meta-analysis of randomized controlled trials. Ann Intern Med 1998;128:89–95.

88. Gorelick PB. The status of alcohol as a risk factor for stroke. Stroke 1989;20:1607–1610.

89. Hillborn M, Kaste M. Alcohol intoxication: a risk factor for primary subarachnoid hemorrhage. Neurology 1982; 32:706–711.

90. Kagan A, Yano K, Rhoads G, et al. Alcohol and cardiovascular disease: the Hawaiian experience. Circulation 1981; 64(Suppl 3):27–31.

91. Bogousslausky J, Van Melle G, Despland PA, Regli F. Alcohol consumption and carotid atherosclerosis in the Lausanne stroke registry. Stroke 1990;21:715–720.

92. Palomaki H, Kaste M. Regular light-to-moderate intake of alcohol and the risk of ischemic stroke. Stroke 1993; 24:1828–1832.

93. Kiechi S, Willeit J, Rungger G, et al. Alcohol consumption and atherosclerosis: what is the relation. Prospective results from the Bruneck Study. Stroke 1998;29:900–907.

94. Gorelick PB, Rodin MB, Langenberg P, et al. Is acute alcohol ingestion a risk factor for ischemic stroke? Stroke 1987;18:359–364.

95. Gorelick PB, Rodin MB, Langengerg P, et al. Weekly alcohol consumption, cigarette smoking, and the risk of ischemic stroke. Neurology 1989;39:339–343.

96. Truelsen T, Gronbaek M, Schnohr P, Boysen G. Intake of beer, wine, and spirits and risk of stroke. The Copenhagen Heart Study. Stroke 1998;29:2467–2472.

97. Hertog MG, Feskens EJ, Hollman PC, et al. Dietary antioxidant flavonoids and risk of coronary heart disease. Lancet 1993;342:1007–1011.

98. Frankel EN, Kanner J, German JB, et al. Inhibition of oxidation of human low-density lipoproteins by phenolic substances in red wine. Lancet 1993;341:454–457.

99. Hillbom M, Haapaniemi H, Juvela S, et al. Recent alcohol consumption, cigarette smoking, and cerebral infarction in young adults. Stroke 1995;26:40–45.

100. Nicolaides A, Kalodicki E, Ramaswami G, et al. The Significance of Cerebral Infarcts on CT Scans in Patients with Transient Ischemic Attacks. In EF Bernstein, AD Callow, AN Nicolaides, EG Shifrin (eds), Cerebral Revascularisation. London: Med-Orion, 1993;159–178.

101. Caplan LR. Significance of Unexpected (Silent) Brain Infarcts. In LR Caplan, EG Shifrin, AN Nicolaides, WS Moore (eds), Cerebrovascular Ischaemia. Investigation and Management. London, Med-Orion, 1996;423–433.

102. Nicolaides AN. Asymptomatic Carotid Stenosis and the Risk of Stroke (the ACSRS Study); Identification of a High Risk Group. In LR Caplan, EG Shifrin, AN Nicolaides, WS Moore (eds), Cerebrovascular Ischaemia. Investigation and Management. London: Med-Orion, 1996;435–441.

103. Wityk RJ, Chang H-M, Rosengart A, et al. Proximal extracranial vertebral artery disease in the New England Medical Center Posterior Circulation Registry. Arch Neurol 1998;55:470–478.

104. Caplan LR. Posterior Circulation Disease. Clinical Findings, Diagnosis, and Management. Boston: Blackwell, 1996.

105. Criqui MH. Peripheral arterial disease and subsequent cardiovascular mortality: a strong and consistent association. Circulation 1990;82:2246–2247.

106. Criqui MH, Langer RD, Fronek A, et al. Mortality over a period of 10 years in patients with peripheral arterial disease. N Engl J Med 1992;326:381–386.

107. Caplan LR. Are terms such as completed stroke or RIND of continued usefulness? Stroke 1983;14:431–433.

108. Caplan LR. TIAs: we need to return to the question, "What is wrong with Mr. Jones?" Neurology 1988;38:791–793.

109. Waxman S, Toole J. Temporal profile resembling TIA in the setting of cerebral infarction. Stroke 1983;14:433–437.

110. Nicolaides A, Zukowski A. The Place of Computerized Tomographic Brain Scanning in the Classification of Ischemic Cerebral Disease. In R Courbier (ed), Basis for a Classification of Cerebral Arterial Disease. Amsterdam: Excerpta Medica, 1985;59–64.

111. Adams HP, Kassell N, Mazuz H. The patient with transient ischemic attacks: is this the time for a new therapeutic approach? Stroke 1984;15:371–375.

112. Collaborative Group for the Study of Stroke in Young Women. Oral contraception and increased risk of cerebral ischemia or thrombosis. N Engl J Med 1973;288:871–878.

113. Handin R. Thromboembolic complications of pregnancy and oral contraceptives. Prog Cardiovasc Dis 1974;16:395–405.

114. Layde P, Beral V, Kay C. Further analyses of mortality in oral contraceptive users. Lancet 1981;1:541–546.

115. Longstreth WT Jr, Swanson PD. Oral contraceptives and stroke. Stroke 1984;15:747–750.

116. Johnston SC, Colford JM, Gress DR. Oral contraceptives and the risk of subarachnoid hemorrhage. A meta-analysis. Neurology 1998;51:411–418.

117. Lidegaard O, Kreiner S. Cerebral thrombosis and oral contraceptives: a case-control study. Contraception 1998;57:303–314.

118. Schwartz SM, Siscovick DS, Longstreth WT Jr, et al. Use of low-dose oral contraceptives and stroke in young women. Ann Intern Med 1997;127:596–603.

119. Petitti DB, Sidney S, Bernstein A, et al. Stroke in users of low-dose oral contraceptives. N Engl J Med 1996;335:8–15.

120. Schwartz SM, Petitti DB, Siscovick DS, et al. Stroke and use of low-dose oral contraceptives in young women. A pooled analysis of two U.S. studies. Stroke 1998;29:2277–2284.

121. Chasan-Taber L, Stampfer MJ. Epidemiology of oral contraceptives and cardiovascular disease. Ann Intern Med 1998;128:467–477.

122. Martinelli I, Sacchi E, Landi G, et al. High risk of cerebral-vein thrombosis in carriers of a prothrombin-gene mutation and in users of oral contraceptives. N Engl J Med 1998;338:1793–1797.

123. Qureshi A, Giles WH, Croft JB, Stern BJ. Number of pregnancies and risk for stroke and stroke subtypes. Arch Neurol 1997;54:203–206.

124. Kittner SJ, Stern BJ, Feeser BR, et al. Pregnancy and the risk of stroke. N Engl J Med 1996;335:768–774.

125. Abbott RD, Behrens GR, Sharp DS, et al. Body mass index and thromboembolic stroke in nonsmoking men in older middle age. The Honolulu Heart Program. Stroke 1994;25:2370–2376.

126. Hubert HB, Feinleib M, McNamara PM. Obesity as an independent risk factor for cardiovascular disease: a 26-year follow-up of participants in the Framingham Heart Study. Circulation 1983;67:768–777.

127. Donahue RP, Abbott RD, Bloom E, et al. Central obesity and coronary heart disease in men. Lancet 1987;1:821–824.

128. Wannamethee G, Shaper AG. Physical activity and stroke in middle-aged men. BMJ 1992;304:597–601.

129. Sacco RL, Gan R, Boden-Albala B, et al. Leisure-time physical activity and ischemic stroke risk. The Northern Manhattan Stroke Study. Stroke 1998;29:380–387.

130. Lindenstrom E, Boysen G, Nyboe J. Lifestyle factors and risk of cerebrovascular disease in women. The Copenhagen City Heart Study. Stroke 1993;24:1468–1472.

131. Agnarsson U, Thorgeirsson G, Sigvaldson H, Sigfusson N. Effects of leisure-time physical activity and ventilatory function on risk for stroke in men: the Reykjavik Study. Ann Intern Med 1999;130:987–990.

132. Choi-Kwon S, Kim JS. Lifestyle factors and risk of stroke in Seoul, South Korea. J Stroke Cerebrovasc Dis 1998;7:414–420.

133. Lee I-M, Paffenbarger RS Jr. Physical activity and stroke incidence. The Harvard Alumni health Study. Stroke 1998;29:2049–2054.

134. Lee I-M, Hennekens CH, Berger K, et al. Exercise and risk of stroke in male physicians. Stroke 1999;30:1–6.

135. Paffenbarger RS Jr, Wing AL, Hyde RT, Jung DL. Physical activity and incidence of hypertension in college alumni. Am J Epidemiol 1983;117:245–257.

136. Paffenbarger RS Jr, Jung DL, Leung RW, Hyde RT. Physical activity and hypertension, an epidemiological view. Ann Med 1991;23:319–327.

137. Hayashi T, Tsumura K, Suematsu C, et al. Walking to work and the risk of hypertension in men: the Osaka Health Survey, Ann Intern Med 1999;130:21–26.

138. Wing S, Casper M, Davis WB, et al. Stroke mortality maps. Stroke 1988;19:1507–1513.

139. Lanska DJ. Geographic distribution of stroke mortality in the United States: 1939–1941 to 1979–1981. Neurology 1993;43:1839–1851.

140. Lanska DJ, Kryscio R. Geographic distribution of hospitalization rates, case fatality, and mortality from stroke in the United States. Neurology 1994;44:1541–1550.

141. Toghi H, Yamanouchi H, Murakami M, et al. Importance of the hematocrit as a risk factor in cerebral infarction. Stroke 1978;9:369–374.

142. Harrison MJG, Pollock S, Thomas D, et al. Hematocrit, hypertension, and smoking in patients with transient ischemic attack and in age and sex matched controls. J Neurol Neurosurg Psychiatry 1982;45:550–551.

143. Di Mascio R, Marchioli R, Vitullo F, Tognoni G. A positive relation between high hemoglobin values and the risk of ischemic stroke. Progetto 3A investigators. Eur Neurol 1996;36:85–88.

144. Harrison MJG, Pollock S, Kendall B, et al. Effect of hematocrit on carotid stenosis and cerebral infarction. Lancet 1981;2:114–115.

145. Thomas DJ, Marshall J, Ross-Russel RW, et al. Effects of hematocrit on cerebral blood flow in man. Lancet 1977;2:940–943.

146. Wilhelmsen L, Svarrdsudd K, Korsan-Bengtsen K, et al. Fibrinogen as a risk factor for stroke and myocardial infarction. N Engl J Med 1984;311:501–505.

147. Drouet L. Fibrinogen: a treatable risk factor. Cerebrovasc Dis 1996;6(Suppl 1):2–6.

148. Kristensen B, Malm J, Nilsson T, et al. Increased fibrinogen levels and aquired hypofibrinolysis in young adults with ischemic stroke. Stroke 1998;29:2261–2267.

149. Grotta J, Ackerman R, Correia J, et al. Whole-blood viscosity parameters and cerebral blood flow. Stroke 1982;13:296–298.

150. Caplan LR. The Blood, Concluding Comments. In LR Caplan (ed), Brain Ischemia, Basic Concepts and Clinical Relevance. London: Springer-Verlag, 1995;121–126.

151. Graham IM, Daly LE, Refsum HM, et al. Plasma homocysteine as a risk factor for vascular disease. The European Concerted Action Project. JAMA 1997;277: 1775–1781.

152. Welch GN, Loscalzo J. Homocysteine and atherothrombosis. N Engl J Med 1998;338:1042–1050.

153. Giles WH, Croft JB, Greenlund KJ, et al. Total homocyst(e)ine concentration and the likelihood of nonfatal stroke. Results from the Third National Health and Nutrition Examination Survey, 1988–1994. Stroke 1998; 29:2473–2477.

154. Selhub J, Jacques PF, Bostom AG, et al. Association between plasma homocysteine concentrations and extracranial carotid-artery stenosis. N Engl J Med 1995;332:286–291.

155. Beamer NB, Coull BM, Clark WM, Wynn M. Microalbuminuria in ischemic stroke. Arch Neurol 1999;56:699–702.

156. Gaede P, Vedel P, Parving H-H, Pederson O. Intensified multifactorial intervention in patients with type 2 diabetes mellitus and micro-albuminuria: the Steno type 2 randomized study. Lancet 1999;353:617–622.

157. Alberts MJ. Genetics of Cerebrovascular Disease. Armonk, NY: Futura, 1999.

158. Wolf PA, D'Agostino RB, Belanger AJ, Kannel WB. Probability of stroke: a risk profile from the Framingham Study. Stroke 1991;22:312–318.

159. Wolff PA, Belanger AJ, D'Agostino RB. Quantifying stroke risk factors and potentials for risk reduction. Cerebrovasc Dis 1993;(Suppl 1):7–14.

160. Yamamoto H, Bogousslavsky J. Mechanisms of second and further strokes. J Neurol Neurosurg Psychiatry 1998; 64:771–776.

161. Caplan LR. Editorial. J Neurol Neurosurg Psychiatry 1998; 64:716.

162. Barnett HJM, Gunton RW, Eliasziw M, et al. North American Symptomatic Carotid Endarterectomy Trial (NASCET) Group. JAMA 2000 (in press).

163. Leonberg SC, Elliot FA. Prevention of recurrent stroke. Stroke 1981;12:731–735.

Chapter 19
Complications in Stroke Patients

Sometimes, the brain injury that develops during a stroke is not the only medical problem the patient, family, and doctor must battle. Strokes, like many other serious medical illnesses, can be followed by a host of other problems. These complications can sometimes cause neurologic deterioration; in other instances, the patient feels worse and the deterioration is falsely attributed to worsening of the stroke. Most of the complications that occur after stroke are medical and not neurologic. Complications are extremely common. In the Randomized Trial of Tirilazad Mesylate in Acute Stroke, 95% of the 279 stroke patients had at least one complication.[1] Complications may occur during hospitalization for acute stroke or may develop during rehabilitation and neurologic recovery. A number of reports and reviews discuss the various complications of stroke, frequencies of occurrence, and prevention and management.[1–7] Tables 19-1 and 19-2 list the frequency of various medical complications found in two series of stroke patients.[1,7]

Complications can be serious and cause death. The most common causes of death in patients with stroke are shown in Table 19-3. Brain edema, cardiac abnormalities, and pulmonary embolism dominate during the first week.[8] Pneumonia, urinary tract infections, bed sores, phlebothrombosis and pulmonary embolism, gastrointestinal bleeding, contractures, falls, osteopenia, and depression may develop during the first weeks. These problems may continue during recovery and even after patients return home. Randomized trials, analyses, and meta-analyses have all shown that units dedicated solely to the care of stroke patients decrease mortality and morbidity among stroke patients.[9–12] One important function of stroke units and stroke teams is to systematically pursue measures to monitor complications and prevent their occurrence.

Neurologic Complications

Stroke Progression or Recurrence

Deterioration of neurologic functions, including a decrease in the level of consciousness or progression of focal neurologic signs, develops in more than 25% of stroke patients.[6] In the majority of patients, this progression occurs during the first 24–72 hours and is much less common thereafter.[6,13,14] In patients with intracerebral hemorrhages, the deterioration is often caused by continued bleeding.[15–18] In patients with aneurysmal subarachnoid hemorrhage, rebleeding and vasoconstriction with delayed brain ischemia are most often responsible for neurologic deterioration during the 2 weeks after the initial bleed. Progression of brain ischemia is most common in patients with occlusions of large extracranial and intracranial arteries and those with lacunar infarcts. In patients with ischemic strokes, progression of brain ischemia is often related to propagation of thrombi, embolism, and failure of collateral circulation to develop adequately.

A second stroke may develop in the days and weeks after the initial stroke. This may occur while the patient is still in the acute hospital or during rehabilitation. Among 1,273 patients with brain infarcts entered in the Stroke Data Bank, 40 had a stroke recurrence during the 30 days after the index stroke.[19] The likelihood of recurrence depends heavily on the mechanism of the first stroke and

Table 19-1. Most Frequent Important Medical Events Among 279 Stroke Patients in the Control Limb of the Randomized Trial of Tirilazad Mesylate in Acute Stroke

Event	Serious (n)	%	Total (n)	Percentage
Sepsis	3	1	3	1
Cellulitis	2	1	5	2
Congestive heart failure	7	3	30	11
Cardiac arrest	5	2	5	2
Angina, myocardial infarct	4	1	16	6
Deep vein thrombosis	3	1	6	2
Pulmonary embolism	3	1	4	1
Peripheral vascular disorder	2	1	2	1
All pneumonias	13	5	27	10
Aspiration pneumonia alone	8	3	16	6
Dyspnea	3	1	11	4
Pulmonary edema	3	1	9	3
Gastrointestinal bleed	7	3	15	5
Dehydration	3	1	6	2
Hypoxia	2	1	8	3
Urinary tract infection	3	1	30	11

Source: Modified from KC Johnston, JY Li, PD Lyden, et al. Medical and neurological complications of ischemic stroke. Experience from the RANTTAS trial. Stroke 1998;29:447–453.

treatment. Recurrences are most likely to be caused by the same stroke mechanism as the index stroke.[20] Patients with cardiac-origin embolism are at the highest risk for having a second stroke, but different sources of emboli have different rates of recurrence.[21]

Brain Edema

The most lethal complication of stroke is brain edema after large ischemic and hemorrhagic strokes. In stroke units, brain edema, pulmonary embolism, and cardiac abnormalities are the major cause of early death.[6,9,22] An infarct is a rapidly evolving process, whereas brain edema not only varies with time, but also varies in severity in different areas within and surrounding the lesion.[23] The two main components of the edema are: (1) intracellular (cytotoxic) edema, which results from damage to the sodium-potassium pump with failure of the cell to maintain the normal osmotic gradient across its membrane; and (2) extracellular (vasogenic) edema with fluid occupying the interstitial spaces, especially at the edge of infarcts and hemorrhages.

Brain edema may begin within hours, but usually does not become clinically obvious until 1–4 days after the stroke. Ropper and Shafran analyzed the fluctuating clinical course of patients with stroke and brain edema.[24] During the acute presentation, patients were often drowsy. Usually, a subsequent improvement in the level of consciousness occurred and by the second or third day, patients were usually more alert. As brain edema increases, however, patients again become drowsy. In the series of Ropper and Shafran, drowsiness was not the only sign and was accompanied by one or more of the following[24]:

1. Pupillary asymmetry or lack of pupillary response to light—In most patients, the larger pupil was on the side ipsilateral to the brain infarct; pupillary asymmetry varied from 0.5 to 2.0 mm.
2. Periodic breathing patterns.
3. Sixth nerve paresis.
4. Extensor plantar responses on the previously spared side.
5. Papilledema.
6. Headache or vomiting.
7. Bilateral spontaneous extensor posturing.

Table 19-2. Number of Observed Medical Complications Among 100 Consecutive Stroke Patients During Rehabilitation

Medical Complication	Number
Urinary tract infection	44
Musculoskeletal pain	31
Urinary retention	25
Falls	25
Fungal rash	24
Hypotension	19
Diabetes mellitus	16
Hypertension	15
Cardiac arrhythmia	8
Pneumonia	7
Congestive heart failure	6
Angina pectoris	4
Myocardial infarct	0
Thrombophlebitis	4
Pulmonary embolism	0
Other complications	135
Total	**363**

Source: Reprinted with permission from A Dromerick, M Reding. Medical and neurological complications during in-patient stroke rehabilitation. Stroke 1994;25:358–361.

Table 19-3. Causes of Death in Stroke Patients with Supratentorial Lesions

Cause of Death	Infarction Week 1	Infarction Weeks 2–4	Hemorrhage Week 1	Hemorrhage Weeks 2–4
Transtentorial herniation	36	6	42	2
Pneumonia	0	28	1	2
Cardiac	7	17	0	2
Pulmonary embolism	0	4	0	0
Sudden death	2	8	0	0
Septicemia	1	4	0	0
Unknown	0	12	1	3
Brain stem extension (of hematoma)	—	—	1	1
Total	**46**	**79**	**45**	**10**

Source: Reprinted with permission from F Silver, JW Norris, A Lewis, V Hachinski. Early mortality following stroke: a prospective review. Stroke 1984;15:494.

The clinical findings clearly need not follow the typical "central" or "uncal" herniation syndromes described by Plum and Posner.[25]

Computed tomography and magnetic resonance imaging show mass effect from the edema with compression of the lateral ventricles and shift of midline structures. As expected, patients with the largest infarcts and most mass effect have the poorest prognosis. This does not apply, however, to patients with posterior fossa strokes. When intracranial pressure (ICP) monitoring is performed, pressures consistently greater than 15 mm Hg as determined by subarachnoid screw devices are usually fatal.[24] In patients with large cerebellar infarcts and hemorrhages, small amounts of swelling can compress the brain stem, injure its vital structures, and cause a rapidly progressive obstructive hydrocephalus.[26] Computed tomography may show crowding of the perimesencephalic, ambient, and cerebellopontine-angle cisterns and lack of visibility or displacement of the fourth ventricle. The typical syndrome includes headache, vertigo, nausea, vomiting, and ataxia. Drowsiness may start almost immediately, but usually develops during the next

12 hours to 4 days. It is not unusual for a patient with cerebellar infarction to be sent home from the emergency room with the diagnosis of labyrinthitis only to return in 24–48 hours in a coma. This serious mistake can be avoided if the patient's gait is tested at the time of the initial evaluation. Patients with sizable cerebellar hemorrhages and infarcts nearly always cannot walk or have abnormal gaits with veering or leaning to one side. In the presence of increased posterior fossa pressure, suboccipital decompressive surgery or draining cerebrospinal fluid by a shunt can be life saving.[26,27]

In supratentorial lesions, the therapy for increased pressure is twofold. First, physicians avoid factors that can further increase ICP and promote fluid retention. These include unusual head and neck positions, fever, increased central venous pressure, overhydration, hypoxia, hypercapnia, increased mean airway pressure, and agitation. Second, specific measures can be attempted to decrease pressure. Hyperventilation with reduction of the arterial carbon-dioxide tension to between 20 and 34 mm Hg reduces ICP during the short term, but ICP usually returns to pretreatment levels. Infusion of mannitol and glycerol to maintain blood osmolality between 300 and 310 μOsm/liter also decreases intracranial pressure. This osmotic therapy is effective only when the cell endothelium and membranes are intact. Thus, this therapy is not effective within the core of the infarct or for cytotoxic edema, but helps reduce the extracellular edema that surrounds infarcts.[23]

Steroids may also be tried. The effectiveness and mechanism of action of steroids in decreasing ICP are obscure. Steroids may ameliorate the extracellular edema that surrounds the infarct (as they do in brain tumors) or in areas where the cell membrane is not severely damaged. Steroids may also protect against free-radical generation. The efficacy of steroids is in doubt. Increased risk of gastrointestinal bleeding, infections, and exacerbation of diabetes are reported when steroids are used in stroke patients.[28–30] Therefore, I rarely use steroids after ischemic infarction. In occasional patients, especially young individuals, an impressive edema exists despite a relatively small zone of infarction. In this rare situation, steroids can be helpful. In patients with brain hematomas, I use steroids and osmotic agents to reduce pressure. In patients with large infarcts, although steroids occasionally allow survival for the short term, patients remain in disabled states and succumb later from pneumonia or other complications. Thus, I rarely use steroids in patients with massive infarcts. Craniectomy is another important consideration, especially in young patients with swollen cerebral hemispheres and incipient brain herniation. I discuss craniectomy as a decompressive strategy in Chapter 5.

Seizures

Seizures may also follow strokes. As early as 1864, Jackson recognized seizures as a complication that frequently occurred during the recovery phase of stroke.[31] Among 1,000 patients in a data bank collected in Girona, Spain, 50 (5%) patients had epileptic seizures during the first 48 hours after stroke.[32] Patients with brain hemorrhages have seizures more often than those with infarcts. In the Lausanne Stroke Registry, 7% of intracerebral hemorrhage patients had seizures during acute stroke compared with less than 1% of patients with ischemic strokes.[33] In the Harvard Stroke Registry, 6% of patients with hematomas had seizures during acute hospitalization.[34] Subcortical "slit" hemorrhages are most often accompanied by seizures.[35] Among patients with brain infarcts, those patients who have large and hemorrhagic infarcts have the most likelihood of developing seizures.[32,36,37] Patients with lesions that include the cerebral cortex have a much higher frequency of seizures than those whose lesions are only subcortical.[32,36–38] Patients with embolic brain infarcts of cardiac-origin have a much higher frequency of seizures than those who have large artery occlusive disease. Among 770 patients with supratentorial brain infarcts, the presence of cardiac origin brain embolism meant that the patient had a relative risk of 5.14 of developing early seizures compared with patients without cardiac-origin embolism.[37] Post-stroke seizures can occasionally cause worsening of neurologic deficits.[39] Patients who develop early seizures after stroke have a higher in-hospital mortality than those without seizures, probably reflecting the observation that patients with large infarcts are more likely to develop seizures.[40]

Approximately 10% of patients with strokes have seizures at some time after their stroke. In the Seizures after Stroke Study, a prospective, multicenter study among university hospitals in Canada, Australia, Israel, and Italy, 8.3% of stroke patients had seizures.[41] In this series, more than one-half of seizures occurred on the first day. Eighty percent of seizures occurred by the first month.[41] Gupta and colleagues analyzed the timing of post-infarction seizures.[42] In their series of 70 patients with seizures after ischemic strokes, one-third occurred within the first 2 weeks. Ninety percent of the 30 early seizures occurred within the first 24 hours.[42] Nearly three-fourths of seizures occurred within the first year. Only 2% developed more than 2 years after stroke.[42]

The electroencephalogram may have some prognostic value concerning the likelihood of a stroke patient developing a seizure.[43] Patients with periodic, lateralizing, epileptiform discharges are particularly likely to develop seizures. Patients who have focal spikes are also at increased risk, with 78% developing seizures. In patients with focal slowing, diffuse slowing, or normal electroencephalogram records, only 20%, 10%, and 5%, respectively, had seizures.[43] Early seizures are usually focal spells with secondary generalization. Late-onset seizures are more often generalized.[32,42] Patients with cortical infarcts, especially large infarcts with persistent hemiplegia, are most susceptible to post-infarction epilepsy.[38,42] Usually, post-stroke seizures are readily controlled with one anticonvulsant.[42] I do not prescribe prophylactic anticonvulsants in stroke patients. A minority of stroke patients develop seizures. Potential side effects and toxicity of anticonvulsants complicate the care of patients. I use anticonvulsants only after the patient has had a well-documented seizure.

Medical Complications

Pulmonary Embolism

Pulmonary embolism is the most feared and lethal medical complication in stroke patients. The great majority of patients who develop pulmonary embolism have deep vein thrombi in their lower extremities. Some venous thrombi are located in pelvic structures. Among patients in eight trials that studied the effect of treatment with heparin given within the first 3 weeks after ischemic stroke, 54% of control patients developed deep vein thrombosis as detected by systematic iodine-125 (^{125}I) fibrinogen scanning or venography.[6,44] Prophylactic administration of heparin, low-molecular-weight heparin, or heparinoids led to an 81% reduction in deep vein thrombosis as detected by ^{125}I fibrinogen scanning and venography.[44] Patients who harbor deep vein thrombi detected by noninvasive techniques and venography often do not have abnormal physical signs or symptoms.[6,45,46] Patients with severe leg weakness[47] and those with congestive heart failure and atrial fibrillation[48] are most likely to develop deep vein thrombosis. The true frequency of pulmonary emboli is unknown because many are silent. In necropsy series of patients who die during the first week after stroke, pulmonary emboli, although not always the cause of death, are frequently noted by the pathologist. Wijdicks and Scott reviewed the patient records of 33 patients who had pulmonary emboli after strokes during two decades (1976–1995) at the Mayo Clinic.[49] In three patients who died of progressive brain swelling, pulmonary emboli were found in small pulmonary arteries at necropsy. Among the remaining 30 patients, 15 patients had brain infarcts and 15 patients had intracerebral hemorrhages. None received heparin.[49] Pulmonary embolism occurred from days 3 to 120 (median day, 20) after stroke. Pulmonary embolism resulted in sudden death in 15 of the 30 patients.[49] Pleuritic chest pain, dyspnea, tachycardia, and hypoxemia were clinical clues revealing the presence of pulmonary embolism.

I consider all stroke patients at risk for the development of deep venous thrombosis. I pay particular attention to patients who are immobile. Obesity, obtundation, congestive heart failure, paralysis of one or both legs, hypercoagulability, and abulia are risk factors for phlebothrombosis. I keep some patients with acute cerebral ischemia at bed rest to maximize cerebral blood flow. I mobilize all other patients as soon as possible. Physical therapy is started at the bedside. I encourage patients to flex and extend the knees and ankles throughout the day. Support hose or special inflated stockings are often used. Pneumatic sequential compression does reduce the risk of deep venous thrombosis in patients who are immobilized after stroke.[50] Patients who have not had a hemorrhagic stroke and are not on anticoagulants are given low-dose subcutaneous heparin (5,000 units ["mini" heparin] twice per day) or low-molecular-weight heparin.

Patients who have sudden shortness of breath, chest pain, hypotension, hemoptysis, change in respiratory pattern, hypoxemia, agitation, confusion, or other worsening are suspected of having pulmonary embolism. Depending on the index of suspicion, evaluation should include the following tests:

1. Examination of arterial blood gases
2. Chest x-ray
3. Electrocardiogram
4. Noninvasive studies of the venous circulation in the legs[46]
5. Venography, nuclear lung ventilation, and perfusion scans
6. Pulmonary angiography

Patients who develop phlebothrombosis or pulmonary embolism, or both, are treated urgently with intravenous full-dose heparin or low-molecular-weight heparin.

A recent brain hemorrhage contraindicates anticoagulation. Antifibrinolytic therapy with urokinase or streptokinase therapy is also contraindicated in the presence of a recent stroke. If the pulmonary emboli were multiple and life threatening, the patient might require placement of a venous umbrella or other procedure to occlude the venous circulation. Pulmonary embolism remains a vexing problem throughout the rehabilitation process in patients who remain paretic.

Cardiac Abnormalities

Cardiac dysfunction is another frequent accompaniment of stroke. The dysfunctioning heart may be the source of stroke, coexist with stroke, or be the result of stroke.[51] Patients with ischemic and hemorrhagic stroke have been shown at necropsy to have subendocardial hemorrhages and focal regions of necrosis of cardiac muscle cells.[51–55] Electrocardiogram changes consistent with ischemia, elevated creatine-phosphokinase-myoglobin levels, and various cardiac arrhythmias are found in stroke patients even without known previous heart disease.[51,56,57] In some series, one-third to one-half of patients with strokes have serious cardiac rhythm disturbances, including ventricular tachycardia, salvos or couplets of premature ventricular beats greater than 10 premature beats per minute, second- or third-degree heart block, or asystole.[51,55,56,58,59] In control populations matched for age and history of cardiac disease, such arrhythmias are found in only 15%. Mortality has rarely been related to these arrhythmias. Atrial fibrillation can also develop as a sequel to stroke.[60]

Lesions of particular regions of the brain are most likely to be associated with cardiac abnormalities.[51] Three ways that strokes cause secondary cardiac, cardiovascular, and respiratory changes are as follows[51]:

1. Direct involvement of critical structures, such as the cortex of the insula of Reil, hypothalamus, and brain stem nuclei that make up the central autonomic network,[61] which activate autonomic descending fiber pathways to the heart, blood vessels, and lungs.
2. Mass effect with compression of the hypothalamus or brain stem, or both, also activates autonomic pathways.
3. The acute brain lesion and its stress effects stimulate the hypothalamic-pituitary axis triggering the release of catecholamines and corticosteroids.

Electrical stimulation of the anterior part of the brain, including the frontal pole, premotor and motor cortex, cingulate gyri, orbital frontal gyri, insular cortex, anterior part of the temporal lobe, amygdala, and hippocampus are all known to produce pressor or depressor effects on blood pressure or atrial and ventricular arrhythmias.[51,55,62] Stimulation of some of these regions may cause cardiovascular effects because of a nonspecific activation of limbic cortex, which has secondary effects on the hypothalamus, autonomic nervous system, and hypothalamic-pituitary endocrine axis. Stimulation of the insula has a more specific relation to cardiac and cardiovascular functions. After showing that stimulation of the posterior portions of the rat insular cortex had reproducible effects on heart rate and rhythm, Oppenheimer and colleagues stimulated the insular cortex of human epileptic patients.[63,64] They found that electrical stimulation in areas of the left human insular cortex produced bradycardia and reduced blood pressure, whereas stimulation of the right insular cortex elicited tachycardia and increased blood pressure.[63] Strokes that involve the insular cortex may be accompanied by arrhythmias and other cardiovascular effects.

Projections from the cerebral cortex of the frontal lobe sometimes passing through the temporal lobes and thalami are relayed to the hypothalamus and brain stem nuclei, which then project directly to the intermediolateral cell columns of the thoracic spinal cord that control sympathetic nervous system output to the heart. Stimulation of the lateral and posterior portions of the hypothalamus cause the release of large amounts of catecholamines from the adrenal medulla.[55] Sympathetic stimulation mostly increases the rate and force of the heartbeat and dilates coronary arteries, whereas parasympathetic stimulation slows the atrial rate and force of contractions and constricts the coronary arteries.[51] Brain stem compression and direct involvement of the medulla oblongata can lead to vagal discharges, which can cause sinus bradycardia, cardiac arrhythmias, and even cardiac arrest as well as elevation of systolic blood pressure and a fall in diastolic blood pressure. This train of events is the likely explanation of the blood pressure and pulse changes found in patients with increased ICP and brain herniations that were discovered and emphasized by Harvey Cushing. These changes are usually called the *Cushing response.*

When these changes occur during strokes, creatine-phosphokinase elevations tend to be longer lasting than those associated with primary cardiac disease. Elevations may peak at the fifth day and persist until the twelfth day.[57] When levels of norepinephrine, epinephrine, and dopamine are measured in patients with stroke, patients with transient ischemic attacks, and non-stroke controls, the highest levels are found in stroke patients.[65] The next highest levels are found in transient disorders. Normal values occur in the control population.[51,65] Those patients with stroke and the highest creatine-phosphokinase values have the highest levels of norepinephrine. This information suggests that stroke causes an increase in sympathetic tone elevating levels of catecholamines, which in turn cause focal myocardial damage and subsequent arrhythmias.

Patients who have subarachnoid hemorrhage, vertebrobasilar-territory ischemia, and hemorrhages sometimes develop acute pulmonary edema, which is often sudden in onset and sometimes fatal.[51,66] Pulmonary edema is most likely to develop when a sudden-onset and severe increase in ICP occurs. Weir studied the occurrence of pulmonary edema in patients with fatal subarachnoid hemorrhages.[66] The sudden onset of coma was present in 70% of his fatal cases of patients with ruptured aneurysms who developed pulmonary edema. Respiratory symptoms were noted within a short time period after the onset of headache and neurologic symptoms.[66] Weir attributed the occurrence of pulmonary edema to a sudden, severe increase in ICP, which in turn caused massive autonomic stimulation. Experimental data from studies in cats confirm this hypothesis.[67] Myocardial enzyme release and electrocardiogram changes that indicate abnormal wall motion are often accompanied by decreased left ventricular performance in patients with subarachnoid hemorrhage.[68]

Older patients with cerebral hemispheric infarction seem to be at greater risk for cardiac arrhythmias.[59] Heart rate variability is common in patients with cerebral hemispheric and medullary infarcts.[69] All stroke patients require careful attention to the cardiovascular system by clinical examination and laboratory tests. In addition to surveillance for symptoms, clinicians should carefully monitor vital signs, regular cardiovascular examinations, echocardiography, and routine electrocardiograms. In some patients, continuous cardiac monitoring may be needed. Although its efficacy is unproved, propranolol or other beta blockers are theoretically useful in patients with neurogenic cardiac arrhythmias, treating both the arrhythmia and its cause.[59] Propranolol could, however, worsen sinus bradycardia, heart block, and episodes of asystole. In experimental animals, the cardiac rhythm abnormalities secondary to cerebral ischemia can be effectively treated with propranolol and atropine.[70] If rhythm disturbances occur, I treat with standard antiarrhythmics according to suggestions of cardiology consultants.

Swallowing Abnormalities, Aspiration, and Pneumonia

Dysphagia and aspiration are common after stroke. Symptomatic dysphagia is noted in approximately 25–32% of stroke patients.[71,72] Dysphagia and aspiration are especially common in patients who have had bilateral hemispheric strokes or strokes that involve the brain stem.[73,74] So-called silent aspiration is also common when clinicians look for it. Videofluoroscopic studies can detect abnormalities of swallowing in approximately 50% of stroke patients.[74–76] In one study among 128 patients hospitalized for first strokes, 65 (51%) had swallowing abnormalities detected clinically and 82 (64%) had swallowing abnormalities shown by videofluoroscopy.[76] During the next 6 months, 26 patients (20%) had pulmonary infections, among whom 24 had videofluoroscopic swallowing abnormalities when studied during their acute stroke.[76] Physical therapy with guidance in positioning of food within the oral cavity and pharynx, choice of foods, the use of thermal stimulation, and instructions to the patient can be helpful in preventing aspiration. Most patients are able to resume oral feeding within months although feeding tubes may be needed temporarily.

Pneumonia is common after stroke during the immediate and late periods. The true frequency of this complication is unknown. In one retrospective postmortem study of patients dying with cerebrovascular disease, pneumonia was recorded as a complication in 33%.[77] The cause of pneumonia in patients with stroke is probably multifactorial. In a recumbent position, atelectasis and poor mobilization of secretions often occur. Difficulty in swallowing may also lead to aspiration. Coughing and deep breathing may not be done or may be only poorly performed. Chest movements are also decreased on the hemiplegic side.[78,79] Kaldor and Berlin noted that pneumonia is more likely to exist on the hemiparetic side because of the decreased thoracic movements and impaired pulmonary circulation.[80] Respiratory drive and the function of interstitial muscles are often abnormal on the hemiplegic side.[79]

Swallowing examination by a trained team of evaluators is important in any patient with bulbar signs and those who report dysphagia or have abnormalities in swallowing a test dose of water. Swallowing a small cup of water should be a routine part of the examination in stroke patients. Swallowing function should be tested before giving patients oral feedings. Physiotherapy or nursing techniques probably help to prevent pneumonia after stroke. I encourage deep breathing, coughing, frequent turning, and early mobilization of patients. If fever develops despite these measures, the lung should be aggressively evaluated as the potential source of infection.

Metabolic and Nutritional Disorders

Prolonged undernutrition is an important but seldom recognized complication of stroke, especially in elderly patients whose nutritional intake was poor or marginal before their stroke. Finestone and colleagues evaluated the nutritional state of 49 consecutive stroke patients admitted to a rehabilitation unit and found that approximately one-half were malnourished.[81] In another study, the authors correlated serum albumin concentration, an index of nutritional state, and the presence of chronic disease with the frequency of medical complications and found that 79% of patients with an albumin less than 2.9 g/dl had at least one medical complication during rehabilitation.[82] A high serum albumin correlated with good gains in neurologic functional status.[82] Malnutrition can contribute to diminished immune functions, cardiac and gastrointestinal dysfunction, and abnormal bone metabolism. Malnutrition is a factor in the formation and repair of decubitus ulcers.

To help maintain an adequate nutritional state, I give multivitamins and especially thiamine orally if the patient is able, or parenterally. If the patient is unable to eat by the fourth or fifth day, I insert a small nasogastric feeding tube through which nutritional supplements can be given. Prolonged inability to swallow may require the placement of gastric feeding tubes. The use of percutaneous endoscopic gastrostomy (PEG) tubes with maintenance of nutrition has undoubtedly helped many stroke patients maintain reasonable nutritional balance despite dysphagia. Early PEG placement can improve the outcome in stroke patients.[83] Nutrition can be better maintained using PEGs than with nasogastric tube feedings.[83] PEG placement can be managed with rare complications, such as wound infection and gastrointestinal bleeding. In approximately 25% or more of patients, PEG can be removed when swallowing improves.[84]

Fluid, electrolyte, and nutritional abnormalities may also occur during the acute stroke and recovery periods. Approximately 15% of patients with acute stroke develop hyponatremia. Hyponatremia can cause nausea, vomiting, weakness, confusion, and seizures. Joynt et al. posited that post-stroke hyponatremia is usually related to inappropriate secretion of antidiuretic hormone (ADH).[85] They showed that stroke patients often had excess ADH even in the presence of normal serum sodium levels. Although the mechanism of the inappropriate ADH secretion is unknown, Joynt et al. reviewed some of the potential mechanisms, including damage to the anterior hypothalamus, effects on ADH secretion related to recumbency, resetting of osmoreceptors, damage to a more widespread vasopressin neuronal system, increased release of ADH, and secondary stroke-related elevations in serum catecholamines and cortisol.[85] Changes in the levels of atrial natriuretic factor have also been posited to cause abnormalities of serum sodium concentrations.

In hyponatremic patients, volume depletion and overload must be excluded as contributing factors. In the assessment of this problem, it must be remembered that fluid may accumulate in the sacral regions during prolonged bed rest. If volume status is normal, the syndrome of inappropriate ADH secretion can be diagnosed if symptoms, including decreased serum osmolality, continued urinary excretion of sodium, urine less than maximally dilute, normal renal function, and normal thyroid function, exist in addition to hyponatremia. During the acute stroke period, I advise carefully following the patient's volume status by clinical examination; uniform charting of input, output, and daily weights; and monitoring of electrolytes.

Urinary Tract Infections and Urinary Incontinence

The high frequency of urinary tract infections is probably caused by the following two factors. First, an indwelling catheter is often placed to empty the urinary bladder. This foreign body allows for the introduction and growth of bacteria. Whenever possible, continuous catheter drainage should be avoided. Intermittent catheterization using strict sterile techniques is preferable. In some male patients, condom catheters suffice. A Foley catheter should never be used as a convenience for the staff. Second, the functioning of the urinary bladder and external sphincter can be altered by the stroke. Urinary symptoms are common even in patients with uninfected bladders and include urinary urgency, frequency, and retention. Tsuchida et al. documented these symptoms and attempted to establish their relationship to brain lesions.[86] Patients with frontal and internal-capsular lesions showed a hyperactive bladder or uninhibited sphincter relaxation with subsequent urinary frequency or incontinence. Patients with putaminal lesions had hyperactive bladders with usually normal sphincter function. Patients who had urinary retention showed an inactive or hypoactive bladder with an uncoordinated or normal sphincter; localization of the offending lesion could not be accomplished in these patients. Men in the stroke age group are often geriatric and also have large prostates, which can contribute to the obstructive uropathy.

When confronted with patients with abnormal micturition, I survey for and treat bacterial urinary tract infections when present. In addition, I attempt to define other mechanisms that may be operative in causing symptoms, such as inability to reach the commode or urinal because of gait or limb abnormalities, communication difficulty that may make it hard to signal the nurse, and unavailable nursing personnel. Measurement of post-voided residual urine may be all that is needed, but at times cystometrics and imaging of the kidneys and urinary tract are required to define the problem. I encourage frequent voiding during the day and night in an effort to train the bladder. Pharmacotherapy can be used if these maneuvers fail to help alleviate the problem.

Gastrointestinal Bleeding

Physicians have long realized that some patients with stroke and other brain diseases develop gastrointestinal hemorrhage. This problem, usually called *Cushing's ulcers*, *stress ulcers*, or *hemorrhagic gastritis*, can be life threatening when severe. Davenport and colleagues reported that 18 of 607 (3%) stroke patients at their hospital in Edinburgh had gastrointestinal hemorrhages. One-half of the hemorrhages were severe.[87] Most patients had hematemesis or melena, but one patient suddenly developed abdominal pain and hemodynamic shock.[87] Older patients with severe strokes and decreased levels of consciousness are most likely to develop gastrointestinal bleeding. Corticosteroids given for brain edema also increase the risk of stress ulceration in the stomach. Prophylactic use of H_2 antagonists is recommended in patients who have large strokes with reduced awareness.

Immobility and Its Complications

Pressure Decubitus Ulcers

The development of bedsores is an iatrogenic and preventable complication of stroke that significantly hinders the rehabilitation process. Patients who are immobilized, have limited ability to reposition themselves, and do not sense the need to change position are at risk of developing bedsores if not frequently turned and repositioned.[88] Incontinence also increases the risk for developing skin breakdown. The skin should be kept clean and dry, and the patient should be turned frequently. Adequate nutrition should be given. Pressure on anesthetic or immobilized limbs must be avoided. The use of padded heel boots can spare the heels from ulcers. Egg-crate mattresses, waterbeds, or soft cotton padding may help retard the development of sacral pressure sores. Physicians and nursing personnel should periodically examine the entire skin surface looking for any area of early breakdown. Particular attention should be paid to susceptible areas, such as the sacrum, buttocks, heels, elbows, wrists, toes, and occiput. If an ulcer develops, pressure on that area should be totally avoided, special mattresses should be used, and the wound should be dressed and, if necessary, débrided and the skin grafted.

Contractures and Shoulder Pain

Immobility of the limbs and maintenance in fixed, usually flexed positions can lead to fixed contractures at the knees and elbows. Decreased shoulder movement can lead to shoulder pain, frozen shoulders, and the so-called shoulder-hand syndrome. In one study, 36 of 132 (27%) hemiplegic stroke patients developed the shoulder-hand syndrome.[89] The shoulder-hand syndrome is characterized by pain and tenderness when abducting, flexing, and externally rotating the upper arm; pain and swelling over the carpal bones; and edema of the distal hand joints. Severe shoulder weakness, spasticity, and subluxation of the shoulder increase the likelihood of developing shoulder pain and swelling of the upper extremity. Early full range of movement of the shoulder joint is important in preventing this unpleasant and disabling stroke complication. Nonsteroidal anti-inflammatory drugs, such as indomethacin and low-dose corticosteroids, may be helpful in patients who develop shoulder pain. The most important treatment, however, is vigorous physical therapy.[89] Subluxation of the shoulders is another complication of hemiparesis. The weak arm should not be left to hang without support.

Peripheral Nerve Injuries

Peripheral nerve compression is also a hazard in limbs with weakness and reduced sensation. The peroneal nerve is most commonly involved; its compression causes a foot drop. Ulnar palsy caused by compression of the nerve at the elbow is also common, especially in wheelchair-bound patients. Occasionally, patients compress their femoral nerve in relation to local pressure on the groin region while consciousness is reduced. The femoral nerve can also be compressed by retroperitoneal hemorrhages that involve the iliopsoas muscles. The most common cause of these hematomas is anticoagulation. The earliest sign is often a dropped knee jerk on the side of the retroperitoneal hematoma.

Osteopenia and Osteoporosis

Studies of bone mineral densities after stroke have shown that a significant reduction in bone mineral density occurs on the hemiplegic side.[90–93] The causes are multifactorial but include immobilization-induced calcium resorption from bone, sometimes with hypercalcemia; lack of sunlight exposure; poor nutrition with inadequate vitamin D stores; and osteoporosis before the stroke. The hemiosteoporosis is most severe in those patients with severe hemiplegia, especially those that have prolonged immobilization. The reduced bone density predisposes to hip and other fractures, which tend to occur predominantly on the hemiplegic side. Calcium and vitamin D supplements are important prophylactically in patients at risk for this complication. Early mobilization and exposure to sunlight are also important.

Depression and Other Psychological Effects of Stroke

One of the most important and yet frequently overlooked complications of stroke is depression. New personality traits can emerge or old ones become accentuated. The patient may become apathetic, inflexible, rigid, impulsive, insensitive, or indifferent to others; adopt a poor perception of self; or become guilt-ridden, paranoid, or suicidal.

Depression is reported to occur in 26–60% of stroke patients.[94–98] Approximately 20–25% of patients have a major depressive disorder.[97–99] Astrom and colleagues analyzed the prevalence of major depression at various time intervals after stroke and their most important correlations and determinants.[97] Approximately 25% of their stroke patients had a major depression during the acute post-stroke period, and 31% were depressed at 3 months. Acute depression was most frequent in patients with anterior lesions in the left hemisphere, aphasic patients, and those who lived alone. At 1 year, 16% of patients were depressed. Two- and 3-year depression rates were 19% and

29%, respectively. Dependency and lack of social contacts were important determinants of late depression.[97] Patients who have a history of depression before their stroke are also prone to become depressed after a stroke.[98] Others have found that at 6 months after stroke an increased prevalence of symptoms of both major and minor depressive symptoms can be found, increasing from 23% and 20%, respectively, immediately after the stroke to 35% and 26% at 6 months.[99,100] Diagnosis of depression is often difficult because functional psychogenic reactions are hard to separate from organic behavioral changes related to the stroke, such as abulia, aprosodia, impersistence, and anosognosia.[101]

Facial expression, gestures, pauses, loudness, emphasis, and other nonlinguistic aspects give verbal communication an emotive context. Aprosodia is the inability to express or understand the emotive content of spoken language. Patients with right parasylvian strokes may be unable to communicate emotion in spoken language. Thus, an observer might erroneously believe that they are depressed. Binder noted additional factors complicating the recognition of depression.[102] An accurate history may not be available because of aphasia or slowed responses. Vegetative and autonomic signs may also be difficult to interpret. Stroke may suppress appetite, change sleep patterns, or create a pseudobulbar state with rapid shifts from laughing to crying.

Often, sexual function in patients with stroke is ignored. For some patients, stroke may make sexual relations cumbersome and decrease their frequency. The patient and family should be reassured that for most mechanisms of stroke, sex is unlikely to cause a recurrent stroke. Sexual activity should be encouraged in those couples who were sexually active before the stroke, although it may require some creativity on the part of the participants.

Ross and Rush proposed guidelines for the diagnosis of depression.[103] Depression should be considered in patients who are not making expected recovery, are uncooperative in rehabilitation, or lose previously achieved milestones. Emotional outbursts, inflexibility, irritability, insensitivity to others, and suicidal ideations may occur. A flat affect must be distinguished from a depressed affect. Collateral history from friends and caregivers are also needed.

Depression is more common after left- than right-hemisphere strokes.[95,97,101,104–107] In the left hemisphere, the more anteriorly placed infarctions are correlated with a higher frequency of depression.[105,106] When cortical and basal ganglia lesions, infarcts, and hemorrhages affect the left hemisphere anteriorly, they are more likely to be associated with depression than similarly placed right-cerebral lesions.

Finkelstein et al. used the dexamethasone-suppression test to assess patients with mood and vegetative disturbances after stroke.[96] An abnormal test is defined as failure to suppress cortisol secretion in response to exogenously administered dexamethasone. This test is reported to be abnormal in 60–80% of psychiatric patients with endogenous depression. Abnormal dexamethasone suppression tests in patients with stroke were associated with occurrence of moderate to severe mood, sleep, and appetite disturbances.[96]

The causes of late depressive reaction are often unknown. Whether it is a reaction to the loss the patient feels or a result of brain injury is unclear. Injury may result in depletion of noradrenergic neurotransmitters resulting in depression. Nortriptyline, trazodone, and serotonin re-uptake inhibitors are reported to be effective in ameliorating significantly the symptoms of depression in patients with stroke.[101,108–110]

Beyond pharmacologic therapy, clinicians should try to adopt a hopeful and fighting attitude. I encourage activity and independence for the family and patient. Physicians should attempt to promote continued affection, understanding, and respect between the family and patient. I suggest that physicians reassure all involved that efforts are intended to maximize rehabilitation and prevent recurrent stroke. I recommend that physicians promote the patient's self-confidence and emphasize the old adage, "When the going gets tough, the tough get going!"

Caregivers and Their Reactions to the Stroke Patient

Strokes and stroke patients do not live in a vacuum. Strokes cause important ramifications that affect all those who interact with the individual stroke survivor, but most of the burden falls on the family and principal caregiver. Stroke is a disease that hits the whole family constellation, not merely the stroke patient.

Stroke patients who have severe deficits often become dependent on caregivers for daily activities and physical and emotional support. Members of the family must deal with the physical handicaps and, often, new personality traits. If the patient is dependent on family members for care, the main caregiver can develop feelings of entrapment, isolation, anger, and depression. In some families, it seems as if a new dependent child has been thrust on them. Physicians should remember that caregivers are often old and sick and have their own physical and emotional problems.

Researchers have begun to analyze and quantitate burdens perceived by those caring for stroke patients. Researchers have also begun to describe and quantify the emotional and physical consequences of caregiving.[111–114] A Dutch study analyzed the burden of caregiving among 121 partners of patients who were living at home.[113] The investigators interviewed the caregivers 3 years after stroke affected their loved ones. Caregivers reported feeling overwhelmed with responsibility, uncertainty, and worry. They found it difficult to handle the restraints placed on their own social lives and interests.[113] Analysis showed that higher levels of burden were explained by the stroke patient's degree of disability and the amount of care needed. Data also revealed that the caregiver's emotional distress, loneliness, and perception of his or her ability to care for the stroke patient shaped the burden the caregiver felt.[113]

The emotional outcome of stroke on caregivers was analyzed in a Scottish study of 231 stroke patients and their caregivers.[114] Severe emotional distress and depression were common among caregivers. Caregivers were more likely to be depressed if the stroke patient was dependent or emotionally distressed. The caregivers' emotional state in terms of anxiety and depression highly correlated with the emotional state of the stroke patient. Women who cared for male stroke patients had more anxiety and depression than male caregivers. Older caregivers were more depressed than young caregivers.[114] In another study, the proportion of caregivers that were depressed did not diminish over time.[111]

Clearly, care, education, and concern must be addressed to the caregivers and their families as well as the stroke patients.

References

1. Johnston KC, Li JY, Lyden PD, et al. Medical and neurological complications of ischemic stroke: experience from the RANTTAS trial. RANTTAS Investigators. Stroke 1998;29:447–453.
2. Davenport RJ, Dennis MS, Wellwood I, Warlow CP. Complications after acute stroke. Stroke 1996;27:415–420.
3. Smithard DG, O'Neill PA, Park C, et al. Complications and outcome after acute stroke. Stroke 1996;27:1200–1204.
4. Biller J, Patrick JT. Management of medical complications of stroke. J Stroke Cerebrovasc Dis 1997;6:217–220.
5. Zorowitz RD, Tietjen GE. Medical complications after stroke. J Stroke Cerebrovasc Dis 1999;8:192–196.
6. van der Worp HB, Kappelle LJ. Complications of acute ischaemic stroke. Cerebrovasc Dis 1998;8:124–132.
7. Dromerick A, Reding M. Medical and neurological complications during inpatient stroke rehabilitation. Stroke 1994;25:358–361.
8. Silver F, Norris JW, Lewis A, Hachinski V. Early mortality following stroke: a prospective review. Stroke 1984;15:494.
9. Kaste M, Palmomaki H, Sarna S. Where and how should elderly stroke patients be treated? A randomized trial. Stroke 1995;26:249–253.
10. Indredavik B, Slordahl SA, Bakke F, et al. Stroke unit treatment. Long term effects. Stroke 1997;28:1861–1866.
11. Stroke Unit Trialists' Collaboration. Collaborative systematic review of the randomized trials of organised inpatient (stroke unit) care after stroke. BMJ 1997;314:1151–1159.
12. Stroke Unit Trialists' Collaboration. How do stroke units improve patient outcomes? A collaborative systematic review of the randomized trials. Stroke 1997;28:2139–2144.
13. Toni D, Fiorelli M, Gentile M, et al. Progressing neurological deficit secondary to acute ischemic stroke: a study on predictability, pathogenesis, and prognosis. Arch Neurol 1995;52:670–675.
14. Davalos A, Cendra E, Teruel J, et al. Deteriorating ischemic stroke: risk factors and prognosis. Neurology 1990;40:1865–1869.
15. Kelly R, Bryer JR, Scheinberg P, Stokes IV. Active bleeding in hypertensive intracerebral hemorrhage: computed tomography. Neurology 1982;32:852–856.
16. Broderick JP, Brott TG, Tomsick T, et al. Ultra-early evaluation of intracerebral hemorrhage. J Neurosurg 1990;72:195–199.
17. Fujii Y, Tanaka R, Takeuchi S, et al. Hematoma enlargement in spontaneous intracerebral hemorrhage. J Neurosurg 1994;80:51–57.
18. Kazui S, Naritomi H, Yamamoto H, et al. Enlargement of spontaneous intracerebral hemorrhage: incidence and time course. Stroke 1996;27:1783–1787.
19. Sacco RL. Foulkes MA, Mohr JP, et al. Determinants of early recurrence of cerebral infarction. The Stroke Data Bank. Stroke 1989;20:983–989.
20. Yamamoto H, Bogousslavsky J. Mechanisms of second and further strokes. J Neurol Neurosurg Psychiatry 1998;64:771–776.

21. Caplan LR. Brain Embolism. In LR Caplan, JW Hurst, MI Chimowitz, (eds), Clinical Neurocardiology. New York: Marcel Dekker, 1999;35–185.

22. White DB, Norris JW, Hachinski VC, et al. Death in early stroke: causes and mechanisms. Stroke 1979; 10:743.

23. O'Brien MD. Ischemic Cerebral Edema. In LR Caplan (ed), Brain Ischemia. Basic Concepts and Clinical Relevance. London: Springer, 1995;43–50.

24. Ropper AH, Shafran B. Brain edema after stroke. Arch Neurol 1984;41:26–29.

25. Plum F, Posner JB. Diagnosis of Stupor and Coma (3rd ed). Philadelphia: Davis, 1980.

26. Caplan LR. Posterior Circulation Disease. Clinical findings, diagnosis, and management. Boston: Blackwell, 1996.

27. Rieke K, Krieger D, Adams H-P, et al. Therapeutic strategies in space-occupying cerebellar infarction based on clinical, neuroradiological, and neurophysiological data. Cerebrovasc Dis 1993;3:45–55.

28. von Rosen F, Guazzo EP. Increased Intracranial Pressure. In T Brandt, LR Caplan, J Dichgans, et al (eds), Neurological Disorders. Course and Treatment. San Diego: Academic, 1996;521–529.

29. Norris JW. Steroid therapy in acute cerebral infarction. Arch Neurol 1976;33:69–71.

30. Ottonello GA, Primavera A. Gastrointestinal complications of high dose corticosteroid therapy in acute cerebrovascular patients. Stroke 1979;10:208–210.

31. Taylor J. Selected writings of John Hughlings Jackson on epilepsy and epileptiform convulsions, Vol. 1. London: Hodder & Stoughton, 1931:230–235.

32. Davalos A, de Cendra E, Molins A, et al. Epileptic seizures at the onset of stroke. Cerebrovasc Dis 1992;2:327–331.

33. Bogousslavsky J, van Melle G, Regli F. The Lausanne Stroke Registry: analysis of 1000 consecutive patients with first stroke. Stroke 1988;19:1083–1092.

34. Mohr JP, Caplan LR, Melski JW, et al. The Harvard Cooperative Stroke Registry: a prospective registry. Neurology 1978;28:754–762.

35. Caplan LR. General Symptoms and Signs. In CS Kase, LR Caplan (eds), Intracerebral Hemorrhage. Boston: Butterworth–Heinemann, 1994;31–43.

36. Bladin CF. Seizures after stroke. M.D. thesis. University of Melbourne, Australia, 1997.

37. Heuts-van Rank EPM. Seizures following a first cerebral infarct. Risk factors and prognosis. Thesis. Rijksuniversiteit Limberg, Maastricht, Netherlands, 1996.

38. Olsen TS, Hogenhaven H, Thage O. Epilepsy after stroke. Neurology 1987;37:1209–1211.

39. Bogousslavsky J, Martin R, Regli F, et al. Persistent worsening of stroke sequelae after delayed seizures. Arch Neurol 1992;49:385–388.

40. Arboix A, Comes E, Massons J, et al. Relevance of early seizures for in-hospital mortality in acute cerebrovascular disease. Neurology 1996;47:1429–1435.

41. Bladin CF, Johnston PJ, Smuraloska L, et al. What causes seizures after stroke? Stroke 1994;25:245.

42. Gupta SR, Naheedey MH, Elias D, Rubino F. Postinfarction seizures: a clinical study. Stroke 1988;19:1477–1481.

43. Holmes GL. The electroencephalogram as a predictor of seizures following cerebral infarction. Clin Electroencephalogr 1980;11:83–86.

44. Sandercock PAG, van den Belt AGM, Lindley RI, Slattery J. Antithrombotic therapy in acute ischaemic stroke:an overview of the completed randomised trials. J Neurol Neurosurg Psychiatry 1993;56:17–25.

45. Warlow C, Ogston D, Douglas AS. Deep venous thrombosis of the legs after stroke. BMJ 1976;1:1178–1183.

46. Kearon C, Julian JA, Math JM, et al. Noninvasive diagnosis of deep venous thrombosis. Ann Intern Med 1998;128: 663–677.

47. Landi G, D'Angelo A, Boccardi E, Candelise L, et al. Venous thromboembolism in acute stroke: prognostic importance of hypercoagulability. Arch Neurol 1992;49: 279–283.

48. Noel P, Gregoire F, Capon A, Lehrert P. Atrial fibrillation as a risk factor for deep venous thrombosis and pulmonary emboli in stroke patients. Stroke 1991;22:760–762.

49. Wijdicks EFM, Scott JP. Pulmonary embolism associated with acute stroke. Mayo Clin Proc 1997;72:297–300.

50. Kamran SI, Downey D, Ruff RL. Pneumatic sequential compression reduces the risk of deep vein thrombosis in stroke patients. Neurology 1998;50:1683–1688.

51. Caplan LR, Hurst JW. Cardiac and cardiovascular findings in patients with nervous system diseases—Brain diseases—Stroke. In LR Caplan, JW Hurst, MI Chimowitz (eds), Clinical Neurocardiology. New York: Marcel Dekker, 1999;303–312.

52. Norris JW, Kolin A, Hachinski VC. Focal myocardial lesions in stroke. Stroke 1980;11:130.

53. Connor RC. Focal myocytolysis and fuchsinophilic degeneration of the myocardium of patients dying with various brain lesions. Ann N Y Acad Sci 1969;156:261–270.

54. Samuels M. "Voodoo" death revisited: the modern lessons of neurocardiology. Neurologist 1997;3:293–304.

55. Ali AS, Levine SR. Heart and Brain Relationships. In LR Caplan (ed), Brain Ischemia, Basic Concepts and Clinical Relevance. London: Springer, 1995;317–328.

56. Rolak LA, Rokey R. Electrocardiographic Features. In LA Rolak, R Rokey (eds), Coronary and Cerebrovascular Disease. A Practical Guide. Mt Kisco, NY: Futura, 1990; 139–197.

57. Puleo P. Cardiac Enzyme Assessment. In LA Rolak, R Rokey (eds), Coronary and Cerebrovascular Disease. A Practical Guide. Mt Kisco, NY: Futura, 1990;199–216.

58. Myers MG, Norris JW, Hachinski VC, et al. Cardiac sequelae of acute stroke. Stroke 1982;13:838–842.

59. Mikolich JR, Jacobs WC, Fletcher GF. Cardiac arrhythmias in patients with acute cerebrovascular accidents. JAMA 1981;246:1314–1317.

60. Vingerhoets F, Bogousslavsky J, Regli F, Van Melle G. Atrial fibrillation after acute stroke. Stroke 1993;24:26–30.

61. Benarroch EE. The central autonomic network: functional organization, dysfunction, and perspective. Mayo Clin Proc 1993;68:988–1001.

62. Talman WT. Cardiovascular regulation and lesions of the central nervous system. Ann Neurol 1985;18:1–12.

63. Oppenheimer SM, Cechetto DF, Hachinski VC. Cerebrogenic cardiac arrythmias. Cerebral electrocardiographic

influences and their role in sudden death. Arch Neurol 1990;47:513–519.

64. Oppenheimer SM, Hopkins DA. Suprabulbar Neural Regulation of the Heart. In JA Armour, JL Ardell (eds), Neurocardiology. New York: Oxford University Press, 1994; 309–341.

65. Myers MS, Norris JW, Hachinski VC, et al. Plasma norepinephrine in stroke. Stroke 1981;12:200–204.

66. Weir BK. Pulmonary edema folllowing fatal aneurysmal rupture. J Neureosurg 1978;49:502–507.

67. Hoff JT, Nishimura M. Experimental neurogenic pulmonary edema in cats. J Neurosurg 1978;18:383–389.

68. Mayer SA, Lin J, Homma S, et al. Myocardial injury and left ventricular performance after subarachnoid hemorrhage. Stroke 1999;30:780–786.

69. Korpelainen JT, Sotaniemi KA, Makkallio A, et al. Dynamic behavior of heart rate in ischemic stroke. Stroke 1999;30:1008–1013.

70. Weidler DJ, Das SK, Sodeman TM. Cardiac arrhythmias secondary to acute cerebral ischemia: prevention by autonomic blockade. Circulation 1976;53(Suppl 2):102.

71. Horner J, Massey EW. Silent aspiration following stroke. Neurology 1988;38:317–319.

72. Groher ME, Bukatman R. The prevalence of swallowing disorders in two teaching hospitals. Dysphagia 1986;1:3–6.

73. Horner J, Massey EW, Brazer SR. Aspiration in bilateral stroke patients. Neurology 1990;40:1686–1688.

74. Alberts MJ, Horner J. Dysphagia and Aspiration Syndromes. In J Bogousslavsky, LR Caplan (eds), Stroke Syndromes. Cambridge: Cambridge University Press, 1995;213–222.

75. Horner J, Massey EW, Risler JE, et al. Aspiration following stroke: clinical correlates and outcome. Neurology 1988;38:1359–1362.

76. Mann G, Dip PG, Hankey GJ, Cameron D. Swallowing function after stroke. Prognosis and prognostic factors at 6 months. Stroke 1999;30:744–748.

77. Mulley GP. Pneumonia, stroke, and laterality. Lancet 1981;1:1051.

78. Fluck DC. Chest movements in hemiplegia. Clin Sci 1966;31:383–388.

79. Przedborski S, Brunko E, Hubert M, et al. The effect of acute hemiplegia on intercostal muscle activity. Neurology 1988;38:1882–1884.

80. Kaldor A, Berlin I. Pneumonia, stroke, and laterality. Lancet 1981;1:843.

81. Finestone HM, Green-Finestone LS, Wilson ES, Teasell RW. Malnutrition in stroke patients on the rehabilitation service and at follow-up. Prevalence and predictors. Arch Phys Med Rehabil 1995;76:310–316.

82. Aptaker RI, Roth EJ, Reichhardt G, et al. Serum albumin level as a predictor of geriatric stroke rehabilitation outcome. Arch Phys Med Rehabil 1994;75:80–84.

83. Norton B, Homer-Ward M, Donnelly MT, et al. A randomized prospective comparison of percutaneous endoscopic gastrostomy and nasogastric tube feedings after acute dysphagic stroke. BMJ 1996;312:13–16.

84. Wijdicks EFM, McMahon MM. Percutaneous endoscopic gastrostomy after acute stroke: complications and outcome. Cerebrovasc Dis 1999;9:109–111.

85. Joynt RJ, Feibel JH, Sladek CM. Antidiuretic hormone levels in stroke patients. Ann Neurol 1981;9:182–184.

86. Tsuchida S, Noto H, Yamaguchi D, et al. Urodynamic studies on hemiplegia patients after cerebrovascular accident. Urology 1983;21:315–318.

87. Davenport RJ, Dennis MS, Warlow CP. Gastrointestinal hemorrhage after acute stroke. Stroke 1996;27:421–424.

88. Smith DM. Pressure ulcers in the nursing home. Ann Intern Med 1995;123:433–442.

89. Braus DF, Krauss JK, Strobel J. The shoulder-hand syndrome after stroke: a prospective clinical trial. Ann Neurol 1994;36:728–733.

90. Sato Y, Maruoka H, Oizumi K. Amelioration of hemiplegia-associated osteopenia more than 4 years after stroke by 1 alpha-hydroxyvitamin D_3 and calcium supplementation. Stroke 1997;28:736–739.

91. Sato Y, Kuno H, Kaji M, et al. Increased bone resorption during the first year after stroke. Stroke 1998;29:1373–1377.

92. Sato Y, Fujimatsu Y, Honda Y, et al. Accelerated bone remodeling in patients with poststroke hemiplegia. J Stroke Cerebrovasc Dis 1998;7:58–62.

93. Ramnemark A, Nyberg L, Lorentzon R, et al. Hemiosteoporosis after severe stroke, independent of changes in body composition and weight. Stroke 1999;30:755–760.

94. Feibel JH, Springer CJ. Depression and failure to resume social activities after stroke. Arch Phys Med Rehabil 1982;63:276–277.

95. Robinson RG, Szetela B. Mood change following left hemisphere brain injury. Ann Neurol 1981;9:447–453.

96. Finkelstein S, Benowitz LI, Baldessarini RJ, et al. Mood, vegetative disturbances, and dexamethasone suppression test after stroke. Ann Neurol 1982;12:463–468.

97. Astrom M, Adolfdon R, Asplund K. Major depression in stroke patients. A 3-year longitudinal study. Stroke 1993;24:976–982.

98. Pohjasvaara T, Leppavuori A, Siira I, et al. Frequency and clinical determinants of poststroke depression. Stroke 1998;29:2311–2317.

99. Robinson RG, Price TR. Poststroke depressive disorders: a follow-up study of 103 patients. Stroke 1982;13:635–641.

100. Robinson RG, Starr LB, Price TR. A two-year longitudinal study of mood disorders following stroke. Br J Psychiatry 1984;144:256–262.

101. Ghika-Schmid F, Bogousslavsky J. Affective disorders following stroke. Eur Neurol 1997;38:75–81.

102. Binder LM. Emotional problems after stroke. Stroke 1984;15:174–177.

103. Ross ED, Rush AJ. Diagnosis and neuroanatomical correlates of depression in brain-damaged patients. Arch Gen Psychiatry 1981;38:1344–1354.

104. Robinson RG, Starr LB, Kubos K, et al. A two-year longitudinal study of poststroke mood disorders: findings during the initial evaluation. Stroke 1983;14:736–741.

105. Robinson RG, Kubos KL, Starr LB, et al. Mood disorders in stroke patients: importance of location of lesion. Brian 1984;107:81–93.

106. Robinson RG, Kubos KL, Starr LB, et al. Mood changes in stroke patients: relationship to lesion location. Compr Psychiatry 1983;24:555–566.

107. Herrmann M, Bartels C, Schumacher M, Wallesch C-W. Poststroke depression. Is there a pathoanatomic correlate for depression in the postacute stage of stroke? Stroke 1995;26:850–856.
108. Lipsey JR, Robinson RG, Pearlson GD, et al. Nortriptyline treatment of poststroke depression: a double-blind study. Lancet 1984;1:297–300.
109. Reding JJ, Orto LA, Winter SW, et al. Antidepressant therapy after stroke: a double blind trial. Arch Neurol 1986;43:763–765.
110. Andersen G, Vestergaard K, Lauritzen L. Effective treatment of post-stroke depression with the selective reuptake inhibitor citalopram. Stroke 1994;25:1099–1104.
111. Wade DT, Legh-Smith J, Langton-Hewer R. Effects of living with and looking after survivers of a stroke. BMJ 1986;293:418–420.
112. Anderson CS, Linto J, Stewart-Wynne EG. A population-based assessment of the impact and burden of caregiving for long-term stroke survivors. Stroke 1995;26:843–849.
113. Scholte op Reimer WJ, de Haan RJ, Rijnders PT, et al. The burden of caregiving in partners of long-term stroke survivors. Stroke 1998;29:1605–1611.
114. Dennis M, O'Rourke S, Lewis S, et al. A quantitative study of the emotional outcome of people caring for stroke survivors. Stroke 1998;29:1867–1872.

Chapter 20
Rehabilitation

Rehabilitation services are quite different from most traditional medical and surgical units and the process is unfamiliar to many physicians. Rehabilitation has a different emphasis and goal than traditional medicine. Rehabilitation focuses on recovery and adaptation to loss of neurologic function. In contrast, traditional medicine has a pathologic and pathophysiologic emphasis. The goal of traditional medical care is to prevent and treat disease. Rehabilitation is usually performed in buildings or units separated from acute-care hospital and neurologic facilities. Personnel include a much higher ratio of nonphysician to physician staff members. Although a physician usually captains the team, the role of other paramedical personnel is more important than in most acute-care units. Rehabilitation units have a slower pace, longer patient stays, and, at times, different reimbursement rules for third-party payers.

Rehabilitation encourages and relies heavily on family involvement and the education of patients and families. Rehabilitation uses a lot of equipment, such as braces, walking aids, and parallel bars, which are foreign to most medical units. Parts of rehabilitation units look more like gymnasiums, exercise areas, workshops, or schools than standard medical wards.

Because of this perceived strangeness, many physicians are reluctant to refer their patients to rehabilitation facilities. Thus, many patients who should have rehabilitation do not receive it. I believe that rehabilitation for stroke patients is important but underused. In some patients, rehabilitation training can make the difference between a vegetative, bedridden existence in a nursing home and a productive life in society. Immobile patients discharged directly home or to nursing homes and not mobilized during the first months after stroke are unlikely to become more active later. A bed or bed-and-chair existence is physically and psychologically destructive. If the same immobile patients are admitted to rehabilitation units and successfully trained to sit and walk, the probability is high that they can remain self-reliant and increase their activities and independence during the ensuing months. Time is of the essence; training must occur in the weeks after the stroke. Major recovery from stroke takes place during the first 3–6 months. Only small numbers of patients show dramatic improvement during the next 18 months.[1,2] The push from managed-care personnel to get patients out of acute hospitals sicker and quicker means that many patients who are transferred to rehabilitation units require more acute care than they did in the past. The high cost of in-patient rehabilitation programs has led managed-care payers to offer therapy programs in the patients' homes, nursing homes, or as outpatients instead of at rehabilitation facilities.[3]

Recovery After Stroke

Loss of functions is often described as *impairments*, *disabilities*, and *handicaps*. The World Health Organization has defined these terms as follows[4]:

1. Impairment—Any loss or abnormality of psychological, physiologic, or anatomic structure or function.

2. Disability—Any restriction or lack of ability resulting from impairment to perform an activity in the manner or within the range considered normal for a human being.

3. Handicap—A disadvantage for a given individual resulting from an impairment or disability that limits or prevents the fulfillment of a role that is normal for that individual.

During rehabilitation, stroke patients are trained to minimize any handicaps that relate to the neurologic impairments that follow stroke.

Rehabilitation should be considered in terms of the general process of stroke recovery. Rehabilitation occurs during the first weeks and months after stroke onset. Natural recovery mechanisms occur at the same time. Much of the recovery is natural, although most patients are inclined to give complete credit for their improvement to various therapies that they receive during rehabilitation.

Recovery of neurologic function is complex and depends on a number of factors.[5] Some factors relate to the nature and severity of the stroke mechanism. For example, patients with brain hemorrhages recover at a different rate and extent than patients with infarcts of comparable size and location. In many patients, ischemia is transient. Portions of the ischemic zone can return to normal without leaving permanent damage. Positron emission tomography scans and magnetic resonance imaging diffusion and perfusion scanning often show regions of brain tissue that are underperfused acutely but return to normal after reperfusion. Neuroanatomic factors play a major role. The location and size of the infarct or hemorrhage are important as are the lobes and brain regions that are spared.[5,6]

Function-related factors are also important. Limitations of some neurologic functions are easier to overcome or adapt to than other functions. Most patients adapt to a hemianopia that results from an occipital-lobe lesion, but it is more difficult for patients to overcome visual neglect from a parietal-lobe lesion. In the circumstance of an occipital-lobe lesion, the patient is aware of the visual-field deficit and can learn to adapt or compensate for it. Patients with parietal-lobe lesions have more difficulty perceiving and understanding the nature of their visual deficit and are often less able to cope. A visual-field deficit is usually less disabling than hemiparesis. Constructional apraxia is less of a handicap than aphasia. Some neurologic functions are subserved by networks of regions that interact together, whereas other functions are more strictly localized to one or two brain sites. A lesion in the visual cortex-striate region (Brodmann's area 17) involving both banks of the calcarine fissure invariably causes a hemianopia. No other regions exist that subserve identical visual function. Attention to the contralateral side of visual space is a more complex function subserved by the frontal and parietal lobes, with strong thalamic and limbic input and also some involvement of basal-ganglionic structures.[7] A lesion that involves one of these regions might temporarily disrupt attentional functions but usually does not cause persistent neglect. Some functions seem to reside in several different regions. In case of injury to one region, the function is assumed by other spared regions. Patients with persistent lesions in Broca's area often regain excellent speech after a temporary period of mutism.[8,9] Positron emission tomography scanning and functional magnetic resonance imaging studies show which regions are activated in individual patients who recover functions after brain infarcts and hemorrhages.[10]

Individual patient- and character-related factors exist that heavily influence recovery. Some individuals are "survivors" and have the intelligence, determination, and character to succeed under adverse circumstances. Past personal accomplishments, flexibility, and attitudes are important determinants of functional recovery and ability to adapt to a disability. Also important are medical comorbidity. The presence of significant heart disease, pulmonary abnormalities, arthritis, and other diseases and conditions impact heavily on the patient's physical ability to pursue rehabilitation with vigor. Environment-related factors should be considered by physicians. Does the patient have a competent caregiver who will prod, cajole, and motivate the patient to do better? Are sufficient economic resources available? What floor does the patient live on? Is an elevator available in the building? Are stores, restaurants, movie theaters, and recreational and social activities within easy access for the patient? Are family members and friends nearby? Are they supportive and helpful? The answers to these queries are seldom noted in hospital charts but are just as important for meaningful recovery as the nature and severity of the neurologic signs.

Goals and Activities within Rehabilitation Units

In the ideal rehabilitation facility, a number of goals should be pursued concurrently.[3,11,12] Methods used to treat acute stroke and preventive strategies emphasized at the acute-care facility should be continued. This means that physicians and nurses at the rehabilitation facility should become fully knowledgeable about the causative stroke mechanism and treatments used to minimize the deficit and prevent worsening and stroke recurrence. Many patients are sent to rehabilitation units with incomplete evaluations at acute-care facilities. Investigations of the causative cardio-cerebrovascular-hematologic causes of stroke must be pursued further while the patient is being rehabilitated. Control of stroke risk factors, such as cessation of smoking and appropriate diet, should be continued at the rehabilitation unit.

Nurses and physicians in rehabilitation units must monitor the occurrence of stroke complications and use strategies to prevent them.[3,11,12] Chapter 19 is devoted to stroke complications. Probably one of the major explanations for the success of stroke units is their focus on systematically watching for and treating complications that develop. Mobilization and physical therapy help prevent phlebothrombosis, contractures, and bed sores. Therapy can also ameliorate dysphagia and help prevent aspiration and pneumonia. Attention to micturition can help prevent urinary tract infections and urosepsis.

The process of evaluating the nature and severity of various neurologic, medical, and psychological dysfunctions and disabilities should begin shortly after the patient is transferred to the rehabilitation unit.[13] The outcome of rehabilitation can often be predicted by analysis of a number of variables related to the neurologic deficits found.[13] Motor functions of the limbs, micturition, swallowing, gait, speech, perception, cognitive and behavioral abilities, psychological reactions, and intelligence should be assessed. Recognition of impairments and disabilities is the first step in devising strategies and programs to train the stroke patient to overcome and adapt to any dysfunctions found and prevent the development of further handicaps.

Strokes do not just affect the individual stroke patient. Stroke is a disease that affects the patient's family, friends, and environment. The caregiver, family, and friends play a major role in reintegrating the patient back into his or her home and social environment. Educating and training caregivers are important during the rehabilitation process. Caregivers should be instructed on the nature of the stroke patient's dysfunctions and strategies used to deal with these impairments.

During rehabilitation, strategies are devised to reintegrate the patient back to his or her home. This often entails evaluation of the home and suggestions to make the home environment safer for the patient. For example, if the patient customarily slept on the second floor and the kitchen, television, and living and dining rooms are on the first floor, it might be simpler to create a sleeping area for the patient on the first floor to facilitate eating and daily activities. Showers may need to be made safer and more readily usable. Social agencies may need to be mobilized for the care and support of the patient. Visiting nurses, therapists, homemakers, and food delivery services may need to be consulted when patients return to their homes.

Perhaps most important is the spirit and milieu of the unit. Personnel must possess an optimistic outlook accompanied with understanding. Planning should be practical, and the goals must be realistic. The use of equipment, strategies, and programs that help patients and caregivers recognize and deal with disabilities is helpful.

Rehabilitation Team and Their Work

The general theme of stroke rehabilitation is a disability-oriented, multidisciplinary team approach. Team members include the patient, patient's family, primary-care physician, neurologist, physical therapist, occupational therapist, speech therapist, social worker, and rehabilitation nurse. Members of the team should meet regularly to identify specific rehabilitation goals, strategies for their attainment, and methods of implementation. These team members educate and train patients and family members in their areas of expertise. Ideally, the team rehabilitation process should begin early in the course of the acute stroke so improvement in quality of life can be achieved as early as possible.

Physicians involved in rehabilitation come from a variety of disciplines. Physiatrists, internists, orthopedists, rheumatologists, geriatricians, and cardiologists are sometimes placed in charge of rehabilitation units, wards, or services within these units. Neurologists are gradually becoming more active in rehabilitation departments and units. The role of the physician differs within rehabilitation units from the traditional role of the doctor in an acute-care facility.[3] The physician directs the team. They evaluate and prognosticate. These physicians interact with the team of therapists about compensatory physical and cognitive strategies and assist devices. They try various drug interventions to treat pain, spasticity, and cognitive and mood disorders. These physicians serve as administrative brokers to gather the resources and services that the patients and their families need.[3]

Rehabilitation nurses are key members of the team. Often, one nurse acts to coordinate physician orders and integrate the various strategies used in the rehabilitation process. Nurses must often adopt an attitude unusual in the nursing profession. A nurse is usually the provider of direct care. On a rehabilitation unit, however, the nurse must often sit back and let the patient accomplish tasks at hand, providing teaching, encouragement, and help as needed. Extreme patience is required. Nurses must synthesize the recommendations of other team members and directly apply these ideas to the everyday care of patients. Nurses also monitor and direct treatment for medical complications that might occur during rehabilitation.

The physical therapist's main function is training the patient for ambulation. Balancing, weight-shifting techniques, parallel bars, various orthotics, and quad canes are used. Severe weakness in a lower extremity does not preclude ambulation. Often, a patient is unable to lift his or her leg from the bed yet eventually becomes ambulatory. Increased extensor tone combined with minimal bracing permits walking. Even before ambulation training begins, physical therapists perform range-of-motion, strengthening, and endurance exercises. In addition, physical therapists can help provide appropriate supporting apparatus, such as lap boards, chair-arm supports, and swings. Range-of-motion exercises are passive and active and should be performed at least four times daily. Patients can use the normal arm to passively move the paralyzed extremity through a full range of motion. These exercises help prevent deconditioning, excessive spasticity, joint contractures, and peripheral edema. Range-of-motion exercises combined

with upper-extremity support are the keys to preventing a painful shoulder caused by subluxation or spasticity. Both the family and nursing staff should take active roles using the recommendations of the physical therapist for remobilization throughout the day.

Occupational therapists perform upper-extremity retraining with particular attention to teaching practical activities of daily living. Patients and therapists work on improving fine-motor skills so activities such as feeding, dressing, personal hygiene, and cooking can be accomplished. These skills allow the development of independent function. Often, special devices, including a reacher, utensil holder, specially placed rails or handles, commodes, tub benches, or handheld showers, are used. An occupational therapist can customize these techniques and physical changes in the home to adapt to the patient's deficits.

Speech therapists work to improve communication skills. The goal is to facilitate communication early in the patient's rehabilitation. The methods may be verbal or nonverbal, using spoken or written words, gestures, or word boards. The boards may contain letters that patients point to for spelling words or may contain words or pictures to designate needs or wishes. Computer programs are often helpful for facilitating communication skills. Often, therapists can develop techniques of nonverbal communication for severely aphasic patients so their needs can be met and feelings of isolation eliminated. During the first 3 months after a stroke, much spontaneous language recovery occurs. Beyond 3 months, the therapist's role is to enhance further recovery of language function. Physicians should not accept a nihilistic attitude toward speech therapy. I advise physicians to start aphasic patients on a comprehensive program of speech therapy early during the course of treatment. Physicians should continue to pursue a vigorous course of treatment in most patients, withholding treatment only in patients who are demented or severely globally aphasic. Speech therapists also help evaluate and treat dysarthria and dysphagia, breath control, and articulation. Speech therapists can often suggest types of foods, liquids, and eating techniques that might be best tolerated by patients.

Next to the patient, the family has the most difficult task. Usually medically unsophisticated, family members must learn new skills from rehabilitation team members and directly supervise the care of the stroke patient. The family's questions and concerns should be carefully addressed by each team member. It is often useful for the family member most directly involved in home care to spend a few days at the hospital to effectively acquire the necessary skills. Once patients return home, continued contact with the team is crucial so progress can be monitored, new problems identified, and solutions implemented. This contact may be in the form of visits to the home or appointments at the rehabilitation unit with individual team members.

Patient Selection

Although rehabilitation is important, not all stroke patients benefit. If every stroke patient were referred, rehabilitation facilities would be swamped and the cost to taxpayers would greatly increase, whereas effective retraining for those who may benefit most would suffer from dilution. Selection of appropriate patients is important. Patients who are already ambulatory and have only slight or temporary deficits do not need to stay in a rehabilitation unit; they do well on their own or with outpatient care. The patient who is stuporous, completely immobile, or has severe right-hemisphere dysfunction does not usually benefit from rehabilitation. Most observers agree that the middle group between these two extremes is the appropriate target for rehabilitative care. How should this group be identified? What factors should be considered in making the triage decision?

Patients of all ages can be offered rehabilitation. By decade, no difference in outcome has been shown; substantial recovery is noted in all age groups.[14,15] Those patients who have serious cognitive impairment or severe underlying medical illness may be unable to participate in effective rehabilitation programs; these patients are either unable to learn compensatory techniques or tolerate the physical activity required. Aphasia, however, does not preclude stroke rehabilitation. When outcome is measured by performance of daily activities, ability to walk, and discharge disposition, no difference is found between aphasic and nonaphasic patients referred for rehabilitation.[15–18] Higher cortical-function abnormalities other than aphasia, such as perceptual abnormalities, anosog-

nosia, aprosodia, neglect, impersistence, reduplicative paramnesia, and prosopagnosia, may make rehabilitation more difficult but not impossible. These cognitive abnormalities tend to improve with time, allowing the stroke rehabilitation process to proceed.[5]

Neurologic findings, such as limb paralysis, are prognostically important,[3,13,19] but neurologic disability and accompanying medical illness are not the only factors that predict outcome. A host of nonmedical social, psychological, and environmental factors are of equal or even greater importance. Two of the most accurate prognostic predictors in patients with head trauma are (1) presence of a "significant other" to help the patient and (2) whether the patient had a job before the injury.

Similarly, a number of seemingly mundane factors apply when deciding on treatment for a stroke patient. What was the patient's prestroke level of capability? Does the patient have financial support to help with special equipment, transportation, and so forth? Does the patient have a car or access to other transportation? Does the patient have someone at home who is motivated, capable, and available to help and encourage recovery? [20] Does the home have stairs or a bathroom on every floor? Is "Meals on Wheels" or a store that delivers and takes telephone orders accessible to the patient? What community services are available? These prognostic factors and others must be considered to offer rehabilitation to those who will benefit most. I believe that when prognosis is uncertain, the patient should be given the benefit of the doubt. A trial period of rehabilitation should be offered.

Use of Rehabilitation

Stroke units and rehabilitation services share a common focus on stroke patients, a multidisciplinary team approach, and emphasis on maximizing functional recovery. Strategies and methods of rehabilitation vary greatly between units and have changed over time. Descriptions of the methods, techniques, and aids used during rehabilitation are far beyond the scope of this book and beyond the knowledge and expertise of the author. Excellent chapters and monographs devoted entirely to this subject exist elsewhere.[3,11,12,14,21,22] Stroke units and rehabilitation services exist in different locations, some within acute-care hospitals and others in free-standing hospitals apart from acute-care facilities.

Stroke units and facilities have been studied in a number of trials.[3,23–32] These trials suggest that the milieu and greater frequency and intensity of rehabilitation services in dedicated stroke and rehabilitation units lead to better outcomes. Mortality is reduced. More patients return home and less patients are transferred to chronic hospitals and nursing homes. Short- and long-term functional outcomes are also improved. Doubt that stroke units work no longer exists.[3,23–32] Some trials have studied the use of various techniques and strategies for specific functions, such as recovery of hemiplegic gait,[33] improvement in upper-extremity function,[34] recovery from aphasia,[35] and management of spatial neglect.[36] Other trials study the effects of specific strategies on general functional outcome (e.g., the effect of sensory stimulation on outcome of patients with severe stroke-related hemiparesis).[37]

Ottenbacher and Jannell performed a meta-analysis of trials and studies conducted between 1960 and 1990.[28] The analysis included patients who had a stroke-related hemiparesis who were given rehabilitation services in a design that compared at least two groups or conditions for change in a quantifiable functional measure. Outcomes studied included gait, hand functions, activities of daily living, response times, and visual perceptual functions. From 173 statistical evaluations performed on 3,717 patients studied in these trials, the meta-analysis showed that the average patient who received a program that included focused stroke rehabilitation or a particular procedure performed better than approximately 65% of patients in the comparison groups.[3,28] Greater effects of treatment were obtained when rehabilitation was performed early. Younger patients tended to do better than older patients.

Why do stroke units perform better than non-dedicated units? The reasons are probably multifactorial and include such difficult-to-quantify ingredients as attitude, milieu, caring, education, multidisciplinary approach, and systematic attention to routines and details.

Coordination of Acute and Long-Term Care

To be optimally successful, rehabilitation should be fully integrated with traditional medical care.

Therapy should begin as early as possible while the patient is still on the acute medical or neurologic unit. Physicians, nurses, and other personnel must be involved. Therapy should not be completely delegated to physical and occupational therapists. The therapy should not should not be limited to the 30 minutes or so patients typically spend each day with therapists. Passive and active range-of-motion exercises and other physical therapy should be encouraged by ward personnel. If the patient goes to a rehabilitation unit, the acute-care team should continue to follow the patient whenever possible. Acute medical problems do not suddenly disappear when the patient is transferred. Subsequent strokes and medical complications are common among recuperating patients.

The patient receives mixed signals if treatment and advice begun on the acute service are not followed through at the rehabilitation unit. The patient may have been persuaded by a doctor on the acute-care unit who advised the need for a low-salt, low-cholesterol diet, only to be served butter, cream, and eggs on the rehabilitation unit. Medical treatment and surveillance should be continued during rehabilitation and afterward. Similarly, when the patient leaves the rehabilitation unit, the physician must continue to emphasize the need to carry out various rehabilitation techniques. After treatment in the acute-care center and rehabilitation facilities, patients usually return to the care of their principal care physician, most likely an internist or family practitioner. The primary-care physician must be kept up-to-date with the patient's findings, current treatment decisions, and recommendations so they can continue medical treatment and retraining procedures and strategies. Rehabilitation and traditional medical care should be intertwined and overlapped, not seen by the patient as unrelated phases with one consultation succeeding the other.

Pitfalls of Exaggerated Emphasis on Physical Therapy

I have been impressed with the frequency after discharge of a phenomenon that I have referred to as the *hyper-PT* or *hyper–physical therapy syndrome*. Patients affected by this syndrome continue to intensively strive to improve hand, arm, or limb function and return these functions to normal. Instead of expending energy on readapting to their former lifestyle, which probably does not require absolutely normal function, they continue to exercise and focus attention on their limb dysfunction. These patients exchange a practical, reachable goal (a return to all prior activities) for an impractical, unreachable, and unimportant goal (a return to premorbid strength). Many patients also attribute their recovery to physical therapy and are fearful of stopping or decreasing it. Much of their energy and time are taken up in going to and from therapy, doing therapy at home, and resting after therapy is over. These individuals have little time and energy left for living. Patients should be gradually weaned from physical therapy at the appropriate time and be encouraged to adapt to their deficit, turning attention away from limb impairment toward enjoyment of life.

Loss of self-image and oversensitivity to minor disabilities are other common problems. Sometimes, exposure to others who have regained full prestroke activities despite unresolved neurologic deficits is of great help to patients.

References

1. Andrew K, Brocklehurst JC, Richard B, et al. The rate of recovery from stroke and its measurement. Rehab Med 1981;3:155–161.
2. Katz S, Ford AB, Chinn AB, et al. Prognosis after stroke: II. Long-term course of 159 patients. Medicine (Baltimore) 1966;45:236–246.
3. Dobkin, BH. Neurologic Rehabilitation. Philadelphia: Davis, 1996.
4. World Health Organization. WHO International Classification of Impairments, Disabilities, and Handicaps: A Manual of Classification Relating to the Consequences of Disease. Geneva: World Health Organization, 1980.
5. Caplan LR, Hier DB. Recovery from Right Hemisphere Stroke. In R Corbier (ed), Basis for a Classification of Cerebral Arterial Diseases. Amsterdam: Excerpta Medica, 1985;163–171.
6. Hier DB, Mondlock J, Caplan LR. Recovery of behavioral abnormalities after right hemisphere stroke. Neurology 1983;33:345–350.
7. Mesulam M. From sensation to cognition. Brain 1998; 121:1013–1052.
8. Mohr JP, Pessin MS, Finkelstein S, et al. Broca aphasia; pathological and clinical aspects. Neurology 1978;28: 311–324.
9. Alexander M, Naeser M, Palumbo C. Broca's area aphasia. Neurology 1990;40:353–362.
10. Weiler C, Chollet F, Frackowiak RSJ. Physiological Aspects of Recovery from Stroke. In M Ginsberg, J Bogousslavsky (eds), Cerebrovascular Disease: Patho-

physiology, Diagnosis, and Management. Malden, MA: Blackwell, 1998;2057–2067.
11. U.S. Department of Health and Human Services. Poststroke rehabilitation. Clinical practice guideline. Number 16. Rockville, MD: Public Health Service-Agency for Health Care Policy and Research, 1995.
12. Miyai I, Reding MJ. Stroke Recovery and Rehabilitation. In M Ginsberg, J Bogousslavsky (eds), Cerebrovascular Disease: Pathophysiology, Diagnosis, and Management, Vol 2. Malden, MA: Blackwell, 1998;2043–2056.
13. Alexander M. Stroke rehabilitation outcome: a potential use of predictive variables to establish levels of care. Stroke 1994;25:128–134.
14. Feigenson JS. Neurological Rehabilitation. In AB Baker (ed), Clinical Neurology. New York: Harper & Row, 1983; 1–66.
15. Feigenson JS, McDowell FH, Meese P, et al. Factors influencing outcome and length of stay in a stroke rehabilitation unit: I. Analysis of 248 unscreened patients—medical and function prognostic indication. Stroke 1977;8:651–656.
16. Feigenson JS, McCarthy ML, Greenberg SD, et al. Factors influencing outcome and length of stay in a stroke rehabilitation unit: II. Comparison of 318 screened and 248 unscreened patients. Stroke 1977;8:657–662.
17. Feigenson JS, McCarthy ML, Meese P, et al. Stroke rehabilitation: factors predicting outcome and length of stay—an overview. N Y State J Med 1977;77:1426–1430.
18. Nicholas M, Helm-Estabrooks N, Ward-Lonergan J, et al. Evolution of severe aphasia in the first two years post onset. Arch Phys Med Rehabil 1993;74:830–836.
19. Taub N, Wolfe C, Richardson E, et al. Predicting the disability of first-time stroke sufferers at 1 year. Stroke 1994; 25:352–357.
20. DeJong G, Branch LG. Predicting the stroke patient's ability to live independently. Stroke 1982;13:648–655.
21. Kaplan PE, Cerullo LJ. Stroke Rehabilitation. Boston: Butterworth–Heinemann, 1986.
22. Ozer MN, Materson RS, Caplan LR. Management of Persons with Stroke. St. Louis: Mosby, 1994.
23. Garraway W, Aktar A, Hockey L, et al. Management of acute stroke in the elderly: follow-up of a controlled trial. BMJ 1980;2:827–829.
24. Wood-Dauphinee S, Shapiro S, Bass E, et al. A randomized trial of team care following stroke. Stroke 1984;15: 864–872.
25. Strand T, Asplund K, Eriksson S, et al. A non-intensive stroke unit reduces functional disability and the need for long-term hospitalization. Stroke 1985;17:377–381.
26. Indredavik B, Bakke F, Solberg R, et al. Benefit of a stroke unit: a randomized controlled trial. Stroke 1991;22: 1026–1031.
27. Kalra L, Dale P, Crome P. Improving stroke rehabilitation: a controlled trial. Stroke 1993;24:1462–1467.
28. Ottenbacher KJ, Jannell S. The results of clinical trials in stroke rehabilitation research. Arch Neurol 1993;50:37–44.
29. Kaste M, Palmomaki H, Sarna S. Where and how should elderly stroke patients be treated? a randomized trial. Stroke 1995;26:249–253.
30. Indredavik B, Slordahl SA, Bakke F, et al. Stroke unit treatment. Long term effects. Stroke 1997;28:1861–1866.

31. Stroke Unit Trialists' Collaboration. Collaborative systematic review of the randomized trials of organized in-patient (stroke unit) care after stroke. BMJ 1997;314:1151–1159.

32. Stroke Unit Trialists' Collaboration. How do stroke units improve patient outcomes? A collaborative systematic review of the randomized trials. Stroke 1997;28:2139–2144.

33. Colborne G, Olney S, Griffin M. Feedback of ankle and soleus electromyography in the rehabilitation of hemiplegic gait. Arch Phys Med Rehabil 1993;74:1100–1106.

34. Nakayama H, Jorgenson H, Raaschou H, et al. Recovery of upper extremity function in stroke patients. The Copenhagen Stroke Study. Arch Phys Med Rehabil 1994;75;394–398.

35. Shewan C, Kertesz A. Effects of speech and language treatment on recovery from aphasia. Brain Lang 1984;23:272–299.

36. Halligan P, Marshall J. Spatial neglect. Position papers on theory and practise. Neuropsych Rehabil 1994;4:103–230.

37. Johansson K, Lindgren I, Widner H, et al. Can sensory stimulation improve the functional outcome in stroke patients? Neurology 1993;43:2189–2192.

Index